D0875606

HIV-1: MOLECULAR BIOLOGY AND PATHOGENESIS

VIRAL MECHANISMS, Second Edition

HIV-1: MOLECULAR BIOLOGY AND PATHOGENESIS

VIRAL MECHANISMS, Second Edition

The First of a Two-Volume Set

Edited by

Kuan-Teh Jeang

Molecular Virology Section
LMM, NIAID, NIH
Bethesda, Maryland

ADVANCES IN
PHARMACOLOGY

VOLUME 55

AMSTERDAM • BOSTON • HEIDELBERG • LONDON
NEW YORK • OXFORD • PARIS • SAN DIEGO
SAN FRANCISCO • SINGAPORE • SYDNEY • TOKYO
Academic Press is an imprint of Elsevier

ELSEVIER

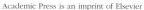

Academic Press is an imprint of Elsevier
525 B Street, Suite 1900, San Diego, California 92101-4495, USA
84 Theobald's Road, London WC1X 8RR, UK

This book is printed on acid-free paper. ∞

For all information on all Elsevier Academic Press publications
visit our Web site at www.books.elsevier.com

ISBN-13: 978-0-12-373610-9

PRINTED IN THE UNITED STATES OF AMERICA
07 08 09 10 9 8 7 6 5 4 3 2 1

"This book is dedicated by Kuan-Teh Jeang to Diane, David, John and Diana Jeang."

Contents

HIV-1 RNA Packaging

Andrew M. L. Lever

Structure and Function of the HIV Envelope Glycoprotein as Entry Mediator, Vaccine Immunogen, and Target for Inhibitors

Ponraj Prabakaran, Antony S. Dimitrov, Timothy R. Fouts, and Dimiter S. Dimitrov

HIV-1 Reverse Transcription: Close Encounters Between the Viral Genome and a Cellular tRNA

Truus E. M. Abbink and Ben Berkhout

Transcription of HIV: Tat and Cellular Chromatin

Anne Gatignol

Posttranscriptional Control of HIV-1 and Other Retroviruses and Its Practical Applications

Barbara K. Felber, Andrei S. Zolotukhin, and George N. Pavlakis

HIV Accessory Genes Vif and Vpu

Klaus Strebel

Interactions of HIV-1 Viral Protein R with Host Cell Proteins

Richard Y. Zhao, Robert T. Elder, and Michael Bukrinsky

HIV-1 Protease: Structure, Dynamics, and Inhibition

John M. Louis, Rieko Ishima, Dennis A. Torchia, and Irene T. Weber

Properties, Functions, and Drug Targeting of the Multifunctional Nucleocapsid Protein of the *Human Immunodeficiency Virus*

Jean-Luc Darlix, José Luis Garrido, Nelly Morellet, Yves Mély, and Hugues de Rocquigny

Human Immunodeficiency Virus Type I Assembly, Release, and Maturation

Catherine S. Adamson and Eric O. Freed

Role of Nef in HIV-1 Replication and Pathogenesis

John L. Foster and J. Victor Garcia

Treatment Implications of the Latent Reservoir for HIV-1

Susan Peterson, Alison P. Reid, Scott Kim, and Robert F. Siliciano

RNA Interference and HIV-1

Man Lung Yeung, Yamina Bennasser, Shu-Yun Le, and Kuan-Teh Jeang

Contributors

Numbers in parentheses indicate the pages on which the authors' contributions begin.

Truus E. M. Abbink (99) Laboratory of Experimental Virology, Department of Medical Microbiology, Center for Infection and Immunity Amsterdam (CINIMA), Academic Medical Center of the University of Amsterdam, Meibergdreef 15, 1105 AZ Amsterdam, The Netherlands

Catherine S. Adamson (347) Virus-Cell Interaction Section, HIV Drug Resistance Program, National Cancer Institute, Frederick, Maryland 21702

Yamina Bennasser (427) Molecular Virology Section, Laboratory of Molecular Microbiology, National Institute of Allergy and Infectious Diseases, National Institutes of Health, Bethesda, Maryland 20892

Ben Berkhout (99) Laboratory of Experimental Virology, Department of Medical Microbiology, Center for Infection and Immunity Amsterdam (CINIMA), Academic Medical Center of the University of Amsterdam, Meibergdreef 15, 1105 AZ Amsterdam, The Netherlands

Michael Bukrinsky (233) Department of Microbiology, Immunology, and Tropical Medicine, The George Washington University, Washington, District of Columbia 20037

Jean-Luc Darlix (299) LaboRetro, Unité INSERM de Virologie Humaine, IFR128, ENS Sciences de Lyon, 46 allée d'Italie, 69364 Lyon, France

Hugues de Rocquigny (299) Institut Gilbert Laustriat, Pharmacologie et Physico-Chimie des Interactions, Cellulaires et Moléculaires, UMR 7034 CNRS, Faculté de Pharmacie, Université Louis Pasteur, Strasbourg 1, 74, Route du Rhin, 67401 ILLKIRCH Cedex, France

Antony S. Dimitrov (33) Profectus BioSciences, Inc., Techcenter at UMBC, Baltimore, Maryland 21227

Dimiter S. Dimitrov (33) Protein Interactions Group, CCRNP, CCR, NCI-Frederick, NIH Frederick, Maryland 21702

Robert T. Elder (233) Department of Pediatrics and Children's Memorial Research Center, Northwestern University Feinberg School of Medicine, Chicago, Illinois 60614

Barbara K. Felber (161) Human Retrovirus Pathogenesis Section, Vaccine Branch, Center for Cancer Research, National Cancer Institute-Frederick, Frederick, Maryland 21702

John L. Foster (389) Department of Internal Medicine, University of Texas Southwestern Medical Center, Dallas, Texas 75390

Timothy R. Fouts (33) Profectus BioSciences, Inc., Techcenter at UMBC, Baltimore, Maryland 21227

Eric O. Freed (347) Virus-Cell Interaction Section, HIV Drug Resistance Program, National Cancer Institute, Frederick, Maryland 21702

Robert C. Gallo (XVII) Institute of Human Virology and Division of Basic Science, University of Maryland Biotechnology Institute, Baltimore, Maryland 21201

J. Victor Garcia (389) Department of Internal Medicine, University of Texas Southwestern Medical Center, Dallas, Texas 75390

José Luis Garrido (299) LaboRetro, Unité INSERM de Virologie Humaine, IFR128, ENS Sciences de Lyon, 46 allée d'Italie, 69364 Lyon, France

Anne Gatignol (137) Virus-Cell Interactions Laboratory, Lady Davis Institute for Medical Research, Department of Microbiology & Immunology and Experimental Medicine, McGill University, Montréal, Québec, Canada

Rieko Ishima (261) Department of Structural Biology, School of Medicine, University of Pittsburgh, Pittsburgh, Pennsylvania 15260

Kuan-Teh Jeang (427) Molecular Virology Section, Laboratory of Molecular Microbiology, National Institute of Allergy and Infectious Diseases, National Institutes of Health, Bethesda, Maryland 20892

Scott Kim (411) Department of Medicine, Johns Hopkins University School of Medicine, Baltimore, Maryland 21205

Shu-Yun Le (427) Center for Cancer Research Nanobiology Program, NCI Center for Cancer Research, NCI, National Insitutes of Health, Frederick, Maryland 21702

Andrew M. L. Lever (1) Department of Medicine, University of Cambridge, Addenbrooke's Hospital, Cambridge CB2 2QQ, United Kingdom

John M. Louis (261) Laboratory of Chemical Physics, National Institute of Diabetes, Digestive and Kidney Diseases, National Institutes of Health, Bethesda, Maryland 20892

Yves Mély (299) Institut Gilbert Laustriat, Pharmacologie et Physico-Chimie des Interactions, Cellulaires et Moléculaires, UMR 7034 CNRS, Faculté de Pharmacie, Université Louis Pasteur, Strasbourg 1, 74, Route du Rhin, 67401 ILLKIRCH Cedex, France

Nelly Morellet (299) Unité de Pharmacologie Chimique et Génétique, INSERM U640-CNRS UMR 8151, UFR des Sciences Pharmaceutiques et Biologiques, 4, avenue de l'observatoire, 75270 Paris Cedex 06, France

George N. Pavlakis (161) Human Retrovirus Section, Vaccine Branch, Center for Cancer Research, National Cancer Institute-Frederick, Frederick, Maryland 21702

Susan Peterson (411) Department of Medicine, Johns Hopkins University School of Medicine, Baltimore, Maryland 21205

Ponraj Prabakaran (33) Protein Interactions Group, CCRNP, CCR, NCI-Frederick, NIH, Frederick, Maryland 21702

Alison P. Reid (411) Department of Medicine, Johns Hopkins University School of Medicine, Baltimore, Maryland 21205

Robert F. Siliciano (411) Department of Medicine, Johns Hopkins University School of Medicine, Baltimore, Maryland 21205

Klaus Strebel (199) Laboratory of Molecular Microbiology, National Institute of Allergy and Infectious Diseases, National Institutes of Health, 4/312, Bethesda, Maryland 20892

Dennis A. Torchia (261) Molecular Structural Biology Unit, National Institute of Dental and Craniofacial Research, National Institutes of Health, Bethesda, Maryland 20892

Irene T. Weber (261) Department of Biology, Molecular Basis of Disease Program, Georgia State University, Atlanta, Georgia 30303

Man Lung Yeung (427) Molecular Virology Section, Laboratory of Molecular Microbiology, National Institute of Allergy and Infectious Diseases, National Institutes of Health, Bethesda, Maryland 20892

Richard Y. Zhao (233) Department of Pediatrics and Children's Memorial Research Center, Northwestern University Feinberg School of Medicine, Chicago, Illinois 60614; Department of Microbiology-Immunology and Department of Pathology, University of Maryland School of Medicine, Baltimore, Maryland 21201

Andrei S. Zolotukhin (161) Human Retrovirus Pathogenesis Section, Vaccine Branch, Center for Cancer Research, National Cancer Institute-Frederick, Frederick, Maryland 21702

Preface

Some months ago while in Europe, I saw a presentation on HIV/AIDS that was repeatedly shown on CNN. While overall it served a very positive function in that it enhanced awareness of the problem and helped disseminate correct information on the status of the epidemic, the risks of HIV transmission, and some aspects of HIV therapy, I was nonetheless struck by the oft-stated advertisement that the "show" was composed of HIV/AIDS experts handling a give and take with members of the audience. Yet, to my knowledge not even one member of the group of experts was a scientist. At the closure of this program, one panelist, a movie star, stated that HIV/AIDS would be solved by people coming together (or something close to this comment), and that it was not the science. I may be completely wrong, but his words sounded so "politically correct," pro-"solidarity," and all such things (whatever they mean), and at least so minimally near to science and to an understanding of how progress really occurs, that it gave me chills.

I am worried. As science and technology progress faster and faster, we have developed an enormous gap between science and our technical culture and the population at large, perhaps even to the point of occasional anti-science and hostility. As others have noted, it has been a little over 200 years since educated people such as Benjamin Franklin and Thomas Jefferson could do serious science and/or inventions as a hobby. A major portion of the population could understand them. Consider how remote that is today for a politician and for the mass of society. Are we doing enough to educate a broader mass of society? Can we do much better or is it now simply too complex and specialized? I do not know the answers, but it is a cause for pondering and for trying to improve our communications.

Going back to the remarks of the movie star and considering the topic of this book, should not we at least try to make it abundantly clear that not 50%, 70%, or 90%, but virtually 100% of *all* fundamental, conceptual, and *practical* (including diagnosis, prognosis, and therapy) advances in

HIV/AIDS research came out of basic science, and precisely from studies of HIV molecular biology and pathogenesis? Perhaps we can make three exceptions: (1) the early (1981–1982) epidemiological studies (chiefly those driven by James Curran and his coworkers) did define risk groups and patterns of how the disease spreads, (2) the clinicians gave us key information that there was a significant decline in CD4+ T cells, and (3) the early isolations of HIV. However, even in the last two of these three putative exceptions, we must still recognize some role of basic science (albeit not of HIV molecular biology or pathogenesis). After all, CD4 measurements required earlier discovery of this cell surface molecule by monoclonal antibodies, and HIV isolations required first a surrogate marker for presence of a retrovirus, namely precision assays for reverse transcriptase and second growth of primary T cells with IL-2. Of course, both reverse transcriptase (1970) and IL-2 (1976) came out of basic research.

It is unnecessary to detail here the subsequent advances that had major practical impact, namely the linkage of HIV to AIDS (causation), the development of the HIV blood test, and the development of effective anti-HIV therapy, which came entirely from basic research on HIV molecular biology/immunology: (1) the permanent cell line production of HIV was a prerequisite for sufficient HIV proteins for the test; (2) the ELISA, but especially the western blot (adopted for the first time from its use in basic research to a confirmatory blood test); (3) the cell line was also to prove to be valuable if not essential for drug screening, for example AZT story. We can also add that targeting reverse transcriptase and the HIV protease in therapy, obviously also came out of earlier molecular biological studies on animal retroviruses, HTLV-1 and HTLV-2, and finally on HIV. As to future therapy, we know that targeting integrase as well as blocking HIV entry are already here or on the horizon and, of course, these therapeutic approaches are completely dependent on detailed knowledge gained from molecular biological studies on integration of the DNA provirus (the former) and on the steps of HIV cell entry (the later).

We can also imagine that future treatments may interfere with the chronic activation state of many HIV infected people, and our awareness of the importance of activation in HIV progression came directly from studies of HIV/SIV pathogenesis.

We have known for some time that the kind of HIV one gets infected with can be "practically" important—beginning with the West African seroepidemiological studies of Essex and colleagues, a significantly different HIV was eventually defined (HIV-2), and we all know it is far less pathogenic and less infectious. Molecular analysis of a wide range of HIV isolates has helped define the epidemic, sort out some differences in therapeutic sensitivity, subtle and occasionally not so subtle differences in pathogenicity, and awareness of major differences in responses to vaccines. Finally, all current vaccines are based at least in part on HIV molecular biology.

Books like this one are needed by us, but we should also try to see if we can provide understandable summaries for a much wider audience. I hope the publishers and editor will agree.

Robert C. Gallo

Andrew M. L. Lever

Department of Medicine, University of Cambridge, Addenbrooke's Hospital
Cambridge CB2 2QQ, United Kingdom

HIV-1 RNA Packaging

I. Chapter Overview

RNA encapsidation by retroviruses is a remarkable process by which the virus negotiates trafficking of a minority species of mRNA through a particular cellular pathway to become its genome. During this, in the case of HIV, it may first be translated before being selected by the viral Gag protein, highly specifically, from the cellular background pool of mRNAs. These processes involve recognition of RNA secondary and tertiary structures and an RNA–RNA intermolecular interaction to package a diploid dimeric RNA genome. RNA transport and encapsidation involves cellular chaperone proteins of which, as yet, few have been identified. Better understood is the structural detail of the interaction between the viral RNA and the Gag protein. This process requires flexibility and conformational change in the

Advances in Pharmacology, Volume 55
Copyright © 2000, 2007, Elsevier Inc. All rights reserved.

1054-3589/07 $35.00
DOI: 10.1016/S1054-3589(07)55001-5

RNA and reflects the fact that transport from transcriptional site to virion likely involves the genomic RNA adopting a number of different structures to display the relevant stage-specific *cis*-acting signals. The specificity of this process and the virus-specific nature of RNA export from a cell make these processes attractive therapeutic targets.

II. Introduction

The process of encapsidating the genomic RNA of HIV within the viral particle has become better understood in the past 5 years; however, there is still a great deal of the "black box" about it. As the emphasis in studying viral replication switches from the functions of isolated viral components to the interactions of these with the much more numerous cellular factors, it has become clear that in RNA packaging, just as with viral assembly, more than Gag alone is required. Packaging is not merely defined as the affinity of the interaction between Gag protein and a specialized region of the viral RNA—the packaging signal (psi or Ψ). In previous chapter 1 of volume 48 on this subject (Lever, 2000) in this series, the concept of a "packaging pathway" was ventured in which the viral RNA had to negotiate a very specific route from transcription through to the budding virus in order to be packaged successfully. This concept is now better substantiated for packaging and for other aspects of viral export (Swanson *et al.*, 2004). For RNA encapsidation there are more data on how the pathway begins, some of the chaperones involved (Fig. 1), the physical route taken, and the nature of the RNA–protein interaction involved. These may involve changes in the structure of the RNA as it proceeds through the cell depending on optimizing its various *cis*-acting functions at appropriate times. There still remain many incompletely answered questions which were posed in the previous chapter including the role of RNA dimerization in packaging (Greatorex, 2004; Russell *et al.*, 2004). Where does it occur, how does it happen, and how essential it is? The exact definition of the minimal sequences required for RNA encapsidation in HIV still eludes us. Although pragmatic approaches in optimizing lentivirus-based vectors have given us a minimal functional packaging region, no one would claim that it is the minimal packaging signal; however, as proposed below, since packaging may involve control of RNA trafficking as well as binding to Gag, there may be several RNA regions involved as was suggested by several early studies (Berkowitz *et al.*, 1995a; McBride and Panganiban, 1996). This chapter aims to analyze the data that pertain to particular parts of the packaging pathway. Some caveats are mentioned above, an even larger one being that what has been shown in one retrovirus does not necessarily apply to another; so where other retroviral systems are cited because of the absence of corresponding data from HIV,

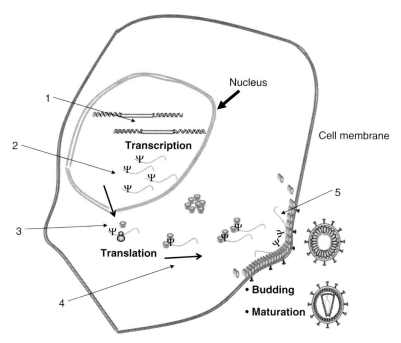

FIGURE 1   Factors affecting packaging—the packaging pathway. Aspects of RNA encapsidation in HIV: (1) proximity of transcription may increase copackaging of heterologous genomes as dimers; (2) transport proteins including Rev and hnRNPA2 influence trafficking and nuclear export route; (3) Gag–RNA interaction occurs initially in a perinuclear/centrosomal site; (4) cotranslational packaging with Gag protein binding to the UTR and sequestering the RNA for transport to the cell membrane facilitated by cellular protein ligands; and (5) RNA dimerization and RNA-assisted particle assembly and export.

it may or may not be the same for HIV. The chapter is divided into two sections: first, the route of RNA export and second, the structural and molecular biology of the Gag–RNA interaction which generates packaging specificity.

As a basic framework it can be stated that retroviruses package their genome with high specificity, despite the relative paucity of this RNA (1% or less) as a component of the capped, polyadenylated mRNAs present within an infected cell. Two copies are packaged which at some stage become linked through a dimer linkage site. The protein responsible for the capture is the uncleaved Gag polyprotein precursor and this recognizes structures formed in the viral RNA created by complex folding using Watson–Crick and noncanonical base pairing. RNA dimers within the particle may be homo- or heterodimers partly depending on the number of transcriptionally active viruses within the infected cell.

III. The Packaging Pathway ────────────────────

A. Transcription and Packaging

HIV is known to integrate preferentially in gene-rich regions of the genome (Schroder *et al.*, 2002). Recombination can occur during reverse transcription between copackaged heterodimers (Katz and Skalka, 1990). This occurs at an unusually high rate in HIV-1 and is probably a major source of sequence diversity in HIV (Rhodes *et al.*, 2003). There have been to date no studies in HIV examining the site of integration and its effect on packaging. In murine (Kharytonchyk *et al.*, 2005) and avian (Rasmussen and Pedersen, 2006) retroviruses, experimental evidence suggests that RNAs transcribed from integrated proviruses, which are physically close in the genome, are more likely to be packaged as heterodimers than are genomic RNAs from those which are physically distant. Thus even at this stage the trafficking of the RNA within the cell is to some extent decided. There is no evidence that the nature of the integration site influences whether an RNA is packaged other than it being transcriptionally active or not.

B. RNA Transport from the Nucleus

As yet there are limited data as to the route that the viral RNA will take after transcription and what the important chaperones are. In *Rous sarcoma virus* (RSV), accumulating evidence suggests that some of the viral Gag protein may return from the cytoplasm into the nucleus (Scheifele *et al.*, 2002) to capture the genomic RNA. There is no evidence that this is common to other retroviruses and indeed there is evidence to the contrary in HIV. Although the Matrix region of HIV-1 Gag has a nuclear localization signal (Bukrinsky *et al.*, 1993) and HIV Gag has been identified in the nucleus, it may have been passively imported by binding to shuttling RNAs or proteins; it has recently been suggested to have an additional role in regulating splicing through binding PRP4 and blocking phosphorylation of SF2 (Bennett *et al.*, 2004).

As an unspliced RNA containing instability sequences which favor nuclear retention and splicing, genomic RNA depends on Rev and its RNA response element the Rev responsive element (RRE) for nuclear export (Cullen, 1992). Rev acts through the CRM1 pathway (Neville *et al.*, 1997) but there may be additional chaperones specific for viral RNA. Rev and the RRE also seem to have a role in enhancing packaging (Anson and Fuller, 2003; Lucke *et al.*, 2005; Richardson *et al.*, 1993). In comparative studies of nuclear export of RNA, alternative export systems such as the constitutive transport element of D-type viruses and the woodchuck posttranscriptional response element are as good as the Rev–RRE system in delivering RNA to the cytoplasm but more gets encapsidated using the Rev–RRE system

(Anson and Fuller, 2003; Lucke *et al.*, 2005). Rev can bind to an RNA loop in the packaging signal region which has a structure closely mimicking the RRE-binding site (Gallego *et al.*, 2003). Mutation of this loop impairs RNA trafficking out of the nucleus (Greatorex *et al.*, 2006).

The RNA-binding protein Staufen (Mouland *et al.*, 2000) may be a ligand for RNA capture and transport. Staufen is better known for its role in RNA localization in *Drosophila* embryos (St Johnston *et al.*, 1991). Staufen binds helical RNA duplexes but without sequence specificity (Wickham *et al.*, 1999). Other cellular proteins have been implicated in retroviral RNA transport (Cochrane *et al.*, 2006).

Subcellular localization studies using confocal microscopy have suggested that RNA may be trafficked out of the nucleus under the influence of hnRNPA2 (Mouland *et al.*, 2000) and arrive at a perinuclear site. The same protein may be involved in transport from this region (Levesque *et al.*, 2006). These have been supported by further confocal and fluorescence resonance energy transfer (FRET)-based studies which implicate the centrosome as the site at which RNA–protein interaction first occurs in packaging (Poole *et al.*, 2005) and also from recent work on Gag trafficking (Perlman and Resh, 2006) showing Gag going through the centrosome *en route* to the cell membrane. D-type viruses such as *Mason-Pfizer monkey virus* have been shown to assemble at this site (Sfakianos *et al.*, 2003). Centrosomal localization of Gag in HIV-1 was dependent on the presence of an intact packaging signal in the coding RNA (Poole *et al.*, 2005), adding to evidence that packaging may involve specific targeting of the RNA to an appropriate cellular site for encapsidation to occur. Thus, a packaging signal may be a subcellular localization signal as well as a Gag-binding site perhaps explaining some of the conflicting data in packaging studies where there are disparities between the degree of inhibition of Gag/RNA binding and the degree of packaging defect produced by certain mutations.

C. Translation and Packaging

At or after the centrosome, the RNA has two options since the genomic RNA of HIV and other retroviruses is bifunctional. It encodes the Gag and Gag/Pol polyproteins as well as functioning as the viral genome. RNA packaging in HIV is preferentially cotranslational. This was first shown categorically for HIV-2 (Griffin *et al.*, 2001; Kaye and Lever, 1999) in which the packaging signal is found upstream (Kaye and Lever, 1998; McCann and Lever, 1997) of the major splice donor (SD) and thus is present on all genomic and subgenomic species. Cross-packaging by HIV-1 Gag confirmed that the spliced HIV-2 RNA had a competent packaging signal yet it is excluded from the native HIV-2 particle. Selectivity was shown to be achieved both by cotranslational packaging and by a relative paucity of available Gag protein (Griffin *et al.*, 2001) minimizing the opportunity for packaging of other psi-containing mRNAs *in trans*. This mechanism contrasts strikingly with the situation in murine leukemia viruses (MuLV) in which it was shown that actinomycin D treatment of virus producing cells led to continued virus production but a loss of genomic RNA content of the virions (Levin and Rosenak, 1976). This implied that genomic RNA that is being translated is not available for subsequent encapsidation. (Another interpretation would be that a cellular factor in limited supply and essential for encapsidation had also been depleted by the actinomycin treatment.) The MuLV system was more recently reexamined using RNase protection in a time course assay analogous to the previous work. This confirmed the inability of translating RNA to be packaged under these circumstances. In HIV by contrast using either actinomycin D or leptomycin B (which rather than blocking transcription, inhibits nuclear export of RNA by interfering with Rev/CRM1 function), the genomic RNA was persistently incorporated into virions implying that the translating and packaging RNA pools were one and the same (Dorman and Lever, 2000). A similar conclusion was reached by a second series of experiments with the additional finding that despite there being a common RNA pool, translation was not an essential prerequisite to packaging (Butsch and Boris-Lawrie, 2000). Later published work generated results implying that HIV-1 also packaged RNA cotranslationally (Liang *et al.*, 2002; Poon *et al.*, 2002); however, more recently further experiments have verified earlier findings (Kaye and Lever, 1999) that *in vivo* HIV can package RNA *in trans* (Nikolaitchik *et al.*, 2006), that is, HIV-1 Gag protein is capable of binding to and encapsidating noncognate RNA containing a packaging signal, something which HIV-2 appears to do much less readily *in vivo* if the Gag is expressed from a psi-containing RNA (Griffin *et al.*, 2001; Strappe *et al.*, 2005).

Cotranslational packaging is a plausible strategy for retroviruses to maintain specificity yet it must be remembered that in general *trans* packaging has been largely studied in overexpression or vector systems in which packaging specificity itself may be less rigorous. However, the very existence of the vast sequence diversity of HIV, much of which has been attributed to recombination, speaks to the fact that packaging of heterodimeric RNA originating from two proviruses in the same cell must be a frequent event or must give rise to advantageous recombinants at a significant frequency. There is evidence that HIV has a greater propensity to package heterodimers than do murine retroviruses (Flynn *et al.*, 2004).

D. Translation and Packaging: Controlling the Balance

Cotranslational packaging poses a further problem for the virus since there will inevitably be competition for the RNA between Gag and the ribosome. This is exacerbated by the proximity of the packaging signal, where Gag binds, and the Gag initiation codon, where the ribosome subunits will assemble. Debate continues as to whether translation initiation in HIV occurs through scanning (Yilmaz *et al.*, 2006) or through an internal ribosome entry site (IRES) (Buck *et al.*, 2001). Some evidence suggests that the ribosome has scanned all or part of the 5′ UTR since an artificially introduced upstream in frame AUG can be used to produce an N-terminally extended protein (Miele *et al.*, 1996). Our own studies suggest that the IRES activity in HIV-1 is relatively weak (Anderson and Lever, personal observations). Even if an IRES does exist and is functional during particular periods of the cell cycle as has been suggested (Brasey *et al.*, 2003), competition between the arriving 40S ribosomal subunit and the Gag protein binding to psi will still occur. In RSV, Gag-mediated inhibition of expression of an RSV psi-containing vector has supported the concept that Gag can compete with the ribosome successfully by binding to the leader region (Sonstegard and Hackett, 1996); however, in RSV if Gag does capture the genome in the nucleus, it is not a useful comparator. In HIV, we have recently shown that competition between translation and packaging does occur, *in vitro* and *in vivo*, and that as the concentration of Gag rises, the rate of translation initially also rises through an as yet unexplained enhancing mechanism but with increasing Gag, it subsequently declines consistent with exclusion of the ribosome by the Gag protein assembling on the RNA (Fig. 2). The reproducible quantitative effect suggests that there are a critical number of Gag proteins needed to bind to the RNA to block scanning (Anderson and Lever, 2006); the stoichiometry is consistent with the leader being completely coated with Gag. Once this has occurred it acts as a switch leading to encapsidation.

E. Cross-Packaging Between Primate Lentiviruses

HIV-1 viral proteins have been shown to package HIV-1, HIV-2 (Kaye and Lever, 1999), and SIV (Rizvi and Panganiban, 1993) psi-containing RNAs, whereas HIV-2 is not only unable to package HIV-1 RNA but also fails to pick up *in trans* HIV-2 (Kaye and Lever, 1999) psi-containing vectors in the same cell. Unexpectedly, SIV, which in many ways resembles HIV-2 in the position of its packaging sequence upstream of the SD (Strappe *et al.*, 2003), behaves more like HIV-1 in being able to capture HIV-2 psi-containing RNA *in trans* as efficiently as it captures its own genome (Strappe *et al.*, 2005). The findings indicate that there is cross-recognition of packaging signals which must therefore, despite sequence dissimilarity, have three-dimensional structural homology. The inability of HIV-2 to cross package any primate lentiviral RNA *in trans* points either at a subcellular localization phenomenon or perhaps that HIV-2 has a strong preference for preformed RNA dimers, whereas HIV-1 and SIV can capture monomeric genomes. The P2/SP1 peptide of Gag may be an important influence on this reciprocity as discussed below.

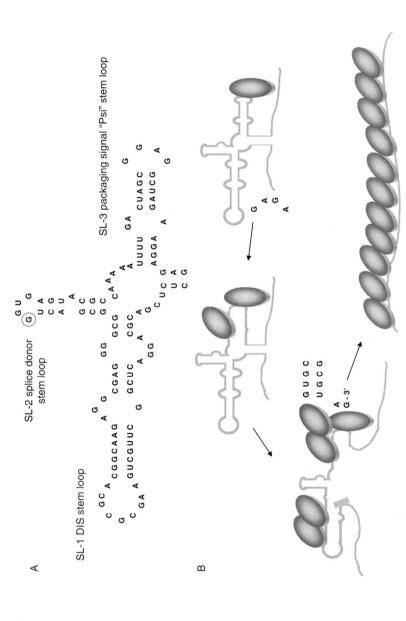

FIGURE 2 (A) Model of RNA secondary structure of the core packaging signal in HIV-1 showing major stem loops. (B) Schematic of RNA capture by Gag through binding to high-affinity sites followed by assembly of Gag on leader.

F. Trafficking to the Cell Membrane and the Budding Virus Particle

Other than the circumstantial evidence quoted above we do not know how many Gag proteins bind to the genome prior to transport to the cell membrane, although it seems unlikely that the complete coating of the 9-kb RNA with Gag occurs. A nucleoprotein complex with a smaller number of Gag proteins forming, with their captured RNA, a trafficking signal is an attractive option.

In other retroviruses, subcellular tracking studies have identified complexes of Gag (Basyuk *et al.*, 2003), RNA, and Env protein trafficking together associated with late endosomal markers. Other chapters will describe viral budding and assembly in more detail.

G. Viral Assembly

It is plausible and supported by some experimental evidence that RNA, but not necessarily the genome, has a structural "scaffolding" role in aiding viral assembly (Cimarelli *et al.*, 2000; Muriaux *et al.*, 2001). This is supported by recent *in vitro* assembly data indicating that RNA may trigger assembly even when present in trace amounts (Ulbrich *et al.*, 2006). Formation of a Gag dimer appears to be a critical stage (Alfadhli *et al.*, 2005) with substitution of the RNA-binding site by a protein dimerization site leading to equally efficient particle assembly. Since particles can be obtained from cells in which the viral RNA has a deleted packaging signal, it is clear that psi alone is not essential for viral assembly. However, the genome has been suggested to have an additional structural role after assembly (Wang and Aldovini, 2002).

How the RNA capture is coordinated with assembly of the viral Gag and Gag/Pol polyproteins is not understood. It would be surprising if the system did not favor a situation where the presence of genomic RNA bound to Gag generated viral particles in preference to Gag particles lacking the genome. As yet there is no evidence of specific RNA binding for the endosomal sorting complex required for transport (ESCRT) family of proteins or other cellular ligands known to be involved in assembly.

IV. RNA/Protein Recognition for Encapsidation: Molecular and Structural Biology _____

Packaging of genomic retroviral RNA depends on structural motifs in the RNA rather than simple sequence recognition. A signal necessary for packaging HIV-1 was identified when deletion of 19 bases from a region between the major 5′ SD and the Gag initiation codon led to a phenotype of normal protein production and viral particle release but with virions containing 5% or less of the normal level of genomic RNA (Lever *et al.*, 1989). Confirmation of this finding followed swiftly (Aldovini and Young, 1990; Clavel and Orenstein, 1990) and mutational analysis identified the zinc finger motifs of the nucleocapsid (NC) region of Gag as critical in this process as had been described in other retroviruses. Certain mutations of the NC region gave a similar phenotype to deletions of the RNA signal (Gorelick *et al.*, 1990).

Notably in many of these studies it was observed that mutations of the RNA or protein gave a packaging defect that was incomplete. This probably reflected the fact that an overexpressed RNA with a defective packaging signal can still gain access to a virion probably through sheer overrepresentation in the cell. However, under these conditions preferential enrichment of genomic RNA in virions relative to spliced RNAs is not seen (Luban and Goff, 1994). Most work has been performed using transient transfection of high expressing constructs, which was often essential in order to generate sufficient viral particles for analysis. The genome is known to comprise only 50% of the total RNA in a virion and a variety of other RNAs have been identified in the virion (Giles *et al.*, 2004). There is evidence of preferential packaging of some cellular RNAs, including the 7 SL RNA, which despite having a similar stem loop to HIV-psi (Zeffman *et al.*, 2000) is captured independently of the RNA-binding region of Gag (Onafuwa-Nuga *et al.*, 2006). RNAs considerably longer than genome length, up to 18 kb, can be encapsidated experimentally, although encapsidation efficiency appears to decline with increasing length (Kumar *et al.*, 2001). tRNAs are present, both those for specific priming of reverse transcription, but also a range of others incorporated randomly (Kleiman *et al.*, 1991; Mak and Kleiman, 1997). Ribosomes themselves have been visualized in retroviral particles defective for genomic RNA (Muriaux *et al.*, 2002). The budding process is probably not rigorously exclusive and an RNA present at a greater than background level will likely be captured nonspecifically by Gag/NC to a level partially reflecting its cellular abundance.

A. Biology of RNA Capture by the Gag Protein

1. Site of the Packaging Signal

In HIV-1, the major psi region is located downstream of the 5′ splice site such that it appears only on the unspliced RNA. In HIV-2 and SIV it is found upstream of the SD. Cotranslational packaging explains the retained specificity. In the latter two, the UTR is significantly longer. The positioning may be influenced by the distance from the 5′ cap site which is similar in all three viruses (Strappe *et al.*, 2003; Fig. 3). It is tempting to speculate that this conservation of RNA sequence length reflects the operation of the molecular

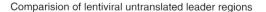

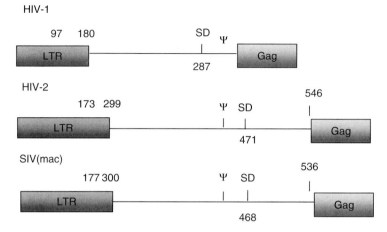

FIGURE 3   Leader sequence diagrams of HIV-1, HIV-2, and SIV showing similarity of packaging signal site relative to transcriptional start site.

"switch" between translation and packaging (and the number of Gag proteins binding to the UTR) described above.

B. Structural RNA Motifs Involved in Packaging HIV RNA

The absence of strong consensus sequences in encapsidation signals implies that the recognition process depends on structural motifs created by intramolecular and possibly intermolecular folding of the RNA and there is evidence for compact folding of the UTR (Berkhout and van Wamel, 2000). A larger complex possibly involving long-range interactions between the poly A sequence and a sequence in the matrix gene (Paillart *et al.*, 2002) may exist. Secondary structural analysis of the HIV leader has been performed using three complementary techniques: biochemical probing to identify double- and single-stranded regions, free energy minimization using computer-based "folding" algorithms, and phylogenetic comparison seeking conserved regions and covariation in base pairing. A daunting number of these analyses have been published (Baudin *et al.*, 1993; Clever and Parslow, 1997; Clever *et al.*, 2002; Damgaard *et al.*, 1998; Harrison and Lever, 1992; Hayashi *et al.*, 1993). Their limitations include the fact that it is not possible to identify biochemically the paired or unpaired nature of every nucleotide and that free energy–based folding programs are based on increasingly sophisticated but still limited parameters and also on nonphysiological conditions of salt and molarity. This has led to controversy over the exact structures since there are often equally plausible models which can be derived from identical data. This has been simultaneously clarified and complicated by the realization that the RNA leader is not a static structure but likely folds into two or possibly more alternative stable structures (Huthoff and Berkhout, 2001). These different forms can be identified *in vitro*, although evidence for them both in infected cells is still lacking (Paillart *et al.*, 2004).

Three stem loops have been reproducibly identified (Clever *et al.*, 1995; Harrison and Lever, 1992) and are generally known by their function or by an SL abbreviation, thus the dimerization loop (SL-1) is upstream of the SD (SL-2) loop and this is 5′ of the packaging signal (psi) or SL-3 stem loop (Fig. 2). Early work suggested that an AU-rich sequence in the leader was important for packaging either alone (Darlix *et al.*, 1990) or in association with SL-2 and/or SL-3 (Sakaguchi *et al.*, 1993). Subsequent work using a vaccinia expression system (Hayashi *et al.*, 1992) implicated the downstream SL-3 region which was later shown to fold into a helix loop structure with a terminal purine tetrad GGAG (G770, G771, G772, G773 numbering from 5′ U3). This motif is accepted as the principal packaging signal (Harrison and Lever, 1992) and is known either as the psi (ψ) loop or stem loop-3 (SL-3) (Clever *et al.*, 1995). Although structures have been published for the upstream SD stem loop (SL-2) (Amarasinghe *et al.*, 2000a,b), there is little evidence that this region contributes significantly to packaging, despite its ability to bind NC protein effectively (Sakaguchi *et al.*, 1993; Shubsda *et al.*, 2002). Similarly, a downstream GNRA motif sometimes termed SL-4 has been modeled (Clever *et al.*, 1995; Kerwood *et al.*, 2001), but it also appears to have little role in packaging and only weak affinity for NC (Amarasinghe *et al.*, 2001). Different regions of the SL-3 stem loop have been implicated as Gag-binding sites in the past but the current consensus is that the purine-rich loop (Sakaguchi *et al.*, 1993) and possibly an internal purine bulge are most important (Zeffman *et al.*, 2000). The terminal tetrad sequence is extremely highly conserved *in vivo* in HIV. However, mutagenesis has demonstrated that alternative loop sequences AAGA (Clever and Parslow, 1997) or GCUA (Russell *et al.*, 2003a) appear to cause no specific packaging deficiency. By contrast, mutations which destabilize the helix completely disrupt packaging (Clever and Parslow, 1997; Harrison *et al.*, 1998), whereas compensatory mutations recreating the helix but with a different sequence can restore it. Mutations that overstabilize the helix loop are strikingly deleterious to RNA/protein binding *in vitro*, particularly those which decrease loop flexibility, for example, creating a GNRA (Paoletti *et al.*, 2002) or UNCG stable terminal tetraloop (Shubsda *et al.*, 2002), implying a lower stability is an intrinsic requirement for function. Intriguingly, protein/RNA affinity studies show that alternative loop sequences (e.g., GGUG) have a higher affinity for NC than the wild-type sequence (Paoletti *et al.*, 2002), thus there are factors other than simply binding affinity determining the conservation of the GGAG loop sequence.

A number of other sequences influence packaging including the TAR stem loop (Harrich *et al.*, 2000; Helga-Maria *et al.*, 1999) and the 5' poly A stem loop in which destabilizing mutations decrease packaging (Das *et al.*, 1997). Structure rather than sequence appears to be critical since compensatory mutations restoring structure restore packaging (Clever *et al.*, 1999). The 5' region of the Gag open reading frame (ORF) has also been implicated in packaging (Luban and Goff, 1994; Parolin *et al.*, 1994). Whatever contributions these make, the SL-3 and the SL-1 region (through RNA dimerization) appear to be the dominant motifs and both are discussed in more detail below.

C. Gag Protein and Packaging

Lentiviruses like other retroviruses mature during and after budding in a process where the viral protease cleaves the Gag and Gag/Pol polyproteins and condensation takes place to produce, in lentiviruses, the typical conical core inside a Matrix-lined spherical envelope. Although the Pol region of the Gag/Pol polyprotein is implicated in encapsidating the primer tRNA required for initiating reverse transcription into the virion (Mak *et al.*, 1994), all the evidence points to the uncleaved Gag proteins as being the ligands which capture the genome. Incorporation of Gag/Pol into particles is in fact dependent on the presence of Gag polyproteins (Kaye and Lever, 1996; Park and Morrow, 1992). Early work identified the basic residues flanking the zinc fingers as important (Poon *et al.*, 1996; Schmalzbauer *et al.*, 1996), and this has been confirmed by the subsequent structural analyses. A number of studies have found that the two zinc fingers of the NC region of Gag (Fig. 4) differ both in their biophysical characteristics notably their electrostatic potential (Khandogin *et al.*, 2003) and that they are not equally important for RNA capture. The first which has a more positive electrostatic potential (and which is more highly conserved) is more critical for function (Dannull *et al.*, 1994; Gorelick *et al.*, 1993). This was supported by early nuclear magnetic resonance (NMR) studies (Demene *et al.*, 1994), although intriguingly mutations of cysteines in the second zinc finger potently impairs genome dimerization (Laughrea *et al.*, 2001). The function of Gag polyprotein as the RNA capture protein was also shown by direct binding assays (Berkowitz and Goff, 1994; Clever *et al.*, 1995) in gel shift (Sakaguchi *et al.*, 1993) and footprinting studies (Damgaard *et al.*, 1998). Gag generally, but not always (Clever *et al.*, 1995), shows greater specific binding to psi than NC (Damgaard *et al.*, 1998) and better annealing properties (Roldan *et al.*, 2004). The "footprint" of Gag(NC) on the leader sequences (Damgaard *et al.*, 1998) demonstrates Gag to have a higher affinity than NC for the terminal psi stem loop, while NC bound more avidly than Gag to the unpaired loop bases in the primer binding site. NC binding to psi is more sensitive to SDS than is Gag (Berkowitz *et al.*, 1993). Single-molecule studies

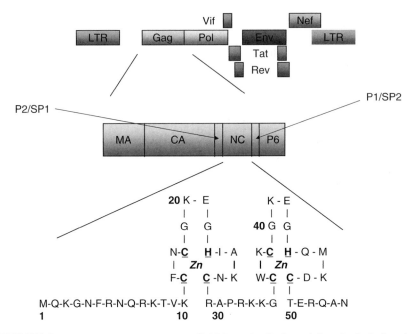

FIGURE 4 HIV gene structure (some small ORFs omitted). Gag subdomains including sites of "spacer" peptides P2/SP1 and P1/SP2 and amino acid sequence of nucleocapsid (NC) region of Gag. CCHC residues coordinating zinc atom are underlined.

examining the relative binding characteristics of NC and Gag also suggest that Gag is superior (Cruceanu *et al.*, 2006). However, the HIV NC in the context of Gag influences specificity as shown by the impaired packaging efficiency of a chimeric Gag protein containing MLV NC in an HIV-1 Gag backbone (Berkowitz *et al.*, 1995b; Zhang and Barklis, 1995). There is evidence for a second RNA-binding site in Matrix but this is probably not nucleotide sequence specific (Lochrie *et al.*, 1997; Ott *et al.*, 2005).

Gag and NC also have roles other than RNA capture and maintaining structural integrity of the virus particle. The functions of NC have recently been reviewed in detail (Levin *et al.*, 2005). It was noted in a number of early mutagenic studies on Gag that mutations producing a relatively modest defect in RNA encapsidation of around 30% (Gorelick *et al.*, 1990) of wild type could give rise to gross defects in replication out of proportion to the RNA level, and it was concluded that perturbing the NC region zinc fingers must be interfering with more than just RNA encapsidation. From many of these it became clear that the nucleic acid chaperone capacity of Gag/NC was involved in a number of processes including reverse transcription and possibly integration of the provirus (Buckman *et al.*, 2003; Feng *et al.*, 1999; Lener *et al.*, 1998; Poljak *et al.*, 2003). This nucleic acid annealing activity was shown to be dependent on peptide domains outside the zinc fingers (De Rocquigny et al., 1992) and unlike for RNA encapsidation (Dannull et al., 1994), the latter were dispensable. Mutation of the CCHC residues to steroid hormone receptor (CCCC) or transcription factor (CCHH) types does not affect RNA binding in vitro (Urbaneja et al., 1999). However, infectivity is severely impaired in the latter. This would be consistent with the zinc fingers fulfilling a dynamic structural role in encapsidation.

Several studies have suggested that the SP1 or P2 spacer peptide of Gag either influences RNA packaging and dimerization (Hill et al., 2002; Shehu-Xhilaga et al., 2001) or conversely that RNA dimerization affects P2 processing (Liang et al., 1999a). Cross-packaging between HIV-1 and HIV-2 is nonreciprocal, HIV-2 failing to capture HIV-1 RNA but a chimera of HIV-2 Gag in which the NC and P2 proteins from HIV-1 have been substituted demonstrates the trans-packaging properties of HIV-1 (Kaye and Lever, 1998). Without the P2 fragment it is much less efficient. The P2 fragment is a critical joining region between CA and NC, and a structure in which matrix and P2 trimers flank dimeric interactions between CA domains has been modeled (Morellet et al., 2005). Mutants in the dimer initiation sequence (DIS) in long-term culture regain wild-type replication kinetics without restoration of a DIS palindrome but rather by mutations in Gag (Liang et al., 1999b) of which those in P2 appear to be critical (Russell et al., 2003), replication being restored, yet without RNA dimerization. Deleterious effects of mutations in SL-3 can also be compensated for by NC and P2 mutation (Rong et al., 2003). P2 clearly has important effects on affinity (Roldan et al., 2004) and on the specificity (Russell et al., 2003b) of RNA capture.

D. Structural Biology of Packaging

The structure of SL-3 has been analyzed by NMR to generate three-dimensional models. Several NMR-based studies have been published (De Guzman et al., 1998; Pappalardo et al., 1998; Zeffman et al., 2000). In one study, the terminal stem with its GGAG loop (nt 770-773) was modeled bound to the NC subfragment of the Gag polyprotein (De Guzman et al., 1998). In all these three studies, the G770 stacks stably on the adjacent base paired C769 with or without the NC protein bound. The first RNA-only study involved the terminal helix loop segment lengthened by three additional base pairs for technical reasons (Pappalardo et al., 1998). Despite the generation of this more stable helix, the structure of the purine loop retains some flexibility with G771 and G773 able to adopt nonstacking positions and with A772 in a space where it could stack on G770 or the first paired G after the loop G774. Homonuclear NMR produced a model in which the G771 alternated between syn and anti conformers. Subsequent multidimensional analysis (Zeffman *et al.*, 2000) showed that the base was in fact in a single conformation intermediate between the two.

On binding to NC the purine loop structure opens dramatically (De Guzman *et al.*, 1998; Zeffman *et al.*, 2000), associated with a change in sugar pucker in G771 from 2'-*endo* to 3'-*endo* and the G771 purine loop inserting into a hydrophobic cleft formed by Trp37 [shown to be critical in earlier binding (Urbaneja *et al.*, 1999) and subsequent (Vuilleumier *et al.*, 1999) fluorescence studies] with Gln45 and Met46 (numbering from the NC initiating methionine). The exocyclic O6 of G771 hydrogen bonds with the NH peptide backbone of Trp37 and Met46, and the H1 proton hydrogen bonds with the CO of Gly35. In the structure where G771 is stably between *syn* and *anti* conformers (Zeffman *et al.*, 2000) A772 stacks on G771, but on protein binding rearranges to allow extensive hydrophobic contacts between the adenine and NC amino acid side chains Ala25, Phe16 [also shown by fluorescence studies (Vuilleumier *et al.*, 1999)], and Asn17, and generates hydrogen bonds with the Arg32 side chain NH which is an unusually well-conserved basic residue only rarely substituted by Lys. Mutations of this Arg cause significant packaging defects (Poon *et al.*, 1996). The fourth base in the loop G773 appears to be the most critical base in the tetraloop for binding affinity to NC (Paoletti *et al.*, 2002). In the protein-free state, it is outside the main structure with its position relatively ill defined. When bound to NC, this base inserts into a hydrophobic cleft formed by the side chains of Val13, Phe16, Ile24, and Ala25. Phe16 and Ala25 backbone NH groups and the Lys14 backbones CO hydrogen bond with the G773 O6 and H1, respectively.

In the extended SL-3 structure a proximal helix is seen with an internal bulge of GA opposite A (Zeffman *et al.*, 2000). The 5' component of the bulge is seen to be highly unstructured with multiple conformations whereas the opposite strand is equally remarkably stable in almost perfect A form hemi-helical structure. These sequences are also highly conserved, and it seems that the intrinsic metastability is a desirable if not essential feature of the internal bulge as well as the terminal purines. The evidence from biochemical structural studies of the RNA in the presence and absence of Gag is that the RNA helices of SL-3 unwind as Gag binds leading to linearization of the RNA with the potential for further assembly of Gag proteins sequentially along the nucleotide chain (Fig. 2) (Zeffman *et al.*, 2000).

The requirement for flexibility of the RNA in binding to Gag and conformational change during assembly seem paramount.

E. Structure of the Dimer Linkage Site RNA

A dimeric RNA is characteristic of retroviruses and the dimeric state is fundamental to recombination. There is evidence that RNA dimerization occurs in stages beginning with a loose dimer, based on interaction between complementary nucleotide sequences which are commonly palindromic, and maturing into a tight complex (Brahic and Vigne, 1975; Laughrea and Jette, 1997). The RNA annealing properties of NC are widely accepted as facilitating maturation of the RNA dimer (Darlix *et al.*, 1990; Feng *et al.*, 1996; Muriaux *et al.*, 1996; Takahashi *et al.*, 2001), but there is also some evidence that the polymerase (Pol) protein is necessary for core maturation and RNA dimerization (Shehu-Xhilaga *et al.*, 2002). Whether this requires direct Pol-RNA interaction is not clear and it may be an effect of Pol on structural maturation of the core which facilitates mature dimer formation. Dimerization and packaging are closely but not inextricably (Laughrea *et al.*, 2001; Sakuragi *et al.*, 2002; Shen *et al.*, 2000) linked. The dimer linkage region may have pure encapsidation functions as mutations in this region may impair packaging somewhat yet virion RNA that is packaged is still dimeric (Berkhout and van Wamel, 1996). Other mutants of the complementary palindromic sequences in the dimer linkage site have even greater effects on packaging yet dimeric RNA is still found in virions, although interstrand affinity is suggested as possibly being lower (Laughrea *et al.*, 1997). *In vitro* studies suggest that the dimerization equilibrium constant is relatively modest 10^5 M(-1) (Shubsda *et al.*, 1999). Insertion of a second DLS into the HIV-1 genome permitting intramolecular bonding to occur leads to encapsidation of RNA monomers (Sakuragi *et al.*, 2001).

Shortening or disruption of the SL-3 region including sequences involved in the extended helix and internal bulge impairs dimerization and packaging (Russell *et al.*, 2003). Mapping of the dimer signal in HIV-1 places it as a component of the packaging signal (Sakuragi *et al.*, 2003), and overall much of the evidence supports a model whereby dimerization is a consequence of the successful capture of the RNA by Gag, although how soon after initial Gag/RNA binding this occurs is still unknown. There is an accepted, although not rigorously proven consensus that the RNA which goes into the budding virion is already dimeric (Rein, 1994). In HIV-2 a functional link between the two processes is also believed to occur (Lanchy *et al.*, 2003), although the sequence of events may differ.

Dimerization of the HIV genomic RNA was originally proposed to involve a region downstream of the major SD (Darlix *et al.*, 1990). However, subsequent work implicated a region 5′ to the SD (Marquet *et al.*, 1994), and it is now believed to occur through an initial loop–loop interaction between the two strands involving complementary palindromic sequences (Paillart *et al.*, 1994; Skripkin *et al.*, 1994) rather than guanine tetrads (Awang and Sen, 1993; Sundquist and Heaphy, 1993). This is the "kissing loop" model and it has become widely accepted with many studies showing the importance of the region 5′ of the major SD in HIV-1 in RNA dimerization (Berkhout and van Wamel, 1996; Haddrick *et al.*, 1996; Laughrea and Jette, 1994; Marquet *et al.*, 1994; Skripkin *et al.*, 1994). The palindromic sequence also enhances recombination within this region of the genome

(Balakrishnan *et al.*, 2001). Mutations of the dimerization region can affect more than one process in the HIV life cycle, and replication defects caused by mutations here cannot be ascribed purely to interference with packaging, for example, there is evidence that proviral DNA synthesis is also affected (Paillart *et al.*, 1996). The terminal palindromic loop of the packaging signal region involved in dimerization is termed either the DIS loop of SL-1 and it has been extensively studied. Some alternative palindrome sequences can substitute effectively for the native sequence (Laughrea *et al.*, 1999). Biochemical probing has produced two-dimensional and putative three-dimensional structures (Jossinet *et al.*, 1999). NMR-derived three-dimensional structure of the "kissing loop" complex involving the intermolecular base pairing has been published which confirmed some of the deductions from the probing that canonical and noncanonical (Paillart *et al.*, 1997) interactions are important but generated novel findings as well (Mujeeb *et al.*, 1998). Subtending the palindrome are three highly conserved purines, almost always adenines, which are essential to the dimerization process. From the first published NMR structure, interstrand canonical base pairing occurs which distorts the two DIS loops into a plane at 90° to the helices and brings the A residues to proximity where they form intermolecular stacks as part of a short triple helix. The strain on the loop is enough apparently to disrupt the closing base pair of the helix. Both NMR and crystallographic studies of the dimer linkage region have since been published by other groups (Ennifar *et al.*, 2001; Kieken *et al.*, 2006). The overall structures are similar, although the crystallographic solution includes a bulged out motif involving the basal adenines leaving a large space in the helix. Both NMR studies produce a bulged in structure which ablates this. It is possible that adjacent stacking artifactually stabilized the bulged out structure in the crystal.

Within the dimer linkage stem loop proximal to the terminal helix is a small bulge with a single G residue opposite an AGG triplet. The bulge is 100% conserved in all HIV-published sequences. The stem between this and the terminal loop has been shown to be critical for dimerization (Shen *et al.*, 2000) as has the stem proximal to it, including the singleton G (Laughrea *et al.*, 1999) and it may in part regulate the two-stage dimerization process (Shen *et al.*, 2001; Takahashi *et al.*, 2000). Structural analysis has produced some divergent results. One NMR study generated a single structure with the singlet G making a mismatched pair with the A stacking on the distal stem and the G doublet stacking on the proximal stem (Lawrence *et al.*, 2003). A second NMR study failed to identify a single conformation for the bulge (Greatorex *et al.*, 2002). A mutant in which two purines had been exchanged, AGG to GGA, generated a stable structure in which triangulated hydrogen bonds across the helix fixed the purines. From this it was inferred that the AGG structure was highly unstable and might adopt alternative confirmations due to the single G resonating between two positions of approximately equal free energy. Subsequent work confirmed that alternative structures exist and that they exchanged readily (Yuan *et al.*, 2003). In this study, a mutant was produced which stabilized one conformation producing a bend in the helix which potentially favored RNA dimerization (Yuan *et al.*, 2003). Thus, another region of highly conserved metastability probably exists in the psi region allowing unwinding of the helix and permitting generation, under appropriate conditions, of a structure which could favor dimer formation and encapsidation. Mutations to GU-rich sequences at the base of the poly A and primer binding site stem loops also affect dimer formation but not local secondary structure, implying that they may be involved in direct intermolecular bonding in the dimer (Russell *et al.*, 2002). In addition, the Tat responsive region (TAR) stem loop contains a palindromic sequence which can self-anneal in the presence of NC protein (Andersen *et al.*, 2004) and it is plausible that this contributes to dimerization after encapsidation. While loop-loop interactions of the terminal SL-1 palindrome are widely accepted as the initiating process in dimerization, what follows this is much less clear. The RNA strands are paired in an antiparallel orientation and theoretically could unwind, and base pair in a complementary bulged helix of some 15–25 base pairs in length (Aci *et al.*, 2005; Bernacchi *et al.*, 2005). NMR structures of an isolated putative helix (Girard *et al.*, 1999) or bulged double helix have been published (Ennifar *et al.*, 1999; Mujeeb *et al.*, 1999; Ulyanov *et al.*, 2006).

F. Conformational Change in the 5′ UTR RNA

As described above, there is ample evidence for small areas of the packaging signal changing conformation during encapsidation. There is also evidence that much larger global changes in structure influence the process. One model in particular postulates an equilibrium between two major species: long distance interaction (LDI) and a branched multiple hairpin (BMH) structure (Huthoff and Berkhout, 2001) (Fig. 5). There is biochemical evidence for these two *in vitro* from the observation of different mobility species of the same RNA. These two structures do not appear to influence the balance between packaging and translation *in vitro* (Abbink *et al.*, 2005). Functionally the model has attractions. The LDI model has the DIS palindrome base paired within a helix reducing the potential for intermolecular dimerization (and possibly packaging?) to occur (Berkhout *et al.*, 2002). The BMH model has the DIS exposed. It also has the packaging signal loop SL-3 extended and accessible, including the extended second helix originally described (Harrison and Lever, 1992). This may be the species that is recognized for encapsidation. The existence of these variants has been challenged, as have the presence of other LDIs in the leader by an *in vivo* study using biochemical probes to interrogate the genome in virions and infected cells (Paillart *et al.*, 2004). In this study, many of the original

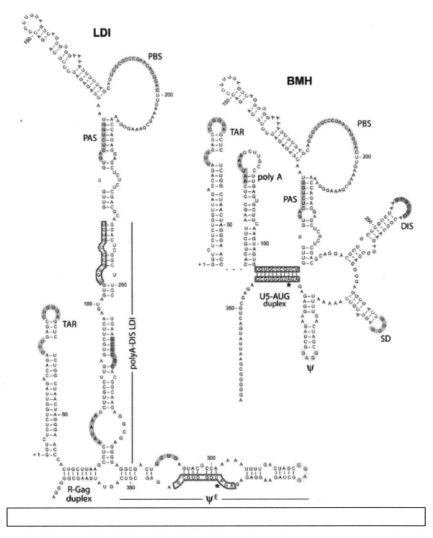

FIGURE 5   Suggested alternative conformations of HIV-1 RNA leader region: long distance interaction (LDI) and branched multiple hairpin (BMH) structures (courtesy of Dr B. Berkhout).

consensus structures were identified but all of the RNA that was detected appeared to be in a structure approximating to the BMH structure. The palindromic sequence involved in dimerization was protected implying that the RNA was already largely dimeric or that the sequence was occluded by other means. We have recently demonstrated that in HIV-2 dimeric RNA can be found in the infected cell although it is not the major unspliced species

(L'Hernault, Greatorex, and Lever, unpublished data), and it is difficult to believe that almost all of the unspliced RNA in the translating pool is dimeric. The disparity between the cellular data and the *in vitro* modeling is unexplained; however, it is notable that the primer extension assays in the *in vivo* work were performed from a 3' primer which exists only in the unspliced RNA and hence their conclusions relate only to the structure of the genomic species. Examination of the BMH/LDI models suggests that the base pairing on which the BMH structure depends would be absent in the spliced messages (Ooms *et al.*, 2004) and hence the 5' region of the LDI model may represent the structure of the 5' end of the singly and multiply spliced RNAs. This has certain logic in that the psi signal and dimerization sites would be optimally presented only in the unspliced RNA.

There is evidence from HIV-2 that spliced and unspliced mRNAs dimerize differently (Lanchy *et al.*, 2004), although paradoxically the genomic RNA forms a less stable dimer than the spliced species. If, as it appears in HIV-2, dimerization and packaging are even more closely linked than in HIV-1, it argues that the dimer that forms has to be one with a specific conformation and that mere dimeric aggregation, however stable, is not the key to successful encapsidation. Dimerization in HIV-2 is a more complex and less well-understood process possibly involving several regions (Lanchy *et al.*, 2003a,b) and more than one palindrome (Lanchy and Lodmell, 2002). Exactly where and when dimers form remains unknown, and this is an area of study in which considerably more work is needed.

V. Conclusions

This chapter has attempted to show what the consensus areas are in RNA packaging in HIV but also to illustrate the yawning gaps in our knowledge. It is never possible to be absolutely comprehensive in such a review and to those authors who believe that their work is incompletely cited, I apologize. A review by definition is one person's view and others may interpret the available data differently. It does seem however that there is an overall model emerging of RNA packaging being, a highly regulated process all the way through from transcription to virus budding. It involves many more cellular ligands than we know at present, and the RNA likely exists in a number of different structures at different time points during its passage through the cell. These structures will change according to the protein ligands that are bound of which, as yet, we know only a few.

As a therapeutic target, RNA encapsidation is extremely attractive. Mutational studies show how sensitive this region is to change and this is reflected in the very high level of sequence conservation of psi. RNA export is also a highly virus-specific process in animal cells and would likely have a wide therapeutic index. Inhibiting packaging would also lead to the release from infected cells of noninfective "empty" virions, which would be effectively a person-specific immunostimulant reflecting the repertoire of virus in that individual. In essence, it would generate a good immune-enhancing "vaccine." For this reason, there have been a number of studies attempting to block packaging therapeutically involving antisense, RNA decoys, ribozymes, RNA interference, and so on (Berkhout, 2004; Chadwick and Lever, 2000; Dorman and Lever, 2001; Joshi *et al.*, 2003; Morris and Rossi, 2006; Nishitsuji *et al.*, 2001) many of which have shown promising results but may be limited by the logistics of translation into a pharmacologic agent. Oligonucleotides can also block packaging (Brown *et al.*, 2005, 2006) and newer conjugated oligos (Ivanova *et al.*, 2006), which may be developed to become orally bioavailable, open up vast new opportunities for interfering with this and many other viral processes.

References

Abbink, T. E., Ooms, M., Haasnoot, P. C., and Berkhout, B. (2005). The HIV-1 leader RNA conformational switch regulates RNA dimerization but does not regulate mRNA translation. *Biochemistry* **44**, 9058–9066.

Aci, S., Mazier, S., and Genest, D. (2005). Conformational pathway for the kissing complex--> extended dimer transition of the SL1 stem-loop from genomic HIV-1 RNA as monitored by targeted molecular dynamics techniques. *J. Mol. Biol.* **351**, 520–530.

Aldovini, A., and Young, R. A. (1990). Mutations of RNA and protein sequences involved in human immunodeficiency virus type 1 packaging result in production of noninfectious virus. *J. Virol.* **64**, 1920–1926.

Alfadhli, A., Dhenub, T. C., Still, A., and Barklis, E. (2005). Analysis of human immunodeficiency virus type 1 Gag dimerization-induced assembly. *J. Virol.* **79**, 14498–14506.

Amarasinghe, G. K., De Guzman, R. N., Turner, R. B., Chancellor, K. J., Wu, Z. R., and Summers, M. F. (2000a). NMR structure of the HIV-1 nucleocapsid protein bound to stem-loop SL2 of the psi-RNA packaging signal. Implications for genome recognition. *J. Mol. Biol.* **301**, 491–511.

Amarasinghe, G. K., De Guzman, R. N., Turner, R. B., and Summers, M. F. (2000b). NMR structure of stem-loop SL2 of the HIV-1 psi RNA packaging signal reveals a novel A-U-A base-triple platform. *J. Mol. Biol.* **299**, 145–156.

Amarasinghe, G. K., Zhou, J., Miskimon, M., Chancellor, K. J., McDonald, J. A., Matthews, A. G., Miller, R. R., Rouse, M. D., and Summers, M. F. (2001). Stem-loop SL4 of the HIV-1 psi RNA packaging signal exhibits weak affinity for the nucleocapsid protein. structural studies and implications for genome recognition. *J. Mol. Biol.* **314**, 961–970.

Anderson, E., and Lever, A. (2006). HIV-1 Gag polyprotein modulates its own translation. *J. Virol.* **80**, 10478–10486.

Andersen, E. S., Contera, S. A., Knudsen, B., Damgaard, C. K., Besenbacher, F., and Kjems, J. (2004). Role of the trans-activation response element in dimerization of HIV-1 RNA. *J. Biol. Chem.* **279**, 22243–22249.

Anson, D. S., and Fuller, M. (2003). Rational development of a HIV-1 gene therapy vector. *J. Gene Med.* **5**, 829–838.

Awang, G., and Sen, D. (1993). Mode of dimerization of HIV-1 genomic RNA. *Biochemistry* **32**, 11453–11457.

Balakrishnan, M., Fay, P. J., and Bambara, R. A. (2001). The kissing hairpin sequence promotes recombination within the HIV-1 5′ leader region. *J. Biol. Chem.* **276**, 36482–36492.

Basyuk, E., Galli, T., Mougel, M., Blanchard, J. M., Sitbon, M., and Bertrand, E. (2003). Retroviral genomic RNAs are transported to the plasma membrane by endosomal vesicles. *Dev. Cell* **5**, 161–174.

Baudin, F., Marquet, R., Isel, C., Darlix, J. L., Ehresmann, B., and Ehresmann, C. (1993). Functional sites in the 5′ region of human immunodeficiency virus type 1 RNA form defined structural domains. *J. Mol. Biol.* **229**, 382–397.

Bennett, E. M., Lever, A. M., and Allen, J. F. (2004). Human immunodeficiency virus type 2 Gag interacts specifically with PRP4, a serine-threonine kinase, and inhibits phosphorylation of splicing factor SF2. *J. Virol.* **78**, 11303–11312.

Berkhout, B. (2004). RNA interference as an antiviral approach: Targeting HIV-1. *Curr. Opin. Mol. Ther.* **6**, 141–145.

Berkhout, B., and van Wamel, J. L. (1996). Role of the DIS hairpin in replication of human immunodeficiency virus type 1. *J. Virol.* **70**, 6723–6732.

Berkhout, B., and van Wamel, J. L. (2000). The leader of the HIV-1 RNA genome forms a compactly folded tertiary structure. *RNA* **6**, 282–295.

Berkhout, B., Ooms, M., Beerens, N., Huthoff, H., Southern, E., and Verhoef, K. (2002). *In vitro* evidence that the untranslated leader of the HIV-1 genome is an RNA checkpoint that regulates multiple functions through conformational changes. *J. Biol. Chem.* **277**, 19967–19975.

Berkowitz, R. D., and Goff, S. P. (1994). Analysis of binding elements in the human immunodeficiency virus type 1 genomic RNA and nucleocapsid protein. *Virology* **202**, 233–246.

Berkowitz, R. D., Luban, J., and Goff, S. P. (1993). Specific binding of human immunodeficiency virus type 1 gag polyprotein and nucleocapsid protein to viral RNAs detected by RNA mobility shift assays. *J. Virol.* **67**, 7190–7200.

Berkowitz, R. D., Hammarskjold, M. L., Helga-Maria, C., Rekosh, D., and Goff, S. P. (1995a). 5′ regions of HIV-1 RNAs are not sufficient for encapsidation: Implications for the HIV-1 packaging signal. *Virology* **212**, 718–723.

Berkowitz, R. D., Ohagen, A., Hoglund, S., and Goff, S. P. (1995b). Retroviral nucleocapsid domains mediate the specific recognition of genomic viral RNAs by chimeric Gag polyproteins during RNA packaging *in vivo*. *J. Virol.* **69**, 6445–6456.

Bernacchi, S., Ennifar, E., Toth, K., Walter, P., Langowski, J., and Dumas, P. (2005). Mechanism of hairpin-duplex conversion for the HIV-1 dimerization initiation site. *J. Biol. Chem.* **280**, 40112–40121.

Brahic, M., and Vigne, R. (1975). Properties of visna virus particles harvested at short time intervals: RNA content, infectivity, and ultrastructure. *J. Virol.* **15**, 1222–1230.

Brasey, A., Lopez-Lastra, M., Ohlmann, T., Beerens, N., Berkhout, B., Darlix, J. L., and Sonenberg, N. (2003). The leader of human immunodeficiency virus type 1 genomic RNA harbors an internal ribosome entry segment that is active during the G2/M phase of the cell cycle. *J. Virol.* **77**, 3939–3949.

Brown, D., Arzumanov, A. A., Turner, J. J., Stetsenko, D. A., Lever, A. M., and Gait, M. J. (2005). Antiviral activity of steric-block oligonucleotides targeting the HIV-1 trans-activation response and packaging signal stem-loop RNAs. *Nucleosides Nucleotides Nucleic Acids* **24**, 393–396.

Brown, D. E., Arzumanov, A., Syed, S., Gait, M. J., and Lever, A. M. (2006). Inhibition of HIV-1 replication by oligonucleotide analogues directed to the packaging signal and trans-activating response region. *Antivir. Chem. Chemother.* **17**, 1–9.

Buck, C. B., Shen, X., Egan, M. A., Pierson, T. C., Walker, C. M., and Siliciano, R. F. (2001). The human immunodeficiency virus type 1 gag gene encodes an internal ribosome entry site. *J. Virol.* **75**, 181–191.

Buckman, J. S., Bosche, W. J., and Gorelick, R. J. (2003). Human immunodeficiency virus type 1 nucleocapsid zn(2+) fingers are required for efficient reverse transcription, initial integration processes, and protection of newly synthesized viral DNA. *J. Virol.* **77**, 1469–1480.

Bukrinsky, M. I., Haggerty, S., Dempsey, M. P., Sharova, N., Adzhubel, A., Spitz, L., Lewis, P., Goldfarb, D., Emerman, M., and Stevenson, M. (1993). A nuclear localization signal within HIV-1 matrix protein that governs infection of non-dividing cells. *Nature* **365**, 666–669.

Butsch, M., and Boris-Lawrie, K. (2000). Translation is not required to generate virion precursor RNA in human immunodeficiency virus type 1-infected T cells. *J. Virol.* **74**, 11531–11537.

Chadwick, D. R., and Lever, A. M. (2000). Antisense RNA sequences targeting the 5′ leader packaging signal region of human immunodeficiency virus type-1 inhibits viral replication at post-transcriptional stages of the life cycle. *Gene Ther.* **7**, 1362–1368.

Cimarelli, A., Sandin, S., Hoglund, S., and Luban, J. (2000). Basic residues in human immunodeficiency virus type 1 nucleocapsid promote virion assembly via interaction with RNA. *J. Virol.* **74**, 3046–3057.

Clavel, F., and Orenstein, J. M. (1990). A mutant of human immunodeficiency virus with reduced RNA packaging and abnormal particle morphology. *J. Virol.* **64**, 5230–5234.

Clever, J., Sassetti, C., and Parslow, T. G. (1995). RNA secondary structure and binding sites for gag gene products in the 5′ packaging signal of human immunodeficiency virus type 1. *J. Virol.* **69**, 2101–2109.

Clever, J. L., and Parslow, T. G. (1997). Mutant human immunodeficiency virus type 1 genomes with defects in RNA dimerization or encapsidation. *J. Virol.* **71**, 3407–3414.

Clever, J. L., Eckstein, D. A., and Parslow, T. G. (1999). Genetic dissociation of the encapsidation and reverse transcription functions in the 5′ R region of human immunodeficiency virus type 1. *J. Virol.* **73**, 101–109.

Clever, J. L., Mirandar, D., Jr., and Parslow, T. G. (2002). RNA structure and packaging signals in the 5′ leader region of the human immunodeficiency virus type 1 genome. *J. Virol.* **76**, 12381–12387.

Cochrane, A. W., McNally, M. T., and Mouland, A. J. (2006). The retrovirus RNA trafficking granule: From birth to maturity. *Retrovirology* **3**, 18.

Cruceanu, M., Urbaneja, M. A., Hixson, C. V., Johnson, D. G., Datta, S. A., Fivash, M. J., Stephen, A. G., Fisher, R. J., Gorelick, R. J., Casas-Finet, J. R., Rein, A., Rouzina, I., *et al.* (2006). Nucleic acid binding and chaperone properties of HIV-1 Gag and nucleocapsid proteins. *Nucleic Acids Res.* **34**, 593–605.

Cullen, B. R. (1992). Mechanism of action of regulatory proteins encoded by complex retroviruses. *Microbiol. Rev.* **56**, 375–394.

Damgaard, C. K., Dyhr-Mikkelsen, H., and Kjems, J. (1998). Mapping the RNA binding sites for human immunodeficiency virus type-1 gag and NC proteins within the complete HIV-1 and -2 untranslated leader regions. *Nucleic Acids Res.* **26**, 3667–3676.

Dannull, J., Surovoy, A., Jung, G., and Moelling, K. (1994). Specific binding of HIV-1 nucleocapsid protein to PSI RNA *in vitro* requires N-terminal zinc finger and flanking basic amino acid residues. *EMBO J.* **13**, 1525–1533.

Darlix, J. L., Gabus, C., Nugeyre, M. T., Clavel, F., and Barre-Sinoussi, F. (1990). Cis elements and trans-acting factors involved in the RNA dimerization of the human immunodeficiency virus HIV-1. *J. Mol. Biol.* **216**, 689–699.

Das, A. T., Klaver, B., Klasens, B. I., van Wamel, J. L., and Berkhout, B. (1997). A conserved hairpin motif in the R-U5 region of the human immunodeficiency virus type 1 RNA genome is essential for replication. *J. Virol.* **71**, 2346–2356.

De Guzman, R. N., Wu, Z. R., Stalling, C. C., Pappalardo, L., Borer, P. N., and Summers, M. F. (1998). Structure of the HIV-1 nucleocapsid protein bound to the SL3 psi-RNA recognition element. *Science* **279**, 384–388.

De Rocquigny, H., Gabus, C., Vincent, A., Fournie-Zaluski, M. C., Roques, B., and Darlix, J. L. (1992). Viral RNA annealing activities of human immunodeficiency virus type 1 nucleocapsid protein require only peptide domains outside the zinc fingers. *Proc. Natl. Acad. Sci. USA* **89**, 6472–6476.

Demene, H., Dong, C. Z., Ottmann, M., Rouyez, M. C., Jullian, N., Morellet, N., Mely, Y., Darlix, J. L., Fournie-Zaluski, M. C., Saragosti, S., and Roques, B. P. (1994). 1H NMR structure and biological studies of the His23-->Cys mutant nucleocapsid protein of HIV-1 indicate that the conformation of the first zinc finger is critical for virus infectivity. *Biochemistry* **33**, 11707–11716.

Dorman, N., and Lever, A. (2000). Comparison of viral genomic RNA sorting mechanisms in human immunodeficiency virus type 1 (HIV-1), HIV-2, and Moloney murine leukemia virus. *J. Virol.* **74**, 11413–11417.

Dorman, N., and Lever, A. M. (2001). RNA-based gene therapy for HIV infection. *HIV Med.* **2**, 114–122.

Ennifar, E., Yusupov, M., Walter, P., Marquet, R., Ehresmann, B., Ehresmann, C., and Dumas, P. (1999). The crystal structure of the dimerization initiation site of genomic HIV-1 RNA reveals an extended duplex with two adenine bulges. *Structure* **7**, 1439–1449.

Ennifar, E., Walter, P., Ehresmann, B., Ehresmann, C., and Dumas, P. (2001). Crystal structures of coaxially stacked kissing complexes of the HIV-1 RNA dimerization initiation site. *Nat. Struct. Biol.* **8**, 1064–1068.

Feng, Y. X., Copeland, T. D., Henderson, L. E., Gorelick, R. J., Bosche, W. J., Levin, J. G., and Rein, A. (1996). HIV-1 nucleocapsid protein induces maturation of dimeric retroviral RNA *in vitro*. *Proc. Natl. Acad. Sci. USA* **93**, 7577–7581.

Feng, Y. X., Campbell, S., Harvin, D., Ehresmann, B., Ehresmann, C., and Rein, A. (1999). The human immunodeficiency virus type 1 Gag polyprotein has nucleic acid chaperone activity: Possible role in dimerization of genomic RNA and placement of tRNA on the primer binding site. *J. Virol.* **73**, 4251–4256.

Flynn, J. A., An, W., King, S. R., and Telesnitsky, A. (2004). Nonrandom dimerization of murine leukemia virus genomic RNAs. *J. Virol.* **78**, 12129–12139.

Gallego, J., Greatorex, J., Zhang, H., Yang, B., Arunachalam, S., Fang, J., Seamons, J., Lea, S., Pomerantz, R. J., and Lever, A. M. (2003). Rev binds specifically to a purine loop in the SL1 region of the HIV-1 leader RNA. *J. Biol. Chem.* **278**, 40385–40391.

Giles, K. E., Caputi, M., and Beemon, K. L. (2004). Packaging and reverse transcription of snRNAs by retroviruses may generate pseudogenes. *RNA* **10**, 299–307.

Girard, F., Barbault, F., Gouyette, C., Huynh-Dinh, T., Paoletti, J., and Lancelot, G. (1999). Dimer initiation sequence of HIV-1Lai genomic RNA: NMR solution structure of the extended duplex. *J. Biomol. Struct. Dyn.* **16**, 1145–1157.

Gorelick, R. J., Nigida, S. M., Jr., Bess, J. W., Jr., Arthur, L. O., Henderson, L. E., and Rein, A. (1990). Noninfectious human immunodeficiency virus type 1 mutants deficient in genomic RNA. *J. Virol.* **64**, 3207–3211.

Gorelick, R. J., Chabot, D. J., Rein, A., Henderson, L. E., and Arthur, L. O. (1993). The two zinc fingers in the human immunodeficiency virus type 1 nucleocapsid protein are not functionally equivalent. *J. Virol.* **67**, 4027–4036.

Greatorex, J. (2004). The retroviral RNA dimer linkage: Different structures may reflect different roles. *Retrovirology* **1**, 22.

Greatorex, J., Gallego, J., Varani, G., and Lever, A. (2002). Structure and stability of wild-type and mutant RNA internal loops from the SL-1 domain of the HIV-1 packaging signal. *J. Mol. Biol.* **322**, 543–557.

Greatorex, J. S., Palmer, E. A., Pomerantz, R. J., Dangerfield, J. A., and Lever, A. M. (2006). Mutation of the Rev-binding loop in the human immunodeficiency virus 1 leader causes a replication defect characterized by altered RNA trafficking and packaging. *J. Gen. Virol.* **87**, 3039–3044.

Griffin, S. D., Allen, J. F., and Lever, A. M. (2001). The major human immunodeficiency virus type 2 (HIV-2) packaging signal is present on all HIV-2 RNA species: Cotranslational RNA encapsidation and limitation of Gag protein confer specificity. *J. Virol.* **75**, 12058–12069.

Haddrick, M., Lear, A. L., Cann, A. J., and Heaphy, S. (1996). Evidence that a kissing loop structure facilitates genomic RNA dimerisation in HIV-1. *J. Mol. Biol.* **259**, 58–68.

Harrich, D., Hooker, C. W., and Parry, E. (2000). The human immunodeficiency virus type 1 TAR RNA upper stem-loop plays distinct roles in reverse transcription and RNA packaging. *J. Virol.* **74**, 5639–5646.

Harrison, G. P., and Lever, A. M. (1992). The human immunodeficiency virus type 1 packaging signal and major splice donor region have a conserved stable secondary structure. *J. Virol.* **66**, 4144–4153.

Harrison, G. P., Miele, G., Hunter, E., and Lever, A. M. (1998). Functional analysis of the core human immunodeficiency virus type 1 packaging signal in a permissive cell line. *J. Virol.* **72**, 5886–5896.

Hayashi, T., Shioda, T., Iwakura, Y., and Shibuta, H. (1992). RNA packaging signal of human immunodeficiency virus type 1. *Virology* **188**, 590–599.

Hayashi, T., Ueno, Y., and Okamoto, T. (1993). Elucidation of a conserved RNA stem-loop structure in the packaging signal of human immunodeficiency virus type 1. *FEBS Lett.* **327**, 213–218.

Helga-Maria, C., Hammarskjold, M. L., and Rekosh, D. (1999). An intact TAR element and cytoplasmic localization are necessary for efficient packaging of human immunodeficiency virus type 1 genomic RNA. *J. Virol.* **73**, 4127–4135.

Hill, M. K., Shehu-Xhilaga, M., Crowe, S. M., and Mak, J. (2002). Proline residues within spacer peptide p1 are important for human immunodeficiency virus type 1 infectivity, protein processing, and genomic RNA dimer stability. *J. Virol.* **76**, 11245–11253.

Huthoff, H., and Berkhout, B. (2001). Two alternating structures of the HIV-1 leader RNA. *RNA* **7**, 143–157.

Ivanova, G., Arzumanov, A., Turner, J., Reigadas, S., Toulmé, J.-J., Brown, D., Lever, A., and Gait, M. (2006). Anti-HIV activity of steric block oligonucleotides. *Ann. NY Acad. Sci.*

Joshi, P. J., Fisher, T. S., and Prasad, V. R. (2003). Anti-HIV inhibitors based on nucleic acids: Emergence of aptamers as potent antivirals. *Curr. Drug Targets Infect. Disord.* **3**, 383–400.

Jossinet, F., Paillart, J. C., Westhof, E., Hermann, T., Skripkin, E., Lodmell, J. S., Ehresmann, C., Ehresmann, B., and Marquet, R. (1999). Dimerization of HIV-1 genomic RNA of subtypes A and B: RNA loop structure and magnesium binding. *RNA* **5**, 1222–1234.

Katz, R. A., and Skalka, A. M. (1990). Generation of diversity in retroviruses. *Annu. Rev. Genet.* **24**, 409–445.

Kaye, J. F., and Lever, A. M. (1996). trans-acting proteins involved in RNA encapsidation and viral assembly in human immunodeficiency virus type 1. *J. Virol.* **70**, 880–886.

Kaye, J. F., and Lever, A. M. (1998). Nonreciprocal packaging of human immunodeficiency virus type 1 and type 2 RNA: A possible role for the p2 domain of Gag in RNA encapsidation. *J. Virol.* **72**, 5877–5885.

Kaye, J. F., and Lever, A. M. (1999). Human immunodeficiency virus types 1 and 2 differ in the predominant mechanism used for selection of genomic RNA for encapsidation. *J. Virol.* **73**, 3023–3031.

Kerwood, D. J., Cavaluzzi, M. J., and Borer, P. N. (2001). Structure of SL4 RNA from the HIV-1 packaging signal. *Biochemistry* **40**, 14518–14529.

Khandogin, J., Musier-Forsyth, K., and York, D. M. (2003). Insights into the regioselectivity and RNA-binding affinity of HIV-1 nucleocapsid protein from linear-scaling quantum methods. *J. Mol. Biol.* **330**, 993–1004.

Kharytonchyk, S. A., Kireyeva, A. I., Osipovich, A. B., and Fomin, I. K. (2005). Evidence for preferential copackaging of Moloney murine leukemia virus genomic RNAs transcribed in the same chromosomal site. *Retrovirology* **2**, 3.

Kieken, F., Paquet, F., Brule, F., Paoletti, J., and Lancelot, G. (2006). A new NMR solution structure of the SL1 HIV-1Lai loop-loop dimer. *Nucleic Acids Res.* **34**, 343–352.

Kleiman, L., Caudry, S., Boulerice, F., Wainberg, M. A., and Parniak, M. A. (1991). Incorporation of tRNA into normal and mutant HIV-1. *Biochem. Biophys. Res. Commun.* **174**, 1272–1280.

Kumar, M., Keller, B., Makalou, N., and Sutton, R. E. (2001). Systematic determination of the packaging limit of lentiviral vectors. *Hum. Gene Ther.* **12**, 1893–1905.

Lanchy, J. M., and Lodmell, J. S. (2002). Alternate usage of two dimerization initiation sites in HIV-2 viral RNA *in vitro*. *J. Mol. Biol.* **319**, 637–648.

Lanchy, J. M., Ivanovitch, J. D., and Lodmell, J. S. (2003a). A structural linkage between the dimerization and encapsidation signals in HIV-2 leader RNA. *RNA* **9**, 1007–1018.

Lanchy, J. M., Rentz, C. A., Ivanovitch, J. D., and Lodmell, J. S. (2003b). Elements located upstream and downstream of the major splice donor site influence the ability of HIV-2 leader RNA to dimerize *in vitro*. *Biochemistry* **42**, 2634–2642.

Lanchy, J. M., Szafran, Q. N., and Lodmell, J. S. (2004). Splicing affects presentation of RNA dimerization signals in HIV-2 *in vitro*. *Nucleic Acids Res.* **32**, 4585–4595.

Laughrea, M., and Jette, L. (1994). A 19-nucleotide sequence upstream of the 5′ major splice donor is part of the dimerization domain of human immunodeficiency virus 1 genomic RNA. *Biochemistry* **33**, 13464–13474.

Laughrea, M., and Jette, L. (1997). HIV-1 genome dimerization: Kissing-loop hairpin dictates whether nucleotides downstream of the 5′ splice junction contribute to loose and tight dimerization of human immunodeficiency virus RNA. *Biochemistry* **36**, 9501–9508.

Laughrea, M., Jette, L., Mak, J., Kleiman, L., Liang, C., and Wainberg, M. A. (1997). Mutations in the kissing-loop hairpin of human immunodeficiency virus type 1 reduce viral infectivity as well as genomic RNA packaging and dimerization. *J. Virol.* **71**, 3397–3406.

Laughrea, M., Shen, N., Jette, L., and Wainberg, M. A. (1999). Variant effects of non-native kissing-loop hairpin palindromes on HIV replication and HIV RNA dimerization: Role of stem-loop B in HIV replication and HIV RNA dimerization. *Biochemistry* **38**, 226–234.

Laughrea, M., Shen, N., Jette, L., Darlix, J. L., Kleiman, L., and Wainberg, M. A. (2001). Role of distal zinc finger of nucleocapsid protein in genomic RNA dimerization of human immunodeficiency virus type 1; no role for the palindrome crowning the R-U5 hairpin. *Virology* **281**, 109–116.

Lawrence, D. C., Stover, C. C., Noznitsky, J., Wu, Z., and Summers, M. F. (2003). Structure of the intact stem and bulge of HIV-1 Psi-RNA stem-loop SL1. *J. Mol. Biol.* **326**, 529–542.

Lener, D., Tanchou, V., Roques, B. P., Le Grice, S. F., and Darlix, J. L. (1998). Involvement of HIV-I nucleocapsid protein in the recruitment of reverse transcriptase into nucleoprotein complexes formed *in vitro*. *J. Biol. Chem.* **273**, 33781–33786.

Lever, A., Gottlinger, H., Haseltine, W., and Sodroski, J. (1989). Identification of a sequence required for efficient packaging of human immunodeficiency virus type 1 RNA into virions. *J. Virol.* **63**, 4085–4087.

Lever, A. M. (2000). HIV RNA packaging and lentivirus-based vectors. *Adv. Pharmacol.* **48**, 1–28.

Levesque, K., Halvorsen, M., Abrahamyan, L., Chatel-Chaix, L., Poupon, V., Gordon, H., Desgroseillers, L., Gatignol, A., and Mouland, A. J. (2006). Trafficking of HIV-1 RNA is mediated by heterogeneous nuclear ribonucleoprotein A2 expression and impacts on viral assembly. *Traffic* 7(9), 1177–1193.

Levin, J. G., Guo, J., Rouzina, I., and Musier-Forsyth, K. (2005). Nucleic acid chaperone activity of HIV-1 nucleocapsid protein: Critical role in reverse transcription and molecular mechanism. *Prog. Nucleic Acid Res. Mol. Biol.* 80, 217–286.

Levin, J. G., and Rosenak, M. J. (1976). Synthesis of murine leukemia virus proteins associated with virions assembled in actinomycin D-treated cells: Evidence for persistence of viral messenger RNA. *Proc. Natl. Acad. Sci. USA* 73, 1154–1158.

Liang, C., Rong, L., Cherry, E., Kleiman, L., Laughrea, M., and Wainberg, M. A. (1999a). Deletion mutagenesis within the dimerization initiation site of human immunodeficiency virus type 1 results in delayed processing of the p2 peptide from precursor proteins. *J. Virol.* 73, 6147–6151.

Liang, C., Rong, L., Quan, Y., Laughrea, M., Kleiman, L., and Wainberg, M. A. (1999b). Mutations within four distinct gag proteins are required to restore replication of human immunodeficiency virus type 1 after deletion mutagenesis within the dimerization initiation site. *J. Virol.* 73, 7014–7020.

Liang, C., Hu, J., Russell, R. S., and Wainberg, M. A. (2002). Translation of Pr55(gag) augments packaging of human immunodeficiency virus type 1 RNA in a cis-acting manner. *AIDS Res. Hum. Retroviruses* 18, 1117–1126.

Lochrie, M. A., Waugh, S., Pratt, D. G., Jr., Clever, J., Parslow, T. G., and Polisky, B. (1997). *In vitro* selection of RNAs that bind to the human immunodeficiency virus type-1 gag polyprotein. *Nucleic Acids Res.* 25, 2902–2910.

Luban, J., and Goff, S. P. (1994). Mutational analysis of cis-acting packaging signals in human immunodeficiency virus type 1 RNA. *J. Virol.* 68, 3784–3793.

Lucke, S., Grunwald, T., and Uberla, K. (2005). Reduced mobilization of Rev-responsive element-deficient lentiviral vectors. *J. Virol.* 79, 9359–9362.

Mak, J., and Kleiman, L. (1997). Primer tRNAs for reverse transcription. *J. Virol.* 71, 8087–8095.

Mak, J., Jiang, M., Wainberg, M. A., Hammarskjold, M. L., Rekosh, D., and Kleiman, L. (1994). Role of Pr160gag-pol in mediating the selective incorporation of tRNA(Lys) into human immunodeficiency virus type 1 particles. *J. Virol.* 68, 2065–2072.

Marquet, R., Paillart, J. C., Skripkin, E., Ehresmann, C., and Ehresmann, B. (1994). Dimerization of human immunodeficiency virus type 1 RNA involves sequences located upstream of the splice donor site. *Nucleic Acids Res.* 22, 145–151.

McBride, M. S., and Panganiban, A. T. (1996). The human immunodeficiency virus type 1 encapsidation site is a multipartite RNA element composed of functional hairpin structures. *J. Virol.* 70, 2963–2973.

McCann, E. M., and Lever, A. M. (1997). Location of cis-acting signals important for RNA encapsidation in the leader sequence of human immunodeficiency virus type 2. *J. Virol.* 71, 4133–4137.

Miele, G., Mouland, A., Harrison, G. P., Cohen, E., and Lever, A. M. (1996). The human immunodeficiency virus type 1 5' packaging signal structure affects translation but does not function as an internal ribosome entry site structure. *J. Virol.* 70, 944–951.

Morellet, N., Druillennec, S., Lenoir, C., Bouaziz, S., and Roques, B. P. (2005). Helical structure determined by NMR of the HIV-1 (345–392) Gag sequence, surrounding p2: Implications for particle assembly and RNA packaging. *Protein Sci.* 14, 375–386.

Morris, K. V., and Rossi, J. J. (2006). Lentiviral-mediated delivery of siRNAs for antiviral therapy. *Gene Ther.* 13, 553–558.

Mouland, A. J., Mercier, J., Luo, M., Bernier, L., DesGroseillers, L., and Cohen, E. A. (2000). The double-stranded RNA-binding protein Staufen is incorporated in human immunodeficiency virus type 1: Evidence for a role in genomic RNA encapsidation. *J. Virol.* 74, 5441–5451.

Mujeeb, A., Clever, J. L., Billeci, T. M., James, T. L., and Parslow, T. G. (1998). Structure of the dimer initiation complex of HIV-1 genomic RNA. *Nat. Struct. Biol.* **5**, 432–436.

Mujeeb, A., Parslow, T. G., Zarrinpar, A., Das, C., and James, T. L. (1999). NMR structure of the mature dimer initiation complex of HIV-1 genomic RNA. *FEBS Lett.* **458**, 387–392.

Muriaux, D., De Rocquigny, H., Roques, B. P., and Paoletti, J. (1996). NCp7 activates HIV-1 Lai RNA dimerization by converting a transient loop-loop complex into a stable dimer. *J. Biol. Chem.* **271**, 33686–33692.

Muriaux, D., Mirro, J., Harvin, D., and Rein, A. (2001). RNA is a structural element in retrovirus particles. *Proc. Natl. Acad. Sci. USA* **98**, 5246–5251.

Muriaux, D., Mirro, J., Nagashima, K., Harvin, D., and Rein, A. (2002). Murine leukemia virus nucleocapsid mutant particles lacking viral RNA encapsidate ribosomes. *J. Virol.* **76**, 11405–11413.

Neville, M., Stutz, F., Lee, L., Davis, L. I., and Rosbash, M. (1997). The importin-beta family member Crm1p bridges the interaction between Rev and the nuclear pore complex during nuclear export. *Curr. Biol.* **7**, 767–775.

Nikolaitchik, O., Rhodes, T. D., Ott, D., and Hu, W.-S. (2006). Effects of mutations in the human immunodeficiency virus type 1 gag gene on RNA packaging and recombination. *J. Virol.* **80**, 4691–4697.

Nishitsuji, H., Tamura, Y., Fuse, T., Habu, Y., Miyano-Kurosaki, N., and Takaku, H. (2001). Inhibition of HIV-1 replication by S'LTR? decoy RNA. *Nucleic Acids Res. Suppl.* (1), 141–142.

Onafuwa-Nuga, A. A., Telesnitsky, A., and King, S. R. (2006). 7SL RNA, but not the 54-kd signal recognition particle protein, is an abundant component of both infectious HIV-1 and minimal virus-like particles. *RNA* **12**, 542–546.

Ooms, M., Huthoff, H., Russell, R., Liang, C., and Berkhout, B. (2004). A riboswitch regulates RNA dimerization and packaging in human immunodeficiency virus type 1 virions. *J. Virol.* **78**, 10814–10819.

Ott, D. E., Coren, L. V., and Gagliardi, T. D. (2005). Redundant roles for nucleocapsid and matrix RNA-binding sequences in human immunodeficiency virus type 1 assembly. *J. Virol.* **79**, 13839–13847.

Paillart, J. C., Marquet, R., Skripkin, E., Ehresmann, B., and Ehresmann, C. (1994). Mutational analysis of the bipartite dimer linkage structure of human immunodeficiency virus type 1 genomic RNA. *J. Biol. Chem.* **269**, 27486–27493.

Paillart, J. C., Berthoux, L., Ottmann, M., Darlix, J. L., Marquet, R., Ehresmann, B., and Ehresmann, C. (1996). A dual role of the putative RNA dimerization initiation site of human immunodeficiency virus type 1 in genomic RNA packaging and proviral DNA synthesis. *J. Virol.* **70**, 8348–8354.

Paillart, J. C., Westhof, E., Ehresmann, C., Ehresmann, B., and Marquet, R. (1997). Non-canonical interactions in a kissing loop complex: The dimerization initiation site of HIV-1 genomic RNA. *J. Mol. Biol.* **270**, 36–49.

Paillart, J. C., Skripkin, E., Ehresmann, B., Ehresmann, C., and Marquet, R. (2002). *In vitro* evidence for a long range pseudoknot in the 5′-untranslated and matrix coding regions of HIV-1 genomic RNA. *J. Biol. Chem.* **277**, 5995–6004.

Paillart, J. C., Dettenhofer, M., Yu, X. F., Ehresmann, C., Ehresmann, B., and Marquet, R. (2004). First snapshots of the HIV-1 RNA structure in infected cells and in virions. *J. Biol. Chem.* **279**, 48397–48403.

Paoletti, A. C., Shubsda, M. F., Hudson, B. S., and Borer, P. N. (2002). Affinities of the nucleocapsid protein for variants of SL3 RNA in HIV-1. *Biochemistry* **41**, 15423–15428.

Pappalardo, L., Kerwood, D. J., Pelczer, I., and Borer, P. N. (1998). Three-dimensional folding of an RNA hairpin required for packaging HIV-1. *J. Mol. Biol.* **282**, 801–818.

Park, J., and Morrow, C. D. (1992). The nonmyristylated Pr160gag-pol polyprotein of human immunodeficiency virus type 1 interacts with Pr55gag and is incorporated into viruslike particles. *J. Virol.* **66**, 6304–6313.

Parolin, C., Dorfman, T., Palu, G., Gottlinger, H., and Sodroski, J. (1994). Analysis in human immunodeficiency virus type 1 vectors of cis-acting sequences that affect gene transfer into human lymphocytes. *J. Virol.* **68**, 3888–3895.

Perlman, M., and Resh, M. D. (2006). Identification of an intracellular trafficking and assembly pathway for HIV-1 gag. *Traffic* **7**, 731–745.

Poljak, L., Batson, S. M., Ficheux, D., Roques, B. P., Darlix, J. L., and Kas, E. (2003). Analysis of NCp7-dependent activation of HIV-1 cDNA integration and its conservation among retroviral nucleocapsid proteins. *J. Mol. Biol.* **329**, 411–421.

Poole, E., Strappe, P., Mok, H. P., Hicks, R., and Lever, A. M. (2005). HIV-1 Gag-RNA interaction occurs at a perinuclear/centrosomal site; analysis by confocal microscopy and FRET. *Traffic* **6**, 741–755.

Poon, D. T., Wu, J., and Aldovini, A. (1996). Charged amino acid residues of human immunodeficiency virus type 1 nucleocapsid p7 protein involved in RNA packaging and infectivity. *J. Virol.* **70**, 6607–6616.

Poon, D. T., Chertova, E. N., and Ott, D. E. (2002). Human immunodeficiency virus type 1 preferentially encapsidates genomic RNAs that encode Pr55(Gag): Functional linkage between translation and RNA packaging. *Virology* **293**, 368–378.

Rasmussen, S. V., and Pedersen, F. S. (2006). Co-localization of gammaretroviral RNAs at their transcription site favours co-packaging. *J. Gen. Virol.* **87**, 2279–2289.

Rein, A. (1994). Retroviral RNA packaging: A review. *Arch. Virol. Suppl.* **9**, 513–522.

Rhodes, T., Wargo, H., and Hu, W. S. (2003). High rates of human immunodeficiency virus type 1 recombination: Near-random segregation of markers one kilobase apart in one round of viral replication. *J. Virol.* **77**, 11193–11200.

Richardson, J. H., Child, L. A., and Lever, A. M. (1993). Packaging of human immunodeficiency virus type 1 RNA requires cis-acting sequences outside the 5' leader region. *J. Virol.* **67**, 3997–4005.

Rizvi, T. A., and Panganiban, A. T. (1993). Simian immunodeficiency virus RNA is efficiently encapsidated by human immunodeficiency virus type 1 particles. *J. Virol.* **67**, 2681–2688.

Roldan, A., Russell, R. S., Marchand, B., Gotte, M., Liang, C., and Wainberg, M. A. (2004). *In vitro* identification and characterization of an early complex linking HIV-1 genomic RNA recognition and Pr55Gag multimerization. *J. Biol. Chem.* **279**, 39886–39894.

Rong, L., Russell, R. S., Hu, J., Laughrea, M., Wainberg, M. A., and Liang, C. (2003). Deletion of stem-loop 3 is compensated by second-site mutations within the Gag protein of human immunodeficiency virus type 1. *Virology* **314**, 221–228.

Russell, R. S., Hu, J., Laughrea, M., Wainberg, M. A., and Liang, C. (2002). Deficient dimerization of human immunodeficiency virus type 1 RNA caused by mutations of the u5 RNA sequences. *Virology* **303**, 152–163.

Russell, R. S., Hu, J., Beriault, V., Mouland, A. J., Laughrea, M., Kleiman, L., Wainberg, M. A., and Liang, C. (2003a). Sequences downstream of the 5' splice donor site are required for both packaging and dimerization of human immunodeficiency virus type 1 RNA. *J. Virol.* **77**, 84–96.

Russell, R. S., Roldan, A., Detorio, M., Hu, J., Wainberg, M. A., and Liang, C. (2003b). Effects of a single amino acid substitution within the p2 region of human immunodeficiency virus type 1 on packaging of spliced viral RNA. *J. Virol.* **77**, 12986–12995.

Russell, R. S., Liang, C., and Wainberg, M. A. (2004). Is HIV-1 RNA dimerization a prerequisite for packaging? Yes, no, probably? *Retrovirology* **1**, 23.

Sakaguchi, K., Zambrano, N., Baldwin, E. T., Shapiro, B. A., Erickson, J. W., Omichinski, J. G., Clore, G. M., Gronenborn, A. M., and Appella, E. (1993). Identification of a binding site for the human immunodeficiency virus type 1 nucleocapsid protein. *Proc. Natl. Acad. Sci. USA* **90**, 5219–5223.

Sakuragi, J., Shioda, T., and Panganiban, A. T. (2001). Duplication of the primary encapsidation and dimer linkage region of human immunodeficiency virus type 1 RNA results in the appearance of monomeric RNA in virions. *J. Virol.* **75**, 2557–2565.

Sakuragi, J., Iwamoto, A., and Shioda, T. (2002). Dissociation of genome dimerization from packaging functions and virion maturation of human immunodeficiency virus type 1. *J. Virol.* **76**, 959–967.

Sakuragi, J., Ueda, S., Iwamoto, A., and Shioda, T. (2003). Possible role of dimerization in human immunodeficiency virus type 1 genome RNA packaging. *J. Virol.* **77**, 4060–4069.

Scheifele, L. Z., Garbitt, R. A., Rhoads, J. D., and Parent, L. J. (2002). Nuclear entry and CRM1-dependent nuclear export of the Rous sarcoma virus Gag polyprotein. *Proc. Natl. Acad. Sci. USA* **99**, 3944–3949.

Schmalzbauer, E., Strack, B., Dannull, J., Guehmann, S., and Moelling, K. (1996). Mutations of basic amino acids of NCp7 of human immunodeficiency virus type 1 affect RNA binding *in vitro*. *J. Virol.* **70**, 771–777.

Schroder, A. R., Shinn, P., Chen, H., Berry, C., Ecker, J. R., and Bushman, F. (2002). HIV-1 integration in the human genome favors active genes and local hotspots. *Cell* **110**, 521–529.

Sfakianos, J. N., LaCasse, R. A., and Hunter, E. (2003). The M-PMV cytoplasmic targeting-retention signal directs nascent Gag polypeptides to a pericentriolar region of the cell. *Traffic* **4**, 660–670.

Shehu-Xhilaga, M., Kraeusslich, H. G., Pettit, S., Swanstrom, R., Lee, J. Y., Marshall, J. A., Crowe, S. M., and Mak, J. (2001). Proteolytic processing of the p2/nucleocapsid cleavage site is critical for human immunodeficiency virus type 1 RNA dimer maturation. *J. Virol.* **75**, 9156–9164.

Shehu-Xhilaga, M., Hill, M., Marshall, J. A., Kappes, J., Crowe, S. M., and Mak, J. (2002). The conformation of the mature dimeric human immunodeficiency virus type 1 RNA genome requires packaging of pol protein. *J. Virol.* **76**, 4331–4340.

Shen, N., Jette, L., Liang, C., Wainberg, M. A., and Laughrea, M. (2000). Impact of human immunodeficiency virus type 1 RNA dimerization on viral infectivity and of stem-loop B on RNA dimerization and reverse transcription and dissociation of dimerization from packaging. *J. Virol.* **74**, 5729–5735.

Shen, N., Jette, L., Wainberg, M. A., and Laughrea, M. (2001). Role of stem B, loop B, and nucleotides next to the primer binding site and the kissing-loop domain in human immunodeficiency virus type 1 replication and genomic-RNA dimerization. *J. Virol.* **75**, 10543–10549.

Shubsda, M. F., McPike, M. P., Goodisman, J., and Dabrowiak, J. C. (1999). Monomer-dimer equilibrium constants of RNA in the dimer initiation site of human immunodeficiency virus type 1. *Biochemistry* **38**, 10147–10157.

Shubsda, M. F., Paoletti, A. C., Hudson, B. S., and Borer, P. N. (2002). Affinities of packaging domain loops in HIV-1 RNA for the nucleocapsid protein. *Biochemistry* **41**, 5276–5282.

Skripkin, E., Paillart, J. C., Marquet, R., Ehresmann, B., and Ehresmann, C. (1994). Identification of the primary site of the human immunodeficiency virus type 1 RNA dimerization in vitro. *Proc. Natl. Acad. Sci. USA* **91**, 4945–4949.

Sonstegard, T. S., and Hackett, P. B. (1996). Autogenous regulation of RNA translation and packaging by Rous sarcoma virus Pr76gag. *J. Virol.* **70**, 6642–6652.

St Johnston, D., Beuchle, D., and Nusslein-Volhard, C. (1991). Staufen, a gene required to localize maternal RNAs in the Drosophila egg. *Cell* **66**, 51–63.

Strappe, P. M., Greatorex, J., Thomas, J., Biswas, P., McCann, E., and Lever, A. M. (2003). The packaging signal of simian immunodeficiency virus is upstream of the major splice donor at a distance from the RNA cap site similar to that of human immunodeficiency virus types 1 and 2. *J. Gen. Virol.* **84**, 2423–2430.

Strappe, P. M., Hampton, D., Brown, D., Cachon-Gonzalez, B., Caldwell, M., Fawcett, J., and Lever, A. (2005). Identification of unique reciprocal and non reciprocal cross packaging relationships between HIV-1, HIV-2 and SIV reveals an efficient SIV/HIV-2 lentiviral vector system with highly favourable features for *in vivo* testing and clinical usage. *Retrovirology* **2**, 55.

Sundquist, W. I., and Heaphy, S. (1993). Evidence for interstrand quadruplex formation in the dimerization of human immunodeficiency virus 1 genomic RNA. *Proc. Natl. Acad. Sci. USA* **90**, 3393–3397.

Swanson, C. M., Puffer, B. A., Ahmad, K. M., Doms, R. W., and Malim, M. H. (2004). Retroviral mRNA nuclear export elements regulate protein function and virion assembly. *EMBO J.* **23**, 2632–2640.

Takahashi, K., Baba, S., Koyanagi, Y., Yamamoto, N., Takaku, H., and Kawai, G. (2001). Two basic regions of NCp7 are sufficient for conformational conversion of HIV-1 dimerization initiation site from kissing-loop dimer to extended-duplex dimer. *J. Biol. Chem.* **276**, 31274–31278.

Takahashi, K. I., Baba, S., Chattopadhyay, P., Koyanagi, Y., Yamamoto, N., Takaku, H., and Kawai, G. (2000). Structural requirement for the two-step dimerization of human immunodeficiency virus type 1 genome. *RNA* **6**, 96–102.

Ulbrich, P., Haubova, S., Nermut, M. V., Hunter, E., Rumlova, M., and Ruml, T. (2006). Distinct roles for nucleic acid in *in vitro* assembly of purified Mason-Pfizer monkey virus CANC proteins. *J. Virol.* **80**, 7089–7099.

Ulyanov, N. B., Mujeeb, A., Du, Z., Tonelli, M., Parslow, T. G., and James, T. L. (2006). NMR structure of the full-length linear dimer of stem-loop-1 RNA in the HIV-1 dimer initiation site. *J. Biol. Chem.* **281**, 16168–16177.

Urbaneja, M. A., Kane, B. P., Johnson, D. G., Gorelick, R. J., Henderson, L. E., and Casas-Finet, J. R. (1999). Binding properties of the human immunodeficiency virus type 1 nucleocapsid protein p7 to a model RNA: Elucidation of the structural determinants for function. *J. Mol. Biol.* **287**, 59–75.

Vuilleumier, C., Bombarda, E., Morellet, N., Gerard, D., Roques, B. P., and Mely, Y. (1999). Nucleic acid sequence discrimination by the HIV-1 nucleocapsid protein NCp7: A fluorescence study. *Biochemistry* **38**, 16816–16825.

Wang, S. W., and Aldovini, A. (2002). RNA incorporation is critical for retroviral particle integrity after cell membrane assembly of Gag complexes. *J. Virol.* **76**, 11853–11865.

Wickham, L., Duchaine, T., Luo, M., Nabi, I. R., and DesGroseillers, L. (1999). Mammalian staufen is a double-stranded-RNA- and tubulin-binding protein which localizes to the rough endoplasmic reticulum. *Mol. Cell. Biol.* **19**, 2220–2230.

Yilmaz, A., Bolinger, C., and Boris-Lawrie, K. (2006). Retrovirus translation initiation: Issues and hypotheses derived from study of HIV-1. *Curr. HIV Res.* **4**, 131–139.

Yuan, Y., Kerwood, D. J., Paoletti, A. C., Shubsda, M. F., and Borer, P. N. (2003). Stem of SL1 RNA in HIV-1: Structure and nucleocapsid protein binding for a 1×3 internal loop. *Biochemistry* **42**, 5259–5269.

Zeffman, A., Hassard, S., Varani, G., and Lever, A. (2000). The major HIV-1 packaging signal is an extended bulged stem loop whose structure is altered on interaction with the Gag polyprotein. *J. Mol. Biol.* **297**, 877–893.

Zhang, Y., and Barklis, E. (1995). Nucleocapsid protein effects on the specificity of retrovirus RNA encapsidation. *J. Virol.* **69**, 5716–5722.

Ponraj Prabakaran*, Antony S. Dimitrov[†], Timothy R. Fouts[†], and Dimiter S. Dimitrov*

*Protein Interactions Group, CCRNP, CCR, NCI-Frederick, NIH
Frederick, Maryland 21702

[†]Profectus BioSciences, Inc., Techcenter at UMBC
Baltimore, Maryland 21227

Structure and Function of the HIV Envelope Glycoprotein as Entry Mediator, Vaccine Immunogen, and Target for Inhibitors

I. Chapter Overview

The HIV envelope glycoprotein (Env) binds to cell surface–associated receptor (CD4) and coreceptor (CCR5 or CXCR4) by one of its two non-covalently associated subunits, gp120. The induced conformational changes activate the other subunit (gp41), which causes fusion of the viral with the plasma cell membranes resulting in delivery of the viral genome into the cell

Advances in Pharmacology, Volume 55
1054-3589/07 $35.00
DOI: 10.1016/S1054-3589(07)55002-7

and initiation of the infection cycle. As the only HIV protein exposed to the environment, the Env is also a major immunogen to which neutralizing antibodies are directed, and a target which is relatively easy to access by inhibitors. A fundamental problem in the development of effective vaccines and inhibitors against HIV is the rapid generation of alterations at high levels of expression during long chronic infection and the resulting significant heterogeneity of the Env. The preservation of the Env function as entry mediator and limitations on size and expression impose restrictions on its variability and lead to existence of conserved structures. In this chapter, we discuss advances in our understanding of the Env structure as related to interactions of conserved Env structures with receptor molecules and antibodies with implications for the design of vaccine immunogens and inhibitors.

II. Introduction

Viral membrane–associated glycoproteins have diverse functions in the life cycle of an enveloped virus (Dimitrov, 2004; Smith and Helenius, 2004). They attach virions to cells by binding to host cell receptors, mediate membrane fusion and some of the subsequent steps of virus entry, direct progeny virion morphogenesis during budding, and in some cases have receptor-destroying enzymatic activity for virion release and prevention of superinfection. HIV is no exception. Its envelope glycoprotein (Env) serves at least two functions that are critical for the HIV replication cycle—binding to a receptor (CD4) and a coreceptor (CCR5 or CXCR4) by using one of its two noncovalently associated subunits, gp120, and fusing the viral with the plasma cell membranes, which is mediated by the other subunit gp41. It is also a major antigen and immunogen to which all known neutralizing antibodies are directed. In this chapter, we focus on advances in our knowledge of the Env structure and function as related to its interaction with CD4, coreceptors, and neutralizing antibodies emphasizing conservation of Env structural elements that could be used in the design of vaccine immunogens and inhibitors. A number of excellent reviews have been published, which can provide more details of various aspects of the Env and serve as a source of additional citations (Broder and Dimitrov, 1996; Burton and Montefiori, 1997; Burton *et al.*, 2005; Dimitrov and Broder, 1997; Douek *et al.*, 2006; Fox *et al.*, 2006; Freedman *et al.*, 2003; Gallo *et al.*, 2003; Hunter and Swanstrom, 1990; Liu and Jiang, 2004; Markovic and Clouse, 2004; Mc Cann *et al.*, 2005; Mitchison and Sattentau, 2005; Pierson and Doms, 2003a; Rawat *et al.*, 2003; Ray and Doms, 2006; Reeves and Doms, 2002; Root and Steger, 2004; Sodroski, 1999; Wyatt and Sodroski, 1998; Zolla-Pazner, 2004).

III. Structure of the Env (gp120–gp41) _____

Like many other viral envelope glycoproteins the HIV Env consists of two subunits, the surface glycoprotein (SU), which is responsible for binding to receptor molecules, and the transmembrane glycoprotein (TM), which mediates fusion of the viral membrane with the plasma cell membrane. Initially synthesized as a nonfusogenic polyprotein precursor, gp160, the Env is cleaved by host cell proteases (furin) into the SU (gp120) and the TM (gp41) subunits, which remain noncovalently associated. We will refer to this complex as gp120-gp41 but will also use interchangeably the abbreviation Env to designate a functional fusogenic HIV envelope glycoprotein. Like other viral envelope glycoproteins the Env is oligomeric; the currently accepted view is that it is a trimer of heterodimers consisting of gp120 and gp41. It is heavily glycosylated resulting in a relatively high molecular weight of about 160 kDa for a monomer, about half of its mass is due to carbohydrates.

A. Primary Structure and Sequence Variation

A monomeric Env molecule consists of about 840–860 amino acids depending on the isolate in which about 480 residues belong to gp120. The sequence analysis of gp120 from various isolates suggests the existence of five relatively conserved regions (C1–C5) and five regions (V1–V5) with significantly higher sequence variability—up to 60–80% (Figs. 1A and 2); (Myers *et al.*, 1994; Starcich *et al.*, 1986). Four of these variable regions (V1–V4) have disulfide bridges at the two ends. The TM glycoprotein (gp41) is more conserved than the SU protein (gp120) as is commonly the case with other viral envelope glycoproteins likely related to its major role in fusion of the viral with the cell membranes. It includes a fusion domain (FD), also known as fusion peptide, which consists of a hydrophobic stretch of about 20 amino acid residues at the N-terminus, two heptad repeats HR1 and HR2, transmembrane domain (TM), three stretches of residues between these four major regions, and a cytoplasmic tail. The FD, the heptad repeats, and the TM are highly conserved. The total number of potential glycosylation sites, most of which are functional, varies for gp120 but is close to 20 and 4 for gp41. The extent of conservation of each of these sites is also variable. The gp41 glycosylation sites are more conserved than those on gp120. The primary structural features of the Env with approximate amino acid numbering are summarized in Fig. 1A.

Phylogenetic analysis of envelope sequences revealed the existence of clusters that are approximately equidistant from one another. These were named clades or subtypes. Initially six clades, [A–F], with the prototypic "North-American/European" strains relabeled subtype B, were found

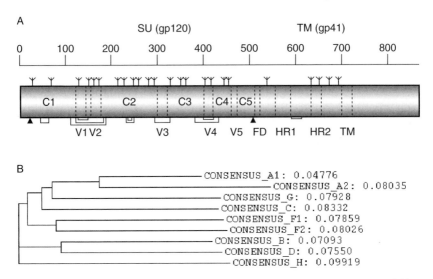

FIGURE I   Primary structure of HIV-1 Env glycoprotein and sequence variations in different regions of the Env lead to several HIV-1 subtypes. (A) A schematic diagram representing different regions of HIV-1 Env glycoprotein. Approximate locations of the cleavage sites (arrowheads), glycosylation sites (branched symbols), constant (C1–C5) and variable (V1–V5) regions, fusion domain (FD), heptad repeats (HR1 and HR2), and transmembrane domain (TM) are shown along with the numbering scheme of amino acids. The cross-linking disulfide bonds connecting various segments are indicated as brackets. (B) The phylogenetic tree constructed by using consensus sequences of HIV-1 M group subtypes A1, A2, B, C, D, F1, F2, G, and H is shown along with evolutionary distances with the maximum value of 0.1.

(Myers *et al.*, 1992). Five of these six Env-based subtypes/clades [A, B, C, D, and F, subtype E″ is now designated as a circulating recombinant form (CRF01_AE)] were also identified from the *gag* gene (Louwagie *et al.*, 1993). Based on phylogenetic comparisons of partial sequences subtypes G to J were added (Janssens *et al.*, 1994; Leitner *et al.*, 1995). These subtypes together were designated as a group called M which stands for "main," distinguishing from the groups O (outlier) (Gurtler *et al.*, 1994) and N (non-M/non-O) (Simon *et al.*, 1998). Figure 1B shows the phylogenetic relationships among the HIV-1 M group members. The tree was constructed by using M group consensus sequences which were downloaded from the HIV Sequence Database, August 2004 (http://www.hiv.lanl.gov). To demonstrate the sequence variations of HIV-1 Env, samples of 100 Env sequences from subtype B and C were obtained from the HIV Sequence Database, aligned, and the amino acid variability at each position was calculated (Korber *et al.*, 1994) (Fig. 2). Note that although the level of variation is very high in the variable regions (up to 60–80%), other regions of the Env are relatively conserved in some cases containing invariant residues. It is tempting to

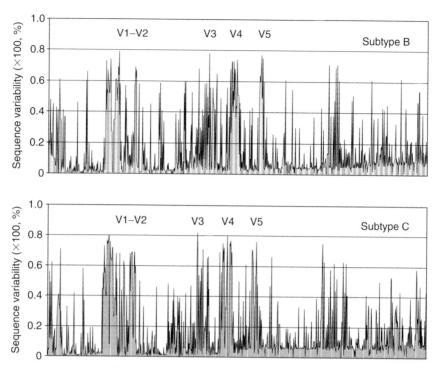

FIGURE 2 Sequence variability at each amino acid position of the Env of prominent HIV-1 subtypes B and C. The x-axes indicate the positions of amino acids as well as allowed gaps from multiple sequence alignments while the y-axes denote the value of sequence variation at each position. The variable loops apparently have larger sequence variations comparing to other portions of the Env (see the text).

speculate that those regions with close to 100% conservation have important functions and if targeted by antibodies or small molecule drugs may not mutate without significant loss of fitness of the virus.

B. Secondary Structure Elements

The Env sequence was used for prediction of its secondary structure by computer modeling. Perhaps the most popular model was developed by Gallaher *et al.* (1989, 1995) before any Env three-dimensional (3D) structures were available. The model predicted predominantly helical structures for gp120 but later the crystal structure analysis of the gp120 revealed mostly β-sheet structures. However, the model correctly predicted essential features of gp41, specifically the two heptad repeats for gp41 that form helical structures. The gp41 model is useful because of lack of available 3D structure of the native gp41. In addition to the prediction of the localization of the heptad repeats, it is also useful for other applications including localization of the antibody epitopes.

C. Tertiary (3D) Structures of gp120 at Atomic Resolution

The determination of the crystal structure of a deglycosylated gp120 core from IIIB complexed with a two-domain fragment from CD4 and the Fab 17b (Figs. 3B, 4B, and 5A and C) at a resolution of 2.5 Å in 1998 by Kwong *et al.* (1998) was a major breakthrough which is still a paradigm for research on the Env structure and function. Later the resolution was improved to 2.2 Å, and the structure of the gp120 core from another (primary) isolate, YU2, was solved (Kwong *et al.*, 2000). The 3D structure of gp120 with any of the variable regions (V1–V5) was not available until recently when the crystal structure of the JR-FL gp120 core with the V3 was determined in complex with CD4 and the broadly neutralizing antibody Fab X5 at 3.5-Å resolution (Fig. 5B) (Huang *et al.*, 2005b). The fully glycosylated unliganded gp120 core structure from an SIV isolate was also recently solved at 4 Å despite resolution-limiting problems (Figs. 3A and 4A). The structural details derived from these four published crystal structures have provided a wealth of information on the interactions with receptors and antibodies as described in more detail below.

The gp120 complexed with CD4 and antibody has a unique fold comprising two domains, inner and outer as designated with respect to the locations of the N- and C-termini which are bridged by a four-stranded antiparallel sheet (Fig. 3B). The inner domain contains two helices and a small five-stranded β-sandwich. The outer domain consists of a six-stranded mixed-directional β-sheet which clamps a helix, $\alpha2$, and a seven-stranded antiparallel β-barrel. The location of the V1–V2 stem is near to the inner domain. The V4 and V5 appear to be stemming out from different regions of the outer domain surface. The recently solved structure of gp120 with the V3 suggests a structured V3, which protrudes 3 nm from the core toward the target membrane (Fig. 5B) (Huang *et al.*, 2005b). The CD4-bound gp120 core structure for three different isolates, IIIB, YU2, and JR-FL, complexed with two different antibodies, 17b and X5, is essentially the same suggesting not only lack of conformational changes induced by antibodies but also that the core structure is preserved for these three isolates. In addition, since the seven disulfide bridges in the core are conserved and buried, one can expect that the major features of the gp120 core as the existence of inner and outer domains joined by a bridging sheet as well as various structural elements including the predominantly β-type of structural elements would be preserved in all HIV isolates. The sequences comprising the inner domain are relatively more conserved than those for the outer domain. The topological structure of gp120 was found compatible with results from biochemical studies. However, the unique two-domain arrangement linked by

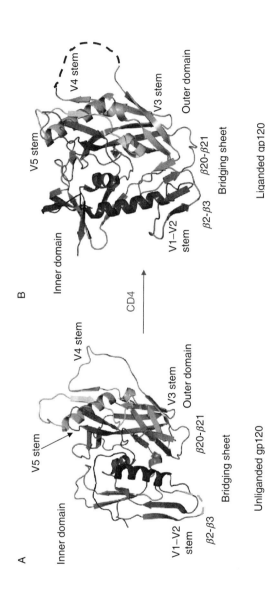

FIGURE 3 Crystal structures of gp120 core in the unliganded and liganded states. (A) Ribbon diagram of the unliganded SIV gp120 core is shown as in the same orientation of the liganded HIV gp120 structure. The color codes are in rainbow representation from colors blue to red for the N- to C-terminus. The positions of variable loops and bridging sheets are labeled. (B) Ribbon diagram depicting the 3D-structure of HIV gp120 core complexed with the first two domains (D1, D2) of CD4 receptor and the Fab fragment of human monoclonal neutralizing antibody 17b (CD4 and 17b are not shown here). The outer domains (in green and yellow) of liganded and unliganded gp120 are relatively conserved while a dramatic change in the inner domain (blue and cyan) occurs. The bridging sheet that connects inner and outer domains is not formed in the unliganded gp120. (See Color Insert.)

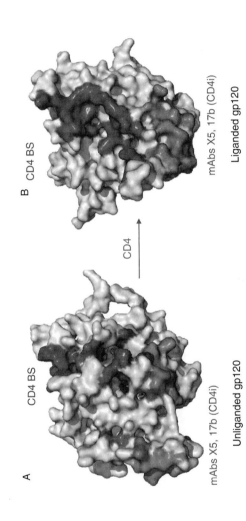

FIGURE 4 Molecular surface diagrams of unliganded (A) and liganded (B) gp120 cores are rendered as viewed from the perspective of CD4 receptor binding. The residues in direct contact with CD4 are in blue; residues contacting the CD4i antibodies, namely, 17b and X5 are in red. The contact residues were selected by limiting interatomic distance of 3.8 Å between gp120 core to the CD4 and CD4i antibodies. (See Color Insert.)

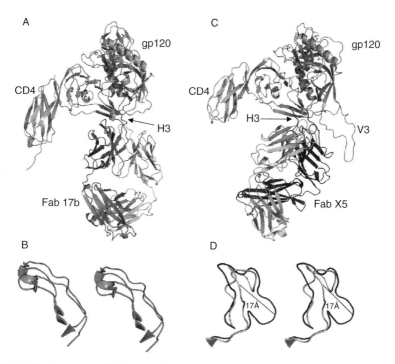

FIGURE 5   Structures of HIV-1 gp120 complexes with CD4 receptor and CD4i antibodies, 17b and X5. (A) HIV-1 gp120 core (green) is bound to the CD4 (orange) and Fab 17b antibody (magenta for heavy and pink for light chains). (B) CDR H3 conformations of antibodies in the free and bound forms are given in stereoviews as crystal structures of 17b and X5 antibodies were available in isolation (PDB codes: 1RZ8 and 1RHH, respectively). (C) HIV-1 gp120 core with an intact V3 (green) is bound to the CD4 (orange) and Fab X5 antibody (blue for heavy and cyan for light chains). CDR H3 loops are labeled and indicated by arrows. The CDR H3 conformations of 17b antibody (C) are similar in free and bound forms. Notably, the H3 of X5 (D) undergoes a large conformational change with the maximum displacement up to 17 Å (blue in bound form and light blue in free form). (See Color Insert.)

a bridging sheet that allows large receptor-induced conformational change has not been anticipated.

The unliganded gp120 (free gp120) has structural arrangements that are remarkably different from those of its CD4-bound form (Fig. 3). The CD4 binding induces large structural changes in the inner domain. Although the overall inner domain structure in the unliganded gp120 is different from that in the CD4-bound gp120 structure, the elements of the secondary gp120 structures are preserved but significantly shuffled and reorganized. Indeed in contrast to the ligand state, the inner domain in the unliganded state is not a single domain but a mixer of distinct substructures—an α-helix, a β-ribbon from one half of the bridging sheet with the V1–V2 stem, and a three-stranded β-sheet with two consecutive strands (Fig. 3A). There are four conserved disulfide bonds in the inner domain that could interlock the structural elements and allow for a large motion with respect to each other. In contrast to the inner domain, the outer domain structure does not change significantly after binding of CD4 except for some local variations as shown for segments colored with green and yellow (Fig. 3). A prominent feature of the unliganded structure is that the bridging sheet is absent and each of its two β-ribbons is displaced up to 20–25 Å. There are two major differences between the unliganded and liganded gp120 structures in relation to CD4 binding. First, the dislocation of the CD4-binding loop with a conserved GGDPE sequence motif, which contacts the complementarity determining region (CDR)2-like loop of CD4. Second, the reorientation of the β20-β21 loop that forms the β-ribbons of the bridging sheet. In addition, both the receptor and coreceptor binding sites are not formed in the unliganded conformation (Fig. 4).

D. 3D Structures of gp41 Fragments

The 3D structure of gp41 in its native state complexed with gp120 is currently unknown. However, several structures of fragments from gp41 have been solved which likely correspond to a postreceptor-binding state. The crystal structures of self-assembled HIV-1 (Chan *et al.*, 1997; Weissenhorn *et al.*, 1997) and SIV (Malashkevich *et al.*, 1998) heptad repeats revealed a six-helix coiled-coil bundle (Fig. 6). This coiled-coil structural feature was previously noted in the hemagglutinin membrane spanning subunit (HA2) (Bullough *et al.*, 1994; Carr and Kim, 1993) and in the TM subunit of Moloney murine leukemia virus (Mo-MLV) (Fass *et al.*, 1996). The heptad repeats HR1 and HR2 are about 40–60 amino acid residues long each with 4–3 hydrophobic repeat sequence and are located between the fusion and the transmembrane domains (Fig. 6A). Complexation of peptides based on these heptad repeats leads to the formation of a thermodynamically stable core of gp41. The gp41 core, the N36–C34 complex, is a six-stranded helical bundle structure consisting of an internal trimeric coiled coil of three N36 helices running parallel to each other, and of external shell of three C34 helices running antiparallel to the N36 helices in a left-handed manner around the central coiled-coil trimer (Fig. 6B). The overall size of the complex in a rectangular shape is about 35 Å in width and 55 Å in height. The 46-residue fragment which connects N36 with C34 is thought to be highly flexible.

The conserved patterns of the amino acid residues in the heptad regions are correlated with the structural and functional properties of the α-helical core structure of gp41. Most of the N-peptide amino acid residues make protein–protein interactions in the internal trimer and form grooves on the

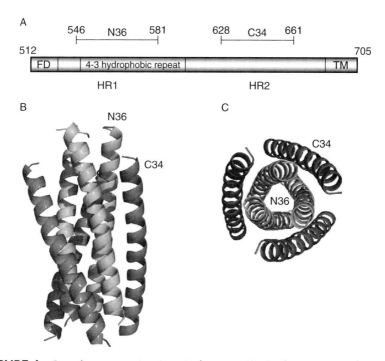

FIGURE 6 Crystal structure trimeric gp41 fragment. (A) A schematic view of gp41 Env showing the locations of functional regions corresponding to the N36 and C34 peptide fragments. (B) The peptides N36–C34 complex forms a stable α-helical domain of six-helix bundle structure. The N36 (green) and C34 (red) helices point to each other in the opposite directions; N36 forms the inner core of the trimeric structure while C34 warps the core. (C) The bottom view of the trimer clearly depicts the arrangement of N36–C34 complex. (See Color Insert.)

surface, which interact with the C-peptide. Thus, N-peptide residues involved in the interactions are highly conserved among HIV-1, HIV-2, and SIV. Similarly, C-peptide residues interacting with N-peptide helices are conserved for a broad range of isolates. A key structural feature on the surface of the N36 trimer is a deep and large cavity which is made up of Leu568, Val570, Trp571, Gly572, and Leu576 resulting in a hydrophobic pocket. This pocket accommodates three protruding hydrophobic residues, Ile635, Trp631, and Trp628, from the C34 helix. All N36 residues forming the cavity are identical between HIV-1 and SIV strains.

The gp41 structure has provided useful information about the membrane fusion mechanism as well as the possibility for its inhibition. Mutations of residues responsible for the gp41 core stabilization affect HIV infectivity and membrane fusion. The positions of some key mutations map to the interaction site between the N36 and C34 helices.

E. Quaternary (Oligomeric) Structure

The oligomeric 3D structure of the Env is critical for our understanding of the mechanisms of entry and neutralization. The structure remains unknown but there are hopes for progress in the near future. Very recently, cryoelectron microscopy (CEM) provided a glimpse of how an oligomeric Env may look like although not at the atomic level of detail. Two different studies depicted somewhat different trimeric Envs and analyzed their distribution on the virion surface (Fig. 7) (Zanetti *et al.*, 2006; Zhu *et al.*, 2006). Zhu *et al.* (2006) described the structural details of an SIV virion at about 3-nm resolution in which an individual Env has three monomers of gp120-gp41 in a tripodlike structure. The overall structure of the Env has two components: "head" and "stalk." The head is mainly composed of gp120 which is supported by the stalk in the form of three separate gp41 legs. The dimension of the trimeric Env derived from this study, 10.5 nm thickness of the head and 1.9 nm vertical length of the legs are comparable to those derived in an earlier study (Zhu *et al.*, 2003). The open tripodlike leg arrangement is also seen in the Env of Mo-MLV (Forster *et al.*, 2005).

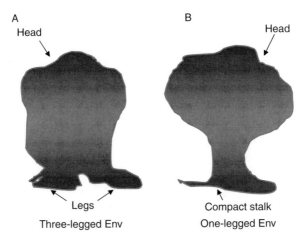

A   B
Head   Head

Legs   Compact stalk
Three-legged Env   One-legged Env

FIGURE 7   Diagrams illustrate 3D structures of Env spikes as revealed from cryoelectron microscopy. (A) The model obtained at ∼3.2-nm resolution by Zhu *et al.* has a head structure comprising trimeric gp120 in three lobes, which is supported by three separate legs in a tripodlike arrangement. The model fitting based on the available gp120 crystal structures suggests carbohydrates on the top; CD4 on the periphery appears closer to the variable loops which may shield the conserved regions of gp120 and gp41. (B) The Env spike model at 2.8-nm resolution as presented by Zanetti *et al.* is similar in having a three-lobed head supported by stalk as seen by Zhu *et al.* but with a subtly different compact stalk with no obvious separation as three legs at the gp41 stem. Model fitting using the gp120 core structures indicates the exposed receptor binding sites, which are protected by the sugars and variable loops. The bridging sheet is either hidden at the trimer-g41 interface or protected by the V3 loop.

The legs are considerably separated and potentially accessible by antibodies. By using gp120 core structures from the liganded and unliganded states, Zhu *et al.* performed docking on the tomograms such that the gp120 appears on the top with sugar-coated facing up and the variable loops along the side of the spike masking critical CD4-binding site (CD4bs). On the transmembrane glycoprotein side, a lower density was observed between the legs of the stem region, where the highly conserved membrane proximal external region (MPER) is located, causing a gap in the surface-rendered model which suggests possible interactions for this region with the plasma membrane. The recent CEM study by Zanetti *et al.* (2006) also focused on the tomographic Env structure of SIV. This study also reveals an Env organization with a three-lobed membrane-distal gp120 trimer and tightly interacting monomers in the gp41 trimer leading to a mushroom-shaped structure with a single stalk. The latter arrangement of the gp41 Env as a single leg contradicts the tripod legs seen by Zhu *et al.* (2006). Possible reasons for the discrepancy in these models could be due to different data collection and image analysis strategies employed (Subramaniam, 2006). It appears that the CEM imaging is still in a developmental stage, and further refinement of methodologies is needed before the results of this promising technology could be accepted with confidence. However, both models provided new levels of structural knowledge to our understanding of the native trimeric Env conformation. Further advancements in CEM imaging or X-ray crystallography at higher resolution and analyzing Env complexes with different monoclonal antibodies (mAbs) recognizing various segments of Env could provide more accurate and complete information.

IV. Env Interactions with CD4 and Coreceptor (CCR5 or CXCR4) Leading to Membrane Fusion

To enter cells, HIV interacts with receptor molecules. Although formally it has not been demonstrated that CD4 and coreceptor are sufficient to mediate membrane fusion after binding to the Env for example, by incorporating them in bilayer membranes and show fusion, it appears that they are the major determinants of the efficiency and kinetics of plasma cell membrane fusion with HIV (Dalgleish *et al.*, 1984; Feng *et al.*, 1996; Klatzmann *et al.*, 1984). Alternative receptors, the most notable being galactosyl ceramide, could mediate fusion of CD4− cells but at very low efficiency, and its biological relevance is not clear (Alfsen and Bomsel, 2002; Harouse *et al.*, 1991; Kensinger *et al.*, 2004). Similarly, CCR5 and CXCR4 are the major biologically important coreceptors, although other chemokine receptors can also serve as coreceptors (Coughlan *et al.*, 2000; Puffer *et al.*, 2000; Sharron *et al.*, 2000). A number of other molecules have been found that could enhance the fusion process mostly by enhancing binding but they are not directly involved in the entry process (Broder and Dimitrov, 1996; Pleskoff *et al.*, 1998). Thus, here we will review advances in our understanding of the Env interactions with CD4 and coreceptor (CCR5 or CXCR4) that are critical for the HIV entry into cells. We will focus mostly on the structural basis of those interactions.

A. CD4 Structure and Biological Function

Human CD4 is a 55–60 kDa type I membrane glycoprotein which consists of 433 amino acids as derived by its cDNA sequence (Littman *et al.*, 1988; Maddon *et al.*, 1985). It contains a 372-residue extracellular portion linked by a hydrophobic transmembrane domain to a 41-residue cytoplasmic tail. The extracellular portion can be divided into four immunoglobulin (Ig)-like domains, designated D1, D2, D3, and D4. Every domain, except D3, contains one disulfide bridge. D1 and D2 are not glycosylated, but D3 and D4 have two N-linked glycosylation sites. The overall shape of the CD4 extracellular portion is rodlike with a length of about 12.5 nm (Kwong *et al.*, 1990). The transmembrane portion is rich in hydrophobic amino acid residues and forms a helical structure. The short cytoplasmic tail of CD4 associates with p56^{lck}—a tyrosine kinase from the *src* family. It contains two cysteins, which are essential for the interaction with lck.

The crystal structure of the first two CD4 domains (D1D2) was first solved for human CD4 (Ryu *et al.*, 1990; Wang *et al.*, 1990), and the structure of the membrane proximal domains (D3D4) was later solved for rat CD4 (Lange *et al.*, 1994). Finally, the crystal structure of the whole extracellular portion of CD4 (four-domain CD4, also known as soluble CD4, sCD4) was solved in 1997 (Wu *et al.*, 1997). Both fragments (D1D2 and D3D4) form rigid, rodlike similar to each other structures. The area buried between the domains allows for a limited flexibility. The first domain, which contains the high-affinity binding site for gp120, is composed of nine β-strands following the Ig fold that resemble in many aspects the structure of the variable (V) domains of an Ig. By analogy with the antibody V domains the nine strands are termed A, B, C, C', C", D, E, F, G; four of them (ABDE) form an antiparallel β-sheet, which is packed against another antiparallel β-sheet formed by CC'C"FG. Also by analogy with the hypervariable CDRs of Ig V domains, the loop between the strands B and C is termed CDR1, that between C' and C" termed CDR2, and that between F and G termed CDR3. However, there are two important differences between D1 of CD4 and an Ig V domain: (1) missing the features of an Ig domain, which are involved in the dimerization with another V domain, and (2) the C'/C" loop (CDR2) protrudes away from the body of the domain; particularly the hydrophobic side chain of F43 is completely exposed to water. That exposure of F43 plays an important role in the interaction with gp120. Domains 1 and 2 have significant overlap, which stabilizes the conformation of the fragment and makes any significant motion at the joint region unlikely. The structure of the fragment from the third and fourth domain of rat CD4 resembles that of the human D1D2 fragment.

The crystal structure of the four-domain sCD4 molecule suggested that the hinge region between the second and the third domain produces variability in structures suggesting flexibility. It was also found that sCD4 forms dimers and that the dimerization occurs by interactions between the D4 domains. In solution, dimerization occurs at relatively high CD4 concentrations (in the millimolar range), which indicates relatively weak interactions and explains why CD4 dimerization has not been observed in gels. However, at the membrane surface, due to the 2D limitation of CD4 motion and restrictions related to the domain structure of the membrane, the CD4 local concentration could be relatively high leading to formation of dimers. A simple estimation shows that for a typical lymphocyte with a radius of several micrometers, membrane thickness 50 nm and about 10^4 surface-associated CD4 molecules, the equivalent bulk CD4 concentration should be in the millimolar range. Earlier observation based on lateral mobility measurements demonstrated that a large portion of membrane-associated CD4 is dimerized or forms higher order complexes (Pal *et al.*, 1991).

The biological function of CD4 was first studied in rat lymphocytes where it was identified in 1977 by using an mAb—W3/25 (Williams *et al.*, 1977). Its human homologue was identified in human T cells by using the mAb T4 (Reinherz *et al.*, 1979). CD4 is expressed on about 60% of peripheral blood T lymphocytes (Reinherz *et al.*, 1979) and in the cells of the monocyte-macrophage lineage including microglial cells and dendritic cells, which are antigen-presenting cells and include Langerhan's cells of the skin and mucous membranes. CD4 plays a central role in the initiation of T cells responses as a coreceptor of the antigen-dependent and class II major histocompatibility complex (MHC)-dependent interactions that initiate T-cell activation through the T-cell receptor (TCR) (Reinherz and Schlossmann, 1980). According to the coreceptor model both CD4 and TCR bind to the same class II molecule, they physically associate on the cell surface on antigen stimulation, the CD4–TCR complex generates a much stronger signal than TCR alone, and the CD4 molecule can transduce a signal. In addition to its central role in activation of T helper cells, CD4 may have other physiological functions. For example, its interaction with IL-16 leads to an increase in intracytoplasmic calcium and inositol trisphosphate, and migratory responses.

B. CD4 Binding to gp120

CD4 binds to gp120 with relatively high (nM) affinity, which is highly variable with the isolate tested and does not significantly depend on the temperature suggesting that the binding is entropy determined. The kinetic constant of sCD4 binding to gp120-gp41 expressing cells depends on temperature suggesting the existence of an energy barrier. The association rate constant at $37\,^\circ$C was determined to be $1.5 \times 10^5\,\mathrm{M}^{-1}\,\mathrm{s}^{-1}$ and the respective dissociation rate constant—$3.3 \times 10^{-4}\,\mathrm{s}^{-1}$ (Dimitrov *et al.*, 1992). The association rate constant decreases with temperature following double hyperbolic dependence with a break at $18\,^\circ$C. At $4\,^\circ$C the association constant value reaches 1.1×10^4, which is a 14-fold decrease in comparison to the value at $37\,^\circ$C. The equilibrium dissociation constant and the rate constants vary for the different experimental systems used to measure them—binding of sCD4 to gp120-gp41 expressing cells or to virions, or binding of gp120 to CD4 expressing cells or to sCD4 in solution, thus reflecting changes in the structure of the Env for different virus isolates and the effect of the oligomeric structure. The essential features of the CD4-gp120 binding process remain consistent to that of binding of two large molecules having binding site areas much smaller than the overall surface area of the molecules—similar to the binding of antibodies to large antigens.

The binding site for gp120 on CD4 was dissected by using mAbs specific for different epitopes of CD4 and by site-directed mutagenesis of CD4. It was localized on the first domain—amino acids 39–52. The X-ray crystallography data showed that the binding epitope is a ridgelike structure formed by the C′ and C″ strands and the loop which connects them, corresponding to the CDR2 of an Ig V domain. At the top of the C′ is a hydrophobic amino acid, F43, which is completely exposed to the water environment and is critical for binding. The exposure of F43 on CD4 suggested that gp120 contains a hydrophobic cleft able to accommodate the protruding F43. The X-ray crystal structure at 2.5-Å resolution of an HIV-1 gp120 core, complexed with a two-domain fragment of human CD4 and an antigen-binding fragment of an antibody that blocks chemokine-receptor binding, revealed a cavity-laden CD4–gp120 interface, a conserved binding site for the chemokine receptor, evidence for a conformational change on CD4 binding, the nature of a CD4-induced (CD4i) antibody epitope, and specific mechanisms for immune evasion (Kwong *et al.*, 1998). A more accurate modeling of less-well-ordered regions provided conclusive identification of the density in the central cavity at the crux of the gp120–CD4 interaction. The structure of a gp120 core from the primary clinical HIV-1 isolate, YU2, compared to that of HXBc2 showed that while CD4 binding is rigid, portions of the gp120 core are conformationally flexible; overall differences are minor, with sequence changes concentrated on a surface expected to be exposed on the envelope oligomer (Kwong *et al.*, 2000). Ongoing crystallographic studies of gp120 are revealing how conserved regions involved in CD4 binding, which are the targets of broadly neutralizing antibodies, are concealed from immune recognition (Kwong, 2006).

Binding of CD4 to gp120-gp41 induces rearrangements in the gp120–gp41 complex resulting in two types of structural changes: (1) dissociation of the CD4–gp120 complex from gp41 (gp120 shedding) and (2) exposure of epitopes on gp120 and gp41 as measured by an increased antibody binding and enhanced cleavage by proteases. While the lack of correlation between sCD4-induced shedding and membrane fusion argues against gp120 shedding as a fusion intermediate, the possibility remains that shedding represents either an abortive pathway of fusion or a final product of the CD4–gp120–gp41 interaction. Despite the lack of knowledge how shedding is involved in fusion, it is clear that it contributes to the irreversible inactivation of HIV-1 by sCD4 as well as by neutralizing antibodies. The results of a recent study indicate that the interactions of membrane-associated oligomeric Env with clusters of membrane-associated CD4 induce conformational changes that after interactions with coreceptors result in the exposure of helical gp41 structure reactive with antibodies, for example, NC-1 (Dimitrov *et al.*, 2005). In a parallel reaction, Env-target complexes dissociate to expose triggered gp120–gp41 on the surface, which further can dissociate to monomers and be inactivated.

C. Interactions of gp120 with Alternative Receptors

Many CD4– cells from neural, epithelial, cervical, and fibroblast origin are infectable by HIV including primary virus isolates. While in some cases the infection still can be mediated by low but undetectable amounts of CD4, in many systems, anti-CD4 mAbs, for example, Leu3A and OKT4A as well as sCD4 cannot inhibit the infection even at high concentration, clearly demonstrating that the infection is mediated by molecules other than CD4. One of the molecules, which have been implicated in mediating the CD4-independent infections, particularly in neural, colon epithelial, and possibly sperm cells is the galactosyl ceramide and its derivatives or structural homologues. These molecules are monohexoside glycolipids inserted in the cellular plasma membranes by two aliphatic chains of their ceramide moieties. They contain one galactose residue in β-glycosidic linkage, which protrudes outside the membrane and is the apparent binding site of gp120 and antibodies. These glycolipids were proposed as alternative HIV receptors based on inhibition of HIV infections by antibodies and binding of gp120 to these galactosyl ceramides as well as the association of greater infectivity with higher expression of those molecules.

Galactosyl ceramides were not detected on lymphoid cells, but are expressed on monocyte-derived macrophages (MDM). Antibodies to them reduce virion binding, but do not inhibit infection in macrophages. Unlike infection of CD4+ cells, infection of CD4– cells is usually of lower efficiency possibly due to inefficiency of the alternative receptor and the small number of cells expressing it. On the background of this inefficient virus spread, detection of inhibition is difficult. It was demonstrated that the inhibition of HIV-1 infection of neural cell lines by anti-galactosyl ceramide antibodies is significant but not complete. However, infection of a colon epithelial cell line (HT29) with such antibodies almost completely prevented infection in contrast to the anti-CD4 antibody Leu3A, which had no effect. Most of the evidence for the proposed role of galactosyl ceramide as an alternative receptor comes from studies of gp120 (gp160) binding to cells expressing galactosyl ceramide or its derivatives. The binding is specific with relatively high affinity—the equilibrium dissociation constant is in the nano-molar range. While the galactose residue in β-glycosidic linkage is the likely site of gp120 binding on the glycolipid, the binding of the receptor to gp120 has not been accurately determined, but may require intact 3D structure because gp120 denaturation prevents binding to galactosyl ceramide. A 193-amino acid fragment from gp120 containing the V3, V4, and V5 regions is probably involved in binding to galactosyl ceramide as shown by generation of infectious chimeric viruses containing that fragment from HIV-1$_{LAI}$, which infects galactosyl ceramide expressing cells, in contrast to HIV-1$_{89.6}$, which does not. The involvement of V3 loop was also shown by anti-V3 loop antibodies, which blocked the binding of galactosyl ceramides to gp120. Interestingly, the preincubation of gp120 with sCD4 caused an increased binding of gp120 to galactosyl ceramide consistent with the model that CD4 induces conformational changes leading to an increased exposure of epitopes including V3 loop. Whether binding to galactosyl ceramide induces conformational changes in gp120–gp41 needs to be clarified. It has been already shown that galactosyl ceramide mediated entry does not require coreceptor, at least not those that help CD4. Other alternative CD4-indepen-dent infection pathways include Fc-receptor- and CR-2-receptor-mediated virus uptake. Those pathways are not efficient and the receptor nature of the participating molecules is not characterized as extensively as for galactosyl ceramide.

While HIV-1 infection is generally not so efficient in CD4– cells, some strains of HIV-2 have the ability to induce rapidly spreading infection and syncytia formation of CD4– cell lines. The highly cytopathic nature of these infections has suggested that these strains are able to utilize an alternative receptor with high efficiency, unlike the case of HIV-1 infecting galactosyl ceramide expressing cells. It was demonstrated that the receptor for an HIV-2 strain, termed HIV-2/vcp, is CXCR4, the coreceptor for the T-cell line tropic HIV-1 isolates (Endres *et al.*, 1996). The HIV-2/vcp strain was derived from the HIV-2/NIH-z isolate and was shown to infect a number of CD4– lymphoid cell lines of T-cell (BC7, HSB, CEMss4-) and B-cell (Daudi, Nalm6) origin, as well as the nonlymphoid rhabdomyosarcoma line RD, which cells are not infectable by HIV-1. The infection with HIV-2/vcp is rapid with extensive cytophatic and formation of syncytial, which cannot be inhibited by anti-CD4 antibodies. In this infection, CXCR4 serves as an alternate receptor, which was supported by three lines of evidence: (1) infection of CD4– cells can be inhibited by 12G5, an anti-CXCR4 specific mAb, (2) cells expressing CXCR4 are able to fuse with HIV-2/vcp-infected cells and support viral infection, and (3) CXCR4 was downregulated by the HIV-2/vcp infection possibly due to direct interaction between the Env and CXCR4 and the Env or other indirect effects. The interaction of the HIV-2/vcp gp120 with CXCR5 involves residues from the CXCR4 N-terminus and the second and third extracellular loops (Lin *et al.*, 2003).

The use of an HIV-1 coreceptor as a primary receptor by isolates of HIV-2 indicates that whether a molecule will serve as a receptor or coreceptor depends on the virus structure. It is another demonstration of the ability of HIV for rapid accommodation to changing environments. It has been hypothesized that CXCR4 and other chemokine receptors could have been initially used as primary receptors for primate lentiviruses and the adaptation of HIV-1 to CD4 is a later event (Dimitrov, 1997; Dimitrov and Broder, 1997).

D. Structure and Biological Function of the Chemokine Receptors CXCR4 and CCR5

Available evidence suggests that biologically important coreceptors for HIV are the chemokine receptors CXCR4 and CCR5 (Berger *et al.*, 1999). They consists of an extracellular N-terminus, an intracellular C-terminus, seven α-helical transmembrane domains with several conserved *Pro* residues, and three intracellular and three extracellular loops composed of hydrophilic amino acids (Dimitrov and Broder, 1997; Dimitrov *et al.*, 1998). Highly conserved cystein residues form disulfide bonds between the first and the second extracellular loops, and between the N-terminus and the third extracellular loop. Both CXCR4 and CCR5 are 352-amino acids long proteins and possess highly acidic N-termini. CXCR4 contains two potential N-linked glycosylation sites—one in the N-terminus, where most G-protein–coupled receptors also contain such sequence motifs and one in the second extracellular loop. CCR5 possesses only one N-linked glycosylation site in the third extracellular loop. The C-termini of both molecules are rich in conserved *Ser* and *Thr* residues and represent potential phosphorylation sites by the family of G-protein–coupled receptor kinases following ligand binding. The highly conserved cysteine residues that are believed to form disulfide bonds may confer a unique barrel shape by bringing the extracellular domains into closer proximity.

E. Env Interactions with CXCR4 and CCR5

CXCR4 can be coimmunoprecipitated with CD4 in the presence of gp120 (Lapham *et al.*, 1996). It can interact with CD4 also in the absence of gp120 (Basmaciogullari *et al.*, 2006; Lapham *et al.*, 1999; Sloane *et al.*, 2005). Gp120 can also interact with CXCR4 in the absence of CD4 but with relatively low affinity—for example, an affinity constant of 86 nM was measured for the interaction between gp120 and CXCR4 expressed on the surface of CD4− neuronal cells (Hesselgesser *et al.*, 1997). Thus, the high-affinity nanomolar CD4–gp120 interaction significantly increases the affinity of CXCR4 to both gp120 and CD4 on complexation. Similar findings were reported for the binding of gp120 to CCR5-expressing cells in the presence of competing radiolabeled chemokines—MIP-1β, MIP-1α, and RANTES (Trkola *et al.*, 1996a; Wu *et al.*, 1996). It was shown that gp120 binding to CCR5 was 100- to 1000-fold enhanced by soluble or cell surface–associated CD4 measured by inhibition of the chemokine binding to CCR5. Antibodies against CD4i epitopes, V3 and V2 loop epitopes, and a C3-V4 epitope on gp120, as well as antibodies to the gp120 binding site on CD4 and to lesser extent on the CDR3-like region of CD4 D1 prevented the enhancement effect. In the absence of CD4 a relatively low-affinity interaction between gp120 and CCR5 can occur. In the absence of gp120 CCR5 similarly to CXCR4 associates with CD4 (Lapham *et al.*, 1999; Staudinger *et al.*, 2003; Xiao *et al.*, 1999). In some cell lines, association of CD4 with CCR5 was not observed (Basmaciogullari *et al.*, 2006).

The 3D structures of gp120 complexes with CXCR4 or CCR5 are currently unknown and therefore the exact localization of the interaction sites is not known. However, a number of studies provided data that allow to approximately localize the binding sites on gp120 and on CXCR4 and CCR5. After the identification of CXCR4 as the long-sought fusion cofactor by E. Berger and associates (Feng *et al.*, 1996), it has been hypothesized that CXCR4 forms a trimolecular complex with CD4 and gp120, and was speculated that the second extracellular loop of CXCR4 is likely to make a contact with gp120 because it is the longest one, and that V3 is likely to be involved in binding to coreceptors because it is a major determinant of the HIV-1 tropism (Dimitrov, 1996). This model proposed a decade ago continues to be essentially correct but much more information has been accumulated that has provided important clues how gp120 interacts with coreceptors and how these interactions could be inhibited. A first indication that the coreceptor N-terminus is important for the interaction with gp120 was obtained in the same study that first reported the discovery of an HIV-1 fusion cofactor—a polyclonal rabbit antiserum to the CXCR4 N-terminus inhibited HIV-1 Env-mediated fusion and virus infection (Feng *et al.*, 1996). Subsequent studies confirmed and extended this initial observation to CCR5 and also discovered the critical role of the coreceptor second extracellular loop in the interaction with gp120. By using chimeras between CCR5 and CCR2b, it was shown that the first 20 amino acids at the N-terminus of CCR5 were critical for coreceptor activity and that the N-terminal domain of CCR5 could confer coreceptor function when placed into the CCR2b background (Rucker *et al.*, 1996). A parallel study obtained similar results utilizing the N-terminus of human CCR5 and the murine CCR5 background

(Atchison *et al.*, 1996). Viruses that use only CCR5 as a coreceptor also interact with the extracellular loops and could tolerate substitution of the N-terminal domain with the corresponding N-terminal domain from divergent chemokine receptors including CCR2b, CCR1, CXCR2, and CXCR4 (Doranz *et al.*, 1997; Rucker *et al.*, 1996). Recently, mAb directed to the second extracellular loop of CCR5 were detected in long-term nonprogressing HIV-1 positive individuals (Pastori *et al.*, 2006). The loss of antibodies in these cases correlated with progression of the disease, which is an indication that the second extracellular loop of CCR5 is a possible target for inhibitors with an *in vivo* efficacy. Changes in individual residues of CCR5 resulted in different effects on Env-mediated fusion by an R5-tropic versus dual-tropic Env, which indicates that HIV-1 isolates differ in the way they interact with their coreceptors—CCR5 restricted viruses can interact with two binding sites on CCR5, one in the N-terminal domain and one in the second extracellular loop, while a dual-tropic Env exhibited a reduced ability to utilize the second extracellular loop and are more sensitive to mutations in the N-terminal domain (Doranz *et al.*, 1997; Rucker *et al.*, 1996). Similarly to CCR5 chimeras, chimeras based on CXCR4 and CXCR2 were examined for their ability to support Env-mediated cell fusion. CXCR4 and CXCR2 share ~35% amino acid identity. In contrast to the observations with CCR5, the N-terminal domain of CXCR4 did not confer coreceptor function to CXCR2 or CCR5 (Lu *et al.*, 1997; Picard *et al.*, 1997). The CXCR4 N-terminus could be substituted by the corresponding region from CXCR2 and still retains the coreceptor function for four of the five examined Env proteins, albeit with lower efficiency than the wild-type CXCR4. Because of this lower efficiency, it was proposed that the N-terminus may be contributing directly to the binding or indirectly by promoting conformation that favors interactions with particular Envs. It was also found that the role of the N-terminus depends on the virus isolate, but does not clearly correlate with the virus tropism. As noted above using an HIV-2 Env as a tool to identify residues of CXCR4 involved in binding to gp120 suggested that both the second and the third extracellular loops of CXCR4 in addition to its N-terminus contribute to the gp120 binding (Lin *et al.*, 2003).

Studies with CCR5 show that 10 variants out of 16 natural CCR5 mutations, described in various human populations, responding to chemokines, are able to act as coreceptors, are efficiently expressed at the cell surface, and bind [(125)I]-MIP-1beta with affinities similar to wtCCR5 (Blanpain *et al.*, 2000). In addition to Delta32 mutations, only C101X is totally unable to mediate entry of HIV-1. The fact that nonfunctional CCR5 alleles are relatively frequent in various human populations reinforces the hypothesis of a selective pressure favoring these alleles (Blanpain *et al.*, 2000). Polymorphisms of the chemokine receptor CCR5 genes have been implicated in HIV disease progression, resistance, or nonprogressive infection. There are two distinct forms of the CCR5 protein, 62 and 42 kDa, that are present in human lymphocytic cells and monkey peripheral blood mononuclear cells. The ratio of these two forms of CCR5 changes with cell growth. Localization studies indicate that the 62-kDa CCR5 resides mainly on the cell membrane and the 42-kDa CCR5 is present solely in the cytoplasm of the cells and therefore cannot function as HIV coreceptor (Suzuki *et al.*, 2002).

The HIV-1 Env and SDF-1α share functional sites on the extracellular domains of CXCR4. Recent data, however, show that there are also four mutations of the second extracellular loop, D182A, D187A, F189A, and P191A, that can reduce HIV-1 entry without impairing either ligand binding or signaling (Tian *et al.*, 2005). Another study shows that CXCR4 can differ both structurally and functionally between cells, with HIV-1 infection and chemotaxis apparently mediated by different isoforms (Sloane *et al.*, 2005). A comparison of wild-type (wt) and dual N-linked glycosylation site, N11A/N176A, mutant CXCR4 expressed in 3T3 and HEK-293 cells demonstrated variability in glycosylation and oligomerization in almost half of the isoforms. Immunoprecipitation of CXCR4 revealed monomer and dimer non-glycosylated forms of 34 and 68 kDa from the N11A/N176A mutant, compared with glycosylated 40 and 47 kDa and 73 and 80 kDa forms from wt. The functional specificity of these isoforms was also demonstrated by the fact that of the 11 different isoforms only an 83 kDa form was found to bind gp120 from HIV-1 IIIB.

F. HIV Entry into Cells Mediated by the Env Interactions with CD4 and Coreceptor

The Env binding to CD4 induces major conformational changes that lead to reorganization of the structural elements comprising the coreceptor binding site (Fig. 4) and enhanced binding to coreceptor (CCR5 or CXCR4) by gp120. The coreceptor binding induces additional conformational changes in gp120 that are transmitted to gp41, which undergoes major conformational changes required for fusion of the viral with the cell membrane. Currently, there are no 3D structures available of the complex of gp120 with coreceptors and the nature of the conformational changes induced by coreceptors in gp120 remains largely unknown. However, several 3D structures of complexes of gp41 fragments are available that are thought to play a major role in the gp41 conformational changes that cause the merging of the viral with the plasma cell membrane. The most prominent of these structures is the so-called six-helix bundle which is thought to be a postfusion structure, a result of conformational changes of a pre-hairpin intermediate (Fig. 6) (Chan and Kim, 1998; Lu *et al.*, 1995; Weissenhorn *et al.*, 1997). It has been suggested that the formation of this six-helix coiled-coil drives the membrane fusion (Markosyan *et al.*, 2003;

Melikyan *et al.*, 2000), although there are indications that six-helix bundles could form prior to fusion (Golding *et al.*, 2002). A parallel pathway is possible that involves the generation of gp41 monomers coexisting with trimers during the fusion process (Dimitrov *et al.*, 2005). The structural basis of the HIV entry mechanism is an active area of research and new exciting developments are expected in the near future.

V. Env Interactions with Antibodies

Infection with HIV or immunization with Env-based immunogens elicits antibodies which can be divided in six major classes in dependence on the location and properties of their epitopes (Choudhry *et al.*, 2006a): (1) antibodies that bind to the region containing the CD4bs on gp120, (2) antibodies binding better to gp120 complexed with CD4 than to gp120 alone (CD4i antibodies), (3) carbohydrate-binding antibodies, (4) gp120 V2- or V3-binding antibodies, (5) gp41 antibodies targeting the MPER, and (6) antibodies binding to other epitopes on gp41. Most of these antibodies are isolate specific. HIV uses various strategies to escape immune responses, including rapid generation of mutants that outpaces the development of neutralizing antibodies (Garber *et al.*, 2004; Richman *et al.*, 2003; Wei *et al.*, 2003) and hiding conserved structures of its envelope glycoprotein (Env) that are important for replication (Burton, 2002; Johnson and Desrosiers, 2002; Poignard *et al.*, 2001; Wei *et al.*, 2003). These conserved structures are hidden by variable loops, extensive glycosylation, transient exposure, occlusion within the oligomer, and conformational masking; thus elicitation of broadly cross-reactive neutralizing antibodies (bcnAbs) *in vivo* is rare and usually occurs after relatively long periods of maturation (Burton and Montefiori, 1997; Zolla-Pazner, 2004). Only several Env-specific human monoclonal antibodies (hmAbs) have been found (Zolla-Pazner, 2004) to exhibit neutralizing activity to primary isolates from different clades, including the anti-gp120 antibodies b12 (Burton *et al.*, 1994; Roben *et al.*, 1994), 2G12 (Sanders *et al.*, 2002; Scanlan *et al.*, 2002; Trkola *et al.*, 1996b), m14 (Zhang *et al.*, 2004b), m18 (Bouma *et al.*, 2003), F105 (Cavacini *et al.*, 1998), 447-52D (Gorny *et al.*, 1992) and Fab X5 (Moulard *et al.*, 2002), and the anti-gp41 antibodies 2F5 (Muster *et al.*, 1993), 4E10 (Stiegler *et al.*, 2001; Zwick *et al.*, 2001) and Fab Z13 (Zwick *et al.*, 2001). Recently, several novel gp41-specific hmAbs were identified that exhibit broad neutralizing activity and bind to conformational epitopes that are distinct from those of 2F5 and 4E10 (Zhang and Dimitrov, 2006; Zhang *et al.*, 2006). These rare cross-reactive antibodies are of particular importance because their epitopes can be used as templates for design of vaccine immunogens and as target for inhibitors. The antibodies themselves have potential as therapeutics. Here we will focus on the latest advances in our understanding of such antibodies targeting gp120 or gp41 mostly from a structural point of view.

A. Antibody Interactions with gp120

The epitopes of many anti-gp120 antibodies have been characterized in the past mostly by site-directed mutagenesis and competitive binding. Here we will focus on two major classes of gp120-specific antibodies that recognize receptor binding sites: CD4bs antibodies which compete with CD4 and so-called CD4i (induced) antibodies that compete with coreceptor for binding to gp120. The binding of the CD4i antibodies to gp120 is typically enhanced to various degrees by complexation of gp120 with CD4.

Perhaps the best-characterized anti-HIV antibody is b12, which binds to gp120s of many (but not all) primary isolates and competes with CD4. Therefore, the b12 epitope significantly overlaps the CD4bs. The structure of IgG1 b12 was determined (Saphire *et al.*, 2001) and biochemical studies were carried out to explore the fine mapping of the interaction of many mAbs including b12 with the CD4bs of gp120 (Pantophlet *et al.*, 2003). Further mutagenesis experiments of b12 and the analysis of its structure identified several residues from the heavy chain CDR3 (H3) and CDR2 (H2) that play a role in the binding to gp120 (Zwick *et al.*, 2003). The unique binding ability of b12 to the gp120 core in a partially stabilized CD4-bound conformation has been recently confirmed by the crystal structure of gp120 core in complex with b12 (Kwong, 2006; Zhou *et al.*, 2007). In addition to the b12 structure, the crystal structures of three other CD4bs antibodies in isolation, m18 (Prabakaran *et al.*, 2006b), F105 (Wilkinson *et al.*, 2005) and m14 (Dimitrov and Ji, 2006), have been recently determined. The major structural feature of these antibodies is the existence of long protruding H3s with hydrophobic residues at the tips. The structures are similar at the bases but vary along the torso and the tip regions related to their differences in specificities and neutralizing activities (Fig. 8). It was thought that the long protruding H3s of the CD4bs antibodies are required to reach cavities on CD4bs on gp120. However, the recently determined structure of a stabilized (in CD4-bound state) gp120 core in complex with Fab b12 suggests that actually the b12 H3 does not contact a cavity (Kwong, 2006), and indeed may not contribute significantly to the contact area directly on the CD4bs on gp120 and to the energy of interactions. It remains to be seen whether this is also true for the other CD4bs antibodies or b12 is unique also in this aspect of its interaction with gp120. The epitopes of these antibodies are likely to share some of the gp120 structures because they overlap with the CD4bs. However, their exact localization is currently unknown except for the b12 epitope that was recently determined by solving the crystal structure of its complex with gp120 stabilized in a conformation corresponding to the CD4-bound gp120 conformation.

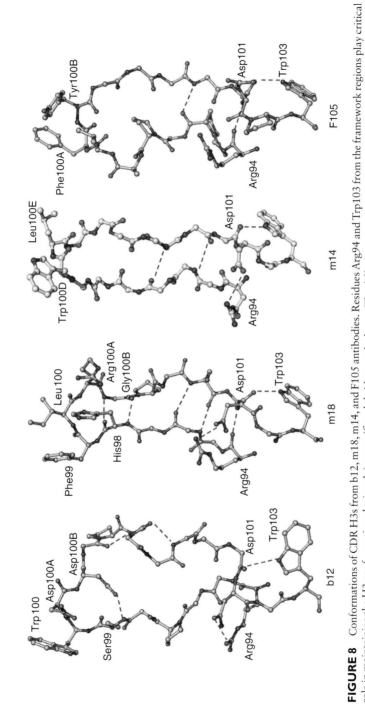

FIGURE 8 Conformations of CDR H3s from b12, m18, m14, and F105 antibodies. Residues Arg94 and Trp103 from the framework regions play critical role in maintaining the H3 conformations by involving specific salt bridges at the bases. The differences in H3 conformations are markedly noticed along the torso and tip regions.

The coreceptor binding site is highly conserved and a target for broadly neutralizing antibodies. The exact localization of the coreceptor binding site on gp120 is not known because of lack of crystal structure of the complex of gp120 with a coreceptor but extensive mutagenesis studies allowed its location around the bridging sheet (Fig. 4). Prior to CD4 binding the elements contributing to the binding site are dispersed over gp120 surface (Fig. 4A) and masked by the V1–V2 variable loops, therefore, are not easily accessible by neutralizing antibodies. The CD4i conformational changes in gp120 lead to the formation of the coreceptor binding site and to enhanced binding of CD4i antibodies which typically compete with the coreceptor for binding to gp120. A number of CD4i antibodies including 17b, X5, 48d, 47e, E51, and 412d recognize highly conserved CD4i epitopes which overlap to various extents with the coreceptor binding site. The epitopes of 17b and X5 are now known after the determination of the gp120 structure complexed with Fab 17b or Fab X5 (Fig. 5).

The epitope of 17b overlaps significantly with the coreceptor binding site. The long H3 dominates the 17b binding to gp120; H2 and residues from the light chain also contribute (Fig. 5A). The antibody–antigen interface for the gp120–17b interactions buries only 455 Å^2 on gp120 and 445 Å^2 on 17b. The epitope spans across the four-stranded bridging sheet (Fig. 5A) and has hydrophobic core flanked by basic residues. Although the 17b paratope is highly acidic, it does not make significant salt bridges with the basic residues of gp120. In the 17b complex structure, a large gap is seen between the V3 base and tips of the light chain. The H3 of 17b appears to be rigid as can be seen only the minor changes between the free (Huang *et al.*, 2004) and bound (Kwong *et al.*, 1998) H3 structures of 17b (Fig. 5B). Importantly, the 17b epitope is well conserved among several HIV-1 isolates. Of the 18 gp120 contact residues, 12 residues are conserved among all HIV-1 isolates (Kwong *et al.*, 1998).

The potent broadly neutralizing CD4i Fab X5 was selected from an immunge phage display antibody library and binds with high-affinity gp120s and gp140s from primary isolates from different clades even in the absence of CD4; however, its binding is significantly (10- to 100-fold) increased in the presence of CD4 (Moulard *et al.*, 2002). Similar to 17b X5 contacts several residues from the bridging sheet but also residues from other regions, which are highly conserved (Fig. 5C, Table I). Notably, the highly conserved Ile423 residue from $\beta 20$, which was previously identified as a hotspot (Darbha *et al.*, 2004), shows a loss of 110 Å^2 in solvent-accessible area on contact with X5. In contrast to 17b, the H3 of X5 undergoes large conformational change on binding to gp120 with the maximum of 17 Å displacement for C_α position at Gly100H (Fig. 5D). This is one of the largest induced fits ever observed for an antibody utilizing the flexibility of its H3 loop. The H3 buries 440 Å^2 of solvent-accessible area when X5 binds to gp120; the corresponding loss for the 17b H3 is only 270 Å^2. The long

TABLE I Comparison of gp120 Epitope Residues from 15 Different Isolates for which scFv m9 Derived from the Fab X5 Antibody Exhibits Potent Neutralization

15 isolates	X5 contacting gp120 residues													
	119	120	122	319	322	323	327	421	422	423	432	434	436	437
2B4C(gp120 in X5 complex)	C	V	L	T	E	I	R	K	Q	I	K	M	A	P
QH0692.42 (B)	C	V	L	A	D	I	R	K	Q	I	K	M	A	P
SF162.LS(B)	C	V	L	A	D	I	R	K	Q	I	K	M	A	P
SC422661.8(B)	C	V	L	–	E	I	R	K	Q	I	K	M	A	P
AC10.0.29(B)	C	V	L	T	D	I	R	K	Q	F	K	M	A	P
PVO.4(B)	C	V	L	A	D	I	R	K	Q	I	K	M	A	P
Q168.a2(A)	C	V	L	A	–	I	R	K	Q	I	Q	I	A	P
Q461.e2(A)	C	V	L	A	D	I	R	K	Q	I	Q	M	A	P
Q769.d22(A)	C	V	L	A	D	I	R	K	Q	I	Q	I	A	P
Q259.d2.17(A)	C	V	L	A	D	I	R	K	Q	I	Q	L	A	P
Q23.17(A)	C	V	L	A	D	I	R	K	Q	I	Q	M	A	P
Du151.2(C)	C	V	L	A	E	I	R	K	Q	I	R	M	A	P
Du422.1(C)	C	V	L	A	E	I	R	K	Q	I	R	M	A	P
Du123.6(C)	C	V	L	A	D	I	R	K	Q	I	R	M	A	P
Du156.12(C)	C	V	L	A	D	I	R	K	Q	I	R	M	A	P
Du172.17(C)	C	V	L	A	D	I	R	K	Q	I	Q	M	A	P
	*	*	*	:	:	*	*	*	*	:	:	:	*	*
Buried surface area (Å)	34.8	33	40	37	48	72	46.6	29.6	38.3	110	53.8	83.9	10	64

Residues forming the epitope are highly conserved as shown by asterisks. The mutation sites with similar amino acids are shown by colons.

highly flexible H3 of X5 may tolerate less-conserved contact residues, for example, Lys432, but at the same time make a tight binding with functional hotspot residues, for example Ile423 as facilitated by the induced fit. This perhaps might contribute to the broad and potent neutralizing ability of the X5. Table I shows a list of 15 different isolates from three major clades (A–C) that were potently neutralized by X5 antibody along with aligned gp120 epitope residues. The gp120 residues that bind to X5 are highly conserved and exposed as marked by asterisks and buried surface areas at the bottom of each epitope residue in Table I. The very long H3 (22 residues) contains four glycines, several charged (mainly acidic from 6 Asp residues) and hydrophobic residues that could reach the parts of CD4i epitopes which are hidden or sterically restricted to other CD4i nonneutralizing antibodies. The acidic surface of the H3 of X5 may mimic the acidic N-terminal portion of CCR5 that is necessary for the gp120 binding. 17b exhibits similar acidic properties due to three Asp and three Glu residues. The gp120 X5 epitope residues at positions Arg327, Lys421, and Lys432 are basic, which are not only compensated by the acidic surface of X5 but also form strong salt bridges. Arg327 and Lys421 are conserved and make direct salt bridges with Asp100G and Asp100D residues of H3, respectively, in the donor–acceptor distances range between 2.6 and 2.9 Å. The less-conserved Lys432 side chain contacts the carbonyl group of the bulky Trp100 which is the perfect candidate for making polar, charged, or stacking interactions with the Lys/Gln/Arg residues at position 432. Though 17b is also acidic no salt bridges are made between gp120 residues and 17b. In addition, the significant role of glycine residues in the H3 of X5 was explored by molecular dynamic simulations. The glycine residues were found to contribute to the H3's flexibility. Taken together, the H3 of X5 appears to be the unique in the mechanism and level of binding activity among known CD4i antibodies. Figure 9A clearly shows how the long H3 of X5 can reach its epitope. An alternative antibody binding mechanism to an exposed receptor binding site of the SARS coronavirus was recently demonstrated (Prabakaran *et al.*, 2006a). The antigen combining site of the anti-SARS Fab m396 forms a canyon to interact with the exposed parts of the receptor binding site (Fig. 9B). It appears that b12 binds to its binding site on gp120 by a mechanism similar to that of Fab m396 and not of Fab X5.

The neutralizing activity of CD4i antibodies could be significantly reduced because of the steric restriction of access to their epitopes. The conserved discontinuous segments of gp120 overlapping with the coreceptor-binding site are recognized by CD4i mAbs, which efficiently bind to gp120 on CD4 binding. But, once the CD4 docks on to the receptor site, the space needed for the antibody binding to its epitope is significantly reduced. It was found that the size restriction effect leads to an inverse correlation between the antibody neutralizing activity and its size (Labrijn *et al.*, 2003). As shown in Fig. 10, the available space between the CD4i

A   B

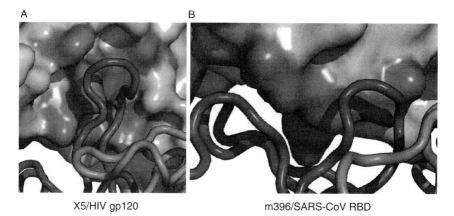

X5/HIV gp120   m396/SARS-CoV RBD

FIGURE 9   Two different antigen-binding sites and binding modes CDRs. (A) In gp120–Fab X5 antibody interaction, the long CDR H3 protrudes into the CD4i binding site. (B) Conversely, in the SARS Env–Fab m396 antibody interaction, the antibody CDRs form like a canyon around the protruding binding site. (See Color Insert.)

epitope and the target cell membrane after CD4 attachment is estimated to be about 85 Å in the highest dimension (Labrijn *et al.*, 2003). While comparing the dimensions of different formats of CD4i antibodies, IgG, Fab, and scFv, as shown in Fig. 10 the antibody fragments in either Fab or scFv are more effective than the whole IgG antibody molecule for getting into the restricted binding site needed for neutralization. However, it should be noted that other factors including avidity effects due to bivalency could contribute to binding. For example, in some cases IgG1 X5 is more potent neutralizer of some isolates than scFv X5 (Labrijn *et al.*, 2003) and *in vivo* could have much greater neutralizing activity due to the effector functions of its Fc.

B. Antibody Interactions with gp41

Two most prominent gp41 antibodies are 2F5 and 4E10, which have been isolated almost two decades ago by H. Katinger and his associates by EBV immortalization of B lymphocytes from an HIV-1-infected individual. On average 2F5 appears to be more potent than 4E10 but 4E10 exhibits broader neutralizing activity when tested in cell line/pseudovirus assays (Binley *et al.*, 2004). 2F5 and 4E10 recognize almost the same contiguous but adjacent segments ELDKWA and NWF[D/N]IT, respectively, in the *Trp*-rich environment of the MPER of gp41 (Fig. 11A). A 36-mer gp41 peptide, DP178 (T20) (aa 638–673) contains the ELDKWA region near to its C-terminal region. This peptide plays an essential role in the fusogenic structure formation and is a potent inhibitor of HIV infection in patients, currently the only entry inhibitor in clinical use. The MPER, which includes

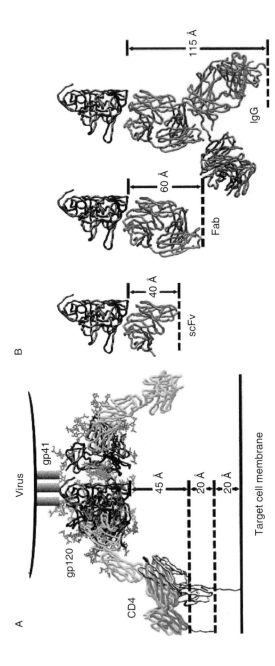

FIGURE 10 Steric restriction of access to CD4i epitopes on CD4 binding. (A) The sketch with molecules shown describes the attachment of HIV-1 from viral membrane to the cell surface CD4 receptor. The binding of CD4 induces conformational changes resulting into the exposure of coreceptor binding site, which is sterically restricted for the CD4i antibodies. Taken into considerations of the dimensions derived from structures of gp120, CD4, and possible flexibility of CD4 molecule, a total distance of about 85 Å between the gp120 and target cell membrane is measured. (B) Dimensions of antibodies in different formats, Fv, Fab, and IgG molecules, are also shown. This clearly shows that CD4i antibodies of scFvs and Fabs have better access to the restricted binding site for competing with the coreceptor than IgGs have. (See Color Insert.)

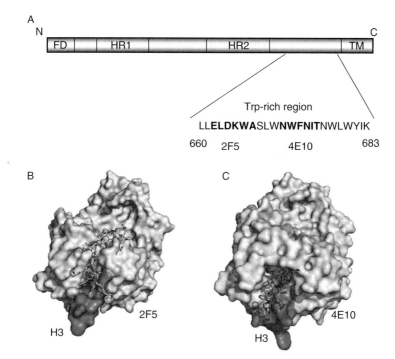

FIGURE 11 Antibody interactions at the membrane-proximal region of gp41. (A) Schematic diagram of gp41 shows the different important regions, FD, fusion domain, HR1, HR2-heptad repeats, and TM, transmembrane domain. The location of membrane-proximal region containing the core 2F5 and 4E10 epitopes on the Trp-rich region of gp41 is indicated along with amino acids sequence. Sequence numbering corresponds to HXB2 scheme. Crystal structures of Fab 2F5 (B) and 4E10 (C) in complex with peptides from the MPER. The H3s of the antibodies are shown in green. (See Color Insert.)

the epitopes of 2F5 and 4E10, is highly conserved and mutations of the hydrophobic residues Trp666, Trp670, and Trp672 in this region largely affect the viral entry. However, attempts to use the MPER for elicitation of 2F5- or 4E10-like antibodies have met limited success. To understand better the interactions of these antibodies with their epitopes, which could provide some clues for development of effective vaccine immunogens, the crystal structures of both 2F5 (Ofek *et al.*, 2004) and 4E10 (Cardoso *et al.*, 2005) complexes with peptides from the MPER have been determined. Below these structures are discussed in detail.

The crystal structure of 2F5 in complex with a 17-mer peptide is shown in Fig. 11B where 2F5 is in surface representation (Ofek *et al.*, 2004). The peptide (residues 654–670) lies at the CDR interface between the heavy and light chains. It is in a relatively extended conformation and spans around

25 Å measured from Glu659 to Trp670 (the leading residues up to Glu659 are disordered in the structure). Two of the three turns, Asp664-Ala667 and Trp666-Leu669, in the 2F5-bound gp41 peptide that belong to type I β-turn are overlapping. Interestingly, three intrapeptide hydrogen bonds constrain the conformations of only six residues from 664 to 669. The total surfaces of 635 Å^2 on 2F5 and 563 Å^2 on the gp41 peptide buried in the antibody–gp41 peptide interactions are typical for an antibody–antigen interaction. Most of the residues between Gln657 and Trp670, except Leu660 and Ser668, directly bind to the antibody. Strikingly the contact region is not only restricted to the CDRs of 2F5, but also includes nonpolymorphic region such as the N-terminus of the light chain. The 2F5 binding site on the peptide is only on one exclusive face which accounts for 41% of the total peptide area available for binding. This indicates that the unbound part of gp41 may interact with other portions of the Env. An analysis of the gp41 peptide surface reveals two major regions: one region which is bound to 2F5 is charged while the other region which is occluded from 2F5 is hydrophobic. The latter property of the surface further suggests for possible protein–protein interactions that occlude from the 2F5 binding. The failures to elicit 2F5-like antibodies by peptides may be related to the lacking of appropriate occlusion. Another hint for the mechanism of 2F5 binding is inferred form the binding mode of the H3 itself. The length of the 2F5 H3 is 22 amino acids which is the same as the length of the H3 of the CD4i antibody X5. Unlike Fab X5, the 2F5 does not make any contact through the H3 tip but only at the base (Fig. 11B, H3 is shown in green). The H3 tip has several hydrophobic residues that present a protruding flat surface. This surface aligns with the hydrophobic indole side chain from Trp670, the terminal residue of the gp41 peptide. The arrangement involving the 2F5 H3 and the gp41 peptide terminal residue in a hydrophobic plane indicates a possibility that the apex of H3 could interact directly with the viral membrane or to accommodate 2F5 to recognize the epitope closer to membrane proximal region. In agreement with other biochemical and NMR studies, it appears that the 2F5 epitope is relatively flexible, probably assuming different conformations depending on the state of gp41. Interestingly, there is no evidence for any access restriction due to size for 2F5.

The interaction of 4E10 with a 13-residue peptide containing the sequence NWFDIT is topologically similar to that of 2F5 with its epitope but differs in details (Cardoso *et al.*, 2005 (Fig. 11C). The 4E10-bound 13-residue peptide has a helical conformation, in contrast to the 2F5-bound peptide, and is similar to the 19-residue peptide structure from the Trp-rich MPER determined by NMR. The key residues Trp672, Phe673, Ile675, and Thr676 appear on the one side of the helix rendering a hydrophobic surface, which interacts with the 4E10 antibody. The residues Trp672 and Phe673 use their side chains to plunge into a hydrophobic pocket created by the CDRs at the antibody-combining site of 4E10.

The total surfaces of 580 and 529 Å^2 are buried on 4E10 and the peptide, respectively, on the binding. The 4E10 H3 does not make any contacts through its tip similarly to 2F5 (Fig. 11B and C). As is in the case of 2F5, this indicates a possibility that the H3 tip contacts the viral membrane or other portions of the ectodomain of the intact virus. In agreement with this possibility is biochemical analysis using Env on proteoliposomes demonstrating enhanced binding of 2F5 and 4E10 in presence of lipid membrane (Ofek *et al.*, 2004). An interesting feature of the 4E10 are the five glycines in the 18-residue long H3, which could certainly contribute to flexibility that may be required for epitope recognition, particularly, two tryptophan residues at the tip, at positions 100 and 100B, to reach the membrane.

These results suggest that conserved and steric constrains-free regions are available as potential epitopes on gp41, for example the epitopes of 2F5 and 4E10. The two antibodies 2F5 and 4E10 share some of the structural features and interaction patterns with the core gp41 epitopes, and also specific features related to their distinct epitopes. How useful will be the information for the MPER structures that are part of their epitopes for the design of effective vaccine immunogens remains to be seen.

Recently, six novel gp41-specific hmAbs were identified that exhibit broad neutralizing activity and bind to conformational epitopes that are distinct from those of 2F5 and 4E10 (Zhang and Dimitrov, 2006; Zhang *et al.*, 2006). They do not compete significantly with 2F5 and 4E10 indicating that the localization of their epitopes is likely outside the MPER. The conserved structures containing these epitopes are being characterized.

C. Mimicry of Receptors by Miniproteins and Antibodies

The conserved CD4bs on gp120 and structurally contiguous segments including the β-hairpin rigid motif of CD4 prompted for the rational design of CD4 mimics that could block the HIV entry (Huang *et al.*, 2005a; Martin *et al.*, 2003a; Vita *et al.*, 1999b; Zhang *et al.*, 1999). The CD4–gp120 binding interactions mainly involve contiguous segments rendered by the CD4 residues 31–35, 40–48, and 58–64 in which about 40% contribution is from the CDR2-like β-hairpin region containing the Phe43 hotspot. A 31-amino acid long CD4 mimic specific for gp120 was initially designed by grafting the major contributor of the CD4-binding component, the CDR2-like loop of CD4 with a major hotspot Phe43, on a small structural scaffold stabilized by a disulfide bond from scorpion toxin charybdotoxin (Drakopoulou *et al.*, 1998). Later, a mini-CD4 protein called CD4M9 with 28 amino acids using the scyllatoxin scaffold was designed, and its three-dimension structure was solved by NMR (Vita *et al.*, 1999b). Based on the structural information derived from the CD4–gp120–17b complex, CD4M9, CD4M32, and CD4M33 miniproteins were designed, and their applications as possible therapeutics were tested by determining several thermodynamic and neutralization parameters. The NMR structure of CD4M9 showed a well-defined β-hairpin with a phenylalanine residue at the position 23, which is equivalent to CDR2 region of CD4, appeared to retain some of the conserved gp120–CD4 interactions in the miniprotein–gp120 docked complex. Finally, the crystal structures of CD4M33 and its analogue F23 in complex with gp120 were determined and the extent of molecular mimicry and neutralization breadth were analyzed (Huang *et al.*, 2005a). In spite of the highly flexible envelope, the conformation of gp120 in these mimic complexes are very similar to that induced by CD4 (Fig. 12). Interestingly, the β-hairpin CD4M33 engages in hydrogen bonding to the strand β15 of gp120 in a similar way as CD4 does. This demonstrates the successful attempt of grafting CD4–gp120 binding interface on to a smaller scaffold. Thermodynamic characterization of gp120 binding to these mimics showed that only half of the associated entropic changes occur compared to CD4 binding. Nonetheless, these mimics induce the same conformational change in gp120 as CD4 that are required for enhanced binding of 17b to gp120. The difference between CD4M33 and F23 mimics is only that the phenyl ring in CD4M33 is replaced with a biphenyl side chain of residue 23. This substitution significantly enhances the structural mimicry of CD4 at this specific position (Huang *et al.*, 2005a). The successful structural mimicry by these miniproteins will prompt researchers to further attempt to design native CD4-like mimics with greater antiviral activity against HIV.

In the giant struggle between the HIV and the immune system, antibodies with unique properties have evolved some of which mimic CD4 and coreceptors but do not induce the same conformational changes as receptors because that could lead to enhancement of infection. In addition, CD4 binds to gp120 through its first domain, which is similar to the V domain of an antibody. For example, the comparison between D1 domain of CD4 and

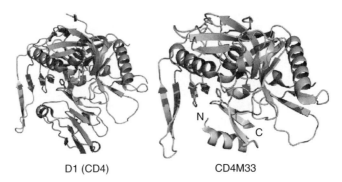

D1 (CD4)   CD4M33

FIGURE 12   Mimicry of receptor CD4 by miniprotein CD4M33. The binding of gp120 (green) to the CD4 (first domain, D1 is only shown) on left and the miniprotein CD4M33 on right are depicted in ribbon diagrams. (See Color Insert.)

VH domain of b12 is shown in Fig. 13A and B. The molecular views were generated by translating the superposition of the two molecules based on the disulfide bridge locations. Tyr53 residue positioned at H2 of b12 as labeled in Fig. 13B was found critical—a Y53G point mutation greatly diminished the binding of b12 to gp120 (Zwick *et al.*, 2003). Based on the footprint data, two fingers, H3 (Trp100) and H2 (Tyr53), were speculated to occupy the hydrophobic pocket on gp120 surface. Since the H2 of b12 is the equivalent of the C′C″ or CDR2-like region of CD4, the b12 could be used as a receptor mimic by further protein engineering of its H2.

The Fab m18 is another CD4bs antibody with broad neutralizing activity which was recently identified (Zhang *et al.*, 2003) and its crystal structure solved (Prabakaran *et al.*, 2006b). Its VH domain that is comparable to D1 of CD4 is shown in Fig. 13C. The most remarkable feature of this antibody is the H3 structure which highly resembles the CDR2-like part of CD4 (Fig. 13D). The m18 H3 adopts not only a β-hairpin but forms a rigid structure with cross-linking hydrogen bonds throughout the torso region of H3, and importantly has a Phe residue at the position 99 analogous to the hotspot Phe43 of CDR2-like loop in CD4. The unexpected structural

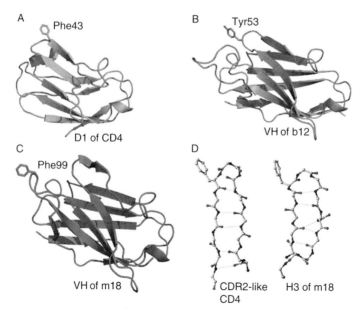

FIGURE 13   Comparisons of CD4 D1 domain with VH domains of CD4bs antibodies b12 and m18. (A) D1 domain CD4 (green) with Phe43 in sticks. (B) VH domain of b12 antibody (cyan) with Tyr53 at the CDR H2 in sticks. (C) VH domain of m18 antibody (blue) with Phe99 at the CDR H2 in sticks. (D) Backbone skeletal views of the CDR2-like region of CD4 and the H3 of m18 indicate a common β-hairpin structure with a phenylalanine residue at the tip.

similarities including hotspot Phe residues and robust β-sheet features observed (Fig. 13D) suggest for possible protein grafting of H3 to mimic the CDR2-like C′C″ of CD4, which might provide a useful strategy for developing antibody-based CD4 mimetic to inhibit HIV entry.

Not only CD4bs antibodies mimic CD4 but also CD4i antibodies, which mostly bind to the coreceptor binding site, mimic certain features of the HIV coreceptors. Unlike the case of CD4 and its mimics, there is no 3D structure available of a coreceptor. However, the crystal structures of several CD4i Fabs were solved and they revealed mechanisms and atomic-level details for three interesting features: posttranslational mimicry of coreceptor by tyrosine sulfation of antibody, an alternative molecular mechanism controlling such sulfation, and highly selective V(H)-gene usage (Choe *et al.*, 2003; Huang *et al.*, 2004). This is another demonstration of the adaptive capabilities of the immune system when confronted by extraordinary viral defenses.

VI. The Env as Vaccine Immunogen and Target for Inhibitors

The development of an effective vaccine against HIV is an international public health priority and the role HIV envelope plays in infection makes it a primary target for such efforts. A multitude of approaches have been attempted that are eloquently summarized in numerous recent reviews (D'Souza *et al.*, 2004; Duerr *et al.*, 2006; Koff *et al.*, 2006; Letvin, 2005; McMichael, 2006; Singh *et al.*, 2005; Slobod *et al.*, 2005; Spearman, 2006; Wang, 2006). From this work, it is clearly possible to create vaccines that induce cellular responses that will protect against disease progression by suppressing viral loads once infection occurs. However, none have been able to achieve the penultimate goal of preventing infection entirely. This goal will require an Env-based vaccine that induces a protective antibody response. Here, we will summarize the prevailing approaches how to use the Env for eliciting broadly neutralizing antibodies and their epitopes as targets for inhibitors with special emphasis on the common challenges.

A. The Relationship Between Viral Neutralization and Protection

A guiding principle of current HIV vaccine efforts is that antibodies that neutralize HIV *in vitro* can protect animals from HIV infection *in vivo*. This principle is based on three observations:

i. In an expanding number of passive challenge studies, macaques treated with mAbs or pooled, high-titered antisera that neutralized *in vitro* were protected from cell-free SHIV virus challenge (Baba *et al.*, 2000;

Emini *et al.*, 1992; Ferrantelli *et al.*, 2003, 2004; Hofmann-Lehmann *et al.*, 2001a,b, 2002; Mascola *et al.*, 1999, 2000, 2003a; Nishimura *et al.*, 2002; Parren *et al.*, 2001; Putkonen *et al.*, 1991; Ruprecht *et al.*, 2001; Shibata *et al.*, 1999; Van Rompay *et al.*, 1998; Zhang *et al.*, 2004a). The antibodies that have demonstrated the best efficacy are IgG1b12, 2G12, 2F5, and HIVIg. Strong cellular responses do not enhance the protection to SHIV challenge provided by passively transferred antibodies (Mascola *et al.*, 2003b).

ii. Second, in natural infection, autologous neutralizing responses exert selective pressure on HIV evolution *in vivo* (Albert *et al.*, 1990; Arendrup *et al.*, 1992; Bradney *et al.*, 1999; Eichberg *et al.*, 1992; Montefiori *et al.*, 1991; Parren *et al.*, 1999; Reitz *et al.*, 1988; Richman *et al.*, 2003; Watkins *et al.*, 1993; Wei *et al.*, 2003). HIV evades this selective pressure by several mechanisms such as introducing new N-linked glycosylation residues to present a protective glycan shield (Back *et al.*, 1994; Chackerian *et al.*, 1997; Derdeyn *et al.*, 2004; Kolchinsky *et al.*, 2001; Quinones-Kochs *et al.*, 2002; Reitter *et al.*, 1998; Wei *et al.*, 2003), conformational or entropic masking of vulnerable epitopes (Kwong *et al.*, 2002), shedding monomeric envelope proteins that enhance the dominance of nonneutralizing epitopes (Burton and Montefiori, 1997), or by simple epitope variation. While it is discouraging that the antibodies cannot control the infection, the observation that HIV has to evade these antibodies suggests that they have an impact.

iii. Long-term nonprogression is associated with the presence of high-titered broadly neutralizing responses (Cao *et al.*, 1995; Cecilia *et al.*, 1999; Hutto *et al.*, 1996; Kloosterboer *et al.*, 2005; Pilgrim *et al.*, 1997; Scarlatti *et al.*, 1996; Zhang *et al.*, 1997). Although others have postulated that this connection is more tenuous (Montefiori *et al.*, 1996) because a direct link between the levels of neutralizing antibodies and disease progression cannot be established (Cecilia *et al.*, 1999), the recent studies connecting evasion with neutralization suggest that perhaps the antibody responses in these patients may be better able to contain the virus long term.

Based on these observations, it is easy to conclude that vaccines that stimulate such neutralizing responses would be highly desirable. Thus, significant efforts have been directed to developing immunogens that induce antibodies with broadly neutralizing specificities.

B. Nonneutralizing Antibodies and Protection?

Antibodies that score positive in an *in vitro* neutralization assay can mediate protection *in vivo*. However, can an antibody that scores negative in such an assay be as effective? The literature suggests that there is a significant subset of these binding but nonneutralizing antibodies that impact HIV disease progression and possibly even transmission. Binding/nonneutralizing antibodies against virus surface glycoproteins have been shown to protect against infection in other virus systems, including *Sindbis virus* (Stanley *et al.*, 1986), *Venezuelan equine encephalomyelitis virus* (Mathews and Roehrig, 1982), herpesvirus (Dix *et al.*, 1981), and vesicular stomatitis virus (Lefrancois, 1984). For HIV, the most compelling evidence of nonneutralizing but protective antibodies comes from tests of DNA/MVA vaccines in macaques. Here, vaccines containing *pol*, *gag*, and *env* sequences (encoding the first 270 amino acid residues of the ADA envelope) afforded stronger protection against mucosal SHIV 89.6P challenge than matched vaccines containing only *gag* and *pol* (Amara *et al.*, 2002). Since the more effective vaccine containing *env* did not raise neutralizing antibodies against the challenge virus, the enhanced protection was attributed to high titers of anti-envelope binding antibodies. A more recent macaque study showed that the viral containment and immune preservation conferred by a DNA/adenovirus vaccine was significantly enhanced by inclusion of chimeric gp140 sequences that were heterologous with respect to the challenge SHIV (Letvin *et al.*, 2004). Although the investigators attributed this protection to cross-reactive cellular responses raised against conserved HIV envelope sequences, this study did not rule out a role for nonneutralizing antibodies. In sum, these nonneutralizing antibodies appear to protect against disease via mechanisms overlooked by conventional *in vitro* viral neutralization assay.

The most common mechanism attributed to "nonneutralizing" control is Fc receptor-mediated or complement-mediated inhibitory or cytolytic activity. For instance, antibody-dependent cell-mediated cytotoxicity (ADCC) (reviewed in Ahmad and Menezes, 1996; Gomez-Roman *et al.*, 2006) has been associated with improved control of viremia and CD4+ counts in HIV-infected patients (Ahmad *et al.*, 2001; Forthal *et al.*, 1999, 2001) and slower disease progression in SIV-infected macaques (Banks *et al.*, 2002). One recent study observed a correlation between ADCC activity and reduced viral load in rhesus macaques after mucosal challenge with SIV (Gomez-Roman *et al.*, 2005). Fc-mediated effector mechanisms have also been attributed to the enhanced neutralizing efficacy of HIV+ or SIV+ serum observed when MDM or immature dendritic cells (iDC) are used as cellular targets instead of activated PBMCs (Holl *et al.*, 2004, 2006a,b). In fact, mAbs that present minimal neutralizing activity in PBMC-based assays can be highly inhibitory in MDM- or iDC-based assays (Holl *et al.*, 2006a). These mAbs recognize portions of the native envelope spike that are exposed on "dead" spikes that are expressed on native virions but are unable to mediate fusion because they are uncleaved or have lost the gp120 portion (Moore *et al.*, 2006; Zanetti *et al.*, 2006; Zhu *et al.*, 2006). How these nonneutralizing antibodies may impact HIV transmission remains unanswered. Although a clear-cut protective mechanism for nonneutralizing anti-HIV antibodies is not established, it is nevertheless prudent to consider Env-based vaccine candidates that may stimulate such inhibitory activities.

C. Antibodies against CD4i Epitopes: Perceptions, Realities, and Opportunities

Humoral responses against gp120 epitopes exposed during viral entry may provide new opportunity for vaccine development. These responses warrant attention because they recognize some of the most conserved and functionally important regions of the HIV envelope. The question at hand is whether these responses (and the antigens that raise them) are worth pursuing as vaccines. Unfortunately, the view of CD4i epitopes as a vaccine target has been colored by the recent findings discussed below.

1. Potency of CD4i Antibodies and CCR5 Expression

Using computational models based on the crystal structure of CD4-bound gp120, it has been suggested that CD4i epitopes are actually occluded during entry (Labrijn *et al.*, 2003). Support for this model was generated by showing that IgG1 X5, which recognizes a CD4i epitope, is profoundly less effective than the smaller Fab or scFv fragments of the same antibody at neutralizing a small panel of primary R5 using isolates (Labrijn *et al.*, 2003). However, for some isolated IgG1 X5 is more potent than the smaller fragments likely due to the avidity effect because of its bivalency. In addition, the neutralizing activities of antibodies to CD4i epitopes are dependent on assay conditions. We have found over 100-fold differences in the levels of CCR5 expression between TZM-bl cell line commonly used in neutralization assays and PHA-activated PBMCs (Choudhry *et al.*, 2006b). Platt *et al.* (1998, 2005) have shown that the entry kinetics of R5 isolates are exquisitely sensitive to the levels of CCR5 expressed on the target cell. In fact, using artificial cell lines as targets, they demonstrated that viruses become increasingly susceptible to entry inhibitors, such as T-20, as the levels of CCR5 drop below $<10^4$ molecules/cell. Binley *et al.* (2004) further emphasized this point by showing that the neutralizing efficacy of Fab X5 is significantly improved in PBMC-based neutralization assays as compared to cell line–based assays. While it is not known how much CCR5 is expressed on the cells initially targeted by HIV, numerous studies have determined the expressed levels of CCR5 on various mucosal and lymphoid tissues to be significantly lower than 10^4 per cell, well in the range that CD4i antibodies may be effective.

2. CD4i Epitopes and HIV/SIV Infection

It is clear that CD4i epitopes are raised during HIV infection, since hmAbs that recognize CD4i epitopes in the coreceptor binding site have been derived from HIV+ persons (Robinson *et al.*, 1992; Xiang *et al.*, 2002a). Last year, it was reported (Decker *et al.*, 2005) that sera from most HIV-infected persons contain antibodies that were extremely potent and cross-reactive in the presence of small amounts of sCD4, which presumably stabilizes the exposure of CD4i epitopes. It was further shown that the titers of broadly neutralizing antibodies that are detected in the CD4-triggered neutralization assay correlated strongly with the abilities of the sera to block the binding of a biotinylated human mAb (19e) to a CD4i epitope on gp120–CD4 complexes in ELISA. These findings have led to the perception that high-tittered responses to CD4i epitopes are found in all HIV-infected persons and are therefore meaningless and irrelevant to vaccine design.

Unfortunately, this perception may be a misinterpretation of these results. First, it was demonstrated that increases in neutralizing potency can be observed in HIV+ serum in the presence of sCD4 (Decker *et al.*, 2005). They also showed that HIV+ sera competed with mAb 19e for binding to gp120–CD4 complexes using an assay that tested percentage blocking with a *single* dilution of serum. Such assays, however, do not demonstrate the presence of a high binding titer of anti-CD4i antibodies. Second, it was proposed that the responses to the highly conserved domains may constrain the breadth of the viral quasispecies that occur during natural infection and drive the evolution of the virus to protect these epitopes (Decker *et al.*, 2005). This hypothesis is consistent with observations from SIVMneCL8 infection of rhesus macaques where the neutralization sensitive and mildly pathogenic strain becomes resistant and highly pathogenic in part by introducing N- and O-linked glycosyl residues in the V1 region that occludes its coreceptor binding (Chackerian *et al.*, 1997; Kimata *et al.*, 1999a,b).

This perception also begs the question whether lead vaccine candidates that are intending to target responses to the CD4-binding domain (CD4BD) should be abandoned given the evidence that responses directed to the CD4BD are highly prevalent in HIV infection and are associated with progression to AIDS (Hioe *et al.*, 2001). CD4BD antibodies have also been shown to inhibit antigen presentation (Hioe *et al.*, 2000, 2001; Tuen *et al.*, 2005). We would argue that in the absence of well-designed safety and animal protection studies that would exclude one epitope or another, it is prudent to consider immunogens designed to effect responses toward any of these epitopes. Therefore, it is reasonable to propose and to test whether a preexisting humoral or mucosal response directed to CD4i epitopes could afford protection against primate lentiviral infection. Several indirect observations from the literature suggest that the answer is yes.

i. Infection of macaques with macrophage tropic SIV strains, such as SIVmac1A11 (Luciw *et al.*, 1992), SIVmac17E-Cl, or SIVmac316 (Puffer *et al.*, 2002), leads to a transient or attenuated viremia. These CD4-independent isolates (Puffer *et al.*, 2002) can generate potent neutralizing responses that may have a role in controlling the observed viremia and in the protection generally observed in subsequent challenge of infected macaques with highly pathogenic SIV strains.

ii. SIV strains that are deficient in either variable loops or specific glycosylation sites that occlude the coreceptor interacting domain in the SIV spike protein are CD4 independent, and highly susceptible to neutralization by SIV immune sera and mAbs that recognize these CD4i epitopes (Johnson *et al.*, 2002, 2003a,b). Attenuated versions of these SIV isolates induce antibody responses capable of neutralizing the "neutralization resistant" SIVmac239 *in vitro* (Reitter *et al.*, 1998), and protecting against SIVmac239 challenge (Mori *et al.*, 2001).

iii. Protection in cohorts of individuals that were exposed to HIV but remain uninfected has been associated with the presence of mucosal or serum antibodies to HIV that, in some studies, exhibited neutralizing activity. In one cohort, this protection was associated with antibody titer to epitopes expressed on CD4–gp120 complexes but not HIV-specific T cell responses (Nguyen *et al.*, 2006).

iv. While passive protection studies have delineated a clear correlation between the neutralizing efficacy of antibodies *in vitro* and their ability to passively protect against SHIV challenge *in vivo*, formulations of polyclonal HIVIg (which contains antibodies to these CD4i epitopes, among others), 2G12, and 2F5 demonstrated protective efficacy from vaginal challenge while similar infusions with mixtures of 2G12, and 2F5 did not (Mascola *et al.*, 2000). This is despite the observations that HIVIg/2G12/2F5 and 2G12/2F5 formulations demonstrated equivalent neutralization titer *in vitro*.

In addition, it appears that fitness during transmission is enhanced if the virus expresses/exposes the coreceptor binding domain on the viral spike. Taken together, we believe the preponderance of evidence suggests that vaccines that target such CD4i epitopes may have provided some level of protection against transmitted virus and logically coincides with ongoing vaccine development efforts in the field.

D. The Hunt for the Right Immunogen

The daunting part of this challenge is the evasive power provided by the sequence diversity of the Env. It was quickly apparent that standard vaccine approaches using killed virus or soluble monomeric gp120 or gp160 as immunogens generated only "type-specific" immunity, and neutralized only the source virus of the immunogen or its very close relatives (Burton *et al.*, 2004). Today, the effort is to identify immunogens or immunization strategies that induce antibody responses that exhibited a broader neutralizing and/or protective phenotype. The immunogen approaches can be grouped in two broad overlapping categories based on whether the respective antibodies target epitopes on the virion spike or epitopes (such as CD4i) that appear during entry.

I. Generating Antibodies That Target the Virion Spike Before Binding to Receptors

Five of the most broadly neutralizing antibodies, 2G12, b12, 447–52D, 2F5, and 4E10, recognize conserved epitopes that are expressed on the viral spike before binding to receptors, leading some investigators to suggest that the optimal vaccine candidate should induce antibodies that preferentially bind to the viral spike (Burton *et al.*, 2004; Fouts *et al.*, 1997; Parren and Burton, 2001). Efforts to reach this goal have focused on the following approaches:

i. Adding or removing *Asn* residues to alter the level of N-linked glyco-sylation that shields the CD4bs. By exposing the deep CD4BS pocket, the hope is the resulting immunogen will induce broadly neutralizing antibodies like b12 (Koch *et al.*, 2003).

ii. Expressing the outer domain of gp120 (Yang *et al.*, 2004). The outer domain is exposed on the envelope spike and contains binding surfaces for 2G12, IgG1b12, and broadly neutralizing anti-V3 loop antibodies.

iii. Expressing soluble forms of the oligomeric envelope trimer to mimic the spike as it appears on the HIV virion. Typically, investigators have expressed these proteins as fusions between gp120 and the ectodomain of gp41 (reviewed in Cho, 2003). These constructs typically generated preparations consisting of mixtures of monomeric and oligomeric forms. Recent efforts have improved consistency and yields of trimeric forms by introducing disulfide links between the proximal domains of gp120 and gp41 (called SOS or SOSIP envelopes) (Beddows *et al.*, 2005; Binley *et al.*, 2000), using envelope genes derived from HIV strains with highly stable spikes (Lian *et al.*, 2005; Sharma *et al.*, 2006; Srivastava *et al.*, 2002; Zhang *et al.*, 2001), creating HIV-SIV envelope chimeras (Center *et al.*, 2004), or fusing the envelope ectodomain to non-HIV sequences that preferentially form trimers (Pancera *et al.*, 2005; Yang *et al.*, 2000, 2002). In an effort to produce soluble spikes with an antigenic profile more consistent with the native virion, investigators have produced the SOS and SOSIP variants in cell lines that overexpress furin, a protease which cleaves gp120–gp41 fusion into its respective domains.

iv. Minimizing the conformational or entropic masking of the conserved neutralizing domains by introducing mutations that restrain the movement of gp120 (Kwong *et al.*, 2002; Xiang *et al.*, 2002b). This concept is derived from studies showing that the binding of broadly neutralizing antibodies such as b12 and 2G12 consistently realized minimal entropic change in gp120. This contrasts sharply with other less effective antibodies such as F105 which generate significantly larger entropic changes. Given the range of movement possible between the inner and outer domains of envelope indicated by the crystal structures, it was proposed that the virus may evade neutralization by using an entropic mask or a conformational barrier that antibodies must overcome to actually bind. Introducing mutations that limit this movement, such as replacing the tryptophan with a serine in position 375, and reduce the entropic requirements for antibody binding may improve the chances of inducing the preferred antibody specificities.

v. Mimicking the high-mannose-type oligosaccharides that are presented on HIV envelope and recognized by 2G12 (reviewed in Wang, 2006). Recently, constructs have been described that mimic the binding site of 2G12 using organic scaffolds decorated with synthetic oligomannose structures. These structures are recognized by 2G12 to varying degrees. The immunogenicity of these constructs has not been described.

vi. Mimicking the MPER of the envelope spike recognized by 2F5 and 4E10 (reviewed in Zwick, 2005). It has been recently appreciated that the lipid membrane and hydrophobic context of the epitope is critical for antibody binding (Haynes et al., 2005a). This observation may explain the dearth of success using peptide-based mimics of the eptiope to induce 2F5- and 4E10-type responses and has rejuvenated efforts to develop new mimics. Several novel constructs have been presented (Brunel et al., 2006; Luo et al., 2006); however, immunogenicity data are limited.

Unfortunately, where they have been evaluated, the immunogen strategies described above typically fail to elicit antibodies capable of neutralizing more than a minor fraction of primary isolates (Beddows et al., 2005; Graham, 2002; Selvarajah et al., 2005). To make matters worse, it was recently hypothesized that B cells responding to MPER epitopes are deleted because the lipid portion of their target epitope is considered "self" (Haynes et al., 2005b). This hypothesis would explain why such responses are so infrequently observed. It also suggests that induction of a response directed to the MPER may require immunogens capable of breaking one's natural tolerance to the cell membrane. Whether IgG1b12 and 2G12 recognized similarly tolerized epitopes is unclear. Certainly, designing vaccine immunogens that would target responses against these epitopes represents a daunting immunological, structural, and potentially, regulatory challenge.

2. Generating Antibodies That Target Entry Intermediates

As summarized earlier, the coreceptor-binding domain is a structure that is highly conserved among HIV, SIV, and HIV-2. This has prompted investigators to develop immunogens that induce antibodies that target this structure. One such immunogen is the gp120–CD4 complex, which forms when the virus attaches to cell surface receptor CD4. Studies in mice, goats, and more recently rhesus macaques have all shown that broadly neutralizing antibody responses are elicited by immunization with various forms of a gp120–CD4 complex (Bower et al., 2004; Celada et al., 1990; Devico et al., 1996; Fouts et al., 2002; Gershoni et al., 1993; Kang et al., 1994). Three groups of immunogens have been developed that attempt to represent gp120–CD4 complex. The first group consists of complexes between soluble envelope protein subunits (gp120) and soluble human CD4 (Bower *et al.*, 2004; Celada *et al.*, 1990; Devico *et al.*, 1996; Fouts *et al.*, 2000, 2002; Gershoni *et al.*, 1993; He *et al.*, 2003; Varadarajan *et al.*, 2005). These immunogens are produced by simply mixing the two soluble components together to allow them to bind and form complexes or expressing the gp120 and sCD4 as a genetically tethered chimeric molecule. An example of such a chimera is the full-length single chain (FLSC) which is genetic fusion between gp120$_{BaL}$ and the D1-D2 domain of CD4 (Fouts *et al.*, 2000). The second group consists of soluble envelope proteins complexed with human mAb, A32 (Liao *et al.*, 2004). A32 binds to an epitope defined by the C1-C4 region on HIV envelope subunit, gp120 and, like CD4, is known to induce the expression of the coreceptor binding domain within gp120 (Liao *et al.*, 2004; Wyatt *et al.*, 1995). Again these complexes are produced by admixing the two components to allow them to bind in solution to form complexes (Liao *et al.*, 2004). The third are complexes between gp120 and a CD4 mimic peptide, CD4M9 (Fouts *et al.*, 2002; Varadarajan *et al.*, 2005; Vita *et al.*, 1999a). Unfortunately, the affinity of the CD4M9 for gp120 is insufficient to permit formation of a stable complex in solution from the two components (Vita *et al.*, 1999a). Stable complexes can be expressed, however, as chimeric fusion protein, SCBaL/M9 (Fouts *et al.*, 2000) or gp120-M9 (Varadarajan *et al.*, 2005), where the gp120$_{BaL}$ or gp120$_{JRFL}$, respectively, are genetically tethered to CD4M9 by a short amino acid linker. Stable complexes have also been created using CD4M33 (Martin *et al.*, 2003b), a modified CD4M9 that exhibits an affinity for gp120 closer to that of CD4 (Huang *et al.*, 2005a). The presumption is that these complexes all exhibit the antigenic features presented when the HIV envelope spike interacts with cell surface CD4. Thus far, only the gp120–CD4 admixed or cross-linked complexes have been shown to elicit neutralizing antibody response. The others are still being evaluated. Whether the resulting neutralizing response arises from the exposure of cryptic epitopes either enhancing their own immunogenicity or alter the immunogenicity of other extant epitopes on gp120 (Celada *et al.*, 1990; DeVico *et al.*, 1995) is still unclear. Either instance would enhance the potential for gp120–CD4 complexes to elicit broadly cross-reactive CD4i antibodies.

Three recent studies have generated rather different results using various forms of gp120–CD4 complex immunogens (He *et al.*, 2003; Liao *et al.*, 2004; Varadarajan *et al.*, 2005). However, these studies suffer from one of either two major flaws. First, they evaluate the immunogenicity of their constructs in animal models (mice or guinea pigs) that are heterologous to the CD4 moiety used in their immunogens (human sCD4). It has been known since 1990, when the first studies of gp120–CD4 complexes appeared, that substantial levels of anti-CD4 antibodies are elicited when the CD4 used in the complex is from a species (i.e., humans) different from the one (i.e., rodents) that is immunized (Celada *et al.*, 1990). Human CD4 is highly immunogenic in rodents and biases responses to a gp120–CD4 complex away from the conserved gp120 epitopes. This obscures the immunogenic properties of the constrained HIV envelope moiety in favor of anti-CD4 responses. That said, two independent reports (Bower *et al.*, 2004; Srivastava *et al.*, 2004) including one single-chain gp120-CD4 immunogen tested in mice (Bower *et al.*, 2004) show that broadly neutralizing antibody fractions can be isolated from animals immunized with heterologous gp120–CD4 complexes that do not recognize CD4.

Second, immunogens which do not truly mimic structure presented by the gp120–CD4 complex were used. One study (Liao *et al.*, 2004) used gp120 conformationally constrained by the A32 mAb as an immunogen. It has been proposed that A32 binds to gp120 in such a way that it is a "CD4 mimic" as judged by the exposure of CD4i epitopes recognized by the mAbs 17b and 48d (Wyatt *et al.*, 1995). Guinea pigs immunized with covalent conjugates of gp120(BaL) and A32 mounted neutralizing antibody responses that were by and large indistinguishable from those elicited by gp120(BaL) alone. We have found that the gp120 conformational changes induced by A32 and CD4 are distinct as judged by differential reactivity with CD4i antibodies such as 19e that recognize epitopes in the bridging sheet of envelope (Fouts *et al.*, unpublished data). Notably, serum antibody responses to this epitope are thought to constrain viral diversity *in vivo* (Decker *et al.*, 2005). This observation may explain why the A32–gp120(BaL) complexes elicited a different pattern of reactivity than our gp120–CD4 complexes.

Other approaches are also being utilized to target the CD4i epitopes. The most common is to remove the hypervariable V1, V2, and/or V3 regions of the envelope that are the primary target of the "type-specific" antibody responses and that shield the conserved neutralizing epitopes (reviewed in Cho, 2003). More recently, investigators have developed constructs derived from the envelope sequences of CD4-independent isolates that have been adapted to grow on cell lines devoid of CD4 (Hoffman *et al.*, 1999; Kolchinsky *et al.*, 2001) or isolated from a patient with high level of broadly neutralizing antibodies (Quinnan *et al.*, 1999; Vujcic and Quinnan, 1995; Zhang *et al.*, 2002). These envelopes contain structural alterations that provide more receptive interactions with the coreceptor such as fewer N-linked glycosylation or shifting the V1–V2 loops.

As the full spectrum and potential of CD4i epitopes is only recently becoming apparent, it is difficult to argue that CD4i epitopes are poor targets for vaccine development (Labrijn *et al.*, 2003). In addition, it is not known whether mAbs specific for CD4i epitopes are protective in passive transfer studies in rhesus macaques. In this regard, until passive transfer studies are carried out using mixtures of mAbs specific for CD4i epitopes and shown to be negative, it is premature to exclude this strategy based on *in vitro* neutralization data alone. It should also be recognized that immunization with gp120–CD4 complexes can dramatically change the immunodominance profile of gp120 (Denisova *et al.*, 1996; Fouts *et al.*, 2002; Kang *et al.*, 1994; Fouts *et al.*, unpublished data), and it is possible that this leads to the immunogenicity of previously silent epitopes that elicit protective responses *in vivo*.

E. The Env as Target for Inhibitors

The entry process for HIV is also a prime target for therapeutics. Early efforts to interfere with entry utilized polyclonal antibody preparations developed from HIV+ patients (HIVIg) or mAbs (2G12, 2F5, 4E10), each of which exhibited exceptional neutralizing capacity *in vitro* (reviewed in Choudhry *et al.*, 2006a). Unfortunately, these preparations did not provide much in the way therapeutic utility despite their safety. When they did impact viral load, the effect was transient with resistant viruses quickly emerging. A key breakthrough came with the licensure of T-20, or enfuvirtide. Targeting the HR1 of gp41 (reviewed in Weiss, 2003), this drug was the first in its class to reach the marketplace and is at the forefront of an army of other inhibitors making their way through clinical development. These drugs generally fall within four broad groups and are being developed for both therapeutic and vaginally or rectally applied microbicidal indications.

i. *Antibodies.* Given their safety record, clinical development of antibodies for HIV therapy continues. Promising new candidates target CD4 and CCR5, attempting to minimize the chances of evasion by targeting cellular receptors instead of the envelope (Dimitrov, 2004).

ii. *Peptides.* This group is populated by Fuzeon and a variety of follow-on candidates, each targeting the helical region of gp41. The main challenge with this group is delivery. Fuzeon requires intramuscular administration twice daily making it a rather unfavorable choice for patients. Newer delivery methods and formulations are being developed that may help solve this problem (Markovic, 2006; Pierson and Doms, 2003a,b).

iii. *Lectins.* A variety of lectins have been shown to inhibit HIV by binding to the mannose structures that cover the envelope spike. These drugs are currently being developed for vaginal or rectal use as microbicides; however, they have potential therapeutic utility (De, 2005; Pierson and Doms, 2003a). Cyanovirin (CV-N) is currently the furthest in clinical development.

iv. *Small compounds.* This group is where the bulk of the new inhibitors fall. Thus far, only Maraviroc, a small molecule antagonist that targets CCR5 has reached Phase III. As a group, these drugs are proving to be highly effective at reducing viral load but are falling out of development because of a variety of safety problems (De, 2005; Kadow *et al.*, 2006; Markovic, 2006; Pierson and Doms, 2003a).

The drugs and their respective targets are eloquently described in many recent reviews some of which are cited above. Given the wealth of research directed to understanding the nuances of HIV entry, we do not anticipate that this pipeline of drug candidates will dry anytime soon.

VII. Conclusions

HIV has evolved a number of strategies to escape host immune surveillance, prominently by modifications to its Env. Latest advances in our understanding of its structure at atomic level of detail promise to provide us with new tools to design effective vaccines and inhibitors. In spite of the significant progress, the contribution to the development of vaccines and therapeutics of the wealth of information about the Env structure is still relatively small. However, current developments promise to revolutionize the way therapeutics and vaccines will be designed in the future. It remains to be seen whether this promise will materialize.

Acknowledgments

We thank the members of our group Protein Interactions, and Anthony DeVico, Robert Blumenthal, Peter Kwong, Xinhua Ji and Hana Golding for helpful discussions. This project was supported by the NIH Intramural AIDS Targeted Antiviral Program (IATAP), the Intramural Research Program of the NIH, National Cancer Institute, Center for Cancer Research, and the Gates Foundation to DSD, and CRADA between NCI and Profectus BioSciences, Inc.

References

Ahmad, A., and Menezes, J. (1996). Antibody-dependent cellular cytotoxicity in HIV infections. *FASEB J.* **10**, 258–266.

Ahmad, R., Sindhu, S. T., Toma, E., Morisset, R., Vincelette, J., Menezes, J., and Ahmad, A. (2001). Evidence for a correlation between antibody-dependent cellular cytotoxicity-mediating anti-HIV-1 antibodies and prognostic predictors of HIV infection. *J. Clin. Immunol.* **21**, 227–233.

Albert, J., Abrahamsson, B., Nagy, K., Aurelius, E., Gaines, H., Nystrom, G., and Fenyo, E. M. (1990). Rapid development of isolate-specific neutralizing antibodies after primary HIV-1 infection and consequent emergence of virus variants which resist neutralization by autologous sera. *AIDS* **4**, 107–112.

Alfsen, A., and Bomsel, M. (2002). HIV-1 gp41 envelope residues 650–685 exposed on native virus act as a lectin to bind epithelial cell galactosyl ceramide. *J. Biol. Chem.* **277**, 25649–25659.

Amara, R. R., Smith, J. M., Staprans, S. I., Montefiori, D. C., Villinger, F., Altman, J. D., O'Neil, S. P., Kozyr, N. L., Xu, Y., Wyatt, L. S., Earl, P. L., Herndon, J. G., et al. (2002). Critical role for Env as well as Gag-Pol in control of a simian-human immunodeficiency virus 89. 6P challenge by a DNA prime/recombinant modified vaccinia virus Ankara vaccine. J. Virol. 76, 6138–6146.

Arendrup, M., Nielsen, C., Hansen, J. E., Pedersen, C., Mathiesen, L., and Nielsen, J. O. (1992). Autologous HIV-1 neutralizing antibodies: Emergence of neutralization-resistant escape virus and subsequent development of escape virus neutralizing antibodies. J. Acquir. Immune Defic. Syndr. 5, 303–307.

Atchison, R. E., Gosling, J., Monteclaro, F. S., Franci, C., Digilio, L., Charo, I. F., and Goldsmith, M. A. (1996). Multiple extracellular elements of CCR5 and HIV-1 entry: Dissociation from response to chemokines. Science 274, 1924–1926.

Baba, T. W., Liska, V., Hofmann-Lehmann, R., Vlasak, J., Xu, W., Ayehunie, S., Cavacini, L. A., Posner, M. R., Katinger, H., Stiegler, G., Bernacky, B. J., Rizvi, T. A., et al. (2000). Human neutralizing monoclonal antibodies of the IgG1 subtype protect against mucosal simian-human immunodeficiency virus infection. Nat. Med. 6, 200–206.

Back, N. K., Smit, L., De Jong, J. J., Keulen, W., Schutten, M., Goudsmit, J., and Tersmette, M. (1994). An N-glycan within the human immunodeficiency virus type 1 gp120 V3 loop affects virus neutralization. Virology 199, 431–438.

Banks, N. D., Kinsey, N., Clements, J., and Hildreth, J. E. (2002). Sustained antibody-dependent cell-mediated cytotoxicity (ADCC) in SIV-infected macaques correlates with delayed progression to AIDS. AIDS Res. Hum. Retroviruses 18, 1197–1205.

Basmaciogullari, S., Pacheco, B., Bour, S., and Sodroski, J. (2006). Specific interaction of CXCR4 with CD4 and CD8alpha: Functional analysis of the CD4/CXCR4 interaction in the context of HIV-1 envelope glycoprotein-mediated membrane fusion. Virology 353, 52–67.

Beddows, S., Schulke, N., Kirschner, M., Barnes, K., Franti, M., Michael, E., Ketas, T., Sanders, R. W., Maddon, P. J., Olson, W. C., and Moore, J. P. (2005). Evaluating the immunogenicity of a disulfide-stabilized, cleaved, trimeric form of the envelope glycoprotein complex of human immunodeficiency virus type 1. J. Virol. 79, 8812–8827.

Berger, E. A., Murphy, P. M., and Farber, J. M. (1999). Chemokine receptors as HIV-1 coreceptors: Roles in viral entry, tropism, and disease. Annu. Rev. Immunol. 17, 657–700.

Binley, J. M., Sanders, R. W., Clas, B., Schuelke, N., Master, A., Guo, Y., Kajumo, F., Anselma, D. J., Maddon, P. J., Olson, W. C., and Moore, J. P. (2000). A recombinant human immunodeficiency virus type 1 envelope glycoprotein complex stabilized by an intermolecular disulfide bond between the gp120 and gp41 subunits is an antigenic mimic of the trimeric virion-associated structure. J. Virol. 74, 627–643.

Binley, J. M., Wrin, T., Korber, B., Zwick, M. B., Wang, M., Chappey, C., Stiegler, G., Kunert, R., Zolla-Pazner, S., Katinger, H., Petropoulos, C. J., and Burton, D. R. (2004). Comprehensive cross-clade neutralization analysis of a panel of anti-human immunodeficiency virus type 1 monoclonal antibodies. J. Virol. 78, 13232–13252.

Blanpain, C., Lee, B., Tackoen, M., Puffer, B., Boom, A., Libert, F., Sharron, M., Wittamer, V., Vassart, G., Doms, R. W., and Parmentier, M. (2000). Multiple nonfunctional alleles of CCR5 are frequent in various human populations. Blood 96, 1638–1645.

Bouma, P., Leavitt, M., Zhang, P. F., Sidorov, I. A., Dimitrov, D. S., and Quinnan, G. V., Jr. (2003). Multiple interactions across the surface of the gp120 core structure determine the global neutralization resistance phenotype of human immunodeficiency virus type 1. J. Virol. 77, 8061–8071.

Bower, J. F., Green, T. D., and Ross, T. M. (2004). DNA vaccines expressing soluble CD4-envelope proteins fused to C3d elicit cross-reactive neutralizing antibodies to HIV-1. Virology 328, 292–300.

Bradney, A. P., Scheer, S., Crawford, J. M., Buchbinder, S. P., and Montefiori, D. C. (1999). Neutralization escape in human immunodeficiency virus type 1-infected long-term nonprogressors. *J. Infect. Dis.* **179**, 1264–1267.

Broder, C. C., and Dimitrov, D. S. (1996). HIV and the 7-transmbembrane domain receptors. *Pathobiology* **64**, 171–179.

Brunel, F. M., Zwick, M. B., Cardoso, R. M., Nelson, J. D., Wilson, I. A., Burton, D. R., and Dawson, P. E. (2006). Structure-function analysis of the epitope for 4E10, a broadly neutralizing human immunodeficiency virus type 1 antibody. *J. Virol.* **80**, 1680–1687.

Bullough, P. A., Hughson, F. M., Skehel, J. J., and Wiley, D. C. (1994). Structure of influenza haemagglutinin at the pH of membrane fusion. *Nature* **371**, 37–43.

Burton, D. R. (2002). Antibodies, viruses and vaccines. *Nat. Rev. Immunol.* **2**, 706–713.

Burton, D. R., and Montefiori, D. C. (1997). The antibody response in HIV-1 infection. *AIDS* **11**(Suppl. A), S87–S98.

Burton, D. R., Pyati, J., Koduri, R., Sharp, S. J., Thornton, G. B., Parren, P. W., Sawyer, L. S., Hendry, R. M., Dunlop, N., Nara, P. L., Lamacchia, M., Garraty, E., *et al.* (1994). Efficient neutralization of primary isolates of HIV-1 by a recombinant human monoclonal antibody. *Science* **266**, 1024–1027.

Burton, D. R., Desrosiers, R. C., Doms, R. W., Koff, W. C., Kwong, P. D., Moore, J. P., Nabel, G. J., Sodroski, J., Wilson, I. A., and Wyatt, R. T. (2004). HIV vaccine design and the neutralizing antibody problem. *Nat. Immunol.* **5**, 233–236.

Burton, D. R., Stanfield, R. L., and Wilson, I. A. (2005). Antibody vs. HIV in a clash of evolutionary titans. *Proc. Natl. Acad. Sci. USA* **102**, 14943–14948.

Cao, Y., Qin, L., Zhang, L., Safrit, J., and Ho, D. D. (1995). Virologic and immunologic characterization of long-term survivors of human immunodeficiency virus type 1 infection [see comments]. *N. Engl. J. Med.* **332**, 201–208.

Cardoso, R. M., Zwick, M. B., Stanfield, R. L., Kunert, R., Binley, J. M., Katinger, H., Burton, D. R., and Wilson, I. A. (2005). Broadly neutralizing anti-HIV antibody 4E10 recognizes a helical conformation of a highly conserved fusion-associated motif in gp41. *Immunity* **22**, 163–173.

Carr, C. M., and Kim, P. S. (1993). A spring-loaded mechanism for the conformational changes of influenza hemagglutinin. *Cell* **73**, 823–832.

Cavacini, L. A., Samore, M. H., Gambertoglio, J., Jackson, B., Duval, M., Wisnewski, A., Hammer, S., Koziel, C., Trapnell, C., and Posner, M. R. (1998). Phase I study of a human monoclonal antibody directed against the CD4-binding site of HIV type 1 glycoprotein 120. *AIDS Res. Hum. Retroviruses* **14**, 545–550.

Cecilia, D., Kleeberger, C., Munoz, A., Giorgi, J. V., and Zolla-Pazner, S. (1999). A longitudinal study of neutralizing antibodies and disease progression in HIV-1-infected subjects. *J. Infect. Dis.* **179**, 1365–1374.

Celada, F., Cambiaggi, C., Maccari, J., Burastero, S., Gregory, T., Patzer, E., Porter, J., McDanal, C., and Matthews, T. (1990). Antibody raised against soluble CD4-rgp120 complex recognizes the CD4 moiety and blocks membrane fusion without inhibiting CD4-gp120 binding. *J. Exp. Med.* **172**, 1143–1150.

Center, R. J., Lebowitz, J., Leapman, R. D., and Moss, B. (2004). Promoting trimerization of soluble human immunodeficiency virus type 1 (HIV-1) Env through the use of HIV-1/simian immunodeficiency virus chimeras. *J. Virol.* **78**, 2265–2276.

Chackerian, B., Rudensey, L. M., and Overbaugh, J. (1997). Specific N-linked and O-linked glycosylation modifications in the envelope V1 domain of simian immunodeficiency virus variants that evolve in the host alter recognition by neutralizing antibodies. *J. Virol.* **71**, 7719–7727.

Chan, D. C., and Kim, P. S. (1998). HIV entry and its inhibition. *Cell* **93**, 681–684.

Chan, D. C., Fass, D., Berger, J. M., and Kim, P. S. (1997). Core structure of gp41 from the HIV envelope glycoprotein. *Cell* **89**, 263–273.

Cho, M. W. (2003). Subunit protein vaccines: Theoretical and practical considerations for HIV-1. *Curr. Mol. Med.* 3, 243–263.

Choe, H., Li, W., Wright, P. L., Vasilieva, N., Venturi, M., Huang, C. C., Grundner, C., Dorfman, T., Zwick, M. B., Wang, L., Rosenberg, E. S., Kwong, P. D., *et al.* (2003). Tyrosine sulfation of human antibodies contributes to recognition of the CCR5 binding region of HIV-1 gp120. *Cell* 114, 161–170.

Choudhry, V., Zhang, M. Y., Dimitrova, D., Prabakaran, P., Dimitrov, A. S., Fouts, T. R., and Dimitrov, D. S. (2006a). Antibody-based inhibitors of HIV infection. *Expert. Opin. Biol. Ther.* 6, 523–531.

Choudhry, V., Zhang, M. Y., Harris, I., Sidorov, I. A., Vu, B., Dimitrov, A. S., Fouts, T., and Dimitrov, D. S. (2006b). Increased efficacy of HIV-1 neutralization by antibodies at low CCR5 surface concentration. *Biochem. Biophys. Res. Commun.* 348, 1107–1115.

Coughlan, C. M., McManus, C. M., Sharron, M., Gao, Z., Murphy, D., Jaffer, S., Choe, W., Chen, W., Hesselgesser, J., Gaylord, H., Kalyuzhny, A., Lee, V. M., *et al.* (2000). Expression of multiple functional chemokine receptors and monocyte chemoattractant protein-1 in human neurons. *Neuroscience* 97, 591–600.

D'Souza, M. P., Allen, M., Sheets, R., and Johnston, M. I. (2004). Current advances in HIV vaccines. *Curr. HIV/AIDS Rep.* 1, 18–24.

Dalgleish, A. G., Beverley, P. C. L., Clapham, P. R., Crawford, D. H., Greaves, M. F., and Weiss, R. A. (1984). The CD4 (T4) antigen is an essential component of the receptor for the AIDS retrovirus. *Nature* 312, 763–767.

Darbha, R., Phogat, S., Labrijn, A. F., Shu, Y., Gu, Y., Andrykovitch, M., Zhang, M. Y., Pantophlet, R., Martin, L., Vita, C., Burton, D. R., Dimitrov, D. S., *et al.* (2004). Crystal structure of the broadly cross-reactive HIV-1-neutralizing Fab X5 and fine mapping of its epitope. *Biochemistry* 43, 1410–1417.

De, C. E. (2005). Emerging anti-HIV drugs. *Expert. Opin. Emerg. Drugs* 10, 241–273.

Decker, J. M., Bibollet-Ruche, F., Wei, X., Wang, S., Levy, D. N., Wang, W., Delaporte, E., Peeters, M., Derdeyn, C. A., Allen, S., Hunter, E., Saag, M. S., *et al.* (2005). Antigenic conservation and immunogenicity of the HIV coreceptor binding site. *J. Exp. Med.* 201, 1407–1419.

Denisova, G., Stern, B., Raviv, D., Zwickel, J., Smorodinsky, N. I., and Gershoni, J. M. (1996). Humoral immune response to immunocomplexed HIV envelope glycoprotein 120. *AIDS Res. Hum. Retroviruses* 12, 901–909.

Derdeyn, C. A., Decker, J. M., Bibollet-Ruche, F., Mokili, J. L., Muldoon, M., Denham, S. A., Heil, M. L., Kasolo, F., Musonda, R., Hahn, B. H., Shaw, G. M., Korber, B. T., *et al.* (2004). Envelope-constrained neutralization-sensitive HIV-1 after heterosexual transmission. *Science* 303, 2019–2022.

Devico, A., Silver, A., Thronton, A. M., Sarngadharan, M. G., and Pal, R. (1996). Covalently crosslinked complexes of human immunodeficiency virus type 1 (HIV-1) gp120 and CD4 receptor elicit a neutralizing immune response that includes antibodies selective for primary virus isolates. *Virology* 218, 258–263.

DeVico, A. L., Rahman, R., Welch, J., Crowley, R., Lusso, P., Sarngadharan, M. G., and Pal, R. (1995). Monoclonal antibodies raised against covalently crosslinked complexes of human immunodeficiency virus type 1 gp120 and CD4 receptor identify a novel complex-dependent epitope on gp 120. *Virology* 211, 583–588.

Dimitrov, A. S., Louis, J. M., Bewley, C. A., Clore, G. M., and Blumenthal, R. (2005). Conformational changes in HIV-1 gp41 in the course of HIV-1 envelope glycoprotein-mediated fusion and inactivation. *Biochemistry* 44, 12471–12479.

Dimitrov, D. S. (1996). Fusin—a place for HIV-1 and T4 cells to meet. Identifying the coreceptor mediating HIV-1 entry raises new hopes in the treatment of AIDS. *Nat. Med.* 2, 640–641.

Dimitrov, D. S. (1997). How do viruses enter cells? The HIV-1 coreceptors teach us a lesson of complexity. *Cell* **91**, 721–730.

Dimitrov, D. S. (2004). Virus entry: Molecular mechanisms and biomedical applications. *Nat. Rev. Microbiol.* **2**, 109–122.

Dimitrov, D. S., and Broder, C. C. (1997). "HIV and Membrane Receptors." Landes Biosciences, Austin, TX.

Dimitrov, D.S., and Ji, X. (2006). Crystal structure of a cross-reactive HIV-1 neutralizing CD4 binding site antibody Fab m14. Personal communication.

Dimitrov, D. S., Hillman, K., Manischewitz, J., Blumenthal, R., and Golding, H. (1992). Kinetics of soluble CD4 binding to cells expressing human immunodeficiency virus type 1 envelope glycoprotein. *J. Virol.* **66**, 132–138.

Dimitrov, D. S., Xiao, X., Chabot, D. J., and Broder, C. C. (1998). HIV coreceptors. *J. Membr. Biol.* **166**, 75–90.

Dix, R. D., Pereira, L., and Baringer, J. R. (1981). Use of monoclonal antibody directed against herpes simplex virus glycoproteins to protect mice against acute virus-induced neurological disease. *Infect. Immun.* **34**, 192–199.

Doranz, B. J., Lu, Z. H., Rucker, J., Zhang, T. Y., Sharron, M., Cen, Y. H., Wang, Z. X., Guo, H. H., Du, J. G., Accavitti, M. A., Doms, R. W., and Peiper, S. C. (1997). Two distinct CCR5 domains can mediate coreceptor usage by human immunodeficiency virus type 1. *J. Virol.* **71**, 6305–6314.

Douek, D. C., Kwong, P. D., and Nabel, G. J. (2006). The rational design of an AIDS vaccine. *Cell* **124**, 677–681.

Drakopoulou, E., Vizzavona, J., and Vita, C. (1998). Engineering a CD4 mimetic inhibiting the binding of the human immunodeficiency virus-1 (HIV-1) envelope glycoprotein gp120 to human lymphocyte CD4 by the transfer of a CD4 functional site to a small natural scaffold. *Lett. Pept. Sci.* **5**, 241–245.

Duerr, A., Wasserheit, J. N., and Corey, L. (2006). HIV vaccines: New frontiers in vaccine development. *Clin. Infect. Dis.* **43**, 500–511.

Eichberg, J. W., Murthy, K. K., Ward, R. H., and Prince, A. M. (1992). Prevention of HIV infection by passive immunization with HIVIg or CD4-IgG. *AIDS Res. Hum. Retroviruses* **8**, 1515–1519.

Emini, E. A., Schleif, W. A., Nunberg, J. H., Conley, A. J., Eda, Y., Tokiyoshi, S., Putney, S. D., Matsushita, S., Cobb, K. E., and Jett, C. M. (1992). Prevention of HIV-1 infection in chimpanzees by gp120 V3 domain-specific monoclonal antibody. *Nature* **355**, 728–730.

Endres, M. J., Clapham, P. R., Marsh, M., Ahuja, M., Turner, J. D., McKnight, A., Thomas, J. F., Stoebenau-Haggarty, B., Choe, S., Vance, P. J., Wells, T. N., Power, C. A., *et al.* (1996). CD4-independent infection by HIV-2 is mediated by fusin/CXCR4. *Cell* **87**, 745–756.

Fass, D., Harrison, S. C., and Kim, P. S. (1996). Retrovirus envelope domain at 1.7 angstrom resolution. *Nat. Struct. Biol.* **3**, 465–469.

Feng, Y., Broder, C. C., Kennedy, P. E., and Berger, E. A. (1996). HIV-1 entry cofactor: Functional cDNA cloning of a seven-transmembrane, G protein-coupled receptor. *Science* **272**, 872–877.

Ferrantelli, F., Hofmann-Lehmann, R., Rasmussen, R. A., Wang, T., Xu, W., Li, P. L., Montefiori, D. C., Cavacini, L. A., Katinger, H., Stiegler, G., Anderson, D. C., McClure, H. M., *et al.* (2003). Post-exposure prophylaxis with human monoclonal antibodies prevented SHIV89. 6P infection or disease in neonatal macaques. *AIDS* **17**, 301–309.

Ferrantelli, F., Rasmussen, R. A., Buckley, K. A., Li, P. L., Wang, T., Montefiori, D. C., Katinger, H., Stiegler, G., Anderson, D. C., McClure, H. M., and Ruprecht, R. M. (2004). Complete protection of neonatal rhesus macaques against oral exposure to pathogenic simian-human immunodeficiency virus by human anti-HIV monoclonal antibodies. *J. Infect. Dis.* **189**, 2167–2173.

Forster, F., Medalia, O., Zauberman, N., Baumeister, W., and Fass, D. (2005). Retrovirus envelope protein complex structure *in situ* studied by cryo-electron tomography. *Proc. Natl. Acad. Sci. USA* **102**, 4729–4734.

Forthal, D. N., Landucci, G., Haubrich, R., Keenan, B., Kuppermann, B. D., Tilles, J. G., and Kaplan, J. (1999). Antibody-dependent cellular cytotoxicity independently predicts survival in severely immunocompromised human immunodeficiency virus-infected patients. *J. Infect. Dis.* **180**, 1338–1341.

Forthal, D. N., Landucci, G., and Keenan, B. (2001). Relationship between antibody-dependent cellular cytotoxicity, plasma HIV type 1 RNA, and CD4+ lymphocyte count. *AIDS Res. Hum. Retroviruses* **17**, 553–561.

Fouts, T., Godfrey, K., Bobb, K., Montefiori, D., Hanson, C. V., Kalyanaraman, V. S., Devico, A., and Pal, R. (2002). Crosslinked HIV-1 envelope-CD4 receptor complexes elicit broadly cross-reactive neutralizing antibodies in rhesus macaques. *Proc. Natl. Acad. Sci. USA* **99**, 11842–11847.

Fouts, T. R., Binley, J. M., Trkola, A., Robinson, J. E., and Moore, J. P. (1997). Neutralization of the human immunodeficiency virus type 1 primary isolate JR-FL by human monoclonal antibodies correlates with antibody binding to the oligomeric form of the envelope glycoprotein complex. *J. Virol.* **71**, 2779–2785.

Fouts, T. R., Tuskan, R., Godfrey, K., Reitz, M., Hone, D., Lewis, G. K., and DeVico, A. L. (2000). Expression and characterization of a single-chain polypeptide analogue of the human immunodeficiency virus type 1 gp120-CD4 receptor complex. *J. Virol.* **74**, 11427–11436.

Fox, T. E., Finnegan, C. M., Blumenthal, R., and Kester, M. (2006). The clinical potential of sphingolipid-based therapeutics. *Cell. Mol. Life Sci.* **63**, 1017–1023.

Freedman, B. D., Liu, Q. H., Del Corno, M., and Collman, R. G. (2003). HIV-1 gp120 chemokine receptor-mediated signaling in human macrophages. *Immunol. Res.* **27**, 261–276.

Gallaher, W. R., Ball, J. M., Garry, R. F., Griffin, M. C., and Montelaro, R. C. (1989). A general model for the transmembrane proteins of HIV and other retroviruses. *AIDS Res. Hum. Retroviruses* **5**, 431–440.

Gallaher, W. R., Ball, J. M., Garry, R. F., Martin-Amedee, A. M., and Montelaro, R. C. (1995). A general model for the surface glycoproteins of HIV and other retroviruses. *AIDS Res. Hum. Retroviruses* **11**, 191–202.

Gallo, S. A., Finnegan, C. M., Viard, M., Raviv, Y., Dimitrov, A., Rawat, S. S., Puri, A., Durell, S., and Blumenthal, R. (2003). The HIV Env-mediated fusion reaction. *Biochim. Biophys. Acta* **1614**, 36–50.

Garber, D. A., Silvestri, G., and Feinberg, M. B. (2004). Prospects for an AIDS vaccine: Three big questions, no easy answers. *Lancet Infect. Dis.* **4**, 397–413.

Gershoni, J. M., Denisova, G., Raviv, D., Smorodinsky, N. I., and Buyaner, D. (1993). HIV binding to its receptor creates specific epitopes for the CD4/gp120 complex. *FASEB J.* **7**, 1185–1187.

Golding, H., Zaitseva, M., de Rosny, E., King, L. R., Manischewitz, J., Sidorov, I., Gorny, M. K., Zolla-Pazner, S., Dimitrov, D. S., and Weiss, C. D. (2002). Dissection of human immunodeficiency virus type 1 entry with neutralizing antibodies to gp41 fusion intermediates. *J. Virol.* **76**, 6780–6790.

Gomez-Roman, V. R., Patterson, L. J., Venzon, D., Liewehr, D., Aldrich, K., Florese, R., and Robert-Guroff, M. (2005). Vaccine-elicited antibodies mediate antibody-dependent cellular cytotoxicity correlated with significantly reduced acute viremia in rhesus macaques challenged with SIVmac251. *J. Immunol.* **174**, 2185–2189.

Gomez-Roman, V. R., Florese, R. H., Patterson, L. J., Peng, B., Venzon, D., Aldrich, K., and Robert-Guroff, M. (2006). A simplified method for the rapid fluorometric assessment of antibody-dependent cell-mediated cytotoxicity. *J. Immunol. Methods* **308**, 53–67.

Gorny, M. K., Conley, A. J., Karwowska, S., Buchbinder, A., Xu, J. Y., Emini, E. A., Koenig, S., and Zolla-Pazner, S. (1992). Neutralization of diverse human immunodeficiency virus type 1 variants by an anti-V3 human monoclonal antibody. *J. Virol.* **66**, 7538–7542.

Graham, B. S. (2002). Clinical trials of HIV vaccines. *Annu. Rev. Med.* **53**, 207–221.

Gurtler, L. G., Hauser, P. H., Eberle, J., von Brunn, A., Knapp, S., Zekeng, L., Tsague, J. M., and Kaptue, L. (1994). A new subtype of human immunodeficiency virus type I (MVP-5180) from Cameroon. *J. Virol.* **68**, 1581–1585.

Harouse, J. M., Bhat, S., Spitalnik, S. L., Laughlin, M., Stefano, K., Silberberg, D. H., and Gonzalez-Scarano, F. (1991). Inhibition of entry of HIV-1 in neural cell lines by antibodies against calactosyl ceramide. *Science* **253**, 320–323.

Haynes, B. F., Fleming, J., StClair, W. E., Katinger, H., Stiegler, G., Kunert, R., Robinson, J., Scearce, R. M., Plonk, K., Staats, H. F., Ortel, T. L., Liao, H. X., *et al.* (2005a). Cardiolipin polyspecific autoreactivity in two broadly neutralizing HIV-1 antibodies. *Science.* **308**, 1096–1908.

Haynes, B. F., Moody, M. A., Verkoczy, L., Kelsoe, G., and Alam, S. M. (2005b). Antibody polyspecificity and neutralization of HIV-1: A hypothesis. *Hum. Antibodies* **14**, 59–67.

He, Y., D'Agostino, P., and Pinter, A. (2003). Analysis of the immunogenic properties of a single-chain polypeptide analogue of the HIV-1 gp120-CD4 complex in transgenic mice that produce human immunoglobulins. *Vaccine* **21**, 4421–4429.

Hesselgesser, J., Halks-Miller, M., DelVecchio, V., Peiper, S. C., Hoxie, J., Kolson, D. L., Taub, D., and Horuk, R. (1997). CD4-independent association between HIV-1 gp120 and CXCR4: Functional chemokine receptors are expressed in human neurons. *Curr. Biol.* **7**, 112–121.

Hioe, C. E., Jones, G. J., Rees, A. D., Ratto-Kim, S., Birx, D., Munz, C., Gorny, M. K., Tuen, M., and Zolla-Pazner, S. (2000). Anti-CD4-binding domain antibodies complexed with HIV type 1 glycoprotein 120 inhibit CD4+ T cell-proliferative responses to glycoprotein 120. *AIDS Res. Hum. Retroviruses* **16**, 893–905.

Hioe, C. E., Tuen, M., Chien, P. C., Jr., Jones, G., Ratto-Kim, S., Norris, P. J., Moretto, W. J., Nixon, D. F., Gorny, M. K., and Zolla-Pazner, S. (2001). Inhibition of human immunodeficiency virus type 1 gp120 presentation to CD4 T cells by antibodies specific for the CD4 binding domain of gp120. *J. Virol.* **75**, 10950–10957.

Hoffman, T. L., LaBranche, C. C., Zhang, W., Canziani, G., Robinson, J., Chaiken, I., Hoxie, J. A., and Doms, R. W. (1999). Stable exposure of the coreceptor-binding site in a CD4-independent HIV-1 envelope protein. *Proc. Natl. Acad. Sci. USA* **96**, 6359–6364.

Hofmann-Lehmann, R., Rasmussen, R. A., Vlasak, J., Smith, B. A., Baba, T. W., Liska, V., Montefiori, D. C., McClure, H. M., Anderson, D. C., Bernacky, B. J., Rizvi, T. A., Schmidt, R., *et al.* (2001a). Passive immunization against oral AIDS virus transmission: An approach to prevent mother-to-infant HIV-1 transmission? *J. Med. Primatol.* **30**, 190–196.

Hofmann-Lehmann, R., Vlasak, J., Rasmussen, R. A., Smith, B. A., Baba, T. W., Liska, V., Ferrantelli, F., Montefiori, D. C., McClure, H. M., Anderson, D. C., Bernacky, B. J., Rizvi, T. A., *et al.* (2001b). Postnatal passive immunization of neonatal macaques with a triple combination of human monoclonal antibodies against oral simian-human immunodeficiency virus challenge. *J. Virol.* **75**, 7470–7480.

Hofmann-Lehmann, R., Vlasak, J., Rasmussen, R. A., Jiang, S., Li, P. L., Baba, T. W., Montefiori, D. C., Bernacky, B. J., Rizvi, T. A., Schmidt, R., Hill, L. R., Keeling, M. E., *et al.* (2002). Postnatal pre- and postexposure passive immunization strategies: Protection of neonatal macaques against oral simian-human immunodeficiency virus challenge. *J. Med. Primatol.* **31**, 109–119.

Holl, V., Hemmerter, S., Burrer, R., Schmidt, S., Bohbot, A., Aubertin, A. M., and Moog, C. (2004). Involvement of Fc gamma RI (CD64) in the mechanism of HIV-1 inhibition by polyclonal IgG purified from infected patients in cultured monocyte-derived macrophages. *J. Immunol.* **173**, 6274–6283.

Holl, V., Peressin, M., Decoville, T., Schmidt, S., Zolla-Pazner, S., Aubertin, A. M., and Moog, C. (2006a). Nonneutralizing antibodies are able to inhibit human immunodeficiency virus type 1 replication in macrophages and immature dendritic cells. *J. Virol.* **80**, 6177–6181.

Holl, V., Peressin, M., Schmidt, S., Decoville, T., Zolla-Pazner, S., Aubertin, A. M., and Moog, C. (2006b). Efficient inhibition of HIV-1 replication in human immature monocyte-derived dendritic cells by purified anti-HIV-1 IgG without induction of maturation. *Blood* **107**, 4466–4474.

Huang, C. C., Venturi, M., Majeed, S., Moore, M. J., Phogat, S., Zhang, M. Y., Dimitrov, D. S., Hendrickson, W. A., Robinson, J., Sodroski, J., Wyatt, R., Choe, H., *et al.* (2004). Structural basis of tyrosine sulfation and VH-gene usage in antibodies that recognize the HIV type 1 coreceptor-binding site on gp120. *Proc. Natl. Acad. Sci. USA* **101**, 2706–2711.

Huang, C. C., Stricher, F., Martin, L., Decker, J. M., Majeed, S., Barthe, P., Hendrickson, W. A., Robinson, J., Roumestand, C., Sodroski, J., Wyatt, R., Shaw, G. M., *et al.* (2005a). Scorpion-toxin mimics of CD4 in complex with human immunodeficiency virus gp120 crystal structures, molecular mimicry, and neutralization breadth. *Structure (Camb.)* **13**, 755–768.

Huang, C. C., Tang, M., Zhang, M. Y., Majeed, S., Montabana, E., Stanfield, R. L., Dimitrov, D. S., Korber, B., Sodroski, J., Wilson, I. A., Wyatt, R., and Kwong, P. D. (2005b). Structure of a V3-containing HIV-1 gp120 core. *Science* **310**, 1025–1028.

Hunter, E., and Swanstrom, R. (1990). Retrovirus envelope glycoproteins. *Curr. Top. Microbiol. Immunol.* **157**, 187–253.

Hutto, C., Zhou, Y., He, J., Geffin, R., Hill, M., Scott, W., and Wood, C. (1996). Longitudinal studies of viral sequence, viral phenotype, and immunologic parameters of human immunodeficiency virus type 1 infection in perinatally infected twins with discordant disease courses. *J. Virol.* **70**, 3589–3598.

Janssens, W., Heyndrickx, L., Fransen, K., Motte, J., Peeters, M., Nkengasong, J. N., Ndumbe, P. M., Delaporte, E., Perret, J. L., Atende, C., *et al.* (1994). Genetic and phylogenetic analysis of env subtypes G and H in central Africa. *AIDS Res. Hum. Retroviruses* **10**, 877–879.

Johnson, W. E., and Desrosiers, R. C. (2002). Viral persistance: HIV's strategies of immune system evasion. *Annu. Rev. Med.* **53**, 499–518.

Johnson, W. E., Morgan, J., Reitter, J., Puffer, B. A., Czajak, S., Doms, R. W., and Desrosiers, R. C. (2002). A replication-competent, neutralization-sensitive variant of simian immunodeficiency virus lacking 100 amino acids of envelope. *J. Virol.* **76**, 2075–2086.

Johnson, W. E., Lifson, J. D., Lang, S. M., Johnson, R. P., and Desrosiers, R. C. (2003a). Importance of B-cell responses for immunological control of variant strains of simian immunodeficiency virus. *J. Virol.* **77**, 375–381.

Johnson, W. E., Sanford, H., Schwall, L., Burton, D. R., Parren, P. W., Robinson, J. E., and Desrosiers, R. C. (2003b). Assorted mutations in the envelope gene of simian immunodeficiency virus lead to loss of neutralization resistance against antibodies representing a broad spectrum of specificities. *J. Virol.* **77**, 9993–10003.

Kadow, J., Wang, H. G., and Lin, P. F. (2006). Small-molecule HIV-1 gp120 inhibitors to prevent HIV-1 entry: An emerging opportunity for drug development. *Curr. Opin. Investig. Drugs* **7**, 721–726.

Kang, C. Y., Hariharan, K., Nara, P. L., Sodroski, J., and Moore, J. P. (1994). Immunization with a soluble CD4-gp120 complex preferentially induces neutralizing anti-human immunodeficiency virus type 1 antibodies directed to conformation-dependent epitopes of gp120. *J. Virol.* **68**, 5854–5862.

Kensinger, R. D., Yowler, B. C., Benesi, A. J., and Schengrund, C. L. (2004). Synthesis of novel, multivalent glycodendrimers as ligands for HIV-1 gp120. *Bioconjug. Chem.* **15**, 349–358.

Kimata, J. T., Gosink, J. J., Kewalramani, V. N., Rudensey, L. M., Littman, D. R., and Overbaugh, J. (1999a). Coreceptor specificity of temporal variants of simian immunodeficiency virus Mne. *J. Virol.* **73**, 1655–1660.

Kimata, J. T., Kuller, L., Anderson, D. B., Dailey, P., and Overbaugh, J. (1999b). Emerging cytopathic and antigenic simian immunodeficiency virus variants influence AIDS progression. *Nat. Med.* **5**, 535–541.

Klatzmann, D., Champagne, E., Chamaret, S., Gruest, J., Guetard, D., Hercend, T., Gluckman, J.-C., and Montagnierce, L. (1984). T-lymphocyte T4 molecule behaves as the receptor for human retrovirus LAV. *Nature* **312**, 767–768.

Kloosterboer, N., Groeneveld, P. H., Jansen, C. A., van der Vorst, T. J., Koning, F., Winkel, C. N., Duits, A. J., Miedema, F., van Baarle, D., van Rij, R. P., Brinkman, K., and Schuitemaker, H. (2005). Natural controlled HIV infection: Preserved HIV-specific immunity despite undetectable replication competent virus. *Virology.* **339**, 70–80.

Koch, M., Pancera, M., Kwong, P. D., Kolchinsky, P., Grundner, C., Wang, L., Hendrickson, W. A., Sodroski, J., and Wyatt, R. (2003). Structure-based, targeted deglycosylation of HIV-1 gp120 and effects on neutralization sensitivity and antibody recognition. *Virology* **313**, 387–400.

Koff, W. C., Johnson, P. R., Watkins, D. I., Burton, D. R., Lifson, J. D., Hasenkrug, K. J., McDermott, A. B., Schultz, A., Zamb, T. J., Boyle, R., and Desrosiers, R. C. (2006). HIV vaccine design: Insights from live attenuated SIV vaccines. *Nat. Immunol.* **7**, 19–23.

Kolchinsky, P., Kiprilov, E., and Sodroski, J. (2001). Increased neutralization sensitivity of CD4-independent human immunodeficiency virus variants. *J. Virol.* **75**, 2041–2050.

Korber, B. T., Kunstman, K. J., Patterson, B. K., Furtado, M., McEvilly, M. M., Levy, R., and Wolinsky, S. M. (1994). Genetic differences between blood- and brain-derived viral sequences from human immunodeficiency virus type 1-infected patients: Evidence of conserved elements in the V3 region of the envelope protein of brain-derived sequences. *J. Virol.* **68**, 7467–7481.

Kwong, P. D. (2006). Functional constraints and antibody recognition of the CD4-binding site on HIV-1 gp120. Fifth International Conference, AIDS Vaccine 06, 29 August–1 September 2006, Amsterdam, the Netherlands.

Kwong, P. D., Ryu, S.-E., Henrickson, W., Axel, R., Sweet, R., Folena-Wasserman, G., and Hensley, P. (1990). Molecular characteristics of recombinant human CD4 as deduced from polymorphic crystals. *Proc. Natl. Acad. Sci. USA* **87**, 6423–6427.

Kwong, P. D., Wyatt, R., Robinson, J., Sweet, R. W., Sodroski, J., and Hendrickson, W. A. (1998). Structure of an HIV gp120 envelope glycoprotein in complex with the CD4 receptor and a neutralizing human antibody. *Nature* **393**, 648–659.

Kwong, P. D., Wyatt, R., Majeed, S., Robinson, J., Sweet, R. W., Sodroski, J., and Hendrickson, W. A. (2000). Structures of HIV-1 gp120 envelope glycoproteins from laboratory-adapted and primary isolates. *Structure* **8**, 1329–1339.

Kwong, P. D., Doyle, M. L., Casper, D. J., Cicala, C., Leavitt, S. A., Majeed, S., Steenbeke, T. D., Venturi, M., Chaiken, I., Fung, M., Katinger, H., Parren, P. W., *et al.* (2002). HIV-1 evades antibody-mediated neutralization through conformational masking of receptor-binding sites. *Nature* **420**, 678–682.

Labrijn, A. F., Poignard, P., Raja, A., Zwick, M. B., Delgado, K., Franti, M., Binley, J., Vivona, V., Grundner, C., Huang, C. C., Venturi, M., Petropoulos, C. J., *et al.* (2003). Access of antibody molecules to the conserved coreceptor binding site on glycoprotein gp120 is sterically restricted on primary human immunodeficiency virus type 1. *J. Virol.* **77**, 10557–10565.

Lange, G., Lewis, S. J., Murshudov, G. N., Dodson, G. G., Moody, P. C., Turkenburg, J. P., Barclay, A. N., and Brady, R. L. (1994). Crystal structure of an extracellular fragment of the rat CD4 receptor containing domains 3 and 4. *Structure* **2**, 469–481.

Lapham, C. K., Ouyang, J., Chandrasekhar, B., Nguyen, N. Y., Dimitrov, D. S., and Golding, H. (1996). Evidence for cell-surface association between fusin and the CD4-gp120 complex in human cell lines. *Science* **274**, 602–605.

Lapham, C. K., Zaitseva, M. B., Lee, S., Romanstseva, T., and Golding, H. (1999). Fusion of monocytes and macrophages with HIV-1 correlates with biochemical properties of CXCR4 and CCR5. *Nat. Med.* **5**, 303–308.

Lefrancois, L. (1984). Protection against lethal viral infection by neutralizing and nonneutralizing monoclonal antibodies: Distinct mechanisms of action *in vivo*. *J. Virol.* **51**, 208–214.

Leitner, T., Alaeus, A., Marquina, S., Lilja, E., Lidman, K., and Albert, J. (1995). Yet another subtype of HIV type 1? *AIDS Res. Hum. Retroviruses* **11**, 995–997.

Letvin, N. L. (2005). Progress toward an HIV vaccine. *Annu. Rev. Med.* **56**, 213–223.

Letvin, N. L., Huang, Y., Chakrabarti, B. K., Xu, L., Seaman, M. S., Beaudry, K., Korioth-Schmitz, B., Yu, F., Rohne, D., Martin, K. L., Miura, A., Kong, W. P., *et al.* (2004). Heterologous envelope immunogens contribute to AIDS vaccine protection in rhesus monkeys. *J. Virol.* **78**, 7490–7497.

Lian, Y., Srivastava, I., Gomez-Roman, V. R., Zur Megede, J., Sun, Y., Kan, E., Hilt, S., Engelbrecht, S., Himathongkham, S., Luciw, P. A., Otten, G., Ulmer, J. B., *et al.* (2005). Evaluation of envelope vaccines derived from the South African subtype C human immunodeficiency virus type 1 TV1 strain. *J. Virol.* **79**, 13338–13349.

Liao, H. X., Alam, S. M., Mascola, J. R., Robinson, J., Ma, B., Montefiori, D. C., Rhein, M., Sutherland, L. L., Scearce, R., and Haynes, B. F. (2004). Immunogenicity of constrained monoclonal antibody A32-human immunodeficiency virus (HIV) Env gp120 complexes compared to that of recombinant HIV type 1 gp120 envelope glycoproteins. *J. Virol.* **78**, 5270–5278.

Lin, G., Baribaud, F., Romano, J., Doms, R. W., and Hoxie, J. A. (2003). Identification of gp120 binding sites on CXCR4 by using CD4-independent human immunodeficiency virus type 2 Env proteins. *J. Virol.* **77**, 931–942.

Littman, D. R., Maddon, P. J., and Axel, R. (1988). Corrected CD4 sequence. *Cell* **55**, 541.

Liu, S., and Jiang, S. (2004). High throughput screening and characterization of HIV-1 entry inhibitors targeting gp41: Theories and techniques. *Curr. Pharm. Des.* **10**, 1827–1843.

Louwagie, J., McCutchan, F. E., Peeters, M., Brennan, T. P., Sanders-Buell, E., Eddy, G. A., van der, G. G., Fransen, K., Gershy-Damet, G. M., Deleys, R., *et al.* (1993). Phylogenetic analysis of gag genes from 70 international HIV-1 isolates provides evidence for multiple genotypes. *AIDS* **7**, 769–780.

Lu, M., Blacklow, S. C., and Kim, P. S. (1995). A trimeric structural domain of the HIV-1 transmembrane glycoprotein. *Nat. Struct. Biol.* **2**, 1075–1082.

Lu, Z., Berson, J. F., Chen, Y., Turner, J. D., Zhang, T., Sharron, M., Jenks, M. H., Wang, Z., Kim, J., Rucker, J., Hoxie, J. A., Peiper, S. C., *et al.* (1997). Evolution of HIV-1 coreceptor usage through interactions with distinct CCR5 and CXCR4 domains. *Proc. Natl. Acad. Sci. USA* **94**, 6426–6431.

Luciw, P. A., Shaw, K. E., Unger, R. E., Planelles, V., Stout, M. W., Lackner, J. E., Pratt-Lowe, E., Leung, N. J., Banapour, B., and Marthas, M. L. (1992). Genetic and biological comparisons of pathogenic and nonpathogenic molecular clones of simian immunodeficiency virus (SIVmac). *AIDS Res. Hum. Retroviruses* **8**, 395–402.

Luo, M., Yuan, F., Liu, Y., Jiang, S., Song, X., Jiang, P., Yin, X., Ding, M., and Deng, H. (2006). Induction of neutralizing antibody against human immunodeficiency virus type 1 (HIV-1) by immunization with gp41 membrane-proximal external region (MPER) fused with porcine endogenous retrovirus (PERV) p15E fragment. *Vaccine* **24**, 435–442.

Maddon, P., Littman, D., Godfrey, M., Maddon, D., Chess, L., and Axel, R. (1985). The isolation and nucleotide sequence of a cDNA encoding the T cell surface protein T4: A new member of the immunoglobulin gene family. *Cell* **42**, 93–104.

Malashkevich, V. N., Chan, D. C., Chutkowski, C. T., and Kim, P. S. (1998). Crystal structure of the simian immunodeficiency virus (SIV) gp41 core: Conserved helical interactions underlie the broad inhibitory activity of gp41 peptides. *Proc. Natl. Acad. Sci. USA* **95**, 9134–9139.

Markosyan, R. M., Cohen, F. S., and Melikyan, G. B. (2003). HIV-1 envelope proteins complete their folding into six-helix bundles immediately after fusion pore formation. *Mol. Biol. Cell* **14**, 926–938.

Markovic, I. (2006). Advances in HIV-1 entry inhibitors: Strategies to interfere with receptor and coreceptor engagement. *Curr. Pharm. Des.* **12**, 1105–1119.

Markovic, I., and Clouse, K. A. (2004). Recent advances in understanding the molecular mechanisms of HIV-1 entry and fusion: Revisiting current targets and considering new options for therapeutic intervention. *Curr. HIV Res.* **2**, 223–234.

Martin, L., Stricher, F., Misse, D., Sironi, F., Pugniere, M., Barthe, P., Prado-Gotor, R., Freulon, I., Magne, X., Roumestand, C., Menez, A., Lusso, P., *et al.* (2003a). Rational design of a CD4 mimic that inhibits HIV-1 entry and exposes cryptic neutralization epitopes. *Nat. Biotechnol.* **21**, 71–76.

Martin, L., Stricher, F., Misse, D., Sironi, F., Pugniere, M., Barthe, P., Prado-Gotor, R., Freulon, I., Magne, X., Roumestand, C., Menez, A., Lusso, P., *et al.* (2003b). Rational design of a CD4 mimic that inhibits HIV-1 entry and exposes cryptic neutralization epitopes. *Nat. Biotechnol.* **21**, 71–76.

Mascola, J. R., Lewis, M. G., Stiegler, G., Harris, D., VanCott, T. C., Hayes, D., Louder, M. K., Brown, C. R., Sapan, C. V., Frankel, S. S., Lu, Y., Robb, M. L., *et al.* (1999). Protection of macaques against pathogenic simian/human immunodefiency virus 89. 6PD by passive transfer of neutralizing antibodies. *J. Virol.* **73**, 4009–4018.

Mascola, J. R., Stiegler, G., VanCott, T. C., Katinger, H., Carpenter, C. B., Hanson, C. E., Beary, H., Hayes, D., Frankel, S. S., Birx, D. L., and Lewis, M. G. (2000). Protection of macaques against vaginal transmission of a pathogenic HIV-1/SIV chimeric virus by passive infusion of neutralizing antibodies. *Nat. Med.* **6**, 207–210.

Mascola, J. R., Lewis, M. G., VanCott, T. C., Stiegler, G., Katinger, H., Seaman, M., Beaudry, K., Barouch, D. H., Korioth-Schmitz, B., Krivulka, G., Sambor, A., Welcher, B., *et al.* (2003a). Cellular immunity elicited by human immunodeficiency virus type 1/simian immunodeficiency virus DNA vaccination does not augment the sterile protection afforded by passive infusion of neutralizing antibodies. *J. Virol.* **77**, 10348–10356.

Mascola, J. R., Lewis, M. G., VanCott, T. C., Stiegler, G., Katinger, H., Seaman, M., Beaudry, K., Barouch, D. H., Korioth-Schmitz, B., Krivulka, G., Sambor, A., Welcher, B., *et al.* (2003b). Cellular immunity elicited by human immunodeficiency virus type 1/simian immunodeficiency virus DNA vaccination does not augment the sterile protection afforded by passive infusion of neutralizing antibodies. *J. Virol.* **77**, 10348–10356.

Mathews, J. H., and Roehrig, J. T. (1982). Determination of the protective epitopes on the glycoproteins of Venezuelan equine encephalomyelitis virus by passive transfer of monoclonal antibodies. *J. Immunol.* **129**, 2763–2767.

Mc Cann, C. M., Song, R. J., and Ruprecht, R. M. (Cann 2005). Antibodies: Can they protect against HIV infection? *Curr. Drug Targets Infect. Disord.* **5**, 95–111.

McMichael, A. J. (2006). HIV vaccines. *Annu. Rev. Immunol.* **24**, 227–255.

Melikyan, G. B., Markosyan, R. M., Hemmati, H., Delmedico, M. K., Lambert, D. M., and Cohen, F. S. (2000). Evidence that the transition of HIV-1 gp41 into a six-helix bundle, not the bundle configuration, induces membrane fusion. *J. Cell Biol.* **151**, 413–423.

Mitchison, N. A., and Sattentau, Q. (2005). Fundamental immunology and what it can teach us about HIV vaccine development. *Curr. Drug Targets Infect. Disord.* 5, 87–93.

Montefiori, D. C., Zhou, I. Y., Barnes, B., Lake, D., Hersh, E. M., Masuho, Y., and Lefkowitz, L. B., Jr. (1991). Homotypic antibody responses to fresh clinical isolates of human immunodeficiency virus. *Virology* 182, 635–643.

Montefiori, D. C., Pantaleo, G., Fink, L. M., Zhou, J. T., Zhou, J. Y., Bilska, M., Miralles, G. D., and Fauci, A. S. (1996). Neutralizing and infection-enhancing antibody responses to human immunodeficiency virus type 1 in long-term nonprogressors. *J. Infect. Dis.* 173, 60–67.

Moore, P. L., Crooks, E. T., Porter, L., Zhu, P., Cayanan, C. S., Grise, H., Corcoran, P., Zwick, M. B., Franti, M., Morris, L., Roux, K. H., Burton, D. R., *et al.* (2006). Nature of nonfunctional envelope proteins on the surface of human immunodeficiency virus type 1. *J. Virol.* 80, 2515–2528.

Mori, K., Yasutomi, Y., Ohgimoto, S., Nakasone, T., Takamura, S., Shioda, T., and Nagai, Y. (2001). Quintuple deglycosylation mutant of simian immunodeficiency virus SIVmac239 in rhesus macaques: Robust primary replication, tightly contained chronic infection, and elicitation of potent immunity against the parental wild-type strain. *J. Virol.* 75, 4023–4028.

Moulard, M., Phogat, S. K., Shu, Y., Labrijn, A. F., Xiao, X. D., Binley, J. M., Zhang, M. Y., Sidorov, I. A., Broder, C. C., Robinson, J., Parren, P. W. H. I., Burton, D. R., *et al.* (2002). Broadly cross-reactive HIV-1-neutralizing human monoclonal Fab selected for binding to gp120-CD4-CCR5 complexes. *Proc. Natl. Acad. Sci. USA* 99, 6913–6918.

Muster, T., Steindl, F., Purtscher, M., Trkola, A., Klima, A., Himmler, G., Ruker, F., and Katinger, H. (1993). A conserved neutralizing epitope on gp41 of human immunodeficiency virus type 1. *J. Virol.* 67, 6642–6647.

Myers, G., MacInnes, K., and Korber, B. (1992). The emergence of simian/human immunodeficiency viruses. *AIDS Res. Hum. Retroviruses* 8, 373–386.

Myers, G., Korber, B., Wain-Hobson, S., Jeang, K. T., Henderson, L. E., and Pavlakis, G. N. (1994). "Human Retroviruses and AIDS: A Compilation and Analysis of Nucleic Acid and Amino Acid Sequences." Los Alamos National Laboratory, Los Alamos, NM.

Nguyen, M., Pean, P., Lopalco, L., Nouhin, J., Phoung, V., Ly, N., Vermisse, P., Henin, Y., Barre-Sinoussi, F., Burastero, S. E., Reynes, J. M., Carcelain, G., *et al.* (2006). HIV-specific antibodies but not T-cell responses are associated with protection in seronegative partners of HIV-1-infected individuals in Cambodia. *J. Acquir. Immune Defic. Syndr.* 42, 412–419.

Nishimura, Y., Igarashi, T., Haigwood, N., Sadjadpour, R., Plishka, R. J., Buckler-White, A., Shibata, R., and Martin, M. A. (2002). Determination of a statistically valid neutralization titer in plasma that confers protection against simian-human immunodeficiency virus challenge following passive transfer of high-titered neutralizing antibodies. *J. Virol.* 76, 2123–2130.

Ofek, G., Tang, M., Sambor, A., Katinger, H., Mascola, J. R., Wyatt, R., and Kwong, P. D. (2004). Structure and mechanistic analysis of the anti-human immunodeficiency virus type 1 antibody 2F5 in complex with its gp41 epitope. *J. Virol.* 78, 10724–10737.

Pal, R., Nair, B. C., Hoke, G. M., Sarngadharan, M. G., and Edidin, M. (1991). Lateral diffusion of CD4 on the surface of a human neoplastic T-cell line probed with a fluorescent derivative of the envelope glycoprotein (gp120) of human immunodeficiency virus type 1 (HIV-1). *J. Cell. Physiol.* 147, 326–332.

Pancera, M., Lebowitz, J., Schon, A., Zhu, P., Freire, E., Kwong, P. D., Roux, K. H., Sodroski, J., and Wyatt, R. (2005). Soluble mimetics of human immunodeficiency virus type 1 viral spikes produced by replacement of the native trimerization domain with a heterologous trimerization motif: Characterization and ligand binding analysis. *J. Virol.* 79, 9954–9969.

Pantophlet, R., Ollmann, S. E., Poignard, P., Parren, P. W., Wilson, I. A., and Burton, D. R. (2003). Fine mapping of the interaction of neutralizing and nonneutralizing monoclonal antibodies with the CD4 binding site of human immunodeficiency virus type 1 gp120. *J. Virol.* 77, 642–658.

Parren, P. W., and Burton, D. R. (2001). The antiviral activity of antibodies *in vitro* and *in vivo*. *Adv. Immunol.* 77, 195–262.

Parren, P. W., Moore, J. P., Burton, D. R., and Sattentau, Q. J. (1999). The neutralizing antibody response to HIV-1: Viral evasion and escape from humoral immunity. *AIDS* 13(suppl. A), S137–S162.

Parren, P. W. H. I., Marx, P. A., Hessell, A. J., Luckay, A., Harouse, J., Cheng-Mayer, C., Moore, J. P., and Burton, D. R. (2001). Antibody protects macaques against vaginal challenge with a pathogenic R5 simian/human immunodeficiency virus at serum levels giving complete neutralization *in vitro*. *J. Virol.* 75, 8340–8347.

Pastori, C., Weiser, B., Barassi, C., Uberti-Foppa, C., Ghezzi, S., Longhi, R., Calori, G., Burger, H., Kemal, K., Poli, G., Lazzarin, A., and Lopalco, L. (2006). Long-lasting CCR5 internalization by antibodies in a subset of long-term nonprogressors: A possible protective effect against disease progression. *Blood* 107, 4825–4833.

Picard, L., Wilkinson, D. A., McKnight, A., Gray, P. W., Hoxie, J. A., Clapham, P. R., and Weiss, R. A. (1997). Role of the amino-terminal extracellular domain of CXCR-4 in human immunodeficiency virus type 1 entry. *Virology* 231, 105–111.

Pierson, T. C., and Doms, R. W. (2003a). HIV-1 entry and its inhibition. *Curr. Top. Microbiol. Immunol.* 281, 1–27.

Pierson, T. C., and Doms, R. W. (2003b). HIV-1 entry inhibitors: New targets, novel therapies. *Immunol. Lett.* 85, 113–118.

Pilgrim, A. K., Pantaleo, G., Cohen, O. J., Fink, L. M., Zhou, J. Y., Zhou, J. T., Bolognesi, D. P., Fauci, A. S., and Montefiori, D. C. (1997). Neutralizing antibody responses to human immunodeficiency virus type 1 in primary infection and long-term-nonprogressive infection. *J. Infect. Dis.* 176, 924–932.

Platt, E. J., Wehrly, K., Kuhmann, S. E., Chesebro, B., and Kabat, D. (1998). Effects of CCR5 and CD4 cell surface concentrations on infections by macrophagetropic isolates of human immunodeficiency virus type 1. *J. Virol.* 72, 2855–2864.

Platt, E. J., Durnin, J. P., and Kabat, D. (2005). Kinetic factors control efficiencies of cell entry, efficacies of entry inhibitors, and mechanisms of adaptation of human immunodeficiency virus. *J. Virol.* 79, 4347–4356.

Pleskoff, O., Treboute, C., and Alizon, M. (1998). The cytomegalovirus-encoded chemokine receptor US28 can enhance cell-cell fusion mediated by different viral proteins. *J. Virol.* 72, 6389–6397.

Poignard, P., Saphire, E. O., Parren, P. W., and Burton, D. R. (2001). Gp120: Biologic aspects of structural features. *Annu. Rev. Immunol.* 19, 253–274.

Prabakaran, P., Gan, J., Feng, Y., Zhu, Z., Choudhry, V., Xiao, X., Ji, X., and Dimitrov, D. S. (2006a). Structure of severe acute respiratory syndrome coronavirus receptor-binding domain complexed with neutralizing antibody. *J. Biol. Chem.* 281, 15829–15836.

Prabakaran, P., Gan, J., Wu, Y. Q., Zhang, M. Y., Dimitrov, D. S., and Ji, X. (2006b). Structural mimicry of CD4 by a cross-reactive HIV-1 neutralizing antibody with CDR-H2 and H3 containing unique motifs. *J. Mol. Biol.* 357, 82–99.

Puffer, B. A., Sharron, M., Coughlan, C. M., Baribaud, F., McManus, C. M., Lee, B., David, J., Price, K., Horuk, R., Tsang, M., and Doms, R. W. (2000). Expression and coreceptor function of APJ for primate immunodeficiency viruses. *Virology* 276, 435–444.

Puffer, B. A., Pohlmann, S., Edinger, A. L., Carlin, D., Sanchez, M. D., Reitter, J., Watry, D. D., Fox, H. S., Desrosiers, R. C., and Doms, R. W. (2002). CD4 independence of simian immunodeficiency virus Envs is associated with macrophage tropism, neutralization sensitivity, and attenuated pathogenicity. *J. Virol.* **76**, 2595–2605.

Putkonen, P., Thorstensson, R., Ghavamzadeh, L., Albert, J., Hild, K., Biberfeld, G., and Norrby, E. (1991). Prevention of HIV-2 and SIVsm infection by passive immunization in cynomolgus monkeys. *Nature* **352**, 436–438.

Quinnan, G. V., Zhang, P. F., Fu, D. W., Dong, M., and Alter, H. J. (1999). Expression and characterization of HIV type 1 envelope protein associated with a broadly reactive neutralizing antibody response. *AIDS Res. Hum. Retroviruses* **15**, 561–570.

Quinones-Kochs, M. I., Buonocore, L., and Rose, J. K. (2002). Role of N-linked glycans in a human immunodeficiency virus envelope glycoprotein: Effects on protein function and the neutralizing antibody response. *J. Virol.* **76**, 4199–4211.

Rawat, S. S., Viard, M., Gallo, S. A., Rein, A., Blumenthal, R., and Puri, A. (2003). Modulation of entry of enveloped viruses by cholesterol and sphingolipids (Review). *Mol. Membr. Biol.* **20**, 243–254.

Ray, N., and Doms, R. W. (2006). HIV-1 coreceptors and their inhibitors. *Curr. Top. Microbiol. Immunol.* **303**, 97–120.

Reeves, J. D., and Doms, R. W. (2002). Human immunodeficiency virus type 2. *J. Gen. Virol.* **83**, 1253–1265.

Reinherz, E. L., and Schlossmann, S. F. (1980). The differentiation and function of human T lymphocytes. *Cell* **19**, 821–827.

Reinherz, E. L., Kung, P. C., Goldstein, G., and Schlossmann, S. F. (1979). Separation of functional subsets of human T cells by a monoclonal antibody. *Proc. Natl. Acad. Sci. USA* **76**, 4061–4065.

Reitter, J. N., Means, R. E., and Desrosiers, R. C. (1998). A role for carbohydrates in immune evasion in AIDS. *Nat. Med.* **4**, 679–684.

Reitz, M. S., Jr., Wilson, C., Naugle, C., Gallo, R. C., and Robert-Guroff, M. (1988). Generation of a neutralization-resistant variant of HIV-1 is due to selection for a point mutation in the envelope gene. *Cell* **54**, 57–63.

Richman, D. D., Wrin, T., Little, S. J., and Petropoulos, C. J. (2003). Rapid evolution of the neutralizing antibody response to HIV type 1 infection. *Proc. Natl. Acad. Sci. USA* **100**, 4144–4149.

Roben, P., Moore, J. P., Thali, M., Sodroski, J., Barbas, C. F., III, and Burton, D. R. (1994). Recognition properties of a panel of human recombinant Fab fragments to the CD4 binding site of gp120 that show differing abilities to neutralize human immunodeficiency virus type 1. *J. Virol.* **68**, 4821–4828.

Robinson, J. E., Yoshiyama, H., Holton, D., Elliott, S., and Ho, D. D. (1992). Distinct antigenic sites on HIV gp120 identified by a panel of human monoclonal antibodies (abstr. Q449). *J. Cell. Biochem.* (Suppl. 16E), 71.

Root, M. J., and Steger, H. K. (2004). HIV-1 gp41 as a target for viral entry inhibition. *Curr. Pharm. Des.* **10**, 1805–1825.

Rucker, J., Samson, M., Doranz, B. J., Libert, F., Berson, J. F., Yi, Y., Smyth, R. J., Collman, R. G., Broder, C. C., Vassart, G., Doms, R. W., and Parmentier, M. (1996). Regions in beta-chemokine receptors CCR5 and CCR2b that determine HIV-1 cofactor specificity. *Cell* **87**, 437–446.

Ruprecht, R. M., Hofmann-Lehmann, R., Smith-Franklin, B. A., Rasmussen, R. A., Liska, V., Vlasak, J., Xu, W., Baba, T. W., Chenine, A. L., Cavacini, L. A., Posner, M. R., Katinger, H., *et al.* (2001). Protection of neonatal macaques against experimental SHIV infection by human neutralizing monoclonal antibodies. *Transfus. Clin. Biol.* **8**, 350–358.

Ryu, S.-E., Kwong, P. D., Truneh, A., Porter, T. G., Arthos, J., Rosenberg, M., Dai, X., Xuong, N., Axel, R., Sweet, R. W., and Hendrickson, W. A. (1990). Crystal structure of an HIV-binding recombinant fragment of human CD4. *Nature* **348**, 419–426.

Sanders, R. W., Venturi, M., Schiffner, L., Kalyanaraman, R., Katinger, H., Lloyd, K. O., Kwong, P. D., and Moore, J. P. (2002). The mannose-dependent epitope for neutralizing antibody 2G12 on human immunodeficiency virus type 1 glycoprotein gp120. *J. Virol.* **76**, 7293–7305.

Saphire, E. O., Parren, P. W., Pantophlet, R., Zwick, M. B., Morris, G. M., Rudd, P. M., Dwek, R. A., Stanfield, R. L., Burton, D. R., and Wilson, I. A. (2001). Crystal structure of a neutralizing human IGG against HIV-1: A template for vaccine design. *Science* **293**, 1155–1159.

Scanlan, C. N., Pantophlet, R., Wormald, M. R., Ollmann, S. E., Stanfield, R., Wilson, I. A., Katinger, H., Dwek, R. A., Rudd, P. M., and Burton, D. R. (2002). The broadly neutralizing anti-human immunodeficiency virus type 1 antibody 2G12 recognizes a cluster of alpha1-->2 mannose residues on the outer face of gp120. *J. Virol.* **76**, 7306–7321.

Scarlatti, G., Leitner, T., Hodara, V., Jansson, M., Karlsson, A., Wahlberg, J., Rossi, P., Uhlen, M., Fenyo, E. M., and Albert, J. (1996). Interplay of HIV-1 phenotype and neutralizing antibody response in pathogenesis of AIDS. *Immunol. Lett.* **51**, 23–28.

Selvarajah, S., Puffer, B., Pantophlet, R., Law, M., Doms, R. W., and Burton, D. R. (2005). Comparing antigenicity and immunogenicity of engineered gp120. *J. Virol.* **79**, 12148–12163.

Sharma, V. A., Kan, E., Sun, Y., Lian, Y., Cisto, J., Frasca, V., Hilt, S., Stamatatos, L., Donnelly, J. J., Ulmer, J. B., Barnett, S. W., and Srivastava, I. K. (2006). Structural characteristics correlate with immune responses induced by HIV envelope glycoprotein vaccines. *Virology.* **352**, 131–144.

Sharron, M., Pohlmann, S., Price, K., Lolis, E., Tsang, M., Kirchhoff, F., Doms, R. W., and Lee, B. (2000). Expression and coreceptor activity of STRL33/Bonzo on primary peripheral blood lymphocytes. *Blood* **96**, 41–49.

Shibata, R., Igarashi, T., Haigwood, N., Buckler-White, A., Ogert, R., Ross, W., Willey, R., Cho, M. W., and Martin, M. A. (1999). Neutralizing antibody directed against the HIV-1 envelope glycoprotein can completely block HIV-1/SIV chimeric virus infections of macaque monkeys. *Nat. Med.* **5**, 204–210.

Simon, F., Mauclere, P., Roques, P., Loussert-Ajaka, I., Muller-Trutwin, M. C., Saragosti, S., Georges-Courbot, M. C., Barre-Sinoussi, F., and Brun-Vezinet, F. (1998). Identification of a new human immunodeficiency virus type 1 distinct from group M and group O. *Nat. Med.* **4**, 1032–1037.

Singh, M., Jeang, K. T., and Smith, S. M. (2005). HIV vaccine development. *Front. Biosci.* **10**, 2064–2081.

Sloane, A. J., Raso, V., Dimitrov, D. S., Xiao, X., Deo, S., Muljadi, N., Restuccia, D., Turville, S., Kearney, C., Broder, C. C., Zoellner, H., Cunningham, A. L., *et al.* (2005). Marked structural and functional heterogeneity in CXCR4: Separation of HIV-1 and SDF-1alpha responses. *Immunol. Cell Biol.* **83**, 129–143.

Slobod, K. S., Bonsignori, M., Brown, S. A., Zhan, X., Stambas, J., and Hurwitz, J. L. (2005). HIV vaccines: Brief review and discussion of future directions. *Expert Rev. Vaccines* **4**, 305–313.

Smith, A. E., and Helenius, A. (2004). How viruses enter animal cells. *Science* **304**, 237–242.

Sodroski, J. G. (1999). HIV-1 entry inhibitors in the side pocket. *Cell* **99**, 243–246.

Spearman, P. (2006). Current progress in the development of HIV vaccines. *Curr. Pharm. Des.* **12**, 1147–1167.

Srivastava, I. K., Stamatatos, L., Legg, H., Kan, E., Fong, A., Coates, S. R., Leung, L., Wininger, M., Donnelly, J. J., Ulmer, J. B., and Barnett, S. W. (2002). Purification and characterization of oligomeric envelope glycoprotein from a primary R5 subtype B human immunodeficiency virus. *J. Virol.* **76**, 2835–2847.

Srivastava, I. K., Ulmer, J. B., and Barnett, S. W. (2004). Neutralizing antibody responses to HIV: Role in protective immunity and challenges for vaccine design. *Expert Rev. Vaccines* **3**, S33–S52.

Stanley, J., Cooper, S. J., and Griffin, D. E. (1986). Monoclonal antibody cure and prophylaxis of lethal Sindbis virus encephalitis in mice. *J. Virol.* **58**, 107–115.

Starcich, B. R., Hahn, B. H., Shaw, G. M., McNeely, P. D., Modrow, S., Wolf, H., Parks, E. S., Parks, W. P., Josephs, S. F., Gallo, R. C., *et al.* (1986). Identification and characterization of conserved and variable regions in the envelope gene of HTLV-III/LAV, the retrovirus of AIDS. *Cell* **45**, 637–648.

Staudinger, R., Phogat, S. K., Xiao, X., Wang, X., Dimitrov, D. S., and Zolla-Pazner, S. (2003). Evidence for CD4-enchanced signaling through the chemokine receptor CCR5. *J. Biol. Chem.* **278**, 10389–10392.

Stiegler, G., Kunert, R., Purtscher, M., Wolbank, S., Voglauer, R., Steindl, F., and Katinger, H. (2001). A potent cross-clade neutralizing human monoclonal antibody against a novel epitope on gp41 of human immunodeficiency virus type 1. *AIDS Res. Hum. Retroviruses* **17**, 1757–1765.

Subramaniam, S. (2006). The SIV surface spike imaged by electron tomography: One leg or three? *PLoS Pathog.* **2**(8), e91.

Suzuki, S., Miyagi, T., Chuang, L. F., Yau, P. M., Doi, R. H., and Chuang, R. Y. (2002). Chemokine receptor CCR5: Polymorphism at protein level. *Biochem. Biophys. Res. Commun.* **296**, 477–483.

Tian, S., Choi, W. T., Liu, D., Pesavento, J., Wang, Y., An, J., Sodroski, J. G., and Huang, Z. (2005). Distinct functional sites for human immunodeficiency virus type 1 and stromal cell-derived factor 1alpha on CXCR4 transmembrane helical domains. *J. Virol.* **79**, 12667–12673.

Trkola, A., Dragic, T., Arthos, J., Binley, J. M., Olson, W. C., Allaway, G. P., Cheng-Mayer, C., Robinson, J., Maddon, P. J., and Moore, J. P. (1996a). CD4-dependent, antibody-sensitive interactions between HIV-1 and its co-receptor CCR-5. *Nature* **384**, 184–187.

Trkola, A., Purtscher, M., Muster, T., Ballaun, C., Buchacher, A., Sullivan, N., Srinivasan, K., Sodroski, J., Moore, J. P., and Katinger, H. (1996b). Human monoclonal antibody 2G12 defines a distinctive neutralization epitope on the gp120 glycoprotein of human immunodeficiency virus type 1. *J. Virol.* **70**, 1100–1108.

Tuen, M., Visciano, M. L., Chien, P. C., Jr., Cohen, S., Chen, P. D., Robinson, J., He, Y., Pinter, A., Gorny, M. K., and Hioe, C. E. (2005). Characterization of antibodies that inhibit HIV gp120 antigen processing and presentation. *Eur. J. Immunol.* **35**, 2541–2551.

Van Rompay, K. K., Berardi, C. J., Dillard, T., Tarara, R. P., Canfield, D. R., Valverde, C. R., Montefiori, D. C., Cole, K. S., Montelaro, R. C., and Miller, C. J. (1998). Passive immunization of newborn rhesus macaques prevents oral simian immunodeficiency virus infection. *J. Infect. Dis.* **177**, 1247–1259.

Varadarajan, R., Sharma, D., Chakraborty, K., Patel, M., Citron, M., Sinha, P., Yadav, R., Rashid, U., Kennedy, S., Eckert, D., Geleziunas, R., Bramhill, D., *et al.* (2005). Characterization of gp120 and its single-chain derivatives, gp120-CD4D12 and gp120-M9: Implications for targeting the CD4i epitope in human immunodeficiency virus vaccine design. *J. Virol.* **79**, 1713–1723.

Vita, C., Drakopoulou, E., Vizzavona, J., Rochette, S., Martin, L., Menez, A., Roumestand, C., Yang, Y. S., Ylisastigui, L., Benjouad, A., and Gluckman, J. C. (1999a). Rational engineering of a miniprotein that reproduces the core of the CD4 site interacting with HIV-1 envelope glycoprotein. *Proc. Natl. Acad. Sci. USA* **96**, 13091–13096.

Vita, C., Drakopoulou, E., Vizzavona, J., Rochette, S., Martin, L., Menez, A., Roumestand, C., Yang, Y. S., Ylisastigui, L., Benjouad, A., and Gluckman, J. C. (1999b). Rational engineering of a miniprotein that reproduces the core of the CD4 site interacting with HIV-1 envelope glycoprotein. *Proc. Natl. Acad. Sci. USA* **96**, 13091–13096.

Vujcic, L. K., and Quinnan, G. V., Jr. (1995). Preparation and characterization of human HIV type 1 neutralizing reference sera. *AIDS Res. Hum. Retroviruses* 11, 783–787.

Wang, J., Yan, Y., Garrett, T. P. J., Liu, J., Rodgers, D. W., Garlick, R. L., Tarr, G. E., Husain, Y., Reinherz, E. L., and Harrison, S. C. (1990). Atomic structure of a fragment of human CD4 containing two immunoglobulin-like domains. *Nature* 348, 411–418.

Wang, L. X. (2006). Toward oligosaccharide- and glycopeptide-based HIV vaccines. *Curr. Opin. Drug Discov. Devel.* 9, 194–206.

Watkins, B. A., Reitz, M. S., Jr., Wilson, C. A., Aldrich, K., Davis, A. E., and Robert-Guroff, M. (1993). Immune escape by human immunodeficiency virus type 1 from neutralizing antibodies: Evidence for multiple pathways. *J. Virol.* 67, 7493–7500.

Wei, X., Decker, J. M., Wang, S., Hui, H., Kappes, J. C., Wu, X., Salazar-Gonzalez, J. F., Salazar, M. G., Kilby, J. M., Saag, M. S., Komarova, N. L., Nowak, M. A., *et al.* (2003). Antibody neutralization and escape by HIV-1. *Nature* 422, 307–312.

Weiss, C. D. (2003). HIV-1 gp41: Mediator of fusion and target for inhibition. *AIDS Rev.* 5, 214–221.

Weissenhorn, W., Dessen, A., Harrison, S. C., Skehel, J. J., and Wiley, D. C. (1997). Atomic structure of the ectodomain from HIV-1 gp41. *Nature* 387, 426–430.

Wilkinson, R. A., Piscitelli, C., Teintze, M., Cavacini, L. A., Posner, M. R., and Lawrence, C. M. (2005). Structure of the Fab fragment of F105, a broadly reactive anti-human immunodeficiency virus (HIV) antibody that recognizes the CD4 binding site of HIV type 1 gp120. *J. Virol.* 79, 13060–13069.

Williams, A. F., Galfre, G., and Milstein, C. (1977). Analysis of cell surfaces by xenogeneic myeloma-hybrid antibodies: Differentiation antigens of rat lymphocytes. *Cell* 12, 663–673.

Wu, H., Kwong, P. D., and Hendrickson, W. A. (1997). Dimeric association and segmental variability in the structure of human CD4. *Nature* 387, 527–530.

Wu, L. J., Gerard, N. P., Wyatt, R., Choe, H., Parolin, C., Ruffing, N., Borsetti, A., Cardoso, A. A., Desjardin, E., Newman, W., Gerard, C., and Sodroski, J. (1996). CD4-induced interaction of primary HIV-1 gp120 glycoproteins with the chemokine receptor CCR-5. *Nature* 384, 179–183.

Wyatt, R., and Sodroski, J. (1998). The HIV-1 envelope glycoproteins: Fusogens, antigens, and immunogens. *Science* 280, 1884–1888.

Wyatt, R., Moore, J., Accola, M., Desjardin, E., Robinson, J., and Sodroski, J. (1995). Involvement of the V1/V2 variable loop structure in the exposure of human immunodeficiency virus type 1 gp120 epitopes induced by receptor binding. *J. Virol.* 69, 5723–5733.

Xiang, S. H., Doka, N., Choudhary, R. K., Sodroski, J., and Robinson, J. E. (2002a). Characterization of CD4-induced epitopes on the HIV type 1 gp120 envelope glycoprotein recognized by neutralizing human monoclonal antibodies. *AIDS Res. Hum. Retroviruses* 18, 1207–1217.

Xiang, S. H., Kwong, P. D., Gupta, R., Rizzuto, C. D., Casper, D. J., Wyatt, R., Wang, L., Hendrickson, W. A., Doyle, M. L., and Sodroski, J. (2002b). Mutagenic stabilization and/or disruption of a CD4-bound state reveals distinct conformations of the human immunodeficiency virus type 1 gp120 envelope glycoprotein. *J. Virol.* 76, 9888–9899.

Xiao, X., Wu, L., Stantchev, T. S., Feng, Y. R., Ugolini, S., Chen, H., Shen, Z., Riley, J. L., Broder, C. C., Sattentau, Q. J., and Dimitrov, D. S. (1999). Constitutive cell surface association between CD4 and CCR5. *Proc. Natl. Acad. Sci. USA* 96, 7496–7501.

Yang, X., Farzan, M., Wyatt, R., and Sodroski, J. (2000). Characterization of stable, soluble trimers containing complete ectodomains of human immunodeficiency virus type 1 envelope glycoproteins. *J. Virol.* 74, 5716–5725.

Yang, X., Lee, J., Mahony, E. M., Kwong, P. D., Wyatt, R., and Sodroski, J. (2002). Highly stable trimers formed by human immunodeficiency virus type 1 envelope glycoproteins fused with the trimeric motif of T4 bacteriophage fibritin. *J. Virol.* **76**, 4634–4642.

Yang, X., Tomov, V., Kurteva, S., Wang, L., Ren, X., Gorny, M. K., Zolla-Pazner, S., and Sodroski, J. (2004). Characterization of the outer domain of the gp120 glycoprotein from human immunodeficiency virus type 1. *J. Virol.* **78**, 12975–12986.

Zanetti, G, Briggs, J. A., Grunewald, K., Sattentau, Q. J., and Fuller, S. D. (2006). Cryo-Electron Tomographic Structure of an Immunodeficiency Virus Envelope Complex *in situ*. *PLoS Pathog.* **2**(8), e83.

Zhang, C. W., Chishti, Y., Hussey, R. E., and Reinherz, E. L. (2001). Expression, purification, and characterization of recombinant HIV gp140. The gp41 ectodomain of HIV or simian immunodeficiency virus is sufficient to maintain the retroviral envelope glycoprotein as a trimer. *J. Biol. Chem.* **276**, 39577–39585.

Zhang, L., Ribeiro, R. M., Mascola, J. R., Lewis, M. G., Stiegler, G., Katinger, H., Perelson, A. S., and Davenport, M. P. (2004a). Effects of antibody on viral kinetics in simian/human immunodeficiency virus infection: Implications for vaccination. *J. Virol.* **78**, 5520–5522.

Zhang, M. Y., and Dimitrov, D. S. (2007). Novel approaches for identification of broadly cross-reactive HIV-1 neutralizing human monoclonal antibodies and improvement of their potency. *Curr. Pharm. Des.* **13**, 203–212.

Zhang, M. Y., Shu, Y., Phogat, S., Xiao, X., Cham, F., Bouma, P., Choudhary, A., Feng, Y. R., Sanz, I., Rybak, S., Broder, C. C., Quinnan, G. V., et al. (2003). Broadly cross-reactive HIV neutralizing human monoclonal antibody Fab selected by sequential antigen panning of a phage display library. *J. Immunol. Methods* **283**, 17–25.

Zhang, M. Y., Xiao, X., Sidorov, I. A., Choudhry, V., Cham, F., Zhang, P. F., Bouma, P., Zwick, M., Choudhary, A., Montefiori, D. C., Broder, C. C., Burton, D. R., et al. (2004b). Identification and characterization of a new cross-reactive human immunodeficiency virus type 1-neutralizing human monoclonal antibody. *J. Virol.* **78**, 9233–9242.

Zhang, M. Y., Choudhry, V., Sidorov, I. A., Tenev, V., Vu, B. K., Choudhary, A., Lu, H., Stiegler, G. M., Katinger, H. W. D., Jiang, S., Broder, C. C., and Dimitrov, D. S. (2006). Selection of a novel gp41-specific HIV-1 neutralizing human antibody by competitive antigen panning. *J. Immunol. Methods* **317**, 21–30.

Zhang, P. F., Bouma, P., Park, E. J., Margolick, J. B., Robinson, J. E., Zolla-Pazner, S., Flora, M. N., and Quinnan, G. V., Jr. (2002). A variable region 3 (V3) mutation determines a global neutralization phenotype and CD4-independent infectivity of a human immunodeficiency virus type 1 envelope associated with a broadly cross-reactive, primary virus-neutralizing antibody response. *J. Virol.* **76**, 644–655.

Zhang, W., Canziani, G., Plugariu, C., Wyatt, R., Sodroski, J., Sweet, R., Kwong, P., Hendrickson, W., and Chaiken, I. (1999). Conformational changes of gp120 in epitopes near the CCR5 binding site are induced by CD4 and a CD4 miniprotein mimetic. *Biochemistry* **38**, 9405–9416.

Zhang, Y. J., Fracasso, C., Fiore, J. R., Bjorndal, A., Angarano, G., Gringeri, A., and Fenyo, E. M. (1997). Augmented serum neutralizing activity against primary human immunodeficiency virus type 1 (HIV-1) isolates in two groups of HIV-1-infected long-term nonprogressors. *J. Infect. Dis.* **176**, 1180–1187.

Zhou, T., Xu, L., Dey, B., Hessel, A. J., Van Ryk, D., Xiang, S. H., Yang, X., Zhang, M. Y., Zwick, M. B., Arthos, J., Burton, D. R., Dimitrov, D. S., et al. (2007). Structural definition of a conserved neutralization epitope on HIV-1 gp120. *Nature* **445**, 732–737.

Zhu, P., Chertova, E., Bess, J., Jr., Lifson, J. D., Arthur, L. O., Liu, J., Taylor, K. A., and Roux, K. H. (2003). Electron tomography analysis of envelope glycoprotein trimers on HIV and simian immunodeficiency virus virions. *Proc. Natl. Acad. Sci. USA* **100**, 15812–15817.

Zhu, P., Liu, J., Bess, J., Jr., Chertova, E., Lifson, J. D., Grise, H., Ofek, G. A., Taylor, K. A., and Roux, K. H. (2006). Distribution and three-dimensional structure of AIDS virus envelope spikes. *Nature* **441**, 847–852.

Zolla-Pazner, S. (2004). Identifying epitopes of HIV-1 that induce protective antibodies. *Nat. Rev. Immunol.* **4**, 199–210.

Zwick, M. B. (2005). The membrane-proximal external region of HIV-1 gp41: A vaccine target worth exploring. *AIDS* **19**, 1725–1737.

Zwick, M. B., Labrijn, A. F., Wang, M., Spenlehauer, C., Saphire, E. O., Binley, J. M., Moore, J. P., Stiegler, G., Katinger, H., Burton, D. R., and Parren, P. W. (2001). Broadly neutralizing antibodies targeted to the membrane-proximal external region of human immunodeficiency virus type 1 glycoprotein gp41. *J. Virol.* **75**, 10892–10905.

Zwick, M. B., Parren, P. W., Saphire, E. O., Church, S., Wang, M., Scott, J. K., Dawson, P. E., Wilson, I. A., and Burton, D. R. (2003). Molecular features of the broadly neutralizing immunoglobulin G1 b12 required for recognition of human immunodeficiency virus type 1 gp120. *J. Virol.* **77**, 5863–5876.

Truus E. M. Abbink and Ben Berkhout

Laboratory of Experimental Virology, Department of Medical Microbiology
Center for Infection and Immunity Amsterdam (CINIMA)
Academic Medical Center of the University of Amsterdam
Meibergdreef 15, 1105 AZ Amsterdam, The Netherlands

HIV-1 Reverse Transcription: Close Encounters Between the Viral Genome and a Cellular tRNA

I. Chapter Overview

Retroviruses differ from other positive-stranded RNA viruses in the process of reverse transcription. This process is an essential step in the viral life cycle as it converts the retroviral genomic RNA into a proviral DNA in a complex, multistep process. In this chapter, we describe in detail the initiation step of reverse transcription. During this step a cellular tRNA primer is placed onto a complementary sequence in the viral genome called the primer-binding site or PBS. The viral enzyme reverse transcriptase (RT)

Advances in Pharmacology, Volume 55
1054-3589/07 $35.00
DOI: 10.1016/S1054-3589(07)55003-9

recognizes this RNA–RNA complex and catalyzes the extension of the 3′ end of the tRNA primer, with the viral RNA (vRNA) acting as template. This initiation step is regulated and most retroviruses are restricted to the use of the cognate, self-tRNA primer. Many years ago, we tried to force *Human immunodeficiency virus type 1* (HIV-1) to use a nonself-tRNA primer by alteration of the PBS. We reasoned that this approach would reveal additional important determinants of primer specificity. Initial attempts failed in our and several other laboratories. Recent insight into additional contacts between the tRNA and the vRNA genome led us to a renewed attempt to change HIV-1 primer specificity. We obtained a replicating HIV-1 variant that uses a nonself tRNA primer. Analysis of this variant confirms the role of multiple determinants of tRNA primer usage.

II. Introduction

In this chapter, we will focus on the initiation step of reverse transcription as performed by HIV-1. In this highly organized process, the cellular tRNA^{Lys3} molecule acts as primer (Fig. 1, indicated by a green frame). No spontaneous switches in tRNA usage by HIV-1 or other retroviruses have been described and attempts to change the identity of the tRNA primer were unsuccessful in the past. These observations indicate that the virus strongly prefers the self-primer, suggesting that a very specific mechanism for primer selection must exist. Indeed, tRNA primers are selectively packaged into virus particles, specifically recognized by the viral RT enzyme, and placed onto the vRNA genome via base pairing to the PBS, thus rendering a specific initiation complex. This chapter will focus primarily on the interaction between the cellular tRNA primer and the vRNA genome. Other aspects that determine primer specificity will be presented more generally. Novel findings have provided new insight into the multiple interactions between the tRNA primer and the vRNA genome. These results have triggered a renewed attempt to change the tRNA usage of HIV-1, thus providing a means to study determinants that specify tRNA usage in more depth. Our results support the model of tRNA primer activation by a vRNA motif. We will specifically discuss the research in our laboratory that led to the identification of this primer activation signal (PAS), which allowed us to successfully switch the tRNA usage of HIV-1.

III. Reverse Transcription

Reverse transcription is the replication step that converts an RNA genome into a proviral DNA copy, a mechanism that is shared by retroviruses, retrotransposons, and hepadnaviruses. The process of reverse transcription is composed of several steps (an overview is presented in Fig. 1).

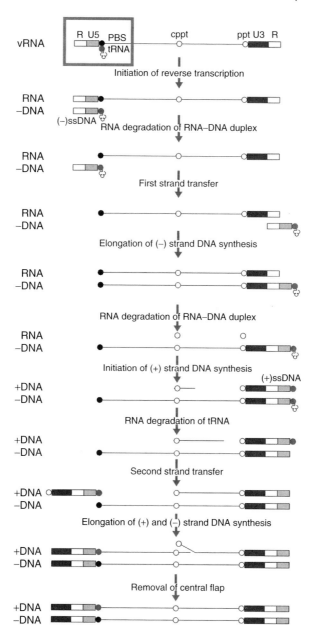

FIGURE I   Mechanism of HIV-1 reverse transcription. The RNA genome contains terminal repeats (5' R and 3' R) that are critical in reverse transcription reaction. The 5' R is followed by the unique U5 element, which is located immediately upstream of the PBS and contains several sequence motifs that regulate reverse transcription. The tRNA^{Lys3} sequence that is complementary to the PBS in the viral genome is indicated by a gray circle with a tRNA loop. This sequence is copied during reverse transcription. The PBS of the viral progeny is thus encoded by the cellular primer and is therefore also marked by a gray circle. The chapter will focus on the initiation step of reverse transcription, indicated by a box at the top left.

The template is the vRNA genome that is flanked by repeat (R) sequences at the 5'- and 3'-termini. The enzymatic reaction is catalyzed by the virion-associated RT (encoded by the *pol* gene, Fig. 2). RT is synthesized as part of the Gag-Pol precursor protein, which is cleaved by the virally encoded protease (PR) into the structural proteins and the replication enzymes RT, PR, and integrase (IN). Processing of the precursor proteins occurs at or

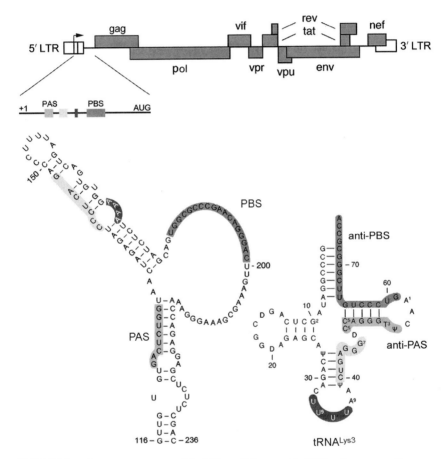

FIGURE 2   The HIV-1 genome and the PBS motif that specify tRNA primer usage. Shown on top is the HIV-1 DNA genome. The 5' LTR is divided in three segments (U3, R, and U5). Transcription starts at the U3-R border (arrow). A close-up of the untranslated leader of the vRNA is shown (from the transcription start site +1 to the gag start codon AUG). Motifs involved in reverse transcription are color-coded and similarly marked in the secondary structure model shown at the bottom. The cloverleaf structure of the tRNA^{Lys3} molecule is also shown. Base modifications in the tRNA molecules are indicated according to standard nomenclature (Sprinzl *et al.*, 1998). Several base-pairing interactions between the primer and the leader have been proposed (color-coded, see text for further details). (See Color Insert.)

soon after the time of virus assembly and budding. Retroviral particles are able to initiate reverse transcription shortly after budding (Arts *et al.*, 1994; Huang *et al.*, 1997; Lori *et al.*, 1992; Oude Essink *et al.*, 1996; Trono, 1992). This suggests that initiation of reverse transcription is restricted until the virus particle has been assembled. The mechanism responsible for this restriction is unknown, but sequence motifs and structures in the viral template have been implicated, as well as low dNTP concentrations inside virus particles (Beerens and Berkhout, 2002a; Beerens *et al.*, 2000b, 2001; Cobrinik *et al.*, 1988, 1991; Cordell *et al.*, 1979; Isel *et al.*, 1995; Liang *et al.*, 1997b).

HIV-1 RT functions as a heterodimer of a 66- and 51-kDa subunit. The first is composed of an RT polymerase domain and an RNaseH domain, and the latter contains only the polymerase domain (Goff, 1990). The p51 subunit results from cleavage of p66 by PR (Di Marzo Veronese *et al.*, 1986; Lightfoote *et al.*, 1986). The polymerization activity has been attributed to the p66 component of the heterodimer (Richter-Cook *et al.*, 1992). As with all DNA polymerases, RT needs a primer with a free 3′-OH group to initiate cDNA synthesis. Although a variety of primer molecules can be used to initiate reverse transcription *in vitro*, all retroviruses use a cellular tRNA molecule (Harada *et al.*, 1975, 1979; Leis *et al.*, 1993; Litvak and Araya, 1982; Mak and Kleiman, 1997; Marquet *et al.*, 1995; Telesnitsky and Goff, 1997). DNA sequence analysis of the proviral genome implicated tRNA^{Lys3} (Fig. 1) as the replication primer for HIV-1 and HIV-2 (Guyader *et al.*, 1987; Wain-Hobson *et al.*, 1985).

A prerequisite for reverse transcription initiation is the formation of a properly folded initiation complex of the viral genome and the tRNA. The 3′-terminal 18 nucleotides (nts) of the tRNA primer base pair with the complementary PBS (position +182 to +199 in Fig. 2) in the viral genome, and the 3′-OH of the tRNA serves to prime template–dependent DNA synthesis (Goff, 1990). The PBS is located close to the 5′ end of the RNA genome in the untranslated leader region (Fig. 2, indicated in green). The tRNA sequence that anneals to the PBS is referred to as anti-PBS (Fig. 1, indicated in green). On annealing, the primer is extended and a cDNA of the 5′ R is synthesized by RT (Fig. 1). This intermediate is termed the minus-strand strong-stop DNA or (−)ssDNA. The RNaseH domain of RT degrades the RNA template that remained annealed to the (−)ssDNA product. Consequently, the (−)ssDNA is released and anneals to the 3′ R region located at the 3′ end of the genome. This step is referred to as the first strand-transfer reaction.

The (−)ssDNA subsequently serves as primer for (−)DNA synthesis. Reverse transcription proceeds and generates a full-length (−)strand cDNA that serves as a template for (+)strand DNA synthesis. RNaseH degrades the RNA template, except for two fragments that resist cleavage: polypurine tracts in the U3 region (3′-PPT) and the center of the template (central PPT, cPPT). The resistant RNA sequences prime (+)strand DNA synthesis, which stops at the first modified base in the tRNA^{Lys3} molecule (Auxilien *et al.*, 1999; Ben Artzi *et al.*, 1996). Thus, the copied 3′-terminal 18 nts of the tRNA end up in the viral progeny, a unique phenomenon in virology (indicated by a red circle in Fig. 1). The tRNA primer is subsequently removed from the (+)ssDNA by RNaseH. A second strand-transfer reaction results in the annealing of (+)ssDNA to the 3′ end of the full-length (−)strand DNA. Reverse transcription proceeds over the (−)strand DNA until it encounters the cPPT-extended (+)strand. Elongation occurs through the cPPT via a mechanism called strand displacement until RT reaches a nearby site (80–100 nts downstream): the central termination sequence. This motif is extremely efficient in terminating HIV-1 RT-catalyzed DNA elongation. Consequently, a double-stranded proviral DNA product is synthesized that is flanked by two long terminal repeats (LTRs) and that contains a discontinuous (+)strand DNA with an ~99-nt DNA flap at its center. This flap sequence is specific for lentiviruses and is important for nuclear import and consequently viral replication in nondividing cells (Charneau *et al.*, 1992, 1994; Hungnes *et al.*, 1992). A cellular endonuclease removes the flap and a DNA ligase completes the continuous double strand (Rumbaugh *et al.*, 1998). The proviral DNA is eventually integrated into the host cell genome by the viral IN protein.

There is one special occasion in which HIV-1 uses a diversity of tRNA molecules as restart primers of reverse transcription. When an excessively stable hairpin structure is introduced in the vRNA genome, virus replication is blocked. Revertants can be selected that delete most of the hairpin structure by a recombination event that uses a variety of tRNA molecules to restart reverse transcription behind the hairpin structure. This mechanism was termed hairpin-induced tRNA-mediated (HITME) recombination (Konstantinova *et al.*, 2006).

IV. Specificity of tRNA Primer Usage

Retroviruses utilize different tRNA primers (Mak and Kleiman, 1997). Avian retroviruses utilize tRNA^{Trp}, whereas the majority of mammalian retroviruses utilize tRNA^{Pro} (e.g., human T-cell leukemia viruses types 1 and 2 and murine leukemia viruses). However, the *Mouse mammary tumor virus* and all lentiviruses, including HIV-1 and HIV-2, utilize tRNA^{Lys3}, whereas tRNA^{Lys1,2} is used by *Mason-Pfizer monkey virus*, *Visna/Maedi virus*, and spumaviruses. Although a variety of primer molecules can be used to initiate reverse transcription, all retroviruses are dedicated to the self-tRNA primer despite an excess of other tRNA molecules in the infected cell (Das *et al.*, 1995; Li *et al.*, 1994; Wakefield *et al.*, 1995). No spontaneous mutations or more gross tRNA switches have been reported. A single point mutation that is recurrently observed at a low incidence in the HIV-1 PBS results from the infrequent usage of a low abundant tRNA^{Lys5} variant (Das et al., 1997, 2005). Primer specificity is however less stringent for murine leukemia viruses compared to other retroviruses (Colicelli and Goff, 1986; Lund et al., 1993; Schwartzberg et al., 1985). Specificity of primer tRNA usage by HIV-1 is imposed at several levels. These mechanisms will be discussed in more detail: selective packaging of tRNA primers into virus particles (Section III.A), specific recognition of the tRNA–vRNA complex by the RT protein (Section III.B), and specific interactions between the tRNA and the viral genome (Section III.C).

A. A tRNA Subset Is Selectively Packaged into HIV-1 Particles

The tRNA primer is selectively packaged into virus particles, resulting in an increased concentration inside the virion compared to the cytoplasm (Jiang et al., 1992, 1993; Mak et al., 1994; Waters and Mullin, 1977). Virus particles without an RNA genome still incorporate the wild-type (wt) set of tRNAs, indicating that the viral genome and interactions between tRNA and vRNA are dispensable in this process (Mak et al., 1994). The RT enzyme, or its precursor Gag-Pol, was initially shown to be involved in selective packaging of the tRNA primers. Selective packaging of tRNAs was affected in virions lacking a functional RT domain (Levin and Seidman, 1981; Mak et al., 1994; Peters and Hu, 1980). For instance, HIV-1 virus-like particles exclusively composed of Gag precursors did not contain wt tRNA levels (Mak et al., 1994). In contrast, PR-deficient virions composed of Gag and Gag-Pol precursor did contain a wt tRNA content, demonstrating the requirement for the Pol region. Apparently, processing of the structural precursor proteins is not required for correct tRNA packaging (Mak et al., 1994). Further investigations revealed that the centrally located thumb domain of RT is indispensable for tRNA^{Lys} incorporation into virus particles (Khorchid et al., 2000).

All tRNA^{Lys} isoacceptors are enriched in HIV-1 virions when compared to other tRNAs. The ratio of tRNA^{Lys3} versus tRNA^{Lys1,2} is the same in cells and virions, with ~8 and 12 molecules, respectively, per particle (Huang et al., 1994). One should keep in mind that tRNAs likely form complexes with proteins in the cytoplasm, such as translation elongation factors or tRNA synthetases, enzymes that carry out tRNA aminoacylation. tRNA^{Lys} molecules are packaged during particle assembly via their interaction with the Gag-Pol precursor and a protein complex composed of the cellular lysyl-tRNA synthetase (LysRS) and the viral Gag protein (Cen et al., 2002; Javanbakht et al., 2003; Jiang et al., 1994; Khorchid et al., 2000; Mak et al., 1994). LysRS engages a specific interaction with the anticodon loop of tRNA^{Lys} isoacceptors on which aminoacylation takes place (Cusack et al., 1996) and this protein has been identified in virus particles (Cen et al., 2001).

The aminoacylation activity of LysRS is not required for tRNA or LysRS incorporation into virions (Cen *et al.*, 2004a). Mutations in the tRNA anticodon loop prohibit tRNA packaging into virus particles, establishing that binding to LysRS is a major determinant for tRNA packaging (Javanbakht *et al.*, 2002). Selective LysRS packaging is observed in virus-like particles exclusively composed of Gag and therefore does not depend on the presence of the Gag-Pol precursor or the tRNA molecule (Cen *et al.*, 2001). LysRS binds tRNA with its N-terminal extension and anticodon-binding domain, whereas it binds Gag with a central motif (Javanbakht *et al.*, 2003). The interacting domains in Gag and LysRS are also involved in formation of homodimers. This homodimerization capacity is not required for the formation of the heterodimeric LysRS–Gag complex (Kovaleski *et al.*, 2006). Altering the level of intracellular LysRS by overexpression or siRNA-mediated silencing results in a concomitantly altered level of $tRNA^{Lys}$ in virus particles, suggesting that LysRS is the limiting factor for $tRNA^{Lys}$ packaging (Cen *et al.*, 2004a; Gabor *et al.*, 2002; Guo *et al.*, 2003).

The presence of other tRNA synthetases in HIV-1 virions has also been analyzed (Cen *et al.*, 2002; Halwani *et al.*, 2004). Eight synthetases (specific for $tRNA^{Lys,Ile,Pro,Trp,Arg,Gln,Met,Tyr}$) were examined, but only LysRS was detected in HIV-1 particles. Approximately 20–25 LysRS and 20 $tRNA^{Lys}$ molecules are present per virus particle, indicating an equimolar stochiometry (Cen *et al.*, 2002). Additionally, *Rous sarcoma virus* particles contain TrpRS and this virus uses $tRNA^{Trp}$ as primer for reverse transcription (Cen *et al.*, 2002; Sawyer and Dahlberg, 1973; Waters and Mullin, 1977). Interestingly, murine leukemia viruses do not package the tRNA synthetase of the priming $tRNA^{Pro}$ species, and these viruses were shown to be less selective in primer use (Colicelli and Goff, 1986; Lund *et al.*, 1993, 2000; Waters and Mullin, 1977). It remains uncertain if tRNA synthetases are packaged into retroviral particles solely because of their interaction with the structural proteins. Additional cellular proteins or cellular compartmentalization may play a role that needs to be addressed. Interestingly, $tRNA^{Lys3}$ is not acylated inside virus particles, probably to allow efficient primer extension by RT (Huang *et al.*, 1994; Rigourd *et al.*, 2003). It is currently unknown whether uncharged or charged tRNAs are incorporated, followed by spontaneous deacylation. It may be worthwhile to analyze the effect of Gag or other virion constituents on LysRS aminoacylation activity or tRNA deacylation.

B. Specific Binding of tRNA and vRNA to RT

The RT domain in Gag-Pol is not only required for selective tRNA packaging, it is also involved in placement of the tRNA primer onto the PBS (Mak *et al.*, 1994; Oude Essink *et al.*, 1995). In addition, HIV-1 RT is strongly committed to the self-$tRNA^{Lys3}$ primer for initiation of reverse transcription (Oude Essink *et al.*, 1996). *In vitro* studies demonstrated a specific interaction of the priming tRNA species with the RT protein (Barat *et al.*, 1989; Haseltine *et al.*, 1977; Oude Essink *et al.*, 1995, 1996; Sarih-Cottin *et al.*, 1992), although a nonspecific tRNA-RT interaction has been reported by others (Delahunty *et al.*, 1994; Kohlstaedt and Steitz, 1992; Sobol *et al.*, 1991). Discrepancies among these studies may be caused by differences in the tRNA source that was studied. Synthetic tRNA^{Lys3} that lacks the base modifications of its natural counterpart were shown to bind RT with reduced affinity and was easily outcompeted by a natural, nonself tRNA molecule (Barat *et al.*, 1991), although this observation is in conflict with other data (Wohrl *et al.*, 1993). Both synthetic and natural tRNA molecules can function as primer for reverse transcription *in vitro*. The overall structure of the L-shaped tRNA seems important for binding to RT, but mapping of the specific tRNA subdomain that is required for this binding has yielded conflicting data.

The connection domain of RT (which is located N-terminal of the RNaseH domain in p66 and constitutes the C-terminal domain of p51) was shown to be critical for tRNA placement on the PBS in virions (Cen *et al.*, 2004b). This observation is supported by biochemical characterization of a similar RT mutant in the Le Grice laboratory (Arts *et al.*, 1996a; Wohrl *et al.*, 1995). Deletion of the p51 C-terminus reduced the binding of heterodimeric RT to tRNA^{Lys3} considerably, whereas it did not affect the catalytic polymerase activity of the enzyme. Initiation of tRNA-mediated reverse transcription was consequently impaired, contrary to DNA- or RNA-oligonucleotide-primed reverse transcription. In addition, RNaseH activity resulted in different cleavage patterns, suggestive of a conformational change in the RT protein. The polymerase domain may be differently positioned with respect to the RNaseH domain in this mutant. This conformational change may result in a less efficient binding of tRNA^{Lys3}. Interestingly, a functional link between the RNaseH domain and tRNA binding has emerged from additional studies. Biochemical studies have provided structural information on the RT-tRNA^{Lys3} complex with an involvement of the RNaseH domain, but no high-resolution picture has emerged from these studies (Dufour *et al.*, 1999; Mishima and Steitz, 1995; Oude Essink *et al.*, 1995; Robert *et al.*, 1990; Wang *et al.*, 2006).

Annealing of the tRNA primer to the PBS requires unwinding of the tRNA acceptor and TψC stems, which occlude the anti-PBS motif. Previous experiments in our laboratory have shown that RT binding facilitates the annealing of tRNA to the PBS (Oude Essink *et al.*, 1995). The temperature at which the tRNA primer was annealed to the viral PBS could be reduced to 37 °C in the presence of RT. Other laboratories have probed the tRNA structure on binding to RT and found no evidence for tRNA melting. The viral template is possibly required for shifting the equilibrium of a closed anti-PBS motif to an open conformation. In addition, the structural nucleocapsid (NC) protein or its precursor Gag has been implicated in placement of the tRNA onto the viral genome (Barat *et al.*, 1993; De Rocquigny *et al.*, 1992; Feng *et al.*, 1999; Fu *et al.*, 1997). HIV-1 NC is a short basic protein with two zinc-finger domains and functions as a nucleic acid chaperone (Darlix *et al.*, 2002; Levin *et al.*, 2005). Like RT, NC seems to destabilize base pairing in tRNA molecules, without complete melting of the structure (Tisne *et al.*, 2001). Addition of a viral template containing a complementary PBS results in RNA–RNA complex formation and significant structural changes in both RNAs. Both basic and zinc-finger domains in NC are required for viral replication and proper annealing/reannealing of the tRNA–vRNA complex. The basic domains have been proposed to destabilize the base pairing in the four-way junction of the tRNA structure and the zinc-finger domains may disrupt tertiary interactions in the tRNA molecule (Hargittai *et al.*, 2001; Tisne *et al.*, 2001).

C. Interactions Between the tRNA Primer and the vRNA Genome

1. PBS Is a Major Determinant in the Viral Template for tRNA Usage

Although selective tRNA incorporation into virus particles and recognition by RT determine primer specificity for HIV-1 to a large extent, these are not the only factors. Viral particles contain a subset of cellular tRNAs, comprising other species than just the primer tRNA species. HIV-1 particles contain $tRNA^{Lys1,2}$ and $tRNA^{Ile}$ (Jiang *et al.*, 1993), but only the $tRNA^{Lys3}$ primer is found in tight association with the vRNA (Jiang *et al.*, 1992, 1993; Mak *et al.*, 1994). As described above, the PBS is dispensable for selective packaging of $tRNA^{Lys3}$ into virus particles, but the PBS is absolutely required for tight annealing of the $tRNA^{Lys3}$ primer (Jiang *et al.*, 1993; Liang *et al.*, 1997c). Partial or complete deletion of the PBS severely compromises viral replication due to the loss of tRNA placement on the viral genome (Das *et al.*, 1995; Liang *et al.*, 1997c). Similar results were obtained in *in vitro* reverse transcription reactions (Huthoff *et al.*, 2003).

To better understand the mechanism of reverse transcription initiation and determinants of primer specificity, we have a long-term interest in the construction of an HIV-1 variant that replicates with tRNA primers other than the natural $tRNA^{Lys3}$. We initially explored this approach by replacing the PBS by sequences that accommodate nonself tRNAs (Das *et al.*, 1995). We reasoned that the PBS is the major determinant of the viral genome for tRNA primer usage and its mutation may enforce nonself tRNA usage. We not only included primers that are used by other retroviruses ($tRNA^{Lys1,2}$, $tRNA^{Pro}$, and $tRNA^{Trp}$) but also $tRNA^{Ile}$ and $tRNA^{Phe}$. A PBS deletion mutant was constructed to serve as a negative control (PBS-), which is replication impaired (Fig. 3A). All mutant viruses showed reduced levels of

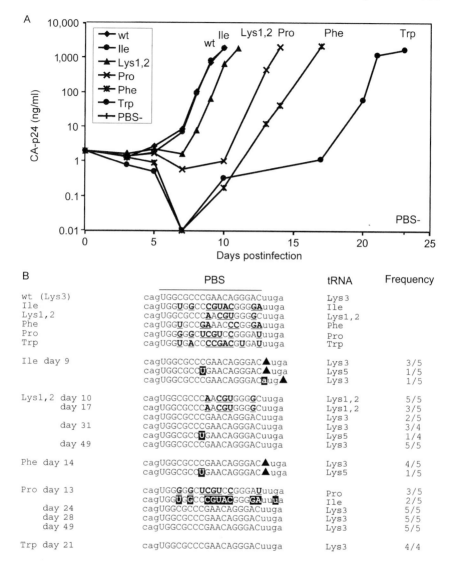

FIGURE 3   Replication and evolution of wt and PBS-mutated HIV-1 viruses. (A) The SupT1 T-cell line was infected with wt and PBS-mutated viruses. Viruses were allowed to replicate for several weeks, and virus production was measured in the culture supernatant at several time points. (B) Proviral DNA was isolated from infected cells at different days postinfection and the PBS sequence was determined. The mutated PBS motifs are shown on top, nucleotides differing from wt are in bold and underlined. The different mutants were followed longitudinally; the changes in the PBS are marked in a black box, a closed triangle represents a deletion, and the frequency within the virus culture is indicated.

viral replication (Fig. 3A). This replication defect did not result from decreased levels of virus production, indicating that the mutant virions are less infectious (Das *et al.*, 1995). The observed order of replication potential is PBS-Lys3 (wt) > PBS-Ile > PBS-Lys1,2 > PBS-Pro > PBS-Phe > PBS-Trp > PBS-. Interestingly, a PBS mutant can revert to the wt sequence in a single round of reverse transcription by annealing of the natural tRNA^{Lys3} primer onto the mutant PBS sequence. On the second strand-transfer, a duplex is formed between a copy of the tRNA^{Lys3} primer (Fig. 1, indicated with a red circle) and a copy of the viral PBS. On completion of reverse transcription, integration in the host genome, and one round of DNA replication, these strands are separated and both wt and PBS-mutated viruses are produced (Berwin and Barklis, 1993; Das *et al.*, 1994; Rhim *et al.*, 1991). Poor replication of the mutant virus will result in outgrowth of the wt virus.

We therefore determined the genotype of the viral progeny. As shown in Fig. 3B, all mutants reverted to the wt PBS-Lys3 sequence. Interestingly, some revertants contained minor sequence alterations immediately downstream of the PBS site (Fig. 3B), which result from misaligned base pairing by the (+)ssDNA on the (−)DNA during the second strand-transfer step of reverse transcription (Das *et al.*, 1995). The PBS-Lys1,2 mutant reverted to the wt PBS-Lys3 sequence relatively slowly. Possibly, HIV-1 replication proceeded more efficiently with tRNA^{Lys1,2} than with other nonself primers. Replication of the PBS-Lys1,2 mutant was indeed more efficient compared to that of the PBS-Phe and PBS-Trp mutants (rapid reversion of the PBS-Ile mutant makes it impossible to accurately assess its replication potential). In addition, we frequently observed a variant PBS-Lys sequence. This variant, with a C189U substitution in the center of the PBS motif, results from the infrequent usage of the low abundant tRNA^{Lys5} variant (Das *et al.*, 1995, 1997).

We also determined the tRNA primer that is annealed to the genomic RNA in virions. The mutant PBS sites were occupied by the corresponding nonself tRNA primers. However, tRNA annealing and extension were strongly decreased in mutant particles compared to wt particles, varying from 3% to 20% of the wt level. This tRNA-priming efficiency correlated reasonably well with the replication rate of the wt and mutant HIV-1 viruses (Das *et al.*, 1995). These results suggest that a change in PBS identity leads to reduced annealing and extension of the nonself tRNA primer, resulting in a lower rate of viral replication. We observed the highest tRNA extension for the wt and PBS-Lys1,2 viruses, suggesting a correlation between the tRNA content of virions and the mechanism of selective tRNA packaging. Overall, changing the PBS to accommodate a nonself primer is not sufficient to force HIV-1 to use a nonself tRNA primer. These results are in agreement with data obtained in other laboratories (Li *et al.*, 1994; Wakefield *et al.*, 1995). Therefore, factors other than the PBS play an important role in the preferential use of the self-tRNA^{Lys3} primer in reverse transcription.

2. Additional Interactions Between the Primer tRNA and the Viral Genome

Determinants of primer specificity other than the PBS are possibly additional contacts between the tRNA^{Lys3} molecule and the HIV-1 genome. Indeed, complementary sequences in the tRNA primer and the vRNA have been identified (Fig. 2, indicated by matching colors). For instance, U5 sequences (positions $+142$ to $+148$) were suggested to interact with the 3' part of the anticodon stem of the tRNA molecule (Fig. 2, indicated in yellow). The role of this interaction was analyzed in *in vitro* reverse transcription assays (Iwatani *et al.*, 2003; Liang *et al.*, 1998). In a previous study, we deleted this RNA sequence (mutant dL, Fig. 4). This mutant shows a threefold defect in reverse transcription *in vitro*, which confirms the results of Iwatani *et al.* (2003). However, the dL mutant virus was not significantly affected in viral replication (Beerens *et al.*, 2001). The importance of the motif in the viral life cycle therefore remains uncertain.

Another interaction between the vRNA genome and tRNA^{Lys3} was analyzed in great detail: the A-rich loop (nts $+168$ to $+171$) in U5 possibly interacts with the U-rich anticodon loop of tRNA^{Lys3} (Fig. 2, indicated in red). The A-rich loop was initially named after its location in the top of a hairpin structure (Baudin *et al.*, 1993; Berkhout, 1996; Isel *et al.*, 1993). However, more recent RNA structure probing led to an adjusted secondary structure model of the PBS domain (Fig. 2). The A-rich sequence is not presented in the terminal loop of a hairpin, but rather forms an internal loop within an extended hairpin (Abbink and Berkhout, 2003; Beerens *et al.*, 2001; Damgaard *et al.*, 2004; Goldschmidt *et al.*, 2003). This tRNA–vRNA interaction was proposed on the basis of extensive biochemical probing experiments and modeling studies (Isel *et al.*, 1995, 1998, 1999). A role for this interaction in reverse transcription was subsequently addressed (Arts *et al.*, 1996a,b; Isel *et al.*, 1995, 1998; Liang *et al.*, 1997a; Voronin and Pathak, 2004; Wakefield and Morrow, 1996; Wakefield *et al.*, 1996). Deletion of the A-rich loop affects initiation and elongation of reverse transcription (Isel *et al.*, 1996; Lanchy *et al.*, 2000; Li *et al.*, 1997c; Liang *et al.*, 1997b, 1998; Zhang *et al.*, 1998). In addition, the deletion affects virus replication, and the A-rich sequence is restored on long-term culturing and virus evolution (Liang *et al.*, 1997b). The combined data suggest that the presence of the A-rich loop enhances reverse transcription initiation, but the motif impairs synthesis of the $(-)$ssDNA due to pausing at the A-rich sequence.

The role of the A-rich loop in primer usage was also addressed by the Morrow group (Dupuy *et al.*, 2003; Kang *et al.*, 1996, 1999; Li *et al.*, 1997a,b,c; Wakefield *et al.*, 1996; Zhang *et al.*, 1996). Simultaneous adaptation of the PBS and the A-rich loop motif to nonself tRNA primers was reasoned to improve the use of nonself tRNAs in reverse transcription and

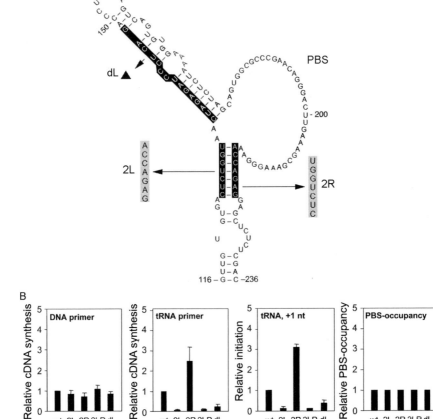

FIGURE 4   Identification of the PAS in the HIV-1 leader. (A) Leader mutants were constructed to study template requirements for tRNA-mediated reverse transcription. Mutant 2L has a 7-nt substitution in the PAS motif and 2R on the opposite site, indicated as complementary PAS (cPAS). The 2L and 2R mutations were combined in the 2LR mutant. Mutant dL has a deletion of nts 134–148. (B) Relative reverse transcription activities of wt and mutant templates. The average activity of the wt template was set at 1. Shown is DNA-primed reverse transcription with the Lys21 primer, tRNA-primed reverse transcription, and tRNA-primed 1-nt incorporation. The PBS-occupancy by the tRNA is also shown.

was examined in the viral context. Such double mutant viruses exhibit a severe replication defect. Variants that use the nonself primers tRNA[His], tRNA[Glu], and tRNA[Lys1,2] were selected on prolonged culturing, although the actual replication capacity of these mutants was recently questioned (Wei *et al.*, 2005). In recent papers from the Morrow group, viral infectivity was addressed more carefully and it appeared that the infectivity was severely hampered by simultaneous mutation of the PBS and the A-rich loop, even in the presence of the second-site reversions identified in long-term culture experiments (Moore-Rigdon *et al.*, 2005; Xu and Morrow, 2006). We previously reasoned that the genetic stability of a crippled virus is difficult to address, since the evolution capacity is determined, among other factors, by the efficiency of viral replication (Berkhout *et al.*, 1997). Consequently, it is uncertain whether the genetic stability of these mutant viruses truly reflects improved nonself tRNA usage or simply an impaired evolutionary power.

In addition, the low replication capacity of the double mutant viruses cannot be solely addressed to defects in reverse transcription initiation. Replication and also reversion analysis are complicated by the fact that the retroviral genome is densely packed with replication signals. For instance, the A-rich loop sequence is an important element for binding of the IN protein and insertion of the proviral HIV-1 DNA into the host chromosome (Esposito and Craigie, 1998). In addition, some of the designed mutants of the Morrow Laboratory harbor an AUG start codon, which likely affects the synthesis of viral proteins and thus viral replication (Das *et al.*, 1998). Finally, important RNA structure motifs other than the A-rich loop are encoded by this domain (Beerens and Berkhout, 2002a; Beerens *et al.*, 2000b, 2001). Destruction and subsequent repair of these structures may explain some of the virus reversion events (Berkhout, 1997). Second-site mutations in other regions of the viral genome that compensate for the switch in tRNA primer have been extensively searched for. However, no such coadaptive changes have been reported thus far (Kang *et al.*, 1996; Zhang *et al.*, 1996).

Unfortunately, the initial biochemical probing studies on the A-rich loop interaction were performed with the HIV-1 MAL isolate. This variant contains an unusual 23-nt duplication, comprising the 3′ part of the PBS and downstream sequences. The duplication is found in a minority of HIV-1 isolates and likely affects the folding of the vRNA template. More recently, the probing studies were repeated with other HIV-1 isolates. From these studies it appeared that the proposed tRNA–vRNA complex, including the A-rich loop interaction, is not formed by the HIV-1 HXB2 prototype (Goldschmidt *et al.*, 2004; Miller *et al.*, 2004). In addition, other members of the *Lentivirus* genus that utilize tRNA^{Lys3} as primer do not possess an A-rich loop in the region 5′ to the PBS, suggesting that the putative A-loop interaction with primer tRNA is not conserved among retroviruses and thus specific for the MAL isolate. The combined observations therefore question the proposed role for the A-rich loop in reverse transcription initiation. Recently, we discovered a novel interaction between the tRNA primer and the vRNA (Fig. 2 indicated in blue) that is conserved among retroviruses. The experiments that led to the identification of this motif and its role in reverse transcription are described in more detail below.

V. Identification of the PAS Motif _____

A. A PAS Motif Resides Upstream of the PBS

Switching tRNA primer usage proved not as simple as initially thought. The PBS is a major but not the only determinant for selective tRNA priming, and additional interactions between the primer and the viral genome are therefore likely. We set out to identify other HIV-1 RNA sequence motifs that are important for reverse transcription and performed a detailed mutational analysis of sequences flanking the PBS (Beerens *et al.*, 2001). We measured the replication capacity of the mutant viruses and analyzed reverse transcription *in vitro* with the mutant RNA templates. These experiments indicated that the U5 region contains a motif that is critical for tRNA^{Lys3}-mediated initiation of reverse transcription, but not for reactions that are initiated by a PBS-bound DNA primer. A second set of mutants was designed to map this HIV-1 RNA motif in more detail, as illustrated in Fig. 4A. More mutants were tested in the original study, but we will focus on the most informative mutants in this chapter. The central stem segment of the PBS domain was mutated by a 7-nt substitution either on the left side in mutant 2L or on the right side in mutant 2R. Mutations 2L and 2R are complementary, and base pairing will be restored in the double mutant 2LR.

We performed *in vitro* reverse transcription reactions with the wt and mutant HIV-1 RNA primed by a DNA oligonucleotide or the natural tRNA^{Lys3} molecule. The efficiency of DNA-primed reverse transcription is equal on all templates (Fig. 4B, DNA primer panel). In contrast, profound differences in cDNA synthesis were observed in tRNA-primed reactions. Mutants 2L and 2LR showed 10-fold reduced tRNA-primed reverse transcription compared with the wt template (Fig. 4B, tRNA panel), whereas mutation 2R enhanced reverse transcription 2.5-fold. These differences in tRNA-primed reverse transcription efficiency on the mutant templates could result from differences in tRNA annealing, initiation, or elongation. To study initiation of tRNA-primed reverse transcription, the reaction was performed in the presence of ^{32}P-dCTP but without the other dNTPs. This will result in the extension of the 76-nt tRNA^{Lys3} primer with 1 nt. The results of the initiation and elongation assay are similar, indicating that the inhibitory effect of 2L and 2LR and the stimulatory effect of 2R are apparent at the level of initiation (Fig. 4B, tRNA, +1nt panel).

The observed differences in initiation efficiency are not caused by different amounts of tRNA primer annealed onto the PBS. We determined the tRNA occupancy of the PBS on the wt and mutant templates. The tRNA primer was annealed onto the template, and this complex was subsequently used for extension of a DNA primer that is positioned downstream of the PBS. We used the *Avian myeloblastosis virus* RT enzyme to selectively extend the DNA primer because this enzyme is unable to extend the tRNA primer (Beerens *et al.*, 2000a; Oude Essink *et al.*, 1996). When the PBS is occupied by the tRNA primer, DNA-primed reverse transcription is blocked by the tRNA to produce a short cDNA. Free RNA templates will produce a full-length cDNA product on the wt template. All templates exclusively yield the stop product, indicating that all templates are fully occupied by the tRNA^{Lys3} primer (Fig. 4B, PBS-occupancy panel).

We refer to this novel motif as the PAS (nts +123 tot +130 of the viral genome). Inactivation of the PAS in mutant 2L inhibits reverse transcription, whereas mutation 2R stimulates initiation, possibly by making the PAS more accessible. Recently, we screened an additional set of 3' truncated HIV-1 RNA templates for reverse transcription activity. Sequences downstream of the PBS were shown to influence the level of initiation of reverse transcription, and these effects reflected RNA structural changes that modulated the accessibility of the PAS motif (Ooms *et al.*, 2007).

B. Strength of the PAS–anti-PAS Interaction Modulates Primer Activation

Mutation of the PAS motif (in 2L and 2LR) impairs virus replication (Beerens *et al.*, 2001). However, faster replicating revertant viruses of 2L were obtained. These variants contain the G127A mutation within the PAS motif. This mutation partially repairs the PAS–anti-PAS interaction, confirming that this interaction is important for virus replication. Indeed, the strength of the PAS–anti-PAS interaction modulates reverse transcription initiation. We introduced mutations in the vRNA template to strengthen or weaken the interaction with the anti-PAS motif in the tRNA^{Lys3} primer (Beerens and Berkhout, 2002b). Stabilization of the PAS–anti-PAS interaction stimulates reverse transcription initiation, whereas destabilization inhibits the reaction. These effects are caused by modulation of the strength of the PAS–anti-PAS interaction, and not by an effect on the PBS stem in the template. There seems to be an optimum in the stability of the PAS–anti-PAS interaction: reverse transcription is inhibited in case the duplex becomes too stable. An excessively stable PAS–anti-PAS interaction may interfere with the correct assembly and/or maturation of the tRNA–vRNA-RT initiation complex (Beerens *et al.*, 2001). In the same study it was tested if modified nucleotides in the tRNA molecule are important for the PAS–anti-PAS interaction. Reverse transcription primed by natural and synthetic tRNA^{Lys3} primers is similarly activated by the PAS mechanism, indicating that the PAS–anti-PAS interaction does not depend on modified nucleotides within the tRNA^{Lys3} molecule (Beerens *et al.*, 2001). Recent studies confirmed the importance of the PAS motif in viral replication and reverse transcription (Voronin and Pathak, 2004; Yuste *et al.*, 2005).

C. The PAS Motif Is Conserved Among Retroviruses

Important proof for the function of the PAS motif is its absolute conservation among all HIV-1 isolates. In fact, similar contacts between the cognate tRNA and vRNA are possible for all retrovirus genera (Beerens and Berkhout, 2002b; Freund et al., 2001; Leis et al., 1993). A similar interaction between a U5 motif in the genome of *Rous sarcoma virus* and the TΨC arm of the tRNA^{Trp} primer was previously analyzed in more detail (Aiyar et al., 1992; Cobrinik et al., 1988, 1991; Leis et al., 1993; Morris et al., 2002). The interaction stimulated initiation of reverse transcription and proved essential for virus replication. These combined results suggest that retroviral reverse transcription is activated by a common mechanism. Interestingly, M-fold analysis of other retroviral sequences indicates that the PAS is usually base paired either to the PBS or to other leader sequences, suggesting that PAS accessibility may regulate reverse transcription in the viral life cycle. Thus, the PAS–anti-PAS interaction has been conserved in evolution, despite diversity in tRNA usage among the different retroviruses. This mechanism may even be more widely conserved, since a PAS-like element was identified for the gypsy retrotransposon that uses tRNA^{Arg} as primer (Beerens and Berkhout, 2002b). These observations indicate that the process of reverse transcription is regulated by a common mechanism in all retroviridae.

VI. Proposed Mechanism of Primer Activation _____

In summary, the PAS motif is not involved in tRNA annealing, but is important for initiation of reverse transcription. These effects are observed exclusively with the natural tRNA^{Lys3} primer and not with a PBS-bound DNA or RNA primer. The PAS sequence is complementary to the TΨC arm of tRNA^{Lys3}. We propose that PAS engages in a base-pairing interaction with this anti-PAS sequence (Fig. 5). In the secondary structure model of the PBS domain, the PAS and PBS motifs are juxtaposed and the PAS sequence is occluded by base pairing. The tRNA^{Lys3} primer anneals to the viral PBS through base pairing with the anti-PBS. Consequently, the acceptor and TΨC stems of the tRNA primer are opened, thus liberating the anti-PAS motif. Next, the PAS motif in the viral template forms a second base-pairing interaction with the tRNA. This renders an RNA–RNA initiation complex that is suitable for reverse transcription. The efficiency of reverse transcription is modulated by the strength of the PAS–anti-PAS interaction. Elongation of reverse transcription will obviously disrupt the PAS–anti-PAS interaction, underlining the transient nature of this base-pairing interaction.

The presence of the PAS enhancer motif that is temporarily repressed by base pairing provides a unique mechanism for regulation of HIV-1 reverse

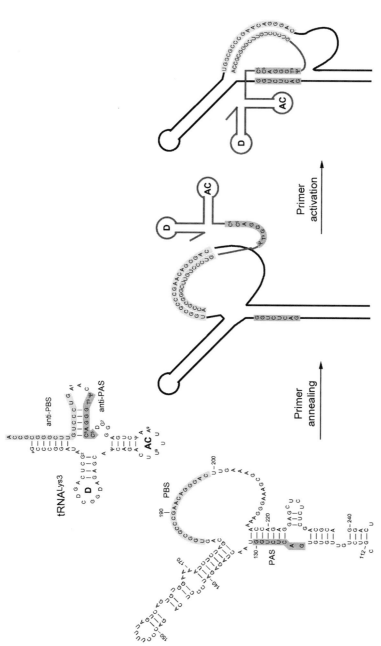

FIGURE 5 Mechanistic model for HIV-1 reverse transcription initiation. The secondary structures of the PBS region of the HIV-1 RNA genome and the tRNA^{Lys3} primer are shown (AC, anticodon loop; D, D loop). The tRNA primer anneals with its 3′-terminal 18 nts to the PBS (PBS and anti-PBS are dark gray). An additional interaction between PAS and anti-PAS (light gray) is required to activate the PBS-bound tRNA primer for reverse transcription.

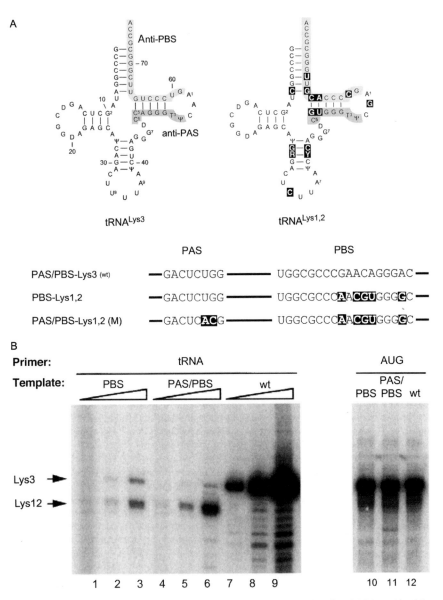

FIGURE 6 *In vitro* switching of HIV-1 tRNA usage. (A) Anti-PBS and anti-PAS motifs of the tRNA[Lys3] and tRNA[Lys1,2] primers are indicated in different shades of gray. tRNA[Lys1,2] nucleotides that differ from tRNA[Lys3] are boxed and marked in bold. The wt and mutant PAS and PBS motifs are shown below. Nucleotides that differ from the wt sequence are marked. (B) The PBS-Lys1,2 (lanes 1–3), the PAS/PBS-Lys1,2 (lanes 4–6) mutant, and wt template (lanes 7–9) were incubated with a calf liver tRNA preparation that contains tRNA[Lys3], tRNA[Lys1,2], and all other tRNA species. We tested three amounts of template RNA (10, 50, and 250 ng). Reverse transcription was initiated from the annealed tRNA primer by addition of ^{32}P-dCTP and

transcription. We speculate that this mechanism may preclude premature reverse transcription in virus-producing cells such that the vRNA genome is copied only after it is appropriately packaged into virions. Although binding of tRNA^{Lys3} to the PBS can occur in virus-producing cells, primer activation requires a structural rearrangement of the tRNA–vRNA complex to establish the PAS–anti-PAS interaction (Fig. 5). It is possible that NC, which acts as an RNA chaperone (Darlix et al., 2002; Levin et al., 2005), mediates this conformational change. Because NC is released from the Gag precursor protein during maturation of virion particles, this mechanism will ensure the precise timing for activation of reverse transcription. tRNA packaging and annealing to the PBS in viral particles is not dependent on Gag processing (Cen et al., 2000), whereas efficient tRNA primer extension is. NC may therefore be essential in controlling an initiation step of reverse transcription that follows these processes, which is consistent with our hypothesis. This regulation may protect the host cell from potentially deleterious unrestricted reverse transcription (Dhellin et al., 1997).

VII. HIV-1 Replication with a Nonself tRNA Primer Confirms the Importance of the PAS Motif

A. Switching tRNA Usage *In Vitro*

As discussed, it proved very difficult to change the identity of the tRNA primer for reverse transcription. Only changing the HIV-1 PBS sequence does not produce a genetically stable virus variant. Because the PAS is involved in tRNA primer activation via a specific base-pairing interaction, we replaced both the PAS and PBS in RNA transcripts with sequences complementary to the nonself tRNA^{Lys1,2} molecules (Fig. 6A). As a control we used the single PBS-Lys1,2 mutant without PAS adaptation. Three concentrations of the wt, PBS-Lys1,2, and PAS/PBS-Lys1,2 templates were incubated with a calf liver tRNA preparation that contains tRNA^{Lys3}, tRNA^{Lys1,2}, and all other tRNA species. The tRNA primer was extended with 1 nt (^{32}P-dCTP) by HIV-1 RT enzyme *in vitro*. The wt template produces an intense tRNA^{Lys3}-primed cDNA, and no tRNA^{Lys1,2} signal is apparent (Fig. 6B, lanes 7–9). The tRNA^{Lys3} signal is significantly reduced on the PBS-Lys1,2 template, and an induced tRNA^{Lys1,2} signal is apparent of approximately similar intensity (Fig. 6B, lanes 1–3). The additional change

---

HIV-1 RT enzyme. This results in the extension of the tRNA primer with 1 nt. The radiolabeled tRNA^{Lys3} product runs slower on the denaturing gel than tRNA^{Lys1,2} due to different base modifications within the tRNA backbone (Das et al., 1995; Oude Essink et al., 1996). The amount of input vRNA was quantified by DNA-primer extension with a DNA primer (AUG primer, lanes 10–12).

of the PAS in the PAS/PBS-Lys1,2 double mutant template markedly increased the tRNA^{Lys1,2} signal, with a concomitant decrease of the tRNA^{Lys3} signal (Fig. 6B, lanes 4–6). The PAS adaptation enhances tRNA^{Lys1,2} usage approximately sixfold. These *in vitro* results demonstrate that the identity of the priming tRNA species can be switched by simultaneous alteration of the PAS and PBS motifs. This observation underscores the role of PAS in reverse transcription initiation. However, the new tRNA^{Lys1,2} primer is used relatively inefficiently ($\sim$5% of tRNA^{Lys3}-usage on the wt template), indicating that other determinants in the mutant template are not optimal for tRNA^{Lys1,2} usage. Still, we pursued the possibility that tRNA usage can be successfully switched by simultaneous adaptations of the PAS and PBS motifs in the viral context.

B. Switching tRNA Usage *In Vivo*

We constructed an HIV-1 variant with the PAS/PBS double mutation to enforce the use of tRNA^{Lys1,2} as replication primer (Fig. 6A). We speculated that the evolutionary jump in primer usage from tRNA^{Lys3} to tRNA^{Lys1,2} would be relatively easy for HIV-1. The two primers are similar and are selectively packaged via the LysRS-dependent mechanism, which does not discriminate among the tRNA^{Lys} isoacceptors. Virus replication of the PAS/PBS double mutant was determined and compared to the wt and the single PBS-Lys1,2 mutant virus (Fig. 7). The ranking order of replication was

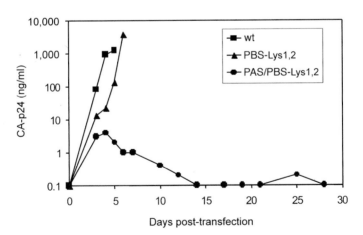

FIGURE 7 Replication capacity of PAS/PBS-Lys1,2 mutant virus. SupT1 cells were transfected with the proviral constructs. CA-p24 production was measured in the culture medium at several days post-transfection. The PBS-Lys1,2 mutant virus was unstable: the PBS reverted to the wt PBS-Lys3 sequence. The PAS/PBS-Lys1,2 virus was severely crippled in replication capacity.

determined as wt>PBS-Lys1,2>PAS/PBS-Lys1,2. The relatively efficient replication and instability of the PBS-Lys1,2 single mutant was reported previously (Das *et al.*, 1995). Addition of the PAS-Lys1,2 mutation severely decreased virus replication and did not rescue replication of the PBS mutant. Rescue would be expected if no other viral factors were implicated in selective tRNA usage. However, several viral factors that closely interact with the tRNA primer may be involved such as the RT enzyme. Thus, other incompatibility problems may not be solved by the imposed usage of a nonself tRNA primer in the PAS/PBS double mutants.

We set out to obtain faster replicating revertant viruses for the PAS/PBS-Lys1,2 mutant. *A priori*, two evolution routes can be envisaged. First, the virus can restore tRNA^{Lys3} usage by reversion to the wt PBS motif. However, priming by tRNA^{Lys3} is inhibited at two levels by the PAS/PBS mutations: tRNA annealing and initiation of reverse transcription. Usage of the new primer is enhanced by these mutations. These combined effects may block the wt-reversion route. Second, the virus can optimize replication with the new tRNA primer, and adaptive changes may thus be acquired in the viral RT enzyme or other cofactors. This latter evolutionary route is very interesting because it may reveal other viral determinants of selective tRNA usage.

We maintained 17 independent cultures with PAS/PBS-Lys1,2 mutants, and break-through replication was monitored within a few weeks in three cultures. Virus was passaged repeatedly and the RNA leader sequence (including the PAS and PBS motifs) was determined for the virus progeny. Partial leader sequences of the revertant PAS/PBS-Lys1,2 viruses are shown in Fig. 8. Three cultures showed signs of replication of PAS/PBS-Lys1,2 revertants. Two variants reverted back to the wt PBS-lys3. The input PAS/PBS-Lys1,2 motifs were maintained in only one culture (L4, Fig. 8). This variant continued to replicate with a tRNA^{Lys1,2} primer up to day 75, but a mixed wt-mutant PBS sequence was detected at day 97. We therefore used the day 47 sample to start a second round of evolution by infecting six fresh SupT1 cell cultures in parallel. All cultures became infected with L4-derived variants that maintained the mutant PBS-Lys1,2 up to day 116. This observation suggests that the L4 viruses acquired at least one adaptive change outside the PBS motif to accommodate tRNA^{Lys1,2} in the second round of evolution. An interesting change was observed within the PAS motif in five out of six revertants (Fig. 8). The mutant PAS-Lys1,2 differs from the wt PAS-Lys3 element at two nucleotide positions. These nucleotides did not revert, but an additional PAS residue was altered (U126C, indicated by R1). In the interaction model presented in Fig. 5, we see that a U-G base pair is replaced by a stronger C-G base pair in the PAS–anti-PAS interaction with tRNA^{Lys1,2} (Fig. 9).

The original L4 revertant did not yet contain the R1 adaptation (Fig. 8). Nevertheless, this virus replicated relatively efficiently, suggesting that at least one other critical mutation must be present elsewhere in the viral

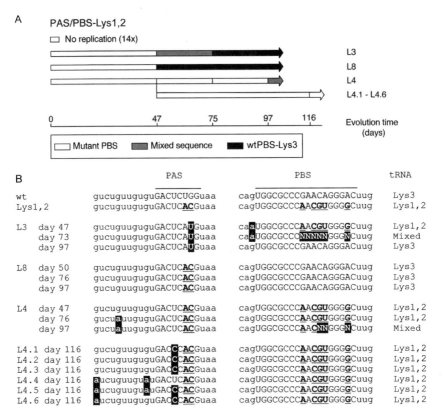

FIGURE 8   Evolution of the PAS/PBS-Lys1,2 mutant M. SupT1 cells were transfected with the molecular clones. Breakthrough replication was observed in some cultures, and virus was cell-free passaged to fresh cells. (A) The identity of the PBS motif is indicated as a function of the evolution time. The input mutant PBS is shown as an open box, the wt revertant as a black box, and mixed wt/revertant sequences as a gray box. (B) The culture number, the day of harvest, and the sequence of the proviral DNA that was isolated from infected cells are listed. The two mutated PAS and PBS nucleotides are indicated in bold and underlined. Nucleotide changes acquired during evolution are in white surrounded by a black box (N indicates a mixed sequence). Mutations in the region just upstream of the PAS that are observed in some cultures may reflect G-to-A hypermutation. These transitions have been described previously for other leader revertant viruses and were therefore not analyzed further (Berkhout *et al.*, 2001). The R1 reversion (U126C) is observed in five out of six L4 cultures at 116 days post-transfection. The R2 reversion in the RNaseH domain (Gly490Glu) was observed in the L4-d47 virus sample.

genome to facilitate reverse transcription primed by the nonself tRNA^{Lys1,2} molecule. We assumed that the L4-d47 virus has a major adaptive change elsewhere in the viral genome that allows efficient tRNA^{Lys1,2} usage. Because no significant changes were present in the leader domain surrounding the PAS/PBS motifs, we sequenced the complete RT gene. One mutation within

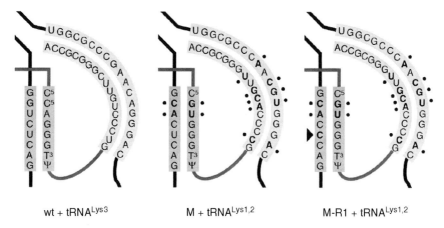

wt + tRNA^{Lys3}   M + tRNA^{Lys1,2}   M-R1 + tRNA^{Lys1,2}

FIGURE 9   The PAS reversion optimizes tRNA annealing. A close-up of the activated template-tRNA initiation complex is shown with the PBS–anti-PBS and PAS–anti-PAS interactions in light and dark gray, respectively (see also Fig. 5). These interactions are indicated for the wt leader with tRNA[Lys3], and for the PAS/PBS-Lys1,2 mutant (M) and the M-R1 revertant with tRNA[Lys1,2]. The sequence differences between wt, M and R1 leader RNA, and the tRNA[Lys3] versus tRNA[Lys1,2] are in bold and marked by dots. The R1 reversion (U126C; indicated by an arrowhead) stabilizes the PAS–anti-PAS interaction (substitution of a weak U-G base pair by a very stable C-G base pair).

the RT gene was identified (indicated by R2), which leads to an amino acid change (G490E) in the RNaseH domain. The mutation was maintained in later samples. The G490 residue is absolutely conserved among virus isolates of all HIV-1 subtypes and of related SIV and HIV-2 viruses that also use tRNA[Lys3] as primer. Interestingly, residue 490 is protruding from the RNaseH domain in the X-ray structure of the RT p51-p66 heterodimer. Thus, residue 490 seems ideally positioned to act as "gatekeeper" for the cleft in between the RNaseH and RT domains. We speculate that part of the tRNA molecule binds in this cleft, which is consistent with previous cross-linking studies (Mishima and Steitz, 1995). These results also imply the RNaseH domain of HIV-1 RT in selective tRNA binding. The combined observations convinced us to look into the PAS and RT reversions in more detail.

C. Role of the PAS and RT Mutations in tRNA[Lys1,2] Primer Usage

We confirmed that the PAS-mutation R1 and the RT-mutation R2 increase the replication of the PAS/PBS-Lys1,2 mutant virus, and stabilize the usage of the tRNA[Lys1,2] primer. The R1 PAS change significantly increased replication of the tRNA[Lys1,2]-using virus, even in the absence of the R2 reversion in RT (Fig. 10). No gross effect of R2 on replication of the

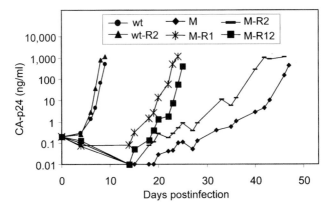

FIGURE 10   Replication of the wt, the PAS/PBS-Lys1,2 mutant, and cloned revertant viruses. SupT1 cells were infected with equal amount of viruses. Virus production was measured in the culture medium for several days. M indicates the original PAS/PBS-Lys1,2 mutant, R1 indicates the U126C reversion in the PAS motif, and R2 indicates the Gly490Glu reversion in the RNaseH domain.

wt and mutant viruses could be observed, but more sensitive virus competition assays indicated the following ranking order: wt $\geq$ wt-R2 $\gg$ M-R1 $\geq$ M-R12 > M-R2 > M. The impact of the R1 mutation on restoration of virus replication is significantly greater than that of the R2 mutation. R1 may also stabilize tRNA^{Lys1,2} usage more potently than R2. R2 did not significantly affect viral replication in a wt and R1 background. Apparently, R2 only stimulates viral replication when the tRNA–vRNA interaction is suboptimal. The R2 mutation in RT was recently tested in the context of other nonself tRNA-using HIV-1 variants, and the results confirm that this adaptation does not stabilize the usage of non-Lys primers in PBS-A-rich loop mutants (Xu and Morrow, 2006). Further *in vitro* studies with recombinant RT may shed more light on the specific role of the RNaseH domain and the R2 mutation in tRNA selection.

To confirm that R1 and R2 can stabilize tRNA^{Lys1,2} usage, we passaged the molecularly cloned M-R1 and M-R12 viruses for over a year. The sequences of the leader RNA and the RT gene were analyzed. Most importantly, all viruses continued to use tRNA^{Lys1,2}. The R1 reversion was maintained in the entire quasispecies population in all cultures. These data suggest that R1 effectively prevents the switch to tRNA^{Lys3}, possibly by improving the use of tRNA^{Lys1,2}. In case the PAS motif is involved in activation of the tRNA primer and not so much in the annealing of the primer onto the PBS, introduction of R1 in the PAS-Lys1,2 motif will result in enhanced primer activation in M-R1 virus particles. We therefore identified the primer that is placed onto the viral PBS inside virus particles. In M and M-R1 virus particles, tRNA^{Lys1,2} was identified as the primer.

The occupancy of the PBS was similar in M, M-R1, and wt viruses. The primer extension defect of the M mutant was corrected by the R1 mutation (Ooms *et al.*, 2007). These data confirm the important role of the PAS motif in primer activation and viral replication.

VIII. Conclusions

Specificity for the tRNA^{Lys3} primer is strictly maintained in HIV-1 evolution. Primer specificity is imposed by at least three mechanisms: selective tRNA packaging into virus particles, specific binding of tRNA to the viral template, and specific contacts between the initiation complex and RT. Therefore, a change in primer usage by HIV-1 requires adaptations in many of its constituents: multiple motifs within the viral leader RNA, and possibly the Gag and RT proteins need to be changed simultaneously. This creates a high genetic barrier for the spontaneous evolution of an altered tRNA primer specificity.

Earlier experiments from several laboratories have shown that altering the PBS sequence alone is not sufficient to stably switch tRNA usage (Das *et al.*, 1995; Li *et al.*, 1994; Wakefield *et al.*, 1995). Additional studies showed that the upstream RNA motif PAS is critically involved in tRNA-primed reverse transcription (Beerens and Berkhout, 2002a; Beerens *et al.*, 2001). The PAS motif exerts its function not by enhancing tRNA annealing to the PBS, but by activating initiation of reverse transcription. The PAS motif engages in a base-pairing interaction with the complementary anti-PAS sequence in the tRNA which likely results in the formation of a higher order RNA structure that is suitable for reverse transcription (Fig. 5). This complex, multistep initiation process allows strict regulation of reverse transcription. By adaptation of both PAS and PBS motifs, the HIV-1 leader could be changed to accommodate the tRNA^{Lys1,2} primer for initiation of reverse transcription *in vitro* (Beerens and Berkhout, 2002b). We also constructed PAS/PBS double mutant viruses that should accommodate tRNA^{Lys1,2} as reverse transcription primer. Since tRNA^{Lys1,2} isoacceptors are selectively packaged via the Gag-Pol–LysRS-tRNA complex, the mutant virus is not expected to encounter difficulties in tRNA^{Lys1,2} packaging. Nevertheless, the mutant virus was severely affected in replication efficiency and it could still revert to a tRNA^{Lys3}-using virus, but acquisition of a second-site reversion in the PAS motif stabilized tRNA^{Lys1,2} usage and improved replication. Fine-tuning of the PAS–anti-PAS interaction strength turns out to be the most decisive change to yield a virus that stably uses tRNA^{Lys1,2}.

The role of the PAS motif in reverse transcription was recently challenged by others (Goldschmidt *et al.*, 2003). These authors reconstructed the 2L, 2R, and 2LR mutants from our initial study and performed reverse transcription and structure probing experiments. In our hands the 2L mutation strongly reduced and the 2R mutation profoundly stimulated reverse transcription initiation. Goldschmidt *et al.* observed an elongation defect of the 2L mutation and no effect of the 2R mutation. Based on structure probing experiments on the naked HIV-1 RNA, aberrant folding of the template rather than inactivation of the PAS sequence was argued to cause the reverse transcription defect of the 2L mutant. We previously addressed this rather complex issue (Huthoff *et al.*, 2003). Careful inspection of the *in vitro* reverse transcription data in the Goldschmidt study reveals a tRNA-specific defect in the synthesis of the first premature cDNA product (which is the best marker for initiation in this assay) on the 2L and 2LR templates that is not observed in RNA oligonucleotide-primed reaction, arguing for a PAS effect. The discrepancy with our results may be caused solely by differences in initiation and elongation; we therefore feel it is of uttermost importance to perform 1 nt-incorporation reactions in case one wants to study reverse transcription initiation. Recent studies in our laboratory show that priming from an RNA oligonucleotide is unaffected by the 2L mutation, confirming the requirement of the PAS motif in tRNA-primed reverse transcription (Ooms *et al.*, 2007). Furthermore, we demonstrated the 2L defect and the 2R upregulation in a physiological setting by analyzing reverse transcription products from the mutant virion particles (Beerens and Berkhout, 2002a). In this chapter, we discussed in detail the wealth of experimental evidence in favor of the importance of the PAS motif in reverse transcription, including the successful switch to tRNA[Lys1,2] usage *in vitro* and *in vivo* by a simultaneous change of the PAS and PBS sequences (Abbink *et al.*, 2004; Beerens and Berkhout, 2002a,b; Beerens *et al.*, 2001). Also the conservation of the PAS motif among all retroviruses strongly supports the role of the PAS enhancer motif.

We demonstrated that the efficiency of reverse transcription can be up- or downregulated by mutations in the HIV-1 PAS element that strengthen or weaken the interaction with the tRNA primer. Furthermore, reverse transcription of the wt HIV-1 template appears restricted by inclusion of the PAS in a repressive RNA secondary structure. This mechanism may preclude premature reverse transcription in the virus-producing cell such that the vRNA genome is copied only after it is appropriately dimerized and packaged in mature virions. Although binding of tRNA[Lys3] to the PBS may occur relatively early in the virus-producing cells, activation of the primer will require a structural rearrangement of the vRNA–tRNA complex to establish the PAS–anti-PAS interaction. This conformational change may be facilitated by NC, which acts as an RNA chaperone. Because NC is only released from the Gag precursor protein during virus maturation, this will ensure the proper timing of initiation of reverse transcription.

Acknowledgments ───────────────────

The authors are particularly grateful to people in the laboratory, past and present, whose work is summarized here: Nancy Beerens, Atze Das, Bep Klaver, Fedde Groot, Marcel Ooms, and Belinda Oude Essink. We thank Marcel Ooms and Joost Haasnoot for critical reading of the chapter and Wim van Est for professional artwork. We thank Judith Levin for discussions. The limited scope of the chapter did not allow us to cite all references, we do apologize to those whose work we may have inadvertently failed to mention. Research in the Berkhout laboratory is supported by the Dutch Organization for Scientific Research (NWO, TOP grant).

References ───────────────────

Abbink, T. E. M., and Berkhout, B. (2003). A novel long distance base-pairing interaction in human immunodeficiency virus type 1 RNA occludes the gag start codon. *J. Biol. Chem.* **278**, 11601–11611.

Abbink, T. E. M., Beerens, N., and Berkhout, B. (2004). Forced selection of a human immunodeficiency virus type 1 variant that uses a non-self tRNA primer for reverse transcription: Involvement of viral RNA sequences and the reverse transcriptase enzyme. *J. Virol.* **78**, 10706–10714.

Aiyar, A., Cobrinik, D., Ge, Z., Kung, H. J., and Leis, J. (1992). Interaction between retroviral U5 RNA and the TΨC loop of the tRNA(Trp) primer is required for efficient initiation of reverse transcription. *J. Virol.* **66**, 2464–2472.

Arts, E. J., Mak, J., Kleiman, L., and Wainberg, M. A. (1994). DNA found in human immunodeficiency virus type 1 particles may not be required for infectivity. *J. Gen. Virol.* **75**, 1605–1613.

Arts, E. J., Ghosh, M., Jacques, P. S., Ehresmann, B., and Le Grice, S. F. J. (1996a). Restoration of tRNALys,3-primed (−)-strand DNA synthesis to an HIV-1 reverse transcriptase mutant with extended tRNAs. *J. Biol. Chem.* **271**, 9054–9061.

Arts, E. J., Stetor, S. R., Li, Y., Rausch, J. W., Howard, K. J., Ehresmann, B., North, T. W., Wohrl, B. M., Goody, R. S., Wainberg, M. A., and Le Grice, S. F. J. (1996b). Initiation of (−) strand DNA synthesis from tRNALys3 on lentiviral RNAs: Implications of specific HIV-1 RNA-tRNALys3 interactions inhibiting primer utilization by retroviral reverse trancriptases. *Proc. Natl. Acad. Sci. USA* **93**, 10063–10068.

Auxilien, S., Keith, G., Le Grice, S. F. J., and Darlix, J.-L. (1999). Role of post-transcriptional modifications of primer tRNALys3 in the fidelity and efficacy of plus strand DNA transfer during HIV-1 reverse transcription. *J. Biol. Chem.* **274**, 4412–4420.

Barat, C., Lullien, V., Schatz, O., Keith, G., Mugeyre, M. T., Grüninger-Leitch, F., Barré-Sinoussi, F., LeGrice, S. F. J., and Darlix, J. L. (1989). HIV-1 reverse transcriptase specifically interacts with the anticodon domain of its cognate primer tRNA. *EMBO J.* **11**, 3279–3285.

Barat, C., Le Grice, S. F., and Darlix, J. L. (1991). Interaction of HIV-1 reverse transcriptase with a synthetic form of its replication primer, tRNA(Lys,3). *Nucleic Acids Res.* **19**, 751–757.

Barat, C., Schatz, O., Le Grice, S., and Darlix, J. L. (1993). Analysis of the interactions of HIV-1 replication primer tRNA(Lys, 3) with nucleocapsid protein and reverse transcriptase. *J. Mol. Biol.* **231**, 185–190.

Baudin, F., Marquet, R., Isel, C., Darlix, J. L., Ehresmann, B., and Ehresmann, C. (1993). Functional sites in the 5′ region of human immunodeficiency virus type 1 RNA form defined structural domains. *J. Mol. Biol.* **229**, 382–397.

Beerens, N., and Berkhout, B. (2002a). The tRNA primer activation signal in the HIV-1 genome is important for initiation and processive elongation of reverse transcription. *J. Virol.* **76**, 2329–2339.

Beerens, N., and Berkhout, B. (2002b). Switching the *in vitro* tRNA usage of HIV-1 by simultaneous adaptation of the PBS and PAS. *RNA* **8**, 357–369.

Beerens, N., Groot, F., and Berkhout, B. (2000a). Stabilization of the U5-leader stem in the HIV-1 RNA genome affects initiation and elongation of reverse transcription. *Nucleic Acids Res.* **28**, 4130–4137.

Beerens, N., Klaver, B., and Berkhout, B. (2000b). A structured RNA motif is involved in the correct placement of the tRNALys3 primer onto the human immunodeficiency virus genome. *J. Virol.* **74**, 2227–2238.

Beerens, N., Groot, F., and Berkhout, B. (2001). Initiation of HIV-1 reverse transcription is regulated by a primer activation signal. *J. Biol. Chem.* **276**, 31247–31256.

Ben Artzi, H., Shemesh, J., Zeelon, E., Amit, B., Kleiman, L., Gorecki, M., and Panet, A. (1996). Molecular analysis of the second template switch during reverse transcription of the HIV RNA template. *Biochemistry* **35**, 10549–10557.

Berkhout, B. (1996). Structure and function of the human immunodeficiency virus leader RNA. *Prog. Nucleic Acid Res. Mol. Biol.* **54**, 1–34.

Berkhout, B. (1997). The primer-binding site on the RNA genome of human and simian immunodeficiency viruses is flanked by an upstream hairpin structure. *Nucleic Acids Res.* **25**, 4013–4017.

Berkhout, B., Klaver, B., and Das, A. T. (1997). Forced evolution of a regulatory RNA helix in the HIV-1 genome. *Nucleic Acids Res.* **25**, 940–947.

Berkhout, B., Das, A. T., and Beerens, N. (2001). HIV-1 RNA editing, hypermutation and error-prone reverse transcription. *Science* **292**, 7.

Berwin, B., and Barklis, E. (1993). Retrovirus-mediated insertion of expressed and non-expressed genes at identical chromosomal locations. *Nucleic Acids Res.* **21**, 2399–2407.

Cen, S., Khorchid, A., Gabor, J., Rong, L., Wainberg, M. A., and Kleiman, L. (2000). Roles of Pr55(gag) and NCp7 in tRNA(3)(Lys) genomic placement and the initiation step of reverse transcription in human immunodeficiency virus type 1. *J. Virol.* **74**, 10796–10800.

Cen, S., Khorchid, A., Javanbakht, H., Gabor, J., Stello, T., Shiba, K., Musier-Forsyth, K., and Kleiman, L. (2001). Incorporation of lysyl-tRNA synthetase into human immunodeficiency virus type 1. *J. Virol.* **75**, 5043–5048.

Cen, S., Javanbakht, H., Kim, S., Shiba, K., Craven, R., Rein, A., Ewalt, K., Schimmel, P., Musier-Forsyth, K., and Kleiman, L. (2002). Retrovirus-specific packaging of aminoacyl-tRNA synthetases with cognate primer tRNAs. *J. Virol.* **76**, 13111–13115.

Cen, S., Javanbakht, H., Niu, M., and Kleiman, L. (2004a). Ability of wild-type and mutant lysyl-tRNA synthetase to facilitate tRNA(Lys) incorporation into human immunodeficiency virus type 1. *J. Virol.* **78**, 1595–1601.

Cen, S., Niu, M., and Kleiman, L. (2004b). The connection domain in reverse transcriptase facilitates the *in vivo* annealing of tRNALys3 to HIV-1 genomic RNA. *Retrovirology* **1**, 33–39.

Charneau, P., Alizon, M., and Clavel, F. (1992). A second origin of DNA plus-strand synthesis is required for optimal human immunodeficiency virus replication. *J. Virol.* **66**, 2814–2820.

Charneau, P., Mirambeau, G., Roux, P., Paulous, S., Buc, H., and Clavel, F. (1994). HIV-1 reverse transcription. A termination step at the center of the genome. *J. Mol. Biol.* **241**, 651–662.

Cobrinik, D., Soskey, L., and Leis, J. (1988). A retroviral RNA secondary structure required for efficient initiation of reverse transcription. *J. Virol.* **62**, 3622–3630.

Cobrinik, D., Aiyar, A., Ge, Z., Katzman, M., Huang, H., and Leis, J. (1991). Overlapping retrovirus U5 sequence elements are required for efficient integration and initiation of reverse transcription. *J. Virol.* **65**, 3864–3872.

Colicelli, J., and Goff, S. P. (1986). Isolation of a recombinant murine leukemia virus utilizing a new primer tRNA. *J. Virol.* **57**, 37–45.

Cordell, B., Swanstrom, R., Goodman, H. M., and Bishop, J. M. (1979). tRNA type as primer for RNA-directed DNA polymerase: Structural determinants of function. *J. Biol. Chem.* **254**, 1866–1874.

Cusack, S., Yaremchuk, A., and Tukalo, M. (1996). The crystal structures of T. thermophilus lysyl-tRNA synthetase complexed with *E. coli* tRNA(Lys) and a T. thermophilus tRNA (Lys) transcript: Anticodon recognition and conformational changes upon binding of a lysyl-adenylate analogue. *EMBO J.* **15**, 6321–6334.

Damgaard, C. K., Andersen, E. S., Knudsen, B., Gorodkin, J., and Kjems, J. (2004). RNA interactions in the 5′ region of the HIV-1 genome. *J. Mol. Biol.* **336**, 369–379.

Darlix, J. L., Lastra, M. L., Mely, Y., and Roques, B. (2002). Nucleocapsid protein chaperoning of nucleic acids at the heart of HIV structure, assembly and cDNA synthesis. *In* "HIV Sequence Compendium 2002" (C. Kuiken, B. Foley, E. Freed, B. Hahn, P. Marx, F. McCutchan, J. Mellors, S. Wolinsky, and B. Korber, Eds.), pp. 69–88. Los Alamos National Laboratory, Theoretical Biology and Biophysics Group, Los Alamos, New Mexico.

Das, A. T., Koken, S. E. C., Oude Essink, B. B., van Wamel, J. L. B., and Berkhout, B. (1994). Human immunodeficiency virus uses tRNA(Lys,3) as primer for reverse transcription in HeLa-CD4+ cells. *FEBS Lett.* **341**, 49–53.

Das, A. T., Klaver, B., and Berkhout, B. (1995). Reduced replication of human immunodeficiency virus type 1 mutants that use reverse transcription primers other than the natural tRNA(3Lys). *J. Virol.* **69**, 3090–3097.

Das, A. T., Klaver, B., and Berkhout, B. (1997). Sequence variation of the HIV primer-binding site suggests the use of an alternative tRNALys molecule in reverse transcription. *J. Gen. Virol.* **78**, 837–840.

Das, A. T., van Dam, A. P., Klaver, B., and Berkhout, B. (1998). Improved envelope function selected by long-term cultivation of a translation-impaired HIV-1 mutant. *Virology* **244**, 552–562.

Das, A. T., Vink, M., and Berkhout, B. (2005). Alternative tRNA priming of human immunodeficiency virus type 1 reverse transcription explains sequence variation in the primer-binding site that has been attributed to APOBEC3G activity. *J. Virol.* **79**, 3179–3181.

De Rocquigny, H., Gabus, C., Vincent, A., Fournie-Zaluski, M.-C., Roques, B., and Darlix, J.-L. (1992). Viral RNA annealing activities of human immunodeficiency virus type 1 nucleocapsid protein require only peptide domains outside the zinc fingers. *Proc. Natl. Acad. Sci. USA* **89**, 6472–6476.

Delahunty, M. D., Wilson, S. H., and Karpel, R. L. (1994). Studies on primer binding of HIV-1 reverse transcriptase using a fluorescent probe. *J. Mol. Biol.* **236**, 469–479.

Dhellin, O., Maestre, J., and Heidmann, T. (1997). Functional differences between the human LINE retrotransposon and retroviral reverse transcriptases for *in vivo* mRNA reverse transcription. *EMBO J.* **16**, 6590–6602.

Di Marzo Veronese, F., Copeland, T. D., DeVico, A. L., Rahman, R., Oroszlan, S., Gallo, R. C., and Sarngadharan, M. G. (1986). Characterization of highly immunogenic p66/p51 as the reverse transcriptase of HTLV-III/LAV. *Science* **231**, 1289–1291.

Dufour, E., Reinbolt, J., Castroviejo, M., Ehresmann, B., Litvak, S., Tarrago-Litvak, L., and Andreola, M.-L. (1999). Cross-linking localization of a HIV-1 reverse transcriptase peptide involved in the binding of primer tRNALys3. *J. Mol. Biol.* **285**, 1339–1346.

Dupuy, L. C., Kelly, N. J., Elgavish, T. E., Harvey, S. C., and Morrow, C. D. (2003). Probing the importance of tRNA anticodon: Human immunodeficiency virus type 1 (HIV-1) RNA genome complementarity with an HIV-1 that selects tRNA(Glu) for replication. *J. Virol.* 77, 8756–8764.

Esposito, D., and Craigie, R. (1998). Sequence specificity of viral end DNA binding by HIV-1 integrase reveals critical regions for protein-DNA interaction. *EMBO J.* 17, 5832–5843.

Feng, Y.-X., Campbell, S., Harvin, D., Ehresmann, B., Ehresmann, C., and Rein, A. (1999). The human immunodeficiency virus type 1 Gag polyprotein has nucleic acid chaperone activity: Possible role in dimerization of genomic RNA and placement of tRNA on the primer binding site. *J. Virol.* 73, 4251–4256.

Freund, F., Boulme, F., Litvak, S., and Tarrago-Litvak, L. (2001). Initiation of HIV-2 reverse transcription: A secondary structure model of the RNA-tRNA(Lys3) duplex. *Nucleic Acids Res.* 29, 2757–2765.

Fu, W., Ortiz-Conde, B. A., Gorelick, R. J., Hughes, S. H., and Rein, A. (1997). Placement of tRNA primer on the primer-binding site requires pol gene expression in avian but not murine retroviruses. *J. Virol.* 71, 6940–6946.

Gabor, J., Cen, S., Javanbakht, H., Niu, M., and Kleiman, L. (2002). Effect of altering the tRNA concentration in human immunodeficiency virus type 1 upon its annealing to viral RNA, Gag-Pol incorporation, and viral infectivity. *J. Virol.* 76, 9096–9102.

Goff, S. P. (1990). Retroviral reverse transcriptase: Synthesis, structure, and function. *J. Acquir. Immune Defic. Syndr.* 3, 817–831.

Goldschmidt, V., Ehresmann, C., Ehresmann, B., and Marquet, R. (2003). Does the HIV-1 primer activation signal interact with tRNA(3)(Lys) during the initiation of reverse transcription? *Nucleic Acids Res.* 31, 850–859.

Goldschmidt, V., Paillart, J. C., Rigourd, M., Ehresmann, B., Aubertin, A. M., Ehresmann, C., and Marquet, R. (2004). Structural variability of the initiation complex of HIV-1 reverse transcription. *J. Biol. Chem.* 279, 35923–35931.

Guo, F., Cen, S., Niu, M., Javanbakht, H., and Kleiman, L. (2003). Specific inhibition of the synthesis of human lysyl-tRNA synthetase results in decreases in tRNA(Lys) incorporation, tRNA(3)(Lys) annealing to viral RNA, and viral infectivity in human immunodeficiency virus type 1. *J. Virol.* 77, 9817–9822.

Guyader, M., Emerman, M., Sonigo, P., Clavel, F., Montagnier, L., and Alizon, M. (1987). Genome organization and transactivation of the human immunodeficiency virus type 2. *Nature* 326, 662–669.

Halwani, R., Cen, S., Javanbakht, H., Saadatmand, J., Kim, S., Shiba, K., and Kleiman, L. (2004). Cellular distribution of Lysyl-tRNA synthetase and its interaction with Gag during human immunodeficiency virus type 1 assembly. *J. Virol.* 78, 7553–7564.

Harada, F., Sawyer, R. C., and Dahlberg, J. E. (1975). A primer ribonucleic acid for initiation of *in vitro* Rous sarcoma virus deoxyribonucleic acid synthesis. *J. Biol. Chem.* 250, 3487–3497.

Harada, F., Peters, G. G., and Dahlberg, J. E. (1979). The primer tRNA for Moloney murine leukemia virus DNA synthesis. Nucleotide sequence and aminoacylation of tRNAPro. *J. Biol. Chem.* 254, 10979–10985.

Hargittai, M. R., Mangla, A. T., Gorelick, R. J., and Musier-Forsyth, K. (2001). HIV-1 nucleocapsid protein zinc finger structures induce tRNA(Lys,3) structural changes but are not critical for primer/template annealing. *J. Mol. Biol.* 312, 985–997.

Haseltine, W. A., Panet, A., Smoler, D., Baltimore, D., Peters, G., Harada, F., and Dahlberg, J. E. (1977). Interaction of tryptophan tRNA and avian myeloblastosis virus reverse transcriptase: Further characterization of the binding reaction. *Biochemistry* 16, 3625–3632.

Huang, Y., Mak, J., Cao, Q., Li, Z., Wainberg, M. A., and Kleiman, L. (1994). Incorporation of excess wild-type and mutant tRNA(3Lys) into human immunodeficiency virus type 1. *J. Virol.* 68, 7676–7683.

Huang, Y., Wang, J., Shalom, A., Li, Z., Khorchid, A., Wainberg, M. A., and Kleiman, L. (1997). Primer tRNALys3 on the viral genome exists in unextended and two-base extended forms within mature human immunodeficiency virus type 1. *J. Virol.* **71**, 726–728.

Hungnes, O., Tjotta, E., and Grinde, B. (1992). Mutations in the central polypurine tract of HIV-1 result in delayed replication. *Virology* **190**, 440–442.

Huthoff, H., Bugala, K., Barciszewski, J., and Berkhout, B. (2003). On the importance of the primer activation signal for initiation of tRNA(lys3)-primed reverse transcription of the HIV-1 RNA genome. *Nucleic Acids Res.* **31**, 5186–5194.

Isel, C., Marquet, R., Keith, G., Ehresmann, C., and Ehresmann, B. (1993). Modified nucleotides of tRNA(3Lys) modulate primer/template loop- loop interaction in the initiation complex of HIV-1 reverse transcription. *J. Biol. Chem.* **268**, 25269–25272.

Isel, C., Ehresmann, C., Keith, G., Ehresmann, B., and Marquet, R. (1995). Initiation of reverse transcription of HIV-1: Secondary structure of the HIV-1 RNA/tRNA(3Lys) (template/primer). *J. Mol. Biol.* **247**, 236–250.

Isel, C., Lanchy, J.-M., Le Grice, S. F. J., Ehresmann, C., Ehresmann, B., and Marquet, R. (1996). Specific initiation and switch to elongation of human immunodeficiency virus type 1 reverse transcriptase require the post-transcriptional modifications of primer tRNALys3. *EMBO J.* **15**, 917–924.

Isel, C., Keith, G., Ehresmann, B., Ehresmann, C., and Marquet, R. (1998). Mutational analysis of the tRNA3Lys/HIV-1 RNA (primer/template) complex. *Nucleic Acids Res.* **26**, 1198–1204.

Isel, C., Westhof, E., Massire, C., Le Grice, S. F. J., Ehresmann, B., Ehresmann, C., and Marquet, R. (1999). Structural basis for the specificity of the initiation of HIV-1 reverse transcription. *EMBO J.* **18**, 1038–1048.

Iwatani, Y., Rosen, A. E., Guo, J., Musier-Forsyth, K., and Levin, J. G. (2003). Efficient initiation of HIV-1 reverse transcription *in vitro*. Requirement for RNA sequences downstream of the primer binding site abrogated by nucleocapsid protein-dependent primer-template interactions. *J. Biol. Chem.* **278**, 14185–14195.

Javanbakht, H., Cen, S., Musier-Forsyth, K., and Kleiman, L. (2002). Correlation between tRNALys3 aminoacylation and its incorporation into HIV-1. *J. Biol. Chem.* **277**, 17389–17396.

Javanbakht, H., Halwani, R., Cen, S., Saadatmand, J., Musier-Forsyth, K., Gottlinger, H., and Kleiman, L. (2003). The Interaction between HIV-1 Gag and Human Lysyl-tRNA Synthetase during Viral Assembly. *J. Biol. Chem.* **278**, 27644–27651.

Jiang, M., Mak, J., Wainberg, M. A., Parniak, M. A., Cohen, E., and Kleiman, L. (1992). Variable tRNA content in HIV-1IIIB. *Biochem. Biophys. Res. Commun.* **185**, 1005–1015.

Jiang, M., Mak, J., Ladha, A., Cohen, E., Klein, M., Rovinski, B., and Kleiman, L. (1993). Identification of tRNAs incorporated into wild-type and mutant human immunodeficiency virus type 1. *J. Virol.* **67**, 3246–3253.

Jiang, M., Mak, J., Huang, Y., and Kleiman, L. (1994). Reverse transcriptase is an important factor for the primer tRNA selection in HIV-1. *Leukemia* **8**(Suppl. 1), S149–S151.

Kang, S.-M., Wakefield, J. K., and Morrow, C. D. (1996). Mutations in both the U5 region and the primer-binding site influence the selection of the tRNA used for the initiation of HIV-1 reverse transcription. *Virology* **222**, 401–414.

Kang, S.-M., Zhang, Z., and Morrow, C. D. (1999). Identification of a human immunodeficiency virus type 1 that stably uses tRNAlys1,2 rather than tRNAlys3 for initiation of reverse transcription. *Virology* **257**, 95–105.

Khorchid, A., Javannbakht, H., Wise, S., Halwani, R., Parniak, M. A., Wainberg, M. A., and Kleiman, L. (2000). Sequences within Pr160gag-pol affecting the selective packaging of primer tRNAlys3 into HIV-1. *J. Mol. Biol.* **299**, 17–26.

Kohlstaedt, L. A., and Steitz, T. A. (1992). Reverse transcriptase of human immuno-deficiency virus can use either human tRNA(3Lys) or *Escherichia coli* tRNA(2Gln) as a primer in an *in vitro* primer-utilization assay. *Proc. Natl. Acad. Sci. USA* **89**, 9652–9656.

Konstantinova, P., de Haan, P., Das, A. T., and Berkhout, B. (2006). Hairpin-induced tRNA-mediated (HITME) recombination in HIV-1. *Nucleic Acids Res.* **34**, 2206–2218.

Kovaleski, B. J., Kennedy, R., Hong, M. K., Datta, S. A., Kleiman, L., Rein, A., and Musier-Forsyth, K. (2006). *In vitro* characterization of the interaction between HIV-1 Gag and human lysyl-tRNA synthetase. *J. Biol. Chem.* **281**, 19449–19456.

Lanchy, J.-M., Isel, C., Keith, G., Le Grice, S. F. J., Ehresmann, C., and Marquet, R. (2000). Dynamics of the HIV-1 reverse transcription complex during initiation of DNA synthesis. *J. Biol. Chem.* **275**, 12306–12312.

Leis, J., Aiyar, A., and Cobrinik, D. (1993). Regulation of initiation of reverse transcription of retroviruses. *In* "Reverse Transcriptase" (A. M. Skalka and S. P. Goff, Eds.), pp. 33–48. Cold Spring Harbor Laboratory Press, Cold Spring Harbor.

Levin, J. G., and Seidman, J. G. (1981). Effect of polymerase mutations on packaging of primer tRNAPro during murine leukemia virus assembly. *J. Virol.* **38**, 403–408.

Levin, J. G., Guo, J., Rouzina, I., and Musier-Forsyth, K. (2005). Nucleic acid chaperone activity of HIV-1 nucleocapsid protein: Critical role in reverse transcription and molecular mechanism. *Prog. Nucleic Acid Res. Mol. Biol.* **80**, 217–286.

Li, X., Mak, J., Arts, E. J., Gu, Z., Kleiman, L., Wainberg, M. A., and Parniak, M. A. (1994). Effects of alterations of primer-binding site sequences on human immunodeficiency virus type 1 replication. *J. Virol.* **68**, 6198–6206.

Li, Y., Kang, S.-M., and Morrow, C. D. (1997a). Stability of HIV type 1 proviral genomes that contain two distinct primer-binding sites. *AIDS Res. Hum. Retroviruses* **13**, 253–262.

Li, Y., Zhang, Z., Kang, S.-M., Buescher, J. L., and Morrow, C. D. (1997b). Insights into the interaction between tRNA and primer binding site from characterization of a unique HIV-1 virus which stabley maintains dual PBS complementarity to tRNAGly and tRNAHis. *Virology* **238**, 273–282.

Li, Y., Zhang, Z., Wakefield, J. K., Kang, S.-M., and Morrow, C. D. (1997c). Nucleotide substitutions within U5 are critical for efficient reverse transcription of human immunodeficiency virus type 1 with a primer binding site complementary to tRNAHis. *J. Virol.* **71**, 6315–6322.

Liang, C., Li, X., Quan, Y., Laughrea, M., Kleiman, L., Hiscott, J., and Wainberg, M. A. (1997a). Sequence elements downstream of theb human immunodeficiency virus type 1 long terminal repeat are required for efficient viral gene transcription. *J. Mol. Biol.* **272**, 167–177.

Liang, C., Li, X., Rong, L., Inouye, P., Quan, Y., Kleiman, L., and Wainberg, M. A. (1997b). The importance of the A-rich loop in human immunodeficiency virus type 1 reverse transcription and infectivity. *J. Virol.* **71**, 5750–5757.

Liang, C., Rong, L., Morin, N., Cherry, E., Huang, Y., Kleiman, L., and Wainberg, M. A. (1997c). The roles of human immunodeficiency virus type 1 Pol protein and the primer binding site in the placement of primer tRNALys3 onto viral genomic RNA. *J. Virol.* **71**, 9075–9086.

Liang, C., Rong, L., Gotte, M., Li, X., Quan, Y., Kleiman, L., and Wainberg, M. A. (1998). Mechanistic studies of early pausing events during initiation of HIV-1 reverse transcription. *J. Biol. Chem.* **273**, 21309–21315.

Lightfoote, M. M., Coligan, J. E., Folks, T. M., Fauci, A. S., Martin, M. A., and Venkatesan, S. (1986). Structural characterization of reverse transcriptase and endonuclease polypep-tides of the acquired immunodeficiency syndrome retrovirus. *J. Virol.* **6016**, 771–775.

Litvak, S., and Araya, A. (1982). Primer transfer RNA in retroviruses. *TIBS* **7**, 361–364.

Lori, F., Veronese, F. D. M., De Vico, A. L., Lusso, P., Reitz, Jr.,M. S., and Gallo, R. C. (1992). Viral DNA carried by human immunodeficiency virus type 1 virions. *J. Virol.* **66**, 5067–5074.

Lund, A. H., Duch, M., Lovmand, J., Jorgensen, P., and Pedersen, F. S. (1993). Mutated primer binding sites interacting with different tRNAs allow efficient murine leukemia virus replication. *J. Virol.* **67**, 7125–7130.

Lund, A. H., Duch, M., and Pedersen, F. S. (2000). Selection of functional tRNA primers and primer binding site sequences from a retroviral combinatorial library: Identification of new functional tRNA primers in murine leukemia virus replication. *Nucleic Acids Res.* **28**, 791–799.

Mak, J., and Kleiman, L. (1997). Primer tRNAs for reverse transcription. *J. Virol.* **71**, 8087–8095.

Mak, J., Jiang, M., Wainberg, M. A., Hammarskjold, M. L., Rekosh, D., and Kleiman, L. (1994). Role of Pr160gag-pol in mediating the selective incorporation of tRNA(Lys) into human immunodeficiency virus type 1 particles. *J. Virol.* **68**, 2065–2072.

Marquet, R., Isel, C., Ehresmann, C., and Ehresmann, B. (1995). tRNAs as primer of reverse transcriptases. *Biochimie* **77**, 113–124.

Miller, J. T., Khvorova, A., Scaringe, S. A., and Le Grice, S. F. (2004). Synthetic tRNALys,3 as the replication primer for the HIV-1HXB2 and HIV-1Mal genomes. *Nucleic Acids Res.* **32**, 4687–4695.

Mishima, Y., and Steitz, J. A. (1995). Site-specific crosslinking of 4-thiouridine-modified human tRNALys3 to reverse transcriptase from human immunodeficiency virus type 1. *EMBO J.* **14**, 2679–2687.

Moore-Rigdon, K. L., Kosloff, B. R., Kirkman, R. L., and Morrow, C. D. (2005). Preferences for the selection of unique tRNA primers revealed from analysis of HIV-1 replication in peripheral blood mononuclear cells. *Retrovirology* **2**, 21–30.

Morris, S., Johnson, M., Stavnezer, E., and Leis, J. (2002). Replication of avian sarcoma virus *in vivo* requires an interaction between the viral RNA and the TpsiC loop of the tRNA (Trp) primer. *J. Virol.* **76**, 7571–7577.

Ooms, M., Cupac, D., Abbink, T. E. M., Huthoff, H., and Berkhout, B. (2007). The availability of the primer activation signal (PAS) affects the efficiency of HIV-1 reverse transcription initiation. *Nucleic Acids Res.* Advance Access Published February 18, 2007, doi: 10.1093/mol bev/msg013.

Oude Essink, B. B., Das, A. T., and Berkhout, B. (1995). Structural requirements for the binding of tRNA Lys3 to reverse transcriptase of the human immunodeficiency virus type 1. *J. Biol. Chem.* **270**, 23867–23874.

Oude Essink, B. B., Das, A. T., and Berkhout, B. (1996). HIV-1 reverse transcriptase discriminates against non-self tRNA primers. *J. Mol. Biol.* **264**, 243–254.

Peters, G. G., and Hu, J. (1980). Reverse transcriptase as the major determinant for selective packaging of tRNA's into avian sarcoma virus particles. *J. Virol.* **36**, 692–700.

Rhim, H., Park, J., and Morrow, C. D. (1991). Deletions in the tRNAlys primer-binding site of human immunodeficiency virus type 1 identify essential regions for reverse transcription. *J. Virol.* **65**, 4555–4564.

Richter-Cook, N. J., Howard, K. J., Cirino, N. M., Wohrl, B. M., and Le Grice, S. F. (1992). Interaction of tRNA(Lys-3) with multiple forms of human immunodeficiency virus reverse transcriptase. *J. Biol. Chem.* **267**, 15952–15957.

Rigourd, M., Bec, G., Benas, P., Le Grice, S. F., Ehresmann, B., Ehresmann, C., and Marquet, R. (2003). Effects of tRNA 3 Lys aminoacylation on the initiation of HIV-1 reverse transcription. *Biochimie* **85**, 521–525.

Robert, D., Sallafranque-Andreola, M. L., Bordier, B., Sarih-Cottin, L., Tarrago-Litvak, L., Graves, P. V., Barr, P. J., Fournier, M., and Litvak, S. (1990). Interactions with tRNA(Lys) induce important structural changes in human immunodeficiency virus reverse transcriptase. *FEBS Lett.* **277**, 239–242.

Rumbaugh, J. A., Fuentes, G. M., and Bambara, R. A. (1998). Processing of an HIV replication intermediate by the human DNA replication enzyme FEN1. *J. Biol. Chem.* **273**, 28740–28745.

Sarih-Cottin, L., Bordier, B., Musier-Forsyth, K., Andreola, M. L., Barr, P. J., and Litvak, S. (1992). Preferential interaction of human immunodeficiency virus reverse transcriptase with two regions of primer tRNA(Lys) as evidenced by footprinting studies and inhibition with synthetic oligoribonucleotides. *J. Mol. Biol.* **226**, 1–6.

Sawyer, R. C., and Dahlberg, J. E. (1973). Small RNAs of Rous sarcoma virus: Characterization by two-dimensional polyacrylamide gel electrophoresis and fingerprint analysis. *J. Virol.* **12**, 1226–1237.

Schwartzberg, P., Colicelli, J., and Goff, S. P. (1985). Recombination between a defective retrovirus and homologous sequences in host DNA: Reversion by patch repair. *J. Virol.* **53**, 719–726.

Sobol, R. W., Suhadolnik, R. J., Kumar, A., Lee, B. J., Hatfield, D. L., and Wilson, S. H. (1991). Localization of a polynucleotide binding region in the HIV-1 reverse transcriptase: Implications for primer binding. *Biochemistry* **30**, 10623–10631.

Sprinzl, M., Horn, C., Brown, M., Ioudovitch, A., and Steinberg, S. (1998). Compilation of tRNA sequences and sequences of tRNA genes. *Nucleic Acids Res.* **26**, 148–153.

Telesnitsky, A., and Goff, S. P. (1997). Reverse transcriptase and the generation of retroviral DNA. *In* "Retroviruses" (J. M. Coffin, S. H. Hughes, and H. E. Varmus, Eds.), pp. 121–160. Cold Spring Harbor Laboratory Press, Cold Spring Harbor.

Tisne, C., Roques, B. P., and Dardel, F. (2001). Heteronuclear NMR studies of the interaction of tRNA(Lys)3 with HIV-1 nucleocapsid protein. *J. Mol. Biol.* **306**, 443–454.

Trono, D. (1992). Partial reverse transcripts in virions from human immunodeficiency and murine leukemia viruses. *J. Virol.* **66**, 4893–4900.

Voronin, Y. A., and Pathak, V. K. (2004). Frequent dual initiation in human immunodeficiency virus-based vectors containing two primer-binding sites: A quantitative *in vivo* assay for function of initiation complexes. *J. Virol.* **78**, 5402–5413.

Wain-Hobson, S., Sonigo, P., Danos, O., Cole, S., and Alizon, M. (1985). Nucleotide sequence of the AIDS virus, LAV. *Cell* **40**, 9–17.

Wakefield, J. K., and Morrow, C. D. (1996). Mutations within the primer binding site of the human immunodeficiency virus type 1 define sequence requirements essential for reverse transcription. *Virology* **220**, 290–298.

Wakefield, J. K., Wolf, A. G., and Morrow, C. D. (1995). Human immunodeficiency virus type 1 can use different tRNAs as primers for reverse transcription but selectively maintains a primer binding site complementary to tRNALys3. *J. Virol.* **69**, 6021–6029.

Wakefield, J. K., Kang, S.-M., and Morrow, C. D. (1996). Construction of a type 1 human immunodeficiency virus that maintains a primer binding site complementary to tRNAHis. *J. Virol.* **70**, 966–975.

Wang, J., Dykes, C., Domoaal, R. A., Koval, C. E., Bambara, R. A., and Demeter, L. M. (2006). The HIV-1 reverse transcriptase mutants G190S and G190A, which confer resistance to non-nucleoside reverse transcriptase inhibitors, demonstrate reductions in RNase H activity and DNA synthesis from tRNA(Lys, 3) that correlate with reductions in replication efficiency. *Virology* **348**, 462–474.

Waters, L. C., and Mullin, B. C. (1977). Transfer RNA in RNA tumor viruses. *Prog. Nucleic Acid Res. Mol. Biol.* **20**, 131–160.

Wei, M., Cen, S., Niu, M., Guo, F., and Kleiman, L. (2005). Defective replication in human immunodeficiency virus type 1 when non-primers are used for reverse transcription. *J. Virol.* **79**, 9081–9087.

Wohrl, B. M., Ehresmann, B., Keith, G., and Le Grice, S. F. (1993). Nuclease footprinting of human immunodeficiency virus reverse transcriptase/tRNA(Lys-3) complexes. *J. Biol. Chem.* **268**, 13617–13624.

Wohrl, B. M., Tantillo, C., Arnold, E., and Le, G. S. (1995). An expanded model of replicating human immunodeficiency virus reverse transcriptase. *Biochemistry* **34**, 5343–5356.

Xu, W., and Morrow, C. D. (2006). The G490E mutation in reverse transcriptase does not impact tRNA primer selection by HIV-1 with altered PBS and A-loop. *Virology* **352**, 380–389.

Yuste, E., Borderia, A. V., Domingo, E., and Lopez-Galindez, C. (2005). Few mutations in the 5′ leader region mediate fitness recovery of debilitated human immunodeficiency type 1 viruses. *J. Virol.* **79**, 5421–5427.

Zhang, Z., Kang, S.-M., LeBlanc, A., Hajduk, S. L., and Morrow, C. D. (1996). Nucleotide sequences within the U5 region of the viral RNA genome are the major determinants for an human immunodeficiency virus type 1 to maintain a primer binding site complementary to tRNAHis. *Virology* **226**, 306–317.

Zhang, Z., Kang, S.-M., Li, Y., and Morrow, C. D. (1998). Genetic analysis of the U5-PBS of a novel HIV-1 reveals multiple interactions between the tRNA and RNA genome required for initiation of reverse transcription. *RNA* **4**, 394–406.

Anne Gatignol

Virus-Cell Interactions Laboratory, Lady Davis Institute for Medical Research, Department of Microbiology & Immunology and Experimental Medicine, McGill University, Montréal, Québec, Canada

Transcription of HIV: Tat and Cellular Chromatin

I. Chapter Overview

Human immunodeficiency virus type 1(HIV-1) provirus is integrated into the cellular chromatin and is structured in nucleosomes. The nucleosomes need to be unfolded to allow transcription to start. The initial nucleosome remodeling occurs by cellular events that activate chromatin-remodeling complexes. The HIV-1 transactivator, Tat, also recruits some of these factors to the promoter, including SWI/SNF, p300/CREB-binding protein (CBP), p300/CBP-associated factor (PCAF), and hGCN5. Tat binds to the positive transcription elongation factor b (P-TEFb), composed of Cyclin T1 (CycT1) and cyclin-dependent kinase 9 (CDK9), and the complex binds to the transactivation

Advances in Pharmacology, Volume 55
1054-3589/07 $35.00
DOI: 10.1016/S1054-3589(07)55004-0

response (TAR) RNA. Tat recruits the TATA-binding protein (TBP), TFIIB, and P-TEFb to the promoter to form an active preinitiation complex (PIC) in which CDK9 hyperphosphorylates the C-terminal domain (CTD) of the RNA polymerase II (RNAPII). This PIC is competent to trigger polymerase departure and active transcriptional elongation. Tat-recruited CDK9 also phosphorylates the DRB sensitivity-inducing factor (DSIF) and the negative elongation factor (NELF), which converts them from negative to positive factors in the elongation process. This activity is maintained from the transcription initiation to the end of the elongation process.

II. Introduction

The production of HIV-1 mRNA from the integrated provirus requires several steps that involve both cellular and viral proteins. The chromatin organized in nucleosomes is transcriptionally inactive and requires cellular events to trigger chromatin remodeling and transcription start. Once some HIV-1 mRNA is made, it is spliced and then exported to the cytoplasm where it is translated into Tat (transactivator of transcription), Rev, and Nef. Tat and Rev then go to the nucleus. Tat exerts its transactivating properties using the chromatin-modeling factors and specific mechanisms that influence both transcription initiation and elongation. As a consequence, the overall mechanism of transcription and transactivation by Tat occurs *in vivo* by sequential steps from chromatin remodeling to transcriptional elongation that requires the involvement of several cellular components.

III. Integrated HIV-1 LTR and Cellular Chromatin

A. Integrated HIV-1 LTR Is Organized in Nucleosomes

Nucleosomes are composed of a 146-bp DNA wrapped around a central histone octamer that constitutes the nucleosome core. Chromatin structure can be altered by chromatin-modifying complexes that facilitate nucleosome unfolding and allow transcription. Some complexes are ATP dependent and contain proteins with a helicase/ATPase domain like the SWI/SNF and the ISWI families. They are involved in nucleosome remodeling by altering histone–DNA interactions (Narlikar *et al.*, 2002; Varga-Weisz and Becker, 2006). Other complexes, composed of histone acetyltransferases (HATs) and histone deacetylases (HDACs), modify nucleosome structure by regulating histone acetylation (Verdone *et al.*, 2005).

After the HIV-1 integrates as DNA in the cellular chromatin, the provirus becomes organized in nucleosomal forms (Fig. 1). The position of nucleosomes in the 5′ LTR has been extensively studied and precisely defined

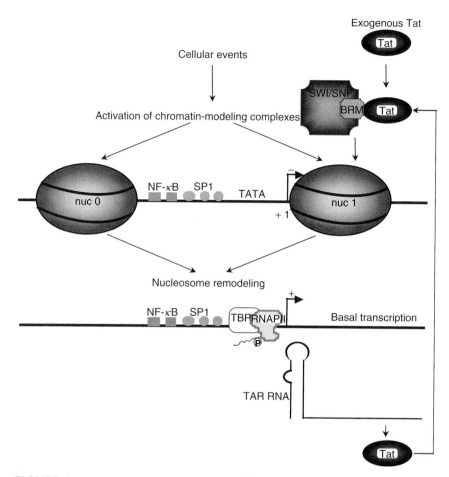

FIGURE 1 Promoter proximal region of the HIV-1 LTR integrated into the chromatin structure and initiation of basal transcription. Nucleosome names and positions are according to Sheridan *et al.* (1997) and Van Lint *et al.* (1996). +1 indicates the transcriptional start site. Cellular events for the initial transcription, or newly synthesized Tat, or exogenous Tat from other infected cells induce the recruitment of chromatin-modeling complexes that will disrupt the nucleosome structure and allow basal transcription.

by the determination of nuclease hypersensitive sites (el Kharroubi and Martin, 1996; el Kharroubi and Verdin, 1994; Pazin *et al.*, 1996; Sheridan *et al.*, 1995, 1997; Van Lint *et al.*, 1994, 1996; Verdin, 1991; Verdin *et al.*, 1993; Widlak *et al.*, 1997). Nucleosomes are barriers to transcription, and nucleosome 1 (nuc 1) of the integrated HIV-1 prevents the assembly of the transcription complex. Nucleosome remodeling by ATP-dependent and histone acetylation complexes triggers basal transcription from the HIV-1 promoter (Pumfery *et al.*, 2003; Quivy and Van Lint, 2002; Van Lint, 2000).

The promoter is then regulated by a large number of transcriptional activators that have access to their DNA-binding sites (Pereira *et al.*, 2000; Rohr *et al.*, 2003). Despite the activity of these factors, the basal transcriptional activity of HIV is very low and the viral transactivator Tat is needed to increase the transcription of the viral genome.

B. Cellular Complexes That Modify Chromatin Structure

The role of chromatin-modifying complexes is to disrupt the nucleosomal structure so that the DNA becomes more accessible to interacting proteins. These complexes belong to two main groups: the ATP-dependent remodeling complexes that alter histone–DNA interactions and proteins that regulate histone acetylation.

I. ATP-Dependent Chromatin-Remodeling Complexes

ATP-dependent chromatin-remodeling complexes consist of 2–12 subunits and their common feature is that they have an ATPase subunit. Subfamilies are defined according to sequences outside of their ATPase domain. In human cells, they are composed of the SWI/SNF, ISWI, and the NURD families. The SWI–SNF complexes, originally found in yeast, are represented by two related complexes in which the BRG1 and the hBRM are the ATPase subunits. Both proteins are involved in chromatin remodeling and muscle gene induction. BRG1 also acts as a tumor suppressor (Becker and Horz, 2002). The ISWI complex was found in *Drosophila*, and its mammalian homologue is SNFL2 in which SNF2h represents the ATPase subunit. ISWI-based complexes can assemble nucleosomes and are involved in heterochromatin replication and transcriptional repression (Fan *et al.*, 2003). The NURD complex combines an ATPase and an HDAC activity and one member, Mi-2, is a dermatomyositis-specific autoantigen (Becker and Horz, 2002). The first two complexes also contribute to higher-order chromatin structure (Varga-Weisz and Becker, 2006).

2. HATs and HDACs

Histone acetylation acts as an activation/repression switch in transcription by regulating DNA accessibility to regulatory proteins. HATs and HDACs catalyze the addition or removal of acetyl residues on lysines located at the N-terminal ends of histones (Gibbons, 2005; Verdone *et al.*, 2005; Yang, 2004). There are three main groups of HATs: the GNAT (Gcn5-related N-acetyltransferases), the p300/CBP, and the MYST families. In human cells, the GNAT includes hGCN5 and the PCAF proteins. Their C-terminal end has a bromodomain that recognizes acetyllysine residues. hGCN5 acetylates nucleosomal histones and is a transcriptional adaptor. PCAF interacts with p300 and CBP and functions as a coactivator in several processes such as myogenesis, nuclear receptor–mediated activation, and growth factor–signaled activation. p300 and CBP are highly homologous and are often referred to as p300/CBP. They stimulate transcription of many genes by interacting with transcription factors. The perturbation of the HAT activity of p300/CBP has been associated with several types of cancers. The MYST family includes several members involved in processes such as DNA replication, DNA repair, and apoptosis. Their dysregulation has been observed in leukemia and sarcoma associated with histone hyperacetylation. These HATs also function as factor acetyltransferases (FATs) by acetylating lysines of non-histone proteins including the HIV-1 transactivator Tat protein. Histone acetylation is reversible, and the removal of acetyl groups is accomplished by HDACs (Sengupta and Seto, 2004). HDACs are enzymes that catalyze the removal of acetyl groups from lysine residues in histone and non-histone proteins. By this activity, they mediate transcriptional repression and silencing. HDAC's hyperactivation is linked to tumorigenesis and cancer development, and HDAC inhibitors are potential anticancer agents (Dokmanovic and Marks, 2005).

C. HIV-1 LTR and Chromatin-Modeling Complexes

The integration of the HIV-1 DNA in human chromatin is not site specific, although it integrates preferentially within active transcription units, but the chromosomal environment influences the level of basal transcriptional activity (Jordan *et al.*, 2001; Lewinski *et al.*, 2005; Schroder *et al.*, 2002). When transcriptionally inactive, basal transcription of the HIV-1 promoter can be enhanced by cytokine activation or phorbol esters that remodel nucleosomes (Henderson *et al.*, 2004; Jordan *et al.*, 2003; Lusic *et al.*, 2003; Verdin *et al.*, 1993). Specifically, activation by phorbol myristate acetate (PMA) destabilizes nuc 1 of HIV-1. On PMA activation, ATF3 transcription factor binds to the AP1-binding site at the nucleosome boundary and then recruits of SWI/SNF (Henderson *et al.*, 2004). Following tetradecanoyl phorbol acetate (TPA) treatment, increased histone acetylation and recruitment of PCAF, CBP, and hGCN5 induced a higher accessibility of DNA in nuc 0, nuc 1, and nuc 2 (Lusic *et al.*, 2003). Therefore, chromatin-remodeling complexes act as a first step on the integrated provirus to destabilize the nucleosomal structure and allow basal transcription. After a threshold amount of RNA is produced, Tat is synthesized and will recruit more chromatin-remodeling factors.

D. Tat and ATP-Dependent Chromatin-Modeling Complexes

Recent data show that Tat also interacts with ATP-dependent chromatin-remodeling complexes. Tat immunoprecipitates with BRM and BRG-1, the ATPase parts of the SWI–SNF complex, and with INI-1 and β-actin from its core component (Agbottah *et al.*, 2006; Ariumi *et al.*, 2006;

Mahmoudi *et al.*, 2006; Treand *et al.*, 2006). Tat recruits these factors to the HIV-1 LTR as shown by chromatin immunoprecipitation (ChIP) that encompasses nuc 1 DNA sequence. These data suggest that Tat brings the SWI–SNF complex to the nucleosome to further increase its transactivating properties. Tat-mediated transactivation is reduced by decreasing BRM, BRG1, or INI-1 expression and enhanced by the overexpression of BRM or INI-1. The activity of these three factors is likely at different steps as BRM interacts only with nonacetylated Tat, whereas BRG-1 interacts only with acetylated Tat. INI-1 activated the LTR in synergy with Tat and p300, but not with a mutated Tat$_{K50,51R}$. The three factors contribute to the recruitment of the SWI–SNF complex to the HIV promoter, to the destabilization of nuc 1, and to the enhancement of HIV-1 transcription (Bukrinsky, 2006).

E. Tat and HAT

TIP60 was originally isolated as a Tat-interacting protein that increases HIV-1 LTR expression (Kamine *et al.*, 1996). It was shown later that it acetylates specific histones, belongs to the MYST family of HATs, and acts as a multifunctional enzyme (Sapountzi *et al.*, 2006; Yamamoto and Horikoshi, 1997). Tat modifies Tip60 activity on MnSOD and mediates its ubiquitination and degradation indicating that the viral protein interferes with cellular processes, but Tip60 does not modify Tat transactivation (Col *et al.*, 2005; Creaven *et al.*, 1999). The TBP-associated factor (TAFs) TAFII250 is also a HAT and binds Tat. This association mediates Tat repression of some promoters including MHC class I (Weissman *et al.*, 1998). Other HATs bind Tat, mediate its acetylation, and increase its transactivating activity on HIV-1 LTR. These are p300/CBP, PCAF, and hGCN5 (Benkirane *et al.*, 1998; Col *et al.*, 2001; Hottiger and Nabel, 1998; Marzio *et al.*, 1998).

IV. The HIV-1 Tat Protein and Its Modifications _____

A. The Tat Protein

The HIV-1 transactivator Tat is a 14-kDa protein encoded by two exons (Fig. 2). Exon 1 encodes amino acids 1–72 and exon 2 encodes amino acids 73–86 or 73–101 depending on the virus strains. Tat can be divided into five domains: domain I (aa 1–20) is located in the N-terminus; mutations in this region do not modify transactivation to a large extent. Domain II has seven highly conserved cysteins, which are important for Tat function. Domain III (aa 40–48) or "core" is essential for transactivation; in this region a single change at K41 abolishes Tat activity. Domain IV (aa 49–72) contains an arginine-rich stretch, which mediates RNA binding and nuclear localization. The first three domains (aa 1–48) represent the activation domain of Tat that

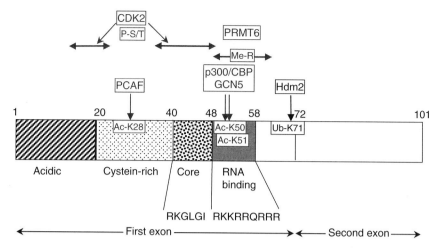

FIGURE 2 Tat structure and its modifications. Tat domains and important amino acids are indicated. Acetylation is mediated by PCAF and p300/CBP and GCN5, phosphorylation by CDK2, methylation by PRMT6, and ubiquitylation by Hdm2 as indicated. When the precise modified amino acid is not known, a horizontal arrow indicates the region where the modification occurs.

functions as a transactivator when linked to region IV or to a heterologous RNA/DNA-binding domain. Tat 66 is sufficient to mediate full transactivation (Kuppuswamy *et al.*, 1989). Domain V, encoded by the second exon contributes to viral infectivity and to other Tat functions (Gatignol and Jeang, 2000; Rana and Jeang, 1999). In contrast to other known transactivators, Tat acts through an RNA target called TAR located in the R region of the LTR. For its function, Tat recruits a cellular kinase that phosphorylates the CTD of the RNAPII, which triggers polymerase departure, promoter clearance, and efficient elongation (Bannwarth and Gatignol, 2005; Barboric and Peterlin, 2005; Brady and Kashanchi, 2005; Brigati *et al.*, 2003; Hetzer *et al.*, 2005). In Tat-mediated transactivation of HIV-1 promoter, the recruitment of cellular proteins and the posttranslational modification of Tat by various enzymes are crucial for its function.

B. Tat-Binding Proteins

Many Tat-binding proteins have been isolated and characterized for their role in Tat-mediated transactivation. The interaction between Tat and the TBP (Kashanchi *et al.*, 1994; Veschambre *et al.*, 1995), TFIIB (Veschambre *et al.*, 1997), TFIIH (Cujec *et al.*, 1997; Garcia-Martinez *et al.*, 1997b), Sp1 (Chun *et al.*, 1998; Jeang *et al.*, 1993; Pagtakhan and Tong-Starksen, 1997), and TAF55 (Chiang and Roeder, 1995) suggest a direct involvement of Tat in the early steps of transactivation during the formation of the PIC.

The best-characterized factor that binds Tat is the P-TEFb that was first characterized as a Tat-associated kinase (TAK; Gold *et al.*, 1998; Herrmann and Rice, 1993, 1995; Mancebo *et al.*, 1997; Yang *et al.*, 1996, 1997; Zhu *et al.*, 1997). P-TEFb is a complex composed of a Cyclin T and the CDK9 (Peng *et al.*, 1998; Price, 2000; Wei *et al.*, 1998). Tat interacts very strongly with CycT1 but not with CDK9. In contrast, CycT1 interacts with both Tat and CDK9 to form the active complex Tat–CycT1–CDK9 (Battisti *et al.*, 2003; Bieniasz *et al.*, 1998; Garber *et al.*, 1998; Wei *et al.*, 1998).

In the absence of Tat, P-TEFb exists in the cell as a large inactive complex composed of 7SK snRNA and MAQ1/HEXIM1 proteins (Michels *et al.*, 2003; Yik *et al.*, 2003). When recruited to a promoter, P-TEFb phosphorylates serines of the RNAPII CTD, the SPT5 subunit of DSIF, and the RD subunit of NELF resulting in the hyperphosphorylation of the RNAPII CTD throughout the transcriptional elongation (Fujinaga *et al.*, 2004; Ivanov *et al.*, 2000).

C. Tat Modifications

1. Tat Acetylation

Tat binding to TAR RNA and its release is regulated by its acetylation by HATs. PCAF acetylates Tat at K28 (Kiernan *et al.*, 1999), but this acetylation releases PCAF from Tat (Bres *et al.*, 2002b). p300/CBP and hGCN5 acetylate Tat at K50 and K51 (Col *et al.*, 2001; Deng *et al.*, 2000; Kaehlcke *et al.*, 2003; Kiernan *et al.*, 1999; Ott *et al.*, 1999). In addition, the bromo-domain of PCAF binds specifically to Ac50Tat and requires Y47 and R53 in Tat (Dorr *et al.*, 2002; Mujtaba *et al.*, 2002). Ac28Tat has an increased affinity for CycT1-CDK9, which enhances the binding of the Tat–P-TEFb complex to TAR RNA (Bres *et al.*, 2002a; Kiernan *et al.*, 1999). In contrast, Ac50Tat or the Ac50Tat–CycT1 complex shows a decreased TAR affinity suggesting a release of Tat–P-TEFb complex from TAR (Bres *et al.*, 2002b; Deng *et al.*, 2000; Kaehlcke *et al.*, 2003; Kiernan *et al.*, 1999).

Tat can also be deacetylated by the activity of the HDAC Sirtuin 1 (Pagans *et al.*, 2005). Evidence that Tat acetylation is important for trans-activation comes from treatment with deacetylase inhibitors that synergize with Tat function and mutations in either K28 or K50 that decrease Tat transactivation and HIV replication (Bres *et al.*, 2002a; Deng *et al.*, 2000; Kiernan *et al.*, 1999; Ott *et al.*, 1999; Roof *et al.*, 2002).

2. Tat Phosphorylation

Tat from HIV-2 but not from HIV-1 is phosphorylated by CDK9 (Herrmann and Rice, 1993) that becomes autophosphorylated upon Tat binding. CDK9 phosphorylation enhances Tat-CycT-CDK9 binding to

TAR RNA (Garber *et al.*, 2000). In contrast, a study shows that CDK2 associated with Cyclin E phosphorylates Tat. Although the precise location of the phosphorylation site is not determined, it requires amino acids 15–24 and 36–49. A decreased CDK2 expression decreases HIV-1 transcription and virus production (Ammosova *et al.*, 2005; Deng *et al.*, 2002). Tat binds to the interferon-induced protein kinase R (PKR) and inhibits its function as a competitive substrate. In turn, Tat is phosphorylated on S62, T64, and S68 by PKR. The mutations in these sites decrease Tat-TAR binding and transactivation of HIV-1 LTR (Brand *et al.*, 1997; Cai *et al.*, 2000; Endo-Munoz *et al.*, 2005; McMillan *et al.*, 1995). Mutational analyses and decreased expression of the kinases suggest a functional importance of the Tat phosphorylation (Ammosova *et al.*, 2005; Endo-Munoz *et al.*, 2005).

3. Tat Methylation

Arginine methylation by protein arginine methyltransferases (PRMTs) regulates several pathways including gene expression (Bedford and Richard, 2005). PRMT6 interacts with and methylates HIV-1 Tat. This methylation occurs in the region between amino acids 49 and 63, which contains 6 arginines. Overexpression of PRMT6 decreases the Tat-mediated transactivated level of HIV-1 LTR, whereas decreased expression of the enzyme increases viral production, suggesting that the methylation of Tat inhibits its activity (Boulanger *et al.*, 2005).

4. Tat Ubiquitination

A ubiquitin-protein ligase, the proto-oncoprotein Hdm2, binds to Tat and mediates its ubiquitination on Lys71. However, this modification does not target Tat to the proteasome for degradation but rather enhances Tat-mediated transactivation (Bres *et al.*, 2003).

The different modifications described above, all have a functional importance in Tat function to different extent. Because Tat truncated to 66 amino acids keeps all of its transactivating activity (Kuppuswamy *et al.*, 1989), modifications in the C-terminal end likely affect transactivation marginally or indirectly but influence primarily other Tat functions. Further studies on these modifications in the various Tat functions will help to elucidate their specific role, but some have already been implicated precisely in the *in vivo* Tat-mediated transactivation steps.

V. Tat-Mediated Transactivation

A dynamic *in vivo* model for Tat-mediated transactivation must include data from transcriptional repression of the chromatinized HIV-1 LTR up to the end of transcriptional elongation and the role of Tat at each step.

A. Initial Production of HIV-1 mRNA

After its entry into the cell, the HIV-1 RNA is reverse transcribed to form DNA that moves to the nucleus *via* the preintegration complex and becomes integrated into the cellular chromatin (Bukrinsky and Haffar, 1999). The integrated HIV-1 LTR is transcriptionally inactive due to the formation of nucleosomes as shown in the proximal promoter (Fig. 1). Nucleosome unfolding is a prerequisite to any transcriptional initiation and this mechanism is accomplished by chromatin-remodeling complexes that modify histone–DNA interactions. These complexes are either activated by cytokines, by chemokines, by various cellular events, or can be recruited by the viral Tat protein after its production (Copeland, 2005; Pumfery *et al.*, 2003). If this first step was to be achieved by Tat, Tat would have to be incorporated into the virus particle, liberated into the cytoplasm, and targeted to the nucleus to exert its activity. Thus far, the Tat protein has been neither observed in the virion (Ott, 1997) nor in the preintegration complex (Bukrinsky and Haffar, 1999), and we have no evidence of its activity during the early steps of HIV replication. Recent data that detect a Tat peptide into the HIV-1 virion (Chertova *et al.*, 2006) may change this view, but awaits studies that would quantify and analyze the functional relevance of this finding. Therefore, it is likely that the initial formation of an open chromatin in the HIV-1 LTR region will be mediated by intra- or extracellular events such as cytokine activation or signal transduction pathways that will activate nucleosome modeling complexes to decrease histone–DNA interactions and activate transcription. These events will trigger transcriptional initiation and the formation of some mRNAs that start with TAR RNA (Copeland, 2005; Pumfery *et al.*, 2003). Some Tat protein will then be produced and will move to the nucleus. It will exert its function on chromatin-modifying complexes and its transactivating properties in the nucleus.

B. Tat Activity on Chromatin-Modifying Complexes

The following steps in Tat activity are exerted either by the newly synthesized Tat or by secreted Tat that has entered a new cell (Noonan and Albini, 2000). Unmodified Tat binds to BRM, the ATPase subunit of the SWI–SNF complex, and the complex contributes to nuc 1 remodeling and promoter activation (Treand *et al.*, 2006). The acetylation of Tat on K50 prevents Tat-BRM binding suggesting an activity before the association between Tat and p300/CBP and hGCN5. It is not known if this recruitment occurs independently from TAR or when Tat is bound to TAR or to CycT1. Considering that nuc 1 encompasses the DNA sequence encoding TAR, if the DNA is completely structured in nucleosomes, no TAR will be present, but if a small part of the chromatin is uncompacted, some TAR-Tat may help bring the complex in the vicinity of nuc 1. Nuc 1 remodeling favors DNA accessibility to the transcription complex.

C. Formation of the TAR RNA–Tat–CycT1–CDK9 Complex

Tat binding to TAR RNA and its release is highly regulated by Tat modifications and its affinity to CycT1-CDK9 (Fig. 3). The newly formed Tat binds PCAF, which generates Ac28Tat that has an increased affinity for CycT1 already bound to CDK9. Tat may co-opt P-TEFb from its inactive storage in 7SK snRNA-MAQ1/HEXIM1 or bind to the free form of P-TEFb present in the cytoplasm. Tat bound to SWI-SNF may also bind P-TEFb to bring the protein modeling complex in proximity to nuc 1. PCAF has a decreased affinity for Ac28Tat, which will induce the dissociation of the complex (Bres *et al.*, 2002b; Kiernan *et al.*, 1999). The Ac28Tat–CycT1–CDK9 complex has an increased affinity for TAR and binds to the low amount of nascent TAR RNA present in the cell. Due to their affinity with Tat, p300/CBP and hGCN5 are recruited at this site and acetylate Tat at K50 and K51 (Col *et al.*, 2001; Deng *et al.*, 2000; Kiernan *et al.*, 1999; Ott *et al.*, 1999). Because Ac50Tat has a decreased affinity for TAR, the p300/CBP-Ac50Tat-P-TEFb is then released from TAR and transferred to the next PIC on the promoter (Bres *et al.*, 2002b; Kaehlcke *et al.*, 2003). It is possible that this dissociation from TAR will also favor a transfer of Tat-SWI/SNF to nuc 1 to open the chromatin (Treand *et al.*, 2006). Some models, mainly based on *in vitro* studies, favor a transfer of Tat–CycT1–CDK9 complex from TAR to the paused elongating complex after TAR (Barboric and Peterlin, 2005; Hetzer *et al.*, 2005; Karn, 1999), but recent data analyzing the factors recruited *in vivo* by Tat at the promoter can only be explained by a transfer of the Tat–CycT1–CDK9 complex from TAR to the transcriptional PIC (Bannwarth and Gatignol, 2005; Brady and Kashanchi, 2005; Lusic *et al.*, 2003; Raha *et al.*, 2005).

D. Tat Activity in the PIC

The role of Tat in the PIC has been deduced from early studies and substantiated by recent studies of *in vivo* models (Bannwarth and Gatignol, 2005; Brady and Kashanchi, 2005; Brigati *et al.*, 2003; Bukrinsky, 2006; Pumfery *et al.*, 2003). Early studies have shown that Tat binds to TBP (Kashanchi *et al.*, 1994; Veschambre *et al.*, 1995), TFIIB (Veschambre *et al.*, 1997), and TAF55 (Chiang and Roeder, 1995), which are part of the PIC (Dahmus, 1996). A direct interaction with TFIIH has also been described (Cujec *et al.*, 1997; Garcia-Martinez *et al.*, 1997b), but not found by others (Battisti *et al.*, 2003; Chen and Zhou, 1999). Kinetic assays show a

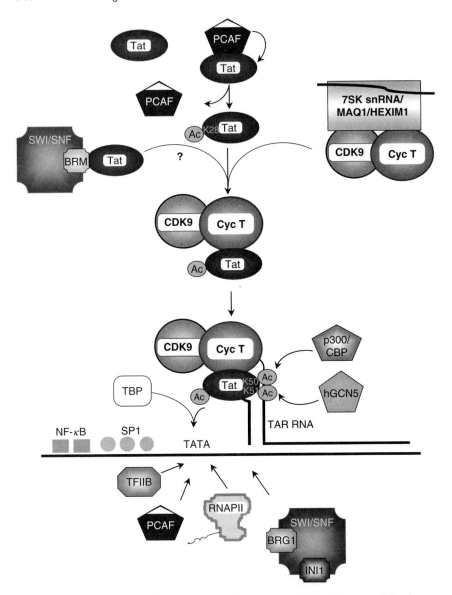

FIGURE 3 Recruitment of the components of a competent PIC by Tat and cellular factors. Tat acetylated in K28 by PCAF binds strongly to CycT-CDK9, and the complex has increased affinity for TAR RNA. Acetylation of Tat by p300/CBP and hGCN5 at K50 and K51 releases the complex from TAR, which contributes to the recruitment of TBP, TFIIB, PCAF, RNAPII, and SWI/SNF at the initiation site.

rapid action of Tat before TAR is made (Jeang and Berkhout, 1992), and functional assays indicate that Sp1 and NF-κB enhance transactivation (Chun *et al.*, 1998; Demarchi *et al.*, 1996, 1999; Jeang *et al.*, 1993; Kamine and Chinnadurai, 1992; Kamine *et al.*, 1991; Liu *et al.*, 1992; Yedavalli *et al.*, 2003).

Several data have shown that the Tat and the P-TEFb complex are present in both the PIC and in the transcription elongation complex (TEC; Garcia-Martinez *et al.*, 1997a; Isel and Karn, 1999; Keen *et al.*, 1996; Ping and Rana, 1999; Zhou *et al.*, 2000). ChIP experiments have shown that Ac50Tat (Kaehlcke *et al.*, 2003) or Ac50/51Tat (Agbottah *et al.*, 2006), but not unacetylated Tat is associated with the HIV-1 promoter *in vivo*, which is in favor of its transfer from TAR to the PIC after acetylation by p300/CBP. Additional ChIP experiments show that p300, CBP, NF-κB p65, and PCAF are recruited early to the HIV-1 promoter upon Tat activation *in vivo* (Lusic *et al.*, 2003; Marzio *et al.*, 1998). When the recruitment of general transcription factors to the promoter was analyzed by ChIP, Tat recruited TBP and TFIIB, but not TFIID as none of the TAFs were detected on the promoter. CycT1 or CDK9 showed the same activity indicating that activators that function via P-TEFb promote the assembly of a transcription complex with TBP and not TFIID (Raha *et al.*, 2005). Consistent with the binding of Ac50Tat to its BRG1 or INI1 subunit (Agbottah *et al.*, 2006; Ariumi *et al.*, 2006; Mahmoudi *et al.*, 2006), SWI/SNF is also recruited by Tat to the chromatin region that encompasses the promoter and nuc 1 (Agbottah *et al.*, 2006). Overall, these data indicate that Tat–CycT1–CDK9 complex bound to TAR recruits TBP and TFIIB for the assembly of the PIC, as well as HATs and SWI/SNF for histone-DNA dissociation (Fig. 4A). Nuc 1 remodeling allows progression of an elongation competent transcription complex.

E. Tat Activity in the Elongation Complex

Tat activity in the elongation complex has been clarified during the last years and is mediated by the activity of Tat-recruited P-TEFb (Bannwarth and Gatignol, 2005; Barboric and Peterlin, 2005; Hetzer *et al.*, 2005). Because no *in vivo* direct evidence of a stalled RNAPII in the absence of Tat has been observed by ChIP, it is very likely that Tat activity on transcriptional elongation is a direct consequence of the formation of a highly competent PIC by the recruitment of Tat-P-TEFb (Raha *et al.*, 2005). The PIC first recruits TFIIH, whose kinase CDK7 hypophosphorylates the RNAPII CTD on Ser5. This step is independent of Tat and will allow the polymerase to synthesize ~15 nt. A coordinated activity between CDK7, released after 14–36 nt and CDK9 brought on the PIC by Tat leads to the hyperphosphorylation of the RNAPII CTD on Ser2 and Ser5 and triggers polymerase departure (Isel and Karn, 1999; Karn, 1999; Zhou *et al.*, 2000, 2001).

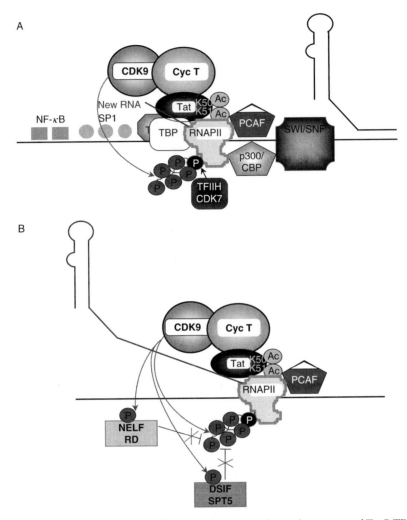

FIGURE 4 Active progression of the transcription complex in the presence of Tat-P-TEFb. (A) Formation of a competent PIC at the HIV promoter. Cellular factors recruited by Tat to the HIV-1 promoter form an active PIC. The complex initiates the transcription of ~15-nt RNA. The phosphorylation of the RNAPII CTD by CDK9 triggers polymerase departure and effective transcription elongation. (B) Transcription elongation complex. The phosphorylation of the RNAPII CTD, NELF, and DSIF by CDK9 is maintained throughout the elongation process.

The RNAPII CTD phosphorylation as well as multiple phosphorylations will be maintained throughout the elongation process by the activity of CDK9 in the Tat–P-TEFb complex (Fig. 4B).

Transcriptional elongation is inhibited by the activity of NELF and by the DSIF that prevents the phosphorylation of the RNAPII CTD. In human,

DSIF is composed of SPT4 and SPT5, whereas NELF is a complex containing five subunits (NELF-A to E) in which NELF-E (also called RD) is an RNA-binding protein (Wada *et al.*, 1998a; Yamaguchi *et al.*, 1999, 2002; Zorio and Bentley, 2001). This inhibition does not affect the RNAPII whose CTD has been hyperphosphorylated by P-TEFb, indicating that the primary function of CDK9 in P-TEFb is to alleviate the negative effects of DSIF and NELF (Wada *et al.*, 1998b; Yamaguchi *et al.*, 1999; Zorio and Bentley, 2001).

The recruitment of P-TEFb by Tat to the PIC promotes the hyperphosphorylation of the RNAPII CTD by CDK9, therefore preventing DSIF and NELF to act against an effective transcription elongation (Kim *et al.*, 2002; Zhou *et al.*, 2000). SPT5 also functions as positive regulator of transcriptional elongation in the context of Tat-mediated transactivation of HIV-1 (Bourgeois *et al.*, 2002; Ivanov *et al.*, 2000; Wu-Baer *et al.*, 1998). SPT5 is phosphorylated by CDK9 during elongation and this mechanism transforms its negative activity into a positive function (Ping and Rana, 2001). SPT5 is also methylated by PRMT1 and PRMT5, but this modification can either enhance or repress HIV-1 gene expression by changing SPT5 association with RNAPII (Kwak *et al.*, 2003).

NELF represses transcription by binding to DSIF–RNAPII complex and RNA (Yamaguchi *et al.*, 2002). The RD/NELF-E subunit of NELF is also phosphorylated by CDK9, which modifies its RNA-binding properties and prevents its repressive activity (Fujinaga *et al.*, 2004). These SPT5 and NELF modifications by CDK9 mediate a switch between transcriptional repression and activation, further enhancing CDK9 activity on the RNAPII CTD phosphorylation (Fujinaga *et al.*, 2004; Kwak *et al.*, 2003; Yamada *et al.*, 2006). This role is confirmed by studies with small interfering (si)RNAs against CDK9 and SPT5, which show that they are required for Tat transactivation and HIV-1 replication (Chiu *et al.*, 2004; Ping *et al.*, 2004). Further studies will help to fully understand their temporal activity in the regulation of HIV transcriptional elongation.

V. Conclusions

The molecular mechanisms leading to active transcription of the HIV-1 integrated DNA have been elucidated in large part. Tat contributes to various steps from chromatin remodeling to the end of transcriptional elongation by the recruitment of a large number of cellular factors. Some discrepancies still remain between the various investigators, who favor more transcriptional initiation or elongation depending on the experimental assays, but the *in vivo* model now reaches a consensus. All studies have contributed to the elucidation of the different *in vivo* steps of transcription and transactivation with Tat recruiting specific factors at each step. Future studies will continue to decipher these complex interactions between the virus and its host.

Acknowledgments _____

The author thanks Dr. Andrew J. Mouland for comments on this chapter. I also thank the members of my laboratory for helpful discussions. The work done in the Gatignol laboratory is supported by the Canadian Institutes of Health Research (CIHR) and the Canadian Foundation for Innovation. The author is the recipient of a Hugh and Helen McPherson Memorial Award.

References _____

Agbottah, E., Deng, L., Dannenberg, L. O., Pumfery, A., and Kashanchi, F. (2006). Effect of SWI/SNF chromatin remodeling complex on HIV-1 Tat activated transcription. *Retrovirology* **3**, 48.

Ammosova, T., Berro, R., Kashanchi, F., and Nekhai, S. (2005). RNA interference directed to CDK2 inhibits HIV-1 transcription. *Virology* **341**, 171–178.

Ariumi, Y., Serhan, F., Turelli, P., Telenti, A., and Trono, D. (2006). The integrase interactor 1 (INI1) proteins facilitate Tat-mediated human immunodeficiency virus type 1 transcription. *Retrovirology* **3**, 47.

Bannwarth, S., and Gatignol, A. (2005). HIV-1 TAR RNA: The target of molecular interactions between the virus and its host. *Curr. HIV Res.* **3**, 61–71.

Barboric, M., and Peterlin, B. M. (2005). A new paradigm in eukaryotic biology: HIV Tat and the control of transcriptional elongation. *PLoS Biol.* **3**, e76.

Battisti, P.-L., Daher, A., Bannwarth, S., Voortman, J., Peden, K. W. C., Hiscott, J., Mouland, A. J., Benarous, R., and Gatignol, A. (2003). Additive activity between the trans-activation response RNA-binding protein, TRBP2, and cyclin T1 on HIV type 1 expression and viral production in murine cells. *AIDS Res. Hum. Retroviruses* **19**, 767–778.

Becker, P. B., and Horz, W. (2002). ATP-dependent nucleosome remodeling. *Annu. Rev. Biochem.* **71**, 247–273.

Bedford, M. T., and Richard, S. (2005). Arginine methylation an emerging regulator of protein function. *Mol. Cell* **18**, 263–272.

Benkirane, M., Chun, R. F., Xiao, H., Ogryzko, V. V., Howard, B. H., Nakatani, Y., and Jeang, K. T. (1998). Activation of integrated provirus requires histone acetyltransferase. p300 and P/CAF are coactivators for HIV-1 Tat. *J. Biol. Chem.* **273**, 24898–24905.

Bieniasz, P. D., Grdina, T. A., Bogerd, H. P., and Cullen, B. R. (1998). Recruitment of a protein complex containing Tat and cyclin T1 to TAR governs the species specificity of HIV-1 Tat. *EMBO J.* **17**, 7056–7065.

Boulanger, M. C., Liang, C., Russell, R. S., Lin, R., Bedford, M. T., Wainberg, M. A., and Richard, S. (2005). Methylation of Tat by PRMT6 regulates human immunodeficiency virus type 1 gene expression. *J. Virol.* **79**, 124–131.

Bourgeois, C. F., Kim, Y. K., Churcher, M. J., West, M. J., and Karn, J. (2002). Spt5 cooperates with human immunodeficiency virus type 1 Tat by preventing premature RNA release at terminator sequences. *Mol. Cell. Biol.* **22**, 1079–1093.

Brady, J., and Kashanchi, F. (2005). Tat gets the "green" light on transcription initiation. *Retrovirology* **2**, 69.

Brand, S. R., Kobayashi, R., and Mathews, M. B. (1997). The Tat protein of human immunodeficiency virus type 1 is a substrate and inhibitor of the interferon-induced, virally activated protein kinase, PKR. *J. Biol. Chem.* **272**, 8388–8395.

Bres, V., Kiernan, R., Emiliani, S., and Benkirane, M. (2002a). Tat acetyl-acceptor lysines are important for human immunodeficiency virus type-1 replication. *J. Biol. Chem.* **277**, 22215–22221.

Bres, V., Tagami, H., Peloponese, J. M., Loret, E., Jeang, K. T., Nakatani, Y., Emiliani, S., Benkirane, M., and Kiernan, R. E. (2002b). Differential acetylation of Tat coordinates its interaction with the co-activators cyclin T1 and PCAF. *EMBO J.* **21**, 6811–6819.

Bres, V., Kiernan, R. E., Linares, L. K., Chable-Bessia, C., Plechakova, O., Treand, C., Emiliani, S., Peloponese, J. M., Jeang, K. T., Coux, O., Scheffner, M., and Benkirane, M. (2003). A non-proteolytic role for ubiquitin in Tat-mediated transactivation of the HIV-1 promoter. *Nat. Cell Biol.* **5**, 754–761.

Brigati, C., Giacca, M., Noonan, D. M., and Albini, A. (2003). HIV Tat, its TARgets and the control of viral gene expression. *FEMS Microbiol. Lett.* **220**, 57–65.

Bukrinsky, M. (2006). SNFing HIV transcription. *Retrovirology* **3**, 49.

Bukrinsky, M. I., and Haffar, O. K. (1999). HIV-1 nuclear import: In search of a leader. *Front. Biosci.* **4**, D772–D781.

Cai, R., Carpick, B., Chun, R. F., Jeang, K.-T., and Williams, B.R (2000). HIV-I TAT inhibits PKR activity by both RNA-dependent and RNA-independent mechanisms. *Arch. Biochem. Biophys.* **373**, 361–367.

Chen, D., and Zhou, Q. (1999). Tat activates human immunodeficiency virus type 1 transcriptional elongation independent of TFIIH kinase. *Mol. Cell. Biol.* **19**, 2863–2871.

Chertova, E., Chertov, O., Coren, L. V., Roser, J. D., Trubey, C. M., Bess, J. W., Jr., Sowder, R. C., II, Barsov, E., Hood, B. L., Fisher, R. J., Nagashima, K., Conrads, T. P., *et al.* (2006). Proteomic and biochemical analysis of purified human immunodeficiency virus type 1 produced from infected monocyte-derived macrophages. *J. Virol.* **80**, 9039–9052.

Chiang, C. M., and Roeder, R. G. (1995). Cloning of an intrinsic human TFIID subunit that interacts with multiple transcriptional activators. *Science* **267**, 531–536.

Chiu, Y. L., Cao, H., Jacque, J. M., Stevenson, M., and Rana, T. M. (2004). Inhibition of human immunodeficiency virus type 1 replication by RNA interference directed against human transcription elongation factor P-TEFb (CDK9/CyclinT1). *J. Virol.* **78**, 2517–2529.

Chun, R. F., Semmes, O. J., Neuveut, C., and Jeang, K.-T. (1998). Modulation of Sp1 phosphorylation by human immunodeficiency virus type 1 Tat. *J. Virol.* **72**, 2615–2629.

Col, E., Caron, C., Seigneurin-Berny, D., Gracia, J., Favier, A., and Khochbin, S. (2001). The histone acetyltransferase, hGCN5, interacts with and acetylates the HIV transactivator, Tat. *J. Biol. Chem.* **276**, 28179–28184.

Col, E., Caron, C., Chable-Bessia, C., Legube, G., Gazzeri, S., Komatsu, Y., Yoshida, M., Benkirane, M., Trouche, D., and Khochbin, S. (2005). HIV-1 Tat targets Tip60 to impair the apoptotic cell response to genotoxic stresses. *EMBO J.* **24**, 2634–2645.

Copeland, K. F. (2005). Modulation of HIV-1 transcription by cytokines and chemokines. *Mini. Rev. Med. Chem.* **5**, 1093–1101.

Creaven, M., Hans, F., Mutskov, V., Col, E., Caron, C., Dimitrov, S., and Khochbin, S. (1999). Control of the histone-acetyltransferase activity of Tip60 by the HIV-1 transactivator protein, Tat. *Biochemistry* **38**, 8826–8830.

Cujec, T. P., Okamoto, H., Fujinaga, K., Meyer, J., Chamberlin, H., Morgan, D. O., and Peterlin, B. M. (1997). The HIV transactivator TAT binds to the CDK-activating kinase and activates the phosphorylation of the carboxy-terminal domain of RNA polymerase II. *Genes Dev.* **11**, 2645–2657.

Dahmus, M. E. (1996). Reversible phosphorylation of the C-terminal domain of RNA polymerase II. *J. Biol. Chem.* **271**, 19009–19012.

Demarchi, F., d'Adda di Fagagna, F., Falaschi, A., and Giacca, M. (1996). Activation of transcription factor NF-kappaB by the Tat protein of human immunodeficiency virus type 1. *J. Virol.* **70**, 4427–4437.

Demarchi, F., Gutierrez, M. I., and Giacca, M. (1999). Human immunodeficiency virus type 1 tat protein activates transcription factor NF-kappaB through the cellular interferon-inducible, double-stranded RNA-dependent protein kinase, PKR. *J. Virol.* **73**, 7080–7086.

Deng, L., de la Fuente, C., Fu, P., Wang, L., Donnelly, R., Wade, J. D., Lambert, P., Li, H., Lee, C. G., and Kashanchi, F. (2000). Acetylation of HIV-1 Tat by CBP/P300 increases transcription of integrated HIV-1 genome and enhances binding to core histones. *Virology* 277, 278–295.

Deng, L., Ammosova, T., Pumfery, A., Kashanchi, F., and Nekhai, S. (2002). HIV-1 Tat interaction with RNA polymerase II C-terminal domain (CTD) and a dynamic association with CDK2 induce CTD phosphorylation and transcription from HIV-1 promoter. *J. Biol. Chem.* 277, 33922–33929.

Dokmanovic, M., and Marks, P. A. (2005). Prospects: Histone deacetylase inhibitors. *J. Cell. Biochem.* 96, 293–304.

Dorr, A., Kiermer, V., Pedal, A., Rackwitz, H. R., Henklein, P., Schubert, U., Zhou, M. M., Verdin, E., and Ott, M. (2002). Transcriptional synergy between Tat and PCAF is dependent on the binding of acetylated Tat to the PCAF bromodomain. *EMBO J.* 21, 2715–2723.

el Kharroubi, A., and Martin, M. A. (1996). cis-acting sequences located downstream of the human immunodeficiency virus type 1 promoter affect its chromatin structure and transcriptional activity. *Mol. Cell. Biol.* 16, 2958–2966.

el Kharroubi, A., and Verdin, E. (1994). Protein-DNA interactions within DNase I-hypersensitive sites located downstream of the HIV-1 promoter. *J. Biol. Chem.* 269, 19916–19924.

Endo-Munoz, L., Warby, T., Harrich, D., and McMillan, N. A. (2005). Phosphorylation of HIV Tat by PKR increases interaction with TAR RNA and enhances transcription. *Virol. J.* 2, 17.

Fan, H. Y., He, X., Kingston, R. E., and Narlikar, G. J. (2003). Distinct strategies to make nucleosomal DNA accessible. *Mol. Cell* 11, 1311–1322.

Fujinaga, K., Irwin, D., Huang, Y., Taube, R., Kurosu, T., and Peterlin, B. M. (2004). Dynamics of human immunodeficiency virus transcription: P-TEFb phosphorylates RD and dissociates negative effectors from the transactivation response element. *Mol. Cell. Biol.* 24, 787–795.

Garber, M. E., Wei, P., KewalRamani, V. N., Mayall, T. P., Herrmann, C. H., Rice, A. P., Littman, D. R., and Jones, K. A. (1998). The interaction between HIV-1 Tat and human cyclin T1 requires zinc and a critical cysteine residue that is not conserved in the murine CycT1 protein. *Genes Dev.* 12, 3512–3527.

Garber, M. E., Mayall, T. P., Suess, E. M., Meisenhelder, J., Thompson, N. E., and Jones, K. A. (2000). CDK9 autophosphorylation regulates high-affinity binding of the human immunodeficiency virus type 1 tat-P-TEFb complex to TAR RNA. *Mol. Cell. Biol.* 20, 6958–6969.

Garcia-Martinez, L. F., Ivanov, D., and Gaynor, R. B. (1997a). Association of Tat with purified HIV-1 and HIV-2 transcription preinitiation complexes. *J. Biol. Chem.* 272, 6951–6958.

Garcia-Martinez, L. F., Mavankal, G., Neveu, J. M., Lane, W. S., Ivanov, D., and Gaynor, R. B. (1997b). Purification of a Tat-associated kinase reveals a TFIIH complex that modulates HIV-1 transcription. *EMBO J.* 16, 2836–2850.

Gatignol, A., and Jeang, K.-T. (2000). Tat as a transcriptional activator and a potential therapeutic target for HIV-1. *In* "Advances in Pharmacology" (K.-T. Jeang, Ed.), pp. 209–227. Academic Press, San Diego, CA, USA and London, UK.

Gibbons, R. J. (2005). Histone modifying and chromatin remodelling enzymes in cancer and dysplastic syndromes. *Hum. Mol. Genet.* 14(Spec. No. 1), R85–R92.

Gold, M. O., Yang, X., Herrmann, C. H., and Rice, A. P. (1998). PITALRE, the catalytic subunit of TAK, is required for human immunodeficiency virus Tat transactivation *in vivo*. *J. Virol.* 72, 4448–4453.

Henderson, A., Holloway, A., Reeves, R., and Tremethick, D. J. (2004). Recruitment of SWI/SNF to the human immunodeficiency virus type 1 promoter. *Mol. Cell. Biol.* 24, 389–397.

Herrmann, C. H., and Rice, A. P. (1993). Specific interaction of the human immunodeficiency virus Tat proteins with a cellular protein kinase. *Virology* 197, 601–608.

Herrmann, C. H., and Rice, A. P. (1995). Lentivirus Tat proteins specifically associate with a cellular protein kinase, TAK, that hyperphosphorylates the carboxyl-terminal domain of the large subunit of RNA polymerase II: Candidate for a Tat cofactor. *J. Virol.* **69**, 1612–1620.

Hetzer, C., Dormeyer, W., Schnolzer, M., and Ott, M. (2005). Decoding Tat: The biology of HIV Tat posttranslational modifications. *Microbes Infect.* 7, 1364–1369.

Hottiger, M. O., and Nabel, G. J. (1998). Interaction of human immunodeficiency virus type 1 Tat with the transcriptional coactivators p300 and CREB binding protein. *J. Virol.* 72, 8252–8256.

Isel, C., and Karn, J. (1999). Direct evidence that HIV-1 Tat stimulates RNA polymerase II carboxyl-terminal domain hyperphosphorylation during transcriptional elongation. *J. Mol. Biol.* **290**, 929–941.

Ivanov, D., Kwak, Y. T., Guo, J., and Gaynor, R. B. (2000). Domains in the SPT5 protein that modulate its transcriptional regulatory properties. *Mol. Cell. Biol.* **20**, 2970–2983.

Jeang, K.-T, Berkhout, B., and Berkhout, B. (1992). Kinetics of HIV-1 long terminal repeat trans-activation. Use of intragenic ribozyme to assess rate-limiting steps. *J. Biol. Chem.* **267**, 17891–17899.

Jeang, K.-T., Chun, R., Lin, N. H., Gatignol, A., Glabe, C. G., and Fan, H. (1993). *In vitro* and *in vivo* binding of human immunodeficiency virus type 1 tat protein and Sp1 transcription factor. *J. Virol.* **67**, 6224–6233.

Jordan, A., Defechereux, P., and Verdin, E. (2001). The site of HIV-1 integration in the human genome determines basal transcriptional activity and response to Tat transactivation. *EMBO J.* **20**, 1726–1738.

Jordan, A., Bisgrove, D., and Verdin, E. (2003). HIV reproducibly establishes a latent infection after acute infection of T cells *in vitro*. *EMBO J.* **22**, 1868–1877.

Kaehlcke, K., Dorr, A., Hetzer-Egger, C., Kiermer, V., Henklein, P., Schnoelzer, M., Loret, E., Cole, P. A., Verdin, E., and Ott, M. (2003). Acetylation of Tat defines a cyclinT1-independent step in HIV transactivation. *Mol. Cell* **12**, 167–176.

Kamine, J., and Chinnadurai, G. (1992). Synergistic activation of the human immunodeficiency virus type 1 promoter by the viral Tat protein and cellular transcription factor Sp1. *J. Virol.* **66**, 3932–3936.

Kamine, J., Subramanian, T., and Chinnadurai, G. (1991). Sp1-dependent activation of a synthetic promoter by human immunodeficiency virus type 1 Tat protein. *Proc. Natl. Acad. Sci. USA* **88**, 8510–8514.

Kamine, J., Elangovan, B., Subramanian, T., Coleman, D., and Chinnadurai, G. (1996). Identification of a cellular protein that specifically interacts with the essential cysteine region of the HIV-1 Tat transactivator. *Virology* **216**, 357–366.

Karn, J. (1999). Tackling Tat. *J. Mol. Biol.* **293**, 235–254.

Kashanchi, F., Piras, G., Radonovich, M. F., Duvall, J. F., Fattaey, A., Chiang, C.-M., Roeder, R. G., and Brady, J. N. (1994). Direct interaction of human TFIID with the HIV-1 transactivator Tat. *Nature* **367**, 295–299.

Keen, N. J., Gait, M. J., and Karn, J. (1996). Human immunodeficiency virus type-1 Tat is an integral component of the activated transcription-elongation complex. *Proc. Natl. Acad. Sci. USA* **93**, 2505–2510.

Kiernan, R. E., Vanhulle, C., Schiltz, L., Adam, E., Xiao, H., Maudoux, F., Calomme, C., Burny, A., Nakatani, Y., Jeang, K. T., Benkirane, M., and Van Lint, C. (1999). HIV-1 tat transcriptional activity is regulated by acetylation. *EMBO J.* **18**, 6106–6118.

Kim, Y. K., Bourgeois, C. F., Isel, C., Churcher, M. J., and Karn, J. (2002). Phosphorylation of the RNA polymerase II carboxyl-terminal domain by CDK9 is directly responsible for human immunodeficiency virus type 1 Tat-activated transcriptional elongation. *Mol. Cell. Biol.* **22**, 4622–4637.

Kuppuswamy, M., Subramanian, T., Srinivasan, A., and Chinnadurai, G. (1989). Multiple functional domains of Tat, the trans-activator of HIV-1, defined by mutational analysis. *Nucleic Acids Res.* **17**, 3551–3561.

Kwak, Y. T., Guo, J., Prajapati, S., Park, K. J., Surabhi, R. M., Miller, B., Gehrig, P., and Gaynor, R. B. (2003). Methylation of SPT5 regulates its interaction with RNA polymerase II and transcriptional elongation properties. *Mol. Cell* **11**, 1055–1066.

Lewinski, M. K., Bisgrove, D., Shinn, P., Chen, H., Hoffmann, C., Hannenhalli, S., Verdin, E., Berry, C. C., Ecker, J. R., and Bushman, F. D. (2005). Genome-wide analysis of chromosomal features repressing human immunodeficiency virus transcription. *J. Virol.* **79**, 6610–6619.

Liu, J., Perkins, N. D., Schmid, R. M., and Nabel, G. J. (1992). Specific NF-kappa B subunits act in concert with Tat to stimulate human immunodeficiency virus type 1 transcription. *J. Virol.* **66**, 3883–3887.

Lusic, M., Marcello, A., Cereseto, A., and Giacca, M. (2003). Regulation of HIV-1 gene expression by histone acetylation and factor recruitment at the LTR promoter. *EMBO J.* **22**, 6550–6561.

Mahmoudi, T., Parra, M., Vries, R. G., Kauder, S. E., Verrijzer, C. P., Ott, M., and Verdin, E. (2006). The SWI/SNF chromatin-remodeling complex is a cofactor for Tat transactivation of the HIV promoter. *J. Biol. Chem.* **281**, 19960–19968.

Mancebo, H. S., Lee, G., Flygare, J., Tomassini, J., Luu, P., Zhu, Y., Peng, J., Blau, C., Hazuda, D., Price, D., and Flores, O. (1997). P-TEFb kinase is required for HIV Tat transcriptional activation *in vivo* and *in vitro*. *Genes Dev.* **11**, 2633–2644.

Marzio, G., Tyagi, M., Gutierrez, M. I., and Giacca, M. (1998). HIV-1 tat transactivator recruits p300 and CREB-binding protein histone acetyltransferases to the viral promoter. *Proc. Natl. Acad. Sci. USA* **95**, 13519–13524.

McMillan, N. A., Chun, R. F., Siderovski, D. P., Galabru, J., Toone, W. M., Samuel, C. E., Mak, T. W., Hovanessian, A. G., Jeang, K.-T., and Williams, B. R. G. (1995). HIV-1 Tat directly interacts with the interferon-induced, double-stranded RNA dependent kinase, PKR. *Virology* **213**, 413–424.

Michels, A. A., Nguyen, V. T., Fraldi, A., Labas, V., Edwards, M., Bonnet, F., Lania, L., and Bensaude, O. (2003). MAQ1 and 7SK RNA interact with CDK9/cyclin T complexes in a transcription-dependent manner. *Mol. Cell. Biol.* **23**, 4859–4869.

Mujtaba, S., He, Y., Zeng, L., Farooq, A., Carlson, J. E., Ott, M., Verdin, E., and Zhou, M. M. (2002). Structural basis of lysine-acetylated HIV-1 Tat recognition by PCAF bromodomain. *Mol. Cell* **9**, 575–586.

Narlikar, G. J., Fan, H. Y., and Kingston, R. E. (2002). Cooperation between complexes that regulate chromatin structure and transcription. *Cell* **108**, 475–487.

Noonan, D., and Albini, A. (2000). From the outside in: Extracellular activities of HIV Tat. *In* "Advances in Pharmacology" (K.-T. Jeang, Ed.), pp. 229–250. Academic Press, San Diego, CA, USA and London, U.K.

Ott, D. E. (1997). Cellular proteins in HIV virions. *Rev. Med. Virol.* **7**, 167–180.

Ott, M., Schnolzer, M., Garnica, J., Fischle, W., Emiliani, S., Rackwitz, H. R., and Verdin, E. (1999). Acetylation of the HIV-1 Tat protein by p300 is important for its transcriptional activity. *Curr. Biol.* **9**, 1489–1492.

Pagans, S., Pedal, A., North, B. J., Kaehlcke, K., Marshall, B. L., Dorr, A., Hetzer-Egger, C., Henklein, P., Frye, R., McBurney, M. W., Hruby, H., Jung, M., *et al.* (2005). SIRT1 regulates HIV transcription via Tat deacetylation. *PLoS Biol.* **3**, e41.

Pagtakhan, A. S., and Tong-Starksen, S. E. (1997). Interactions between Tat of HIV-2 and transcription factor Sp1. *Virology* **238**, 221–230.

Pazin, M. J., Sheridan, P. L., Cannon, K., Cao, Z., Keck, J. G., Kadonaga, J. T., and Jones, K. A. (1996). NF-kappa B-mediated chromatin reconfiguration and transcriptional activation of the HIV-1 enhancer *in vitro. Genes Dev.* 10, 37–49.

Peng, J., Zhu, Y., Milton, J. T., and Price, D. H. (1998). Identification of multiple cyclin subunits of human P-TEFb. *Genes Dev.* 12, 755–762.

Pereira, L. A., Bentley, K., Peeters, A., Churchill, M. J., and Deacon, N. J. (2000). A compilation of cellular transcription factor interactions with the HIV-1 LTR promoter. *Nucleic Acids Res.* 28, 663–668.

Ping, Y. H., and Rana, T. M. (1999). Tat-associated kinase (P-TEFb): A component of transcription preinitiation and elongation complexes. *J. Biol. Chem.* 274, 7399–7404.

Ping, Y. H., and Rana, T. M. (2001). DSIF and NELF interact with RNA polymerase II elongation complex and HIV-1 Tat stimulates P-TEFb-mediated phosphorylation of RNA polymerase II and DSIF during transcription elongation. *J. Biol. Chem.* 276, 12951–12958.

Ping, Y. H., Chu, C. Y., Cao, H., Jacque, J. M., Stevenson, M., and Rana, T. M. (2004). Modulating HIV-1 replication by RNA interference directed against human transcription elongation factor SPT5. *Retrovirology* 1, 46.

Price, D. H. (2000). P-TEFb, a cyclin-dependent kinase controlling elongation by RNA polymerase II. *Mol. Cell. Biol.* 20, 2629–2634.

Pumfery, A., Deng, L., Maddukuri, A., de la Fuente, C., Li, H., Wade, J. D., Lambert, P., Kumar, A., and Kashanchi, F. (2003). Chromatin remodeling and modification during HIV-1 Tat-activated transcription. *Curr. HIV Res.* 1, 343–362.

Quivy, V., and Van Lint, C. (2002). Diversity of acetylation targets and roles in transcriptional regulation: The human immunodeficiency virus type 1 promoter as a model system. *Biochem. Pharmacol.* 64, 925–934.

Raha, T., Cheng, S. W., and Green, M. R. (2005). HIV-1 Tat stimulates transcription complex assembly through recruitment of TBP in the absence of TAFs. *PLoS Biol.* 3, e44.

Rana, T. M., and Jeang, K.-T. (1999). Biochemical and functional interactions between HIV-1 Tat protein and TAR RNA. *Arch. Biochem. Biophys.* 365, 175–185.

Rohr, O., Marban, C., Aunis, D., and Schaeffer, E. (2003). Regulation of HIV-1 gene transcription: From lymphocytes to microglial cells. *J. Leukoc. Biol.* 74, 736–749.

Roof, P., Ricci, M., Genin, P., Montano, M. A., Essex, M., Wainberg, M. A., Gatignol, A., and Hiscott, J. (2002). Differential regulation of HIV-1 clade-specific B, C, and E long terminal repeats by NF-kappaB and the Tat transactivator. *Virology* 296, 77–83.

Sapountzi, V., Logan, I. R., and Robson, C. N. (2006). Cellular functions of TIP60. *Int. J. Biochem. Cell Biol.* 38, 1496–1509.

Schroder, A. R., Shinn, P., Chen, H., Berry, C., Ecker, J. R., and Bushman, F. (2002). HIV-1 integration in the human genome favors active genes and local hotspots. *Cell* 110, 521–529.

Sengupta, N., and Seto, E. (2004). Regulation of histone deacetylase activities. *J. Cell. Biochem.* 93, 57–67.

Sheridan, P. L., Sheline, C. T., Cannon, K., Voz, M. L., Pazin, M. J., Kadonaga, J. T., and Jones, K. A. (1995). Activation of the HIV-1 enhancer by the LEF-1 HMG protein on nucleosome-assembled DNA *in vitro. Genes Dev.* 9, 2090–2104.

Sheridan, P. L., Mayall, T. P., Verdin, E., and Jones, K. A. (1997). Histone acetyltransferases regulate HIV-1 enhancer activity *in vitro. Genes Dev.* 11, 3327–3340.

Treand, C., du Chene, I., Bres, V., Kiernan, R., Benarous, R., Benkirane, M., and Emiliani, S. (2006). Requirement for SWI/SNF chromatin-remodeling complex in Tat-mediated activation of the HIV-1 promoter. *EMBO J.* 25, 1690–1699.

Van Lint, C. (2000). Role of chromatin in HIV-1 transcriptional regulation. *In* "Advances in Pharmacology" (K.-T. Jeang, Ed.), pp. 121–160. Academic Press, San Diego, CA, USA and London, U.K.

Van Lint, C., Ghysdael, J., Paras, P., Jr., Burny, A., and Verdin, E. (1994). A transcriptional regulatory element is associated with a nuclease-hypersensitive site in the pol gene of human immunodeficiency virus type 1. *J. Virol.* **68**, 2632–2648.

Van Lint, C., Emiliani, S., Ott, M., and Verdin, E. (1996). Transcriptional activation and chromatin remodeling of the HIV-1 promoter in response to histone acetylation. *EMBO J.* **15**, 1112–1120.

Varga-Weisz, P. D., and Becker, P. B. (2006). Regulation of higher-order chromatin structures by nucleosome-remodelling factors. *Curr. Opin. Genet. Dev.* **16**, 151–156.

Verdin, E. (1991). DNase I-hypersensitive sites are associated with both long terminal repeats and with the intragenic enhancer of integrated human immunodeficiency virus type 1. *J. Virol.* **65**, 6790–6799.

Verdin, E., Paras, J., and Van Lint, C. (1993). Chromatin disruption in the promoter of human immunodeficiency virus type 1 during transcriptional activation. *EMBO J.* **12**, 3249–3259.

Verdone, L., Caserta, M., and Di Mauro, E. (2005). Role of histone acetylation in the control of gene expression. *Biochem. Cell Biol.* **83**, 344–353.

Veschambre, P., Simard, P., and Jalinot, P. (1995). Evidence for functional interaction between the HIV-1 Tat transactivator and the TATA box binding protein *in vivo. J. Mol. Biol.* **250**, 169–180.

Veschambre, P., Roisin, A., and Jalinot, P. (1997). Biochemical and functional interaction of the human immunodeficiency virus type 1 Tat transactivator with the general transcription factor TFIIB. *J. Gen. Virol.* **78**, 2235–2245.

Wada, T., Takagi, T., Yamaguchi, Y., Ferdous, A., Imai, T., Hirose, S., Sugimoto, S., Yano, K., Hartzog, G. A., Winston, F., Buratowski, S., and Handa, H. (1998a). DSIF, a novel transcription elongation factor that regulates RNA polymerase II processivity, is composed of human Spt4 and Spt5 homologs. *Genes* **12**, 343–356.

Wada, T., Takagi, T., Yamaguchi, Y., Watanabe, D., and Handa, H. (1998b). Evidence that P-TEFb alleviates the negative effect of DSIF on RNA polymerase II-dependent transcription *in vitro. EMBO J.* **17**, 7395–7403.

Wei, P., Garber, M. E., Fang, S. M., Fischer, W. H., and Jones, K. A. (1998). A novel CDK9-associated C-type cyclin interacts directly with HIV-1 Tat and mediates its high-affinity, loop-specific binding to TAR RNA. *Cell* **92**, 451–462.

Weissman, J. D., Brown, J. A., Howcroft, T. K., Hwang, J., Chawla, A., Roche, P. A., Schiltz, L., Nakatani, Y., and Singer, D. S. (1998). HIV-1 tat binds TAFII250 and represses TAFII250-dependent transcription of major histocompatibility class I genes. *Proc. Natl. Acad. Sci. USA* **95**, 11601–11606.

Widlak, P., Gaynor, R. B., and Garrard, W. T. (1997). *In vitro* chromatin assembly of the HIV-1 promoter. ATP-dependent polar repositioning of nucleosomes by Sp1 and NFkappaB. *J. Biol. Chem.* **272**, 17654–17661.

Wu-Baer, F., Lane, W. S., and Gaynor, R. B. (1998). Role of the human homolog of the yeast transcription factor SPT5 in HIV-1 Tat-activation. *J. Mol. Biol.* **277**, 179–197.

Yamada, T., Yamaguchi, Y., Inukai, N., Okamoto, S., Mura, T., and Handa, H. (2006). P-TEFb-mediated phosphorylation of hSpt5 C-terminal repeats is critical for processive transcription elongation. *Mol. Cell* **21**, 227–237.

Yamaguchi, Y., Takagi, T., Wada, T., Yano, K., Furuya, A., Sugimoto, S., Hasegawa, J., and Handa, H. (1999). NELF, a multisubunit complex containing RD, cooperates with DSIF to repress RNA polymerase II elongation. *Cell* **97**, 41–51.

Yamaguchi, Y., Inukai, N., Narita, T., Wada, T., and Handa, H. (2002). Evidence that negative elongation factor represses transcription elongation through binding to a DRB sensitivity-inducing factor/RNA polymerase II complex and RNA. *Mol. Cell. Biol.* **22**, 2918–2927.

Yamamoto, T., and Horikoshi, M. (1997). Novel substrate specificity of the histone acetyltransferase activity of HIV-1-Tat interactive protein Tip60. *J. Biol. Chem.* **272**, 30595–30598.

Yang, X., Herrmann, C. H., and Rice, A. P. (1996). The human immunodeficiency virus Tat proteins specifically associate with TAK *in vivo* and require the carboxyl-terminal domain of RNA polymerase II for function. *J. Virol.* **70**, 4576–4584.

Yang, X., Gold, M. O., Tang, D. N., Lewis, D. E., Aguilar-Cordova, E., Rice, A. P., and Herrmann, C. H. (1997). TAK, an HIV Tat-associated kinase, is a member of the cyclin-dependent family of protein kinases and is induced by activation of peripheral blood lymphocytes and differentiation of promonocytic cell lines. *Proc. Natl. Acad. Sci. USA* **94**, 12331–12336.

Yang, X. J. (2004). The diverse superfamily of lysine acetyltransferases and their roles in leukemia and other diseases. *Nucleic Acids Res.* **32**, 959–976.

Yedavalli, V. S., Benkirane, M., and Jeang, K. T. (2003). Tat and trans-activation-responsive (TAR) RNA-independent induction of HIV-1 long terminal repeat by human and murine cyclin T1 requires Sp1. *J. Biol. Chem.* **278**, 6404–6410.

Yik, J. H., Chen, R., Nishimura, R., Jennings, J. L., Link, A. J., and Zhou, Q. (2003). Inhibition of P-TEFb (CDK9/Cyclin T) kinase and RNA polymerase II transcription by the coordinated actions of HEXIM1 and 7SK snRNA. *Mol. Cell* **12**, 971–982.

Zhou, M., Halanski, M. A., Radonovich, M. F., Kashanchi, F., Peng, J., Price, D. H., and Brady, J. N. (2000). Tat modifies the activity of CDK9 to phosphorylate serine 5 of the RNA polymerase II carboxyl-terminal domain during human immunodeficiency virus type 1 transcription. *Mol. Cell. Biol.* **20**, 5077–5086.

Zhou, M., Nekhai, S., Bharucha, D. C., Kumar, A., Ge, H., Price, D. H., Egly, J. M., and Brady, J. N. (2001). TFIIH inhibits CDK9 phosphorylation during human immunodeficiency virus type 1 transcription. *J. Biol. Chem.* **276**, 44633–44640.

Zhu, Y., Pe'ery, T., Peng, J., Ramanathan, Y., Marshall, N., Marshall, T., Amendt, B., Mathews, M. B., and Price, D. H. (1997). Transcription elongation factor P-TEFb is required for HIV-1 tat transactivation *in vitro*. *Genes Dev.* **11**, 2622–2632.

Zorio, D. A., and Bentley, D. L. (2001). Transcription elongation: The 'Foggy' is liftingellipsis. *Curr. Biol.* **11**, R144–R146.

Barbara K. Felber*, Andrei S. Zolotukhin*, and George N. Pavlakis[†]

*Human Retrovirus Pathogenesis Section, Vaccine Branch, Center for Cancer Research
National Cancer Institute-Frederick, Frederick, Maryland 21702
[†]Human Retrovirus Section, Vaccine Branch, Center for Cancer Research
National Cancer Institute-Frederick, Frederick, Maryland 21702

Posttranscriptional Control of HIV-1 and Other Retroviruses and Its Practical Applications

I. Chapter Overview

Posttranscriptional control is a key step essential for expression of cellular and viral mRNAs. After synthesis, processing (addition of $5'$ cap, $3'$ polyadenylation, splicing), and assembly into ribonucleoprotein complexes (messenger ribonucleoprotein, mRNP), the mRNA is exported into the cytoplasm, which involves complex interactions of the mRNPs with transport receptors and with components of the nuclear pore complex (NPC). Splicing was found to mark mRNA as "export-ready" and plays a critical role in

Advances in Pharmacology, Volume 55

1054-3589/07 $35.00
DOI: 10.1016/S1054-3589(07)55005-2

promoting mRNA transport. Whereas HIV and all the complex retroviruses produce several alternatively spliced mRNAs, only two types of mRNAs are produced from simple retroviruses. The unspliced primary transcript of all retroviruses has to exit the nucleus since it serves as genomic RNA as well as *gag/pol* mRNA. The transport of unspliced RNA to the cytoplasm requires a special export mechanism. Here, we focus on the *cis*-acting viral RNA export elements and the viral and cellular factors promoting export of retroviral mRNAs. Studies on HIV-1 and other complex retroviruses, as well as the simian type D retroviruses and mouse long terminal repeat (LTR) retroelements [intracisternal A-particle (IAP) retroelements] over the past two decades have led to major discoveries on the export mechanisms. These retroviruses utilize distinct RNA export elements such as Rev responsive element (RRE), constitutive transport element (CTE), and RNA transport element (RTE), which represent binding sites for viral (Rev) or cellular (NXF1, RBM15) factors. The identified distinct CRM1 and NXF1 export pathways are also essential for the export of cellular RNAs and proteins. An important practical outcome is the development of the methodology of RNA optimization, which is a widely used approach to achieve high-level gene expression in mammalian cells and is key to the development of efficient vaccine approaches against AIDS as well as for other applications.

II. Introduction

The study of retroviruses, especially HIV-1, has led to major discoveries in the field of mRNA metabolism and transport of macromolecules. Research over the past two decades has revealed that retroviruses depend on an efficient transport mechanism for the nucleocytoplasmic export of their full-length mRNA in its unspliced form, since this transcript encodes the Gag/Pol polyprotein and in addition serves as genomic RNA to be packaged into progeny virions in the cytoplasm (Fig. 1). The export of this

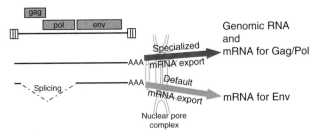

FIGURE 1   Export of the retroviral mRNAs. The unspliced, full-length RNA serves as a genomic RNA and is packaged in the cytoplasm, and it also serves as mRNA encoding Gag/Pol polyprotein. The export of this RNA in its unspliced form requires a specific export mechanism. Env is produced from a spliced mRNA and is transported via the default mRNA export pathway.

RNA in its unspliced form requires a specific export mechanism. Env is produced from a spliced mRNA and is transported via the default mRNA export pathway. Fine-tuned mechanisms control these steps and are essential for the production of infectious virus. An important outcome of this line of research is the discovery of the viral *cis*-acting RNA elements and *trans*-acting factors mediating the export of the unspliced retroviral mRNA as well as the discovery of the two major nuclear export receptors, CRM1 and NXF1 (Fig. 2, Table I). Importantly, CRM1 and NXF1 are essential for the trafficking of cellular proteins and RNAs, and represent distinct export pathways from the nucleus. A summary of the viral and cellular factors and *cis*-acting RNA elements mediating retroviral mRNA export is shown in Table I.

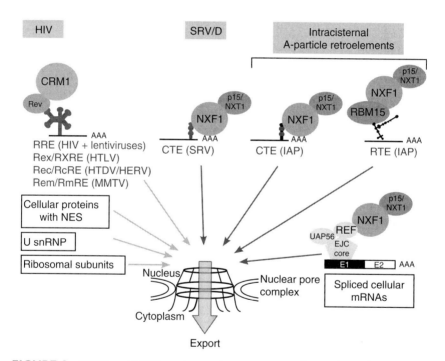

FIGURE 2 CRM1 and NXF1 are key nuclear receptors mediating the nucleocytoplasmic export of viral and cellular macromolecules. The export of HIV RRE-containing mRNAs is mediated via the viral Rev protein and the cellular CRM1 protein. Similarly, the HTLV family of retroviruses, the human endogenous retrovirus HTDV/HERV-K, and MMTV utilize the viral Rex-RXRE, Rec-ReRE, and Rem-RmRE, respectively. The simian-type D retroviruses (SRV-1, SRV-2, and MPMV) and a subgroup of murine endogenous retroelements (intracisternal A-particle retroelement, IAP) use the CTE and CTE-like RNA export elements, respectively, which represent the *cis*-acting binding sites for the cellular NXF1. Another subgroup of IAP contains a distinct RNA export element, RTE, which is tethered via the cellular RMB15 protein to NXF1 export receptor. CRM1 and NXF1 are also nuclear receptors for several cellular proteins and RNAs.

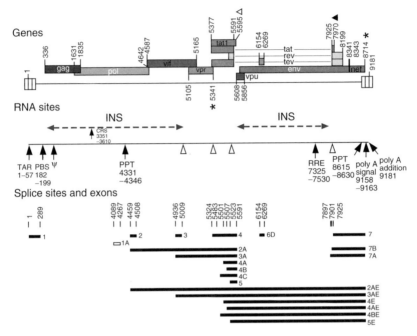

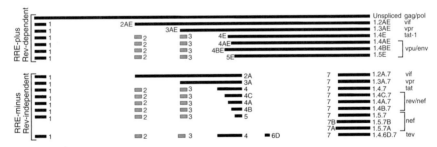

FIGURE 3   A compilation of mRNAs produced by HIV-1. The HIV-1 genome and the different genes are shown. The numbering follows the HIV reference sequence of HXB2 (GenBank accession NC_001802). The numbering marks the beginning and end of the open reading frames (ORFs). The asterisks indicate premature terminator of some ORFs in the HIV strain HXB2 (e.g., vpr 5105-5369; nef 8343-8963). The filled triangle indicates the longer form of Tat found in primary isolates (Opi *et al.*, 2004). The open triangle indicates the terminator of tat-1, produced from mRNAs containing exon 4E, which encodes the first coding exon of *tat* from a partially spliced mRNA. The HIV-1 full-length RNA containing TAR (Tat responsive element), PBS (primer binding site), ψ (packaging signal), PPT (polypurine tract), RRE (Rev-responsive element), polyA signal, and polyadenylation site are shown. The locations of the identified exonic splicing enhancers (ESE, GAR) and silencers (ESE) are indicated with open arrow heads (for recent review see Cochrane *et al.*, 2006). The gray arrows indicate the regions in *gag*, *pol* (Cochrane *et al.*, 1991; Nasioulas *et al.*, 1994; Olsen *et al.*, 1992; Schneider *et al.*, 1997; Schwartz *et al.*, 1992a), *vif* (Rosati, M., G.N.P., and B.K.F., unpublished data), and *env* (including RRE) (Nasioulas *et al.*, 1994) containing experimentally verified INS/CRS elements.

III. HIV-1 Regulation of Gene Expression

Two viral regulatory proteins, Tat and Rev (Fig. 3), have profound effects on virus expression, controlling HIV expression at the transcriptional and posttranscriptional level, respectively. Rev is an essential protein, since Rev-minus virus mutants cannot replicate at all (Feinberg *et al.*, 1986; Sodroski *et al.*, 1986). Similarly, targeting the *rev* mRNA by RNA interference also resulted in inhibiting virus replication (Coburn and Cullen, 2002; Lee *et al.*, 2002). The discovery that the viral Rev protein exports unspliced (and partially spliced) mRNAs (Felber *et al.*, 1989b), and thus promotes the production of structural proteins and infectious virions, opened new opportunities to understand nucleocytoplasmic transport (for reviews see Boris-Lawrie *et al.*, 2001; Cochrane, 2004; Cullen, 2003; Felber and Pavlakis, 1993; Pavlakis and Felber, 1990; Pollard and Malim, 1998; Rosen, 1991).

In the case of HIV-1, mRNA export requires the specific interaction of the viral Rev protein with the *cis*-acting RNA recognition signal, the RRE (Fig. 3) (Bartel *et al.*, 1991; Cochrane *et al.*, 1990a; Cook *et al.*, 1991; Daly *et al.*, 1989; Dayton *et al.*, 1988; Emerman *et al.*, 1989; Felber *et al.*, 1989b; Hadzopoulou-Cladaras *et al.*, 1989; Hammarskjöld *et al.*, 1989; Heaphy *et al.*, 1990; Holland *et al.*, 1990; Malim *et al.*, 1989b; Rosen *et al.*, 1988). RRE is a highly structured RNA element (Fig. 4) embedded within the *env*

TABLE I   Distinct RNA Export Mechanisms Utilized by Retroviruses

Virus	RNA export element	Viral export factor	Cellular export factor	Nuclear receptor
HIV-1	RRE	Rev	N/A	CRM1
HTLV-I	RXRE	Rex	N/A	CRM1
HTDV/HERV-K	RcRE	Rec	N/A	CRM1
MMTV	RmRE	Rem	N/A	CRM1
SRV/D	CTE	N/A	NXF1	NXF1
IAP	CTE$_{IAP}$	N/A	NXF1	NXF1
IAP	RTE	N/A	RBM15	NXF1
RSV	DR	N/A	?	?

N/A, not applicable.

The identified exons and the location of the 5′ and 3′ splice sites are presented (Benko *et al.*, 1990; Neumann *et al.*, 1994; Purcell and Martin, 1993; Salfeld *et al.*, 1990; Schwartz *et al.*, 1990a,b, 1991). A schematic representation of the HIV-1 mRNAs is shown. The mRNAs are composed using a combination of the identified exons. The small exons 2 and 3 (indicated in gray) are found in the multiply spliced mRNAs in combination with the exons 4, 4A, 4B, 4C, and 5. The use of exon 1A has not been detected in infected cells (Lutzelberger *et al.*, 2006). Most of the HIV genes are encoded by several mRNAs. The full-length and partially spliced mRNAs contain RRE and depend on Rev for expression. The multiply spliced mRNA lack RRE and are Rev independent.

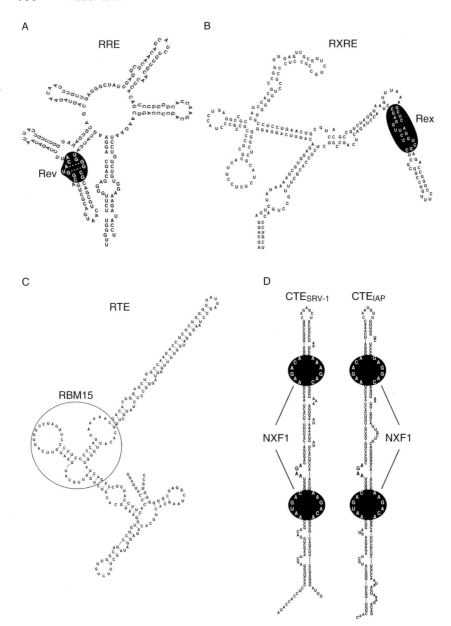

FIGURE 4 Comparison of the RNA export elements used by different retroviruses. Distinct RNA export elements are used by retroviruses [HIV-1 RRE (A), HTLV-I RXRE (B), and SRV-1 CTE (D)] and retroelements [CTE$_{IAP}$ (D) and RTE (C)]. The binding sites for the respective viral or cellular binding factors are indicated.

coding region, and it is present only in the unspliced and partially spliced mRNAs, but is absent from the multiply spliced mRNAs (Fig. 3, bottom panel). In the absence of Rev, the RRE-containing mRNAs are absent from the cytoplasm, and thus no Gag/Pol or Env proteins and no virions are produced (Cochrane *et al.*, 1990a; Dayton *et al.*, 1988; Feinberg *et al.*, 1986; Felber *et al.*, 1989b; Hadzopoulou-Cladaras *et al.*, 1989; Hammarskjöld *et al.*, 1989; Holland *et al.*, 1990, 1992; Malim *et al.*, 1989b; Rosen *et al.*, 1988; Sodroski *et al.*, 1986). Detailed analysis of the subset of the RRE-containing mRNAs in the absence of Rev revealed that they are retained in the nucleus where they either undergo further splicing, thereby increasing the amount of the multiply spliced mRNAs, or they are subjected to degradation (Feinberg *et al.*, 1986; Felber *et al.*, 1989b, 1990; Hadzopoulou-Cladaras *et al.*, 1989; Malim *et al.*, 1989b). Transcomplementation of the Rev-minus HIV with Rev restores export of RRE-containing mRNA as well as virus production. Rev also promotes polysomal association of the RRE-containing mRNAs (Arrigo and Chen, 1991; D'Agostino *et al.*, 1992; Lawrence *et al.*, 1991). Thus, Rev is essential for the nuclear and cytoplasmic trafficking and expression of the RRE-containing mRNAs. In addition to RRE, this subset of viral mRNAs contains nuclear retention signals termed instability sequences (INS) or *cis*-acting repressive signal (CRS) (Cochrane *et al.*, 1991; Hadzopoulou-Cladaras *et al.*, 1989; Nasioulas *et al.*, 1994; Rosen *et al.*, 1988; Schwartz *et al.*, 1992b), which contribute to their poor expression in the absence of Rev (Fig. 3).

IV. Rev and Its Export Receptor CRM1

HIV-1 Rev is produced from a set of multiply spliced mRNAs (Fig. 3). Rev is a small 116-aa nuclear/nucleolar protein (Cochrane *et al.*, 1990b; Cullen *et al.*, 1988; Felber *et al.*, 1989b; Perkins *et al.*, 1989; Venkatesh *et al.*, 1990), and its nucleolar localization is critical for Rev function (Michienzi *et al.*, 2006; Stauber *et al.*, 1995, 1998). Rev was found to shuttle rapidly between the nucleus and cytoplasm (D'Agostino *et al.*, 1995; Kalland *et al.*, 1994; Love *et al.*, 1998; Meyer and Malim, 1994; Neumann *et al.*, 2001; Richard *et al.*, 1994; Stauber *et al.*, 1995; Szilvay *et al.*, 1995; Wolff *et al.*, 2006).

Rev contains four functional determinants: nuclear localization signal (NLS), RNA-binding domain (RBD), oligomerization domain flanking the NLS/RBD, and nuclear export signal (NES) (for reviews see Cochrane, 2004; Hope, 1999; Pavlakis and Felber, 1990; Pollard and Malim, 1998). The NLS and RBD are contained within a conserved arginine-rich N-terminal region spanning amino acids 40–45 (NRRRRW) (Malim *et al.*, 1989a; Perkins *et al.*, 1989). Rev binds to the RRE via a single high-affinity binding site located in stem IIB (Bartel *et al.*, 1991; Heaphy *et al.*, 1990) and multimerizes on the RRE, which is thought to stabilize the protein–RNA

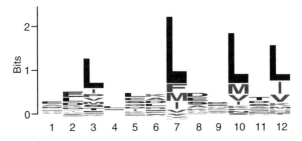

FIGURE 5   A leucine-rich NES motif, common for 80 individual NES sequences from NES database (la Cour *et al.*, 2003), was derived using MEME algorithm (Bailey and Elkan, 1994) and is represented as sequence logo (Schneider and Stephens, 1990). The information content is plotted on *y*-axis (bits), and the leucine residues are shown in black.

complex (Cole *et al.*, 1993; Daelemans *et al.*, 2004; Daly *et al.*, 1993a,b; Jain and Belasco, 2001; Madore *et al.*, 1994; Thomas *et al.*, 1998) (Fig. 4A). Mutations in the multimerization domain, designed not to affect the NLS, abolish nuclear targeting of Rev and render this mutant inactive. Amino acids 75–84 (LPPLERLTLD) represent the core NES, consisting of a leucine-rich sequence (Fischer *et al.*, 1995; Malim *et al.*, 1989a; Mermer *et al.*, 1990; Meyer *et al.*, 1996; Szilvay *et al.*, 1995; Venkatesh and Chinnadurai, 1990) (Fig. 5). Mutations of the leucine residues or insertions/deletions of residues within this core render the protein inactive and also give it a transdominant phenotype, because its localization and RRE-binding ability is not affected.

For nuclear export, Rev binds via NES to the nuclear receptor CRM1/ exportin1, a member of the exportin family (Fornerod *et al.*, 1997; Fukuda *et al.*, 1997; Neville *et al.*, 1997) (Fig. 2). The binding of RanGTP to exportins in the nucleus enables a conformational change allowing strong binding to the export substrate, whereas after translocation into the cytoplasm, the exportin–RanGTP–cargo complexes are destabilized by action of soluble (RanBP1) and NPC-resident (Ran BP2/NUP 358) Ran-binding proteins, as well as by GTP hydrolysis on RanGTP catalyzed by RanGAP (Fried and Kutay, 2003; Mosammaparast and Pemberton, 2004). The NES–CRM1–RanGTP complex binds via CRM1 directly to the FG-repeat determinants of nucleoporins, thereby docking the cargo to the NPC, followed by translocation to the cytoplasm. For Rev complexes, such docking may be initiated by binding via CRM1 to dynamic nucleoporins, for example Nup98, in the nucleoplasm or in the nucleolus, followed by subsequent integration of Nup98 into NPC (Daelemans *et al.*, 2005a; Zolotukhin and Felber, 1999). The interactions of CRM1 with export substrates are facilitated by RanBP3 (Englmeier *et al.*, 2001; Lindsay *et al.*, 2001; Petosa *et al.*, 2004). The use of powerful imaging technology in combination with fluorescence resonance energy transfer (FRET) between fluorescently tagged CRM1 and Rev has provided additional important clues about the mechanistic aspects of Rev trafficking and its interactions with CRM1 and other proteins. Using fluorescence recovery after photobleaching (FRAP), it was shown that CRM1-GFP moves at rates similar to that of free GFP in the nucleoplasm. A slower mobility was detected on the nuclear membrane, consistent with known CRM1 interactions with the NPC (Daelemans *et al.*, 2005a). Although CRM1-GFP is highly mobile in the nucleoplasm, it is not mobile in the nucleoli of Rev-expressing cells, indicating that it is associated with Rev in the nucleolus. Using FRET allowed the direct demonstration of the Rev–CRM1 interaction in the nucleolus. FRET measurements further indicated that Rev is found in multimers in both the nucleolus and the cytoplasm (Daelemans *et al.*, 2004). The Rev-Rev FRET efficiency in the cytoplasm was significantly lower than that in the nucleolus, indicating a different status of Rev in these two compartments. Based on FRET and FRAP measurements, it was proposed that CRM1 is a monomer in the nucleoplasm searching for high-affinity ligands. CRM1 binds to Rev in the nucleolus and moves rapidly to the nuclear pore for exit.

In addition to CRM1 and nucleoporins, several cellular factors such as RNA helicases A (RHA) (Li *et al.*, 1999; Reddy *et al.*, 1999, 2000a), DDX1 (Fang *et al.*, 2004, 2005) and DDX3 (Yedavalli *et al.*, 2004), prothymosin alpha (Kubota *et al.*, 1995), kinesin-like protein REBP (Venkatesh *et al.*, 2003), nucleoporin-like hRIP (Farjot *et al.*, 1999; Fritz and Green, 1996; Fritz *et al.*, 1995; Kiss *et al.*, 2003; Sanchez-Velar *et al.*, 2004; Yu *et al.*, 2005), Sam68 (Li *et al.*, 2002; McLaren *et al.*, 2004; Modem *et al.*, 2005; Reddy *et al.*, 1999, 2000b, 2002), and eIF-5A (Bevec and Hauber, 1997; Elfgang *et al.*, 1999; Hofmann *et al.*, 2001; Liu *et al.*, 1997; Rosorius *et al.*, 1999; Ruhl *et al.*, 1993) were shown to participate at different steps of Rev function such as the interactions with RRE, CRM1, NPC docking, translocation of the Rev-containing mRNP, and cargo release from NPC and perinuclear compartment.

CRM1 is conserved from yeast to humans and mediates the nuclear export of a wide variety of proteins that contain the Rev-like leucine-rich NES, while different NES can vary profoundly in activity (Henderson and Eleftheriou, 2000). It is thought that many NES, including that of Rev, maintain low affinity to CRM1 in order to enable efficient clearance from the receptor in the cytoplasm (reviewed in Kutay and Guttinger, 2005). The CRM1 substrates possess an NES sequence usually conforming to the common consensus (Fig. 4), and include a multitude of shuttling and nuclear-excluded proteins involved in transcription, cell cycle and translation, as well as Rev proteins of all lentiviruses, the Rex proteins of the HTLV family of retroviruses, and the Rev-like proteins Rec of HTDV/HERV-K and Rem of MMTV. A database of experimentally validated NES sequences (NESbase; la Cour *et al.*, 2003) can be found at http://www.cbs.dtu.dk/databases/NESbase.

In addition to its role in protein export, CRM1 is essential for the export of U snRNPs and ribosomal subunits, which is mediated via NES-containing adaptors (Fornerod and Ohno, 2002) (Fig. 2). While CRM1 is clearly dispensable for general mRNA export as seen in various experimental systems and in species ranging from yeast to humans, there could be individual mRNAs such as human IFN-alpha1mRNA (Kimura *et al.*, 2004) and tra-2 mRNA in *Caenorhabditis elegans* (Kuersten *et al.*, 2004) that use CRM1 for export by a yet unknown mechanism.

The CRM1 export pathway is essential in eukaryotes, and some prokaryotic species evolved antibiotics targeting CRM1, in order to eliminate their eukaryotic rivals. Thus, leptomycin B (LMB) (Kudo *et al.*, 1998, 1999; Wolff *et al.*, 1997), a natural product of *Streptomyces* with antifungal activity, binds to CRM1 and inhibits its function. A synthetic compound (Daelemans *et al.*, 2005b) has also been shown to inhibit the CRM1 export pathway by binding to CRM1. The use of these drugs further demonstrated the principle that inhibition of nuclear export of HIV mRNAs completely blocks virus propagation. Because CRM1 inhibition leads to block of nuclear export of essential cargoes, such as U snRNPs, the ribosomal subunits and a series of NES-containing cellular proteins (Fig. 2), these drugs are highly toxic and are not of use against HIV; however, they are excellent tools to understand and dissect the CRM1 export pathway.

V. Posttranscriptional Regulation of Other Complex Retroviruses

Similar posttranscriptional regulation as in HIV-1 was found in all lentiviruses, as well as in human T-cell leukemia virus HTLV-I, where the transport of the unspliced transcript depends on the interaction of the viral Rex protein with the *cis*-acting Rex responsive element RXRE (Fig. 4) (Hidaka *et al.*, 1988; Ingraham *et al.*, 1990; Inoue *et al.*, 1986, 1987; Seiki *et al.*, 1988; for recent review see Younis and Green, 2005); in the human endogenous retrovirus HTDV/HERV-K, which uses the viral Rec protein (previously termed cORF or K-Rev) that interacts with its responsive element RcRE (also termed K-RRE) for export (Bogerd *et al.*, 2000; Lower *et al.*, 1995; Magin *et al.*, 1999, 2000; Yang *et al.*, 1999, 2000); and in the Mouse mammary tumor virus (MMTV) which uses the viral Rem protein that interacts with the *cis*-acting RmRE responsive element (Bar-Sinai *et al.*, 2005; Indik *et al.*, 2005; Mertz *et al.*, 2005) (Fig. 2, Table I). The foamy virus mRNA export mechanism is less well defined (Linial, 1999; Lochelt, 2003; Rethwilm, 2003), and so far there is no evidence that a Rev- or Rex-like export system is used. It is interesting to note, that the respective RTEs are located differentially in different retroviral genomes. In lentiviruses, the RREs are located within *env*, therefore only a subset of the produced mRNAs, the unspliced and the partially spliced species, contain the *cis*-acting binding site for the export factor Rev. In HTLV, HTDV/HERV-K, and MMTV, the *cis*-acting elements (RXRE, RcRE, and RmRE, respectively) are located at the 3′ end overlapping the U3/R of the 3′LTR. Therefore, RXRE, RcRE, and RmRE are present in all the mRNAs, although the fully spliced mRNAs can also be expressed efficiently in the absence of these elements.

Lentiviruses, HTLV, HTDV/HERV-K, and MMTV retroviruses are referred to as "complex," since they encode an array of regulatory and accessory genes in addition to *gag/pol* and *env*. These viruses produce a full-length, unspliced mRNA (encoding *gag/pol* and serving as genomic RNA), a partially spliced (HIV) or singly spliced (HTLV family of retroviruses, HTDV/HERV-K, MMTV) mRNA (encoding *env*), and multiply spliced (HIV) or doubly spliced (HTLV, HTDV/HERV-K, MMTV) mRNAs (encoding regulatory and accessory genes). These additional proteins either are necessary for expression at transcriptional and posttranscriptional level or serve other functions by participating in virus–cell interaction and promoting infectivity.

VI. HIV-I mRNAs Use Multiple Mechanisms to Express Many Proteins from One Transcript

Virus production requires optimal levels of viral precursor RNA and the generation of all virus proteins at levels optimal for particle formation and infectivity. HIV encodes nine genes (Fig. 3). Expression of these proteins from one primary transcript is accomplished by alternative splicing utilizing a combination of the 21 identified exons as well as by the use of bicistronic mRNAs (Vpu/env) and translational frameshifting (i.e., Gag/Pol polyprotein). Therefore, splicing of HIV primary transcript is an essential and highly regulated task, requiring concerted interactions via multiple *cis*-acting splice signals on the HIV primary transcript, which bind to a multitude of factors of the cellular splicing machinery. Such signals and their corresponding binding factors are distinguished as positive or negative acting according to their effect on splicing and ultimately the production and expression of the viral mRNAs (Amendt *et al.*, 1994; Si *et al.*, 1997; Staffa and Cochrane, 1994, 1995; Tange and Kjems, 2001; Tange *et al.*, 2001). The generation of these alternatively spliced mRNA is controlled, in addition to Rev/RRE, via a complex array of splicing enhancers and silencers through their interactions (Fig. 3, locations indicated by open arrow head) with the proteins of the cellular hnRNP A/B family, hnRNP H and the SR family proteins (reviewed in Cochrane *et al.*, 2006; Stoltzfus and Madsen, 2006).

Detailed analysis of HIV splicing revealed the generation of more than 30 mRNAs (Benko *et al.*, 1990; Neumann *et al.*, 1994; Purcell and Martin, 1993; Salfeld *et al.*, 1990; Schwartz *et al.*, 1990a,b, 1991), which are shown in Fig. 3 (bottom panel). The HIV mRNAs fall into three size categories: unspliced, partially spliced (expressing *env, vif, vpu, vpr*), and multiply spliced (expressing *tat, rev, nef*). The unspliced and partially spliced mRNAs contain RRE and depend on Rev for export and expression. The fully spliced mRNAs lack the RRE, are expressed independently of Rev, and are transported from the nucleus via the default mRNA export machinery (utilizing the cellular NXF1 nuclear receptor). The spliced mRNAs are generated by the use of the strong splice donor located 5′ to *gag* (nt 289, Fig. 3) in combination with a series of 3′ splice sites present throughout the precursor mRNA. The presence of a series of 5′ and 3′ splice sites allows for the generation of partially and multiply spliced mRNAs. Although expressed open reading frames (ORFs) are usually preceded by a 3′ splice site, Env is produced only from bistronic *vpu/env* mRNAs. Although several mRNAs produce more than one ORF, it was found that the Tat translation initiation site provides a dominant ribosomal entry site that excludes expression of downstream ORFs (i.e., *rev, env*) by leaky scanning, thus mRNAs (containing exons 4 or 4E) that have Tat as the first ORF express Tat exclusively (Schwartz *et al.*, 1992c). Thus, HIV produces monocistronic (Gag/Pol from the unspliced mRNA and Tat from the exon 4-containing mRNAs) as well as bicistronic mRNAs (using exons 4A, 4B, or 4C for *rev/nef* and exon 5E for *vpu/env*). Thus, there is a great redundancy in that most of the HIV genes are expressed from several mRNAs (Fig. 3), for example, the multiply spliced mRNAs containing exons 4A, 4B, or 4C encode *rev* or the mRNAs containing exon 5 spliced to exons 7, 7A, or 7B encode *nef*. Not all the combinations of exons encode wild-type proteins, for example, splicing of exon 4 to exon 7A or splicing of exons 4A, 4B, or 4C to exon 7A generates Tat and Rev proteins with 8-aa insertions, respectively, but the existence or function of such proteins has not been verified. The small noncoding exons 2 and 3 are present or absent from the multiply spliced species and generate mRNAs with structures like the *tat*-encoding mRNAs 1.4.7, 1.2.4.7, and 1.3.4.7. Taken together, alternative splicing greatly contributes to production of multiple mRNAs encoding a given HIV gene.

Small differences in nucleotide composition of these diverse *cis*-acting signals can have profound effects on splicing, and the levels of individual mRNAs are affected greatly by a few nucleotide substitutions. For example, many HIV-1 isolates express an mRNA that has an additional small exon 6D (Fig. 3) and produces a fusion of Tat-Env-Rev protein, named Tev (Benko *et al.*, 1990; Salfeld *et al.*, 1990), which has both Tat and Rev function (Benko *et al.*, 1990). Another example of splicing variability is the poor expression of *env* due to oversplicing in a molecular HIV clone having a G to A substitution 28 nts upstream of the splice acceptor site SA7 (Paca-Uccaralertkun *et al.*, 2006). This is the region of an identified intron splicing silencer sequence (Damgaard *et al.*, 2002). Interestingly, different HIV isolates also differ in the relative quantities of mRNAs produced (Neumann *et al.*, 1994, 1995; Purcell and Martin, 1993). It has also been proposed recently that some conserved cryptic splice sites (exon 1A) within

HIV *pol* may be important for the regulation of the stability of viral mRNAs (Lutzelberger *et al.*, 2006).

A fine-tuned balance of expression of all the viral mRNAs is essential for the production of infectious virus. The presence of Rev plays a central role in removing mRNAs from the splicing machinery and provides the switch for the production of partially spliced and unspliced transcripts. The multiply spliced mRNA species do not have any problem to be exported using the default mRNA export pathway and they rapidly localize to the cytoplasm after splicing, producing Tat, Rev, and Nef. Except for Tat, Rev, and Nef, all other viral genes are produced from intron-containing mRNAs and are Rev dependent (Fig. 3). A recent study describes the surprising observation that mRNAs encoding the viral regulatory proteins Tat and Rev are retained in the nucleus of infected resting CD4+ T cells (Lassen *et al.*, 2006). Export and expression of such multiply spliced mRNAs was achieved upon over-expression of a cellular RNA-binding protein, the polypyrimidine tract-binding protein (PTB), which was identified to bind these HIV-1 mRNAs. PTB has been implicated in regulating alternative splicing as well as translation (Spellman *et al.*, 2005; Valcarcel and Gebauer, 1997). PTB overexpression in resting CD4+ T cells reversed latency and allowed release of replication-competent HIV-1 without inducing cellular stimulation. These experiments imply regulation of latency at the level of nuclear mRNA export.

VII. Rev-Dependence of HIV-1 mRNAs

In the absence of Rev, the INS/CRS containing HIV-1 mRNAs (Fig. 3) are retained in the nucleus, where they are subjected to either complete splicing or degradation. Rev acts as a molecular switch and increases levels of the RRE-containing mRNAs at the expense of the multiply spliced mRNAs (Felber *et al.*, 1990) and by mediating efficient export and expression of the RRE-containing mRNAs. From this discussion, it is apparent that Rev acts in competition with splicing and rescues unspliced mRNAs for export and translation in the cytoplasm. Interestingly, the Rev–RRE interaction does not affect the expression of a generally well-expressed mRNA. For example, globin pre-mRNA having RRE inserted into its introns or exons is not affected substantially by Rev, and mutation of globin splice sites was necessary to facilitate Rev regulation (Chang and Sharp, 1989). Since globin mRNA is spliced very efficiently, it may not be possible to interfere in this process. Experiments with HIV mRNAs indicated that there are special requirements in these mRNAs making them maximally responsive to Rev. Research from many groups indicates the importance of other *cis*-acting elements in mRNAs that affect the sequence of events leading to processing and transport. It is clear that a large number of nuclear proteins affect the processing of HIV-1 mRNAs. A large family of such factors is related to splicing. HIV-1 splice site arrangement is of course complex, but it also has to be "leaky" or "slow" so that some mRNA can escape splicing. Rev facilitates this escape by linking the unspliced mRNA with the CRM1 exporter, but it is clear that other factors participate in this process by interacting with the mRNA and either affecting its stability and processing or localizing it in sites facilitating Rev function. Certain reports have identified the special properties of some HIV-1 splice sites, which indicate that under certain conditions, 5' splice sites can act as mRNA stabilizers. In the absence of splicing, the 5' splice sites in *env* (splice donor SD5) (Lu *et al.*, 1990) and *pol* (splice donor SD1A) (Lutzelberger *et al.*, 2006) appear to facilitate its rescue by Rev, and the role of U1 snRNA in this process has been recognized.

Although it was proposed that Rev is a direct inhibitor of splicing and that association of splicing components (i.e., U1) is essential for Rev function (Chang and Sharp, 1989; Kjems *et al.*, 1991; Lu *et al.*, 1990), it was also realized that the Rev–RRE interaction could rescue mRNAs that did not go through the splicing pathway (Felber *et al.*, 1989b). For example, subgenomic *gag* and *env* mRNAs, lacking active splice sites, were poorly expressed in the absence of Rev and could be rescued by Rev (Felber *et al.*, 1989b; Nasioulas *et al.*, 1994). This led to the identification of several regions in the *gag*, *pol*, and *env* coding sequences that had a *cis*-acting negative effect on mRNA expression (Cochrane *et al.*, 1991; Nasioulas *et al.*, 1994; Olsen *et al.*, 1992; Schneider *et al.*, 1997; Schwartz *et al.*, 1992a). Sequences able to inhibit expression of mRNA are referred to as INS or CRS and are embedded within the intronic regions (i.e., *gag/pol*, *vif*, and *env*) of HIV-1 mRNAs (Fig. 3). Such elements do not contain any splice sites and they act independent of splicing. It was noted that some INS have an overall higher AU content but no common sequences or structures were identified. Some INS also contain the classical AU-rich elements (AREs) with the signature motif AUUUA (Schneider *et al.*, 1997), which are also found in the 3'UTR of many cytokine and other mRNAs and are responsible for their posttranscriptional control (Shaw and Kamen, 1986; reviewed in Chen and Shyu, 1995; Shim and Karin, 2002) and may contribute to cytoplasmic control of viral mRNAs.

Importantly, functionally analogous nuclear retention signals are found in all lentiviruses, viruses of the HTLV family, RSV, SRV/D, as well as IAP retroelements, suggesting their biological relevance. Several mRNA-binding proteins, including p54nrb/PSF, PTB (hnRNP I), hnRNP A1, and polyadenylate-binding protein 1 (PABP1) were shown to bind specifically to INS elements of HIV-1 *in vitro* (Afonina *et al.*, 1997, 1998; Black *et al.*, 1995, 1996; Najera *et al.*, 1999; Zolotukhin *et al.*, 2003). Of these, PABP1, which normally binds to the polyA tail at 3' end of mRNAs, may act by providing a premature 3'-end definition mark when bound to INS within coding sequences, and thus may cause translation inhibition. Another factor, the p54nrb/PSF heterodimer, is able to shuttle rapidly between paraspeckles, a nuclear domain adjacent to splicing factor compartment, and the nucleoli/

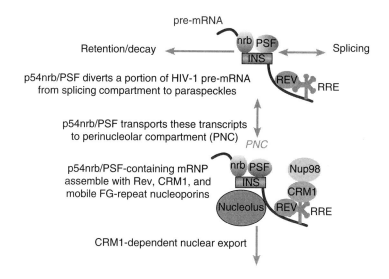

FIGURE 6 Possible mechanism by which p54nrb/PSF acts via INS determinants to sequester HIV-1 transcripts from splicing and to direct them to the CRM1 export route (Zolotukhin *et al.*, 2003). This pathway likely includes the participation of other cellular factors such as proteins identified to bind to the Rev-dependent mRNAs (reviewed in Cochrane *et al.*, 2006).

perinucleolar compartment (PNC) (Dye and Patton, 2001; Fox *et al.*, 2002, 2005; Shav-Tal and Zipori, 2002; Shav-Tal *et al.*, 2005) that is believed to be a crucial site where Rev/CRM1 export is initiated (Daelemans *et al.*, 2005a; Michienzi *et al.*, 2000; Romanov *et al.*, 1997; Zolotukhin and Felber, 1999) (Fig. 6). p54nrb/PSF was proposed to assist Rev to divert the INS-containing transcripts from the splicing route (Zolotukhin *et al.*, 2003), as previously suggested for factors mediating INS function (Afonina *et al.*, 1997, 1998; Berthold and Maldarelli, 1996; Felber *et al.*, 1989b; Mikaelian *et al.*, 1996; Schneider *et al.*, 1997; Schwartz *et al.*, 1992b). Figure 6 shows a model where p54nrb/PSF binds cotranscriptionally to a portion of INS-containing HIV-1 pre-mRNA, physically diverts them from splicing compartment to paraspeckles, and further transports them to the nucleoli/perinucleolar space, where they are assembled with Rev, CRM1, and mobile nucleoporins into export-ready complexes (Zolotukhin *et al.*, 2003).

VIII. Use of RNA Optimization to Achieve High Level of HIV-1 *gag/pol* and *env* Expression Plasmids

Expression of HIV-1 *gag/pol*, *vif*, and *env* requires the viral Rev-RRE regulatory system or alternatively the presence of CTE (Bray *et al.*, 1994; Tabernero *et al.*, 1996) (Rosati and B. K. F., unpublished data), RTE (Nappi *et al.*, 2001), or the RTE-CTE combination (Smulevitch *et al.*, 2006;

see below). Alternatively, altering the nucleotide composition within eight INS regions in the *gag* mRNA (changing 81 of the 1500 nt *gag* gene) without altering the produced protein led to a profound 2-log increase in Gag protein expression in the absence of Rev/RRE (Schneider *et al.*, 1997; Schwartz *et al.*, 1992a). Thus, changes of the nucleotide sequence without altering the amino acid sequence, referred to as RNA or codon optimization, inactivates the INS and CRS and results in high level and Rev-independent production of Gag, Pol, and Env (Graf *et al.*, 2000; Kofman *et al.*, 2003; Kumar *et al.*, 2006; Nasioulas *et al.*, 1994; Rosati *et al.*, 2005; Schneider *et al.*, 1997; Schwartz *et al.*, 1992a). In a recent paper, Graf *et al.* (2006) described the generation of a GFP reporter gene using HIV-like codons which resulted in reduction of GFP expression that can be augmented with the help of the Rev-RRE regulatory system. It is likely that introduction of these global codon changes inadvertently created binding sites of negative-acting factors (reviewed also in Cochrane *et al.*, 2006) analogous to those identified to bind to HIV RNAs or cryptic splice sites. In summary, the discovery of INS and CRS and their effective elimination by RNA optimization has an important practical application, which is the use of such RNA-optimized HIV genes in DNA plasmids or recombinant viral vectors currently used in many vaccine studies in monkeys and humans.

It was speculated that the HIV codons are less adapted to human cells (Grantham *et al.*, 1980), thus HIV mRNAs are poorly expressed due to limitation in the tRNA pool (Haas *et al.*, 1996). It can be argued that changing the codon usage to codons preferred in human cells will increase the translation efficiency, thus resulting in higher protein levels. Several lines of evidence indicate that this hypothesis is not valid: (1) in the presence of Rev, the RRE-containing mRNA produces high levels of protein, despite the "inefficient" codon composition (Cochrane *et al.*, 1990a; Feinberg *et al.*, 1986; Hadzopoulou-Cladaras *et al.*, 1989; Hammarskjöld *et al.*, 1989; Malim and Cullen, 1991; Olsen *et al.*, 1991); (2) INS elements also exerted their downregulatory effect when placed downstream of a reporter coding region, thus they function at the RNA level rather than at translation (Schwartz *et al.*, 1992a,b); (3) changes of few codons (e.g., changes of 69 of 500 codons in *gag*) are sufficient to achieve a >2-log increase in Gag expression (Schneider *et al.*, 1997); (4) efficient expression of HIV *gag* and *env* was obtained from wild-type HIV genes (Chakrabarti *et al.*, 1986; Karacostas *et al.*, 1989) in the absence of Rev-RRE, when expressed from poxvirus vectors such as vaccinia and avipoxviruses (reviewed in Franchini *et al.*, 2004). Poxvirus mRNAs are produced in the cytoplasm and do not enter the nucleus (Moss *et al.*, 1991). Thus, these mRNAs are confined to the cytoplasm, and therefore "escape" the nuclear "experience" and the regulated export process. Taken together, these facts support the model in which INS/CRS elements provide interaction sites for cellular factors that negatively affect the fate of these transcripts in the nuclear compartment, which consequently affects their fate in the cytoplasm. This downregulatory effect can be counteracted either by the presence of posttranscriptional regulatory system (i.e., Rev-RRE, NXF1-CTE, RBM15-RTE) or by removing the negative-acting RNA signals through RNA/codon optimization.

In conclusion, RNA optimization eliminates the negatively-acting elements, thus abolishing interaction with INS-binding cellular factors, rendering the mRNAs Rev independent. This general method of RNA/codon optimization is now used successfully for the optimization of numerous viral and cellular mRNAs and results in great gains in mRNA stability, transport, and expression. Importantly, most of the candidate AIDS vaccines moving toward the clinic incorporate RNA/codon optimization to achieve efficient antigen expression.

IX. Posttranscriptional Control of Simple Retroviruses _____

Simple retroviruses [i.e., simian type D retroviruses (SRV/D), Avian sarcoma/leukosis virus (ASV/ALV), Murine leukemia virus (MuLV)] do not encode additional regulatory or accessory proteins and produce one unspliced and one spliced mRNA. RNA elements essential for nucleocytoplasmic transport of viral mRNAs have been studied in detail for SRV/D [CTE (Bray *et al.*, 1994; Tabernero *et al.*, 1996)] and the ASV/ALV family member RSV [direct repeat element, DR (Ogert and Beemon, 1998; Ogert *et al.*, 1996; Paca *et al.*, 2000)] (Table I). In contrast to HIV, the export of the viral unspliced mRNA is mediated solely by cellular factors, which belong to the conserved RNA export machinery. MuLV contains well-defined signals controlling the generation of the spliced mRNAs (reviewed in Cochrane *et al.*, 2006), but the mechanism used to export its unspliced mRNA is unknown.

For the SRV/D retroviruses, including SRV-1, SRV-2, and MPMV, the RNA export mechanism has been studied in detail. Export of the unspliced SRV/D retrovirus mRNA is mediated by the cellular nuclear export factor 1 (NXF1; previously named TAP) (Grüter *et al.*, 1998), which directly binds to the *cis*-acting constitutive RNA export element (CTE) (Fig. 4D). CTE spans ~170 nts, is located between *env* and the 3'LTR, and is present in both the unspliced mRNA producing Gag/Pol and the singly spliced mRNA encoding Env. Molecular clones of SRV-1 lacking the CTE were found to produce only *env* but not *gag* (Tabernero *et al.*, 1997). Despite the presence of CTE, the singly spliced mRNA does not depend on CTE, and can be exported and expressed independently. In contrast, CTE is essential for the production of Gag/Pol and, hence, for the production of infectious virus.

The CTEs of SRV/D consist of four imperfect direct repeats that represent the core NXF1 binding sites. CTE of SRV-1 and MPMV were shown to fold into an extended stem-loop structure in which these sites are juxtaposed in a mirror-symmetrical fashion within the two internal loops (Fig. 4) (Ernst *et al.*, 1997; Tabernero *et al.*, 1996). Sequence comparison between SRV/D family CTEs shows 88–92% identity, and the nucleotide changes within the stem regions are typically accompanied by compensatory changes maintaining the conserved secondary structure. NXF1 binds to CTE via sequences located in the internal loops and promotes the nucleocytoplasmic export of CTE-containing mRNAs (Grüter *et al.*, 1998). Importantly, NXF1 is essential for cellular mRNA export and defines a general mRNA export pathway that is conserved from yeast to humans (Grüter *et al.*, 1998; Herold *et al.*, 2001; Segref *et al.*, 1997; Tan *et al.*, 2000; Wilkie *et al.*, 2001). Hence, NXF1 is the first cellular protein known to directly mediate mRNA export by providing a direct molecular link between mRNAs and components of the NPC. Thus, although functionally analogous to CRM1, NXF1 identifies a distinct transport pathway (Fig. 2, Table I).

X. NXF1

NXF1 orthologues in eukaryotes share a conserved structural domain architecture including (from the N-terminus) a noncanonical RNP-type RBD, the leucine-rich repeats region (LRR), the NTF2-like domain (sharing structure with NTF2 protein), and the ubiquitin-associated-like domain (UBA-like). Studies of the human NXF1 led to the delineation of functional determinants and signals, which include: (1) A substrate-binding domain comprising RBD and LRR, which exhibits general RNA binding and high-affinity binding to CTE RNA (Braun *et al.*, 1999; Grüter *et al.*, 1998; Liker *et al.*, 2000). This domain contains the regions required for the direct binding to Aly/REF and U2AF35 proteins that serve to facilitate the binding of NXF1 to export-ready mRNAs (Bachi *et al.*, 2000; Stutz *et al.*, 2000; Zolotukhin *et al.*, 2002), and a portion of this domain was shown to be sufficient for the assembly of NXF1 with spliced mRNA (Zolotukhin *et al.*, 2002). Also embedded in this domain is the NLS (Bear *et al.*, 1999) that directs the transportin1-mediated nuclear import (Truant *et al.*, 1999) and an NES that acts via an unknown receptor (Bear *et al.*, 1999), as well as the binding site of microtubule-associated proteins (MAP1A and MAP1B), which are thought to participate in NXF1-dependent cytoplasmic trafficking (Tretyakova *et al.*, 2005; A.S.Z. and B.K.F., unpublished data). (2) The p15/NXT1-binding domain that is structurally similar to nuclear transport factor NTF2 and heterodimerizes with p15/NXT1 cofactor that is also similar to NTF2 (Guzik *et al.*, 2001; Levesque *et al.*, 2001, 2006; Wiegand *et al.*, 2002). This NTF2-like heterodimeric unit acts to recognize the FG-repeats of nucleoporins (Fribourg *et al.*, 2001). (3) The UBA-like domain (Herold *et al.*, 2000) synergizes with p15/NXT1-binding domain to mediate mRNA transport through NPC (Fribourg *et al.*, 2001; Suyama *et al.*, 2000).

NXF1 function is conserved throughout evolution. The human, *C. elegans,* and *Drosophila* NXF1 and the *Saccharomyces cerevisiae* ortho-logue Mex67p are essential for general mRNA export from the nucleus and act as direct export receptors for their mRNA cargo (Braun *et al.,* 1999; Erkmann and Kutay, 2004; Grüter *et al.,* 1998; Herold *et al.,* 2003; Segref *et al.,* 1997; Tan *et al.,* 2000). While retroviruses need to export some of their transcripts before splicing (see above), the export of cellular mRNAs usually occurs after splicing. In case of the retroviral transcripts, NXF1 binds with high affinity directly to CTE, which acts as a constitutive, splicing-independent export mark, mediating the export of CTE-containing mRNA prior to splicing. In contrast, NXF1 is added to the "export-ready" cellular mRNPs as a result of splicing via interactions with cofactors such as exonic junction complex (EJC) components, Aly/REF and Y14/MAGOH (Kataoka *et al.,* 2000, 2001; Strasser and Hurt, 2000; Stutz *et al.,* 2000), as well as with shuttling SR (serine/arginine-rich) splicing factors such as U2AF (Zolotukhin *et al.,* 2002), 9G8, SRp20, and ASF/SF2 (Huang and Steitz, 2001; Huang *et al.,* 2003, 2004; Lai and Tarn, 2004; for reviews see Dreyfuss *et al.,* 1993; Izaurralde, 2002, 2004; Vinciguerra and Stutz, 2004). As part of the export complex, NXF1 interacts with the FG-repeat domains of nucleoporins, a molecular step that is facilitated by the hetero-dimerization of NXF1 with p15/NXT1 (Black *et al.,* 2001; Guzik *et al.,* 2001; Katahira *et al.,* 2002; Levesque *et al.,* 2001; Ossareh-Nazari *et al.,* 2000; Wiegand *et al.,* 2002), and subsequently the NXF1-containing mRNP complex translocates to the cytoplasm by a yet unknown mechanism. Unlike CRM1 and other exportins, NXF1-mediated nucleocytoplasmic transloca-tion is not controlled by Ran GTPase, but instead could be driven by DBP5 RNA helicase that resides at the cytoplasmic face of NPC. Dbp5 is believed to use ATP hydrolysis to assist the NPC translocation of mRNP, when stimulated by its cofactor GLE1 and inositol hexakisphosphate (Cole and Scarcelli, 2006; Weirich *et al.,* 2006). NXF1 further participates in cytoplas-mic trafficking of mRNPs and stably associates with cytoplasmic mRNPs (Zolotukhin *et al.,* 2002) as well as with mRNAs in the polysomal fraction (Jin *et al.,* 2003). Thus, NXF1 participates in the nuclear and cytoplamic trafficking of mRNPs and may also promote translation.

XI. Cellular CTEs

CTEs in SRV/D and in the related murine IAP are highly organized elements consisting of four imperfect direct repeats that constitute the core NXF1 binding sites, which in the secondary RNA structure are juxtaposed within the two internal loops (Fig. 4D). It is therefore possible that the modern CTEs originated from a repeated cellular NXF1-binding sequence that was acquired by ancestral retroviruses and further evolved into a high-affinity

NXF1-binding ligand due to the selective pressure of viral replication. Such a candidate CTE precursor was isolated based on high affinity to NXF1 and consists of multiple 15-nt repeats that are homologous to NXF1-binding motifs in CTE. This element, termed TAP-binding element or TBE, also forms a secondary structure in which these repeat sequences are juxtaposed in a manner similar to NXF1-binding motifs in CTE. Like CTE, TBE is an active nuclear export element. Based on the presence of significant homologies in the regions that are functionally neutral, it was proposed that TBE-like sequences were evolutionary precursors of CTE (Zolotukhin *et al.*, 2001).

An interesting, recent finding is the identification of a cellular CTE-like sequence *Tap*-CTE (Li *et al.*, 2006). This element includes only one of the two NXF1-binding motifs of CTE and resides within the alternatively spliced intron 10 of the human NXF1 gene. NXF1 was shown to act via this CTE to promote the production of a splice variant, which has the CTE-containing intron retained and expresses a truncated NXF1 protein. Importantly, such CTEs are conserved within the NXF1 genes from humans to fish, indicating their functional relevance. Such elements show no evidence of being evolutionary related to TBE (Zolotukhin *et al.*, 2001; A.S.Z. and B.K. F., unpublished data). It is possible that this "cellular" CTE and the viral CTEs emerged independently, as a result of convergent evolution.

XII. Posttranscriptional Control of LTR-Retroelements ⎯⎯⎯

The mouse genome contains thousands of copies of IAP retroelements. These elements contain genes for *gag*, *protease*, and *pol*, a "fossilized" *env* region, and an RNA export element [i.e, CTE-like element (Tabernero *et al.*, 1997) or an RTE (Nappi *et al.*, 2001)] which are flanked by two LTRs. Although most IAPs contain large deletions, intact transposition-competent IAPs have recently been identified (Dewannieux *et al.*, 2004). Our studies showed that the presence of an RNA export element is essential for retrotransposition (A.S.Z. and B.K.F., unpublished data).

Interestingly, on the basis of the presence of posttranscriptional regulatory elements, the murine IAPs can be grouped into two subclasses, indicating a complex evolutionary history. IAPs can carry the CTE-related element CTE_{IAP} (Tabernero *et al.*, 1997) (Fig. 4D), or they carry a distinct element named RTE, which was originally identified by genetic complementation experiments (Nappi *et al.*, 2001) (Fig. 4C). Both CTE_{IAP} and RTE are able to replace Rev/RRE and to rescue virus after insertion into a Rev- and RRE-minus clones of HIV-1 and SIVmac239 (Bray *et al.*, 1994; Nappi *et al.*, 2001; Tabernero *et al.*, 1996, 1997; Valentin *et al.*, 1997; von Gegerfelt and Felber, 1997; von Gegerfelt *et al.*, 2006; Zolotukhin *et al.*, 1994). Thus, these are potent RNA export elements necessary for the transport the full-length IAP mRNA, and they are able substitute for the Rev-RRE export mechanism in HIV and SIV.

A. CTE-Related Element, CTE$_{IAP}$

This 170-nt element shares some identity with the SRV/D CTE and preserves only the overall RNA structure and the sequence of these internal loop regions (Tabernero *et al.*, 1997) (Fig. 4D). The sequences of the double-stranded regions are far divergent but the changes are of compensatory nature, demonstrating that the stem structure and not the sequence of these regions is important for function. The conserved internal loops contain the direct binding sites for the cellular mRNA export factor NXF1 (Grüter *et al.*, 1998). Despite the conservation of the NXF1 binding sites, it was found that CTE$_{IAP}$ is less potent compared to CTE in mediating Rev-dependent reporter gene expression (i.e., HIV Gag). This supports the notion that structural components contribute significantly to the proper positioning of the binding sites within the elements, reminiscent to the findings from mutagenesis studies of RRE, RXRE, and RcRE.

B. RTE

The functional 226-nt RTE RNA element folds into an extended RNA stem structure (Smulevitch *et al.*, 2005) (Fig. 4C). The minimal RTE contains four internal stem loops that are indispensable for function in mammalian cells. RTE is structurally unrelated to the CTE or the CTE$_{IAP}$ (compare Fig. 4C and D). More than 3000 RTE and RTE-related elements were identified in the mouse genome sharing at least 70% sequence identity with the prototype RTE (Nappi *et al.*, 2001). These elements form four subgroups based on their sequence and structure. The predicted key structural features of RTE are preserved among the related elements, consistent with their functional importance. Like CTE, RTE utilizes the cellular mRNA transport machinery and functions in many cell types of different species, indicating that the export factor(s) recognizing RTE are widely expressed and evolutionarily conserved (Nappi *et al.*, 2001). Interestingly, the combination of RTE and CTE in *cis* synergistically increases expression of unstable lentiviral mRNAs, suggesting the NXF1 participates in RTE export (Smulevitch *et al.*, 2006). Recent studies from our laboratories identified the human RNA-binding motif protein 15 (RBM 15) to bind to RTE and to promote export of RTE-containing mRNAs. Interestingly, RBM15 acts as molecular link to tether the RTE-containing mRNAs to the NXF1 pathway (Lindtner *et al.*, 2006).

XIII. Comparison of RNA Export Systems _____

Comparison of the structures of the known *cis*-acting retroviral RNA export elements shows a high degree of complexity with RRE, RXRE, and RcRE being more complex, followed by RTE and then CTE, the simplest stem-loop structure among this group (Fig. 4). Mutagenesis studies of these elements showed that these stem-loop structures are embedded within a tightly structured RNA. Mutagenesis away from the primary binding site(s) for the export factors was often found to eliminate function of the element, probably due to changes in the overall structure. Interestingly, it was found that some of the viral factors cross-activate, for example, HTLV-I Rex can act on HIV-1 RRE (Bogerd et al., 1991; Felber et al., 1989a; Hanly et al., 1989; Itoh et al., 1989; Lewis et al., 1990; Rimsky et al., 1988), but Rev does not act on HTLV-I RXRE (Felber et al., 1989a; Hanly et al., 1989; Rimsky et al., 1988); HTDV/HERV-K Rec acts only on its own RcRE, while HIV Rev and HTLV Rex act also on RcRE (Magin et al., 1999, 2000; Yang et al., 2000); HIV Rev was found to activate the MMTV RmRE (Dangerfield et al., 2005). On the other hand, NXF1 and RBM15 act on their respective elements and not on viral RNA export elements like RRE. In conclusion, there is specificity at the level of protein–RNA interaction. The export factors Rev, Rex, Rec, and Rem tether their respective RNAs to the CRM1 export receptor. In contrast, RBM15 tethers the RTE RNA to the NXF1 receptor, while the CTE RNA is directly recognized by NXF1. Thus, studies of different retroviruses contributed to the identification of two distinct export routes, utilizing CRM1 and NXF1, respectively (Fig. 2, Table I).

XIV. Replacement of Rev Regulation Leads to SIV Attenuation

The understanding of the mechanism of mRNA export and of posttranscriptional regulation of lentivirus expression led to the development of HIV and SIV molecular clones which have Rev/RRE system replaced by the CTE or RTE (Bray et al., 1994; Nappi et al., 2001; Smulevitch et al., 2006; Valentin et al., 1997; von Gegerfelt and Felber, 1997; Zolotukhin et al., 1994). These Rev-independent HIV and SIV clones have altered expression and pathogenicity profiles (Nappi et al., 2001; Valentin et al., 1997; von Gegerfelt and Felber, 1997; von Gegerfelt et al., 1999, 2002, 2006; Zolotukhin et al., 1994). In vivo studies showed that such Rev-independent SIV viruses can propagate in Indian rhesus macaques, infected as neonates or juveniles, but they are nonpathogenic for more that 7 years (von Gegerfelt et al., 1999, 2002, 2006). Moreover, the macaques are chronically infected, but they have very restricted SIV replication (plasma virus loads of less than 100 copies per milliliter), which is controlled by the body's immune system. The lack of development of signs of immune dysfunction in macaques infected by the Rev-independent strains indicates that Rev is a factor essential for the high levels of HIV-1 propagation and for pathogenicity. These data suggest that Rev inhibition, even partial, may have beneficial results and may reduce the pathogenicity of HIV, enabling control of viremia. It is therefore highly desirable to develop drugs able to interfere with Rev function.

XV. Conclusions

Over the past 20 years, research by numerous laboratories has added significantly to our understanding of regulation of expression of retroviruses, and the essential steps governing trafficking of retroviral mRNAs within the nucleus, through the nuclear pore, and in the cytoplasm. This line of research has been instrumental for our understanding of the trafficking of cellular proteins and RNAs. Importantly, we know that there are two distinct export routes, using either CRM1 or NXF1 as nuclear receptors (Fig. 2, Table I). We also have a deep appreciation of the complex interaction between cellular nuclear retention/degradation machinery, splicing, and export mechanisms. Research on retroviruses has been instrumental for the discovery of many of these sophisticated posttranscriptional regulatory steps. Our understanding of the restriction of mRNA expression and the potent tools retroviruses utilize to counteract such nuclear restrictions in order to maximize retroviral mRNA expression, also led to the practical and widely used application of RNA optimization as a powerful approach to obtain high-level of gene expression, essential for many vaccine approaches including HIV.

Acknowledgments

We thank M. Rosati for discussions and T. Jones for editorial assistance.

References

Afonina, E., Neumann, M., and Pavlakis, G. N. (1997). Preferential binding of poly(A)-binding protein 1 to an inhibitory RNA element in the human immunodeficiency virus type 1 gag mRNA. *J. Biol. Chem.* **272**, 2307–2311.

Afonina, E., Stauber, R., and Pavlakis, G. N. (1998). The human Poly(A) binding protein 1 shuttles between the nucleus and the cytoplasm. *J. Biol. Chem.* **273**, 13015–13021.

Amendt, B. A., Hesslein, D., Chang, L., and Stoltzfus, C. M. (1994). Presence of negative and positive cis-acting RNA splicing elements within and flanking the first tat coding exon of human immunodeficiency virus type 1. *Mol. Cell. Biol.* **14**, 3960–3970.

Arrigo, S. J., and Chen, I. S. Y. (1991). Rev is necessary for translation but not cytoplasmic accumulation of HIV-1 *vif, vpr,* and *env/vpu* 2 RNAs. *Genes Dev.* **5**, 808–819.

Bachi, A., Braun, I. C., Rodrigues, J. P., Pante, N., Ribbeck, K., von Kobbe, C., Kutay, U., Wilm, M., Gorlich, D., Carmo-Fonseca, M., and Izaurralde, E. (2000). The C-terminal domain of TAP interacts with the nuclear pore complex and promotes export of specific CTE-bearing RNA substrates. *RNA* **6**, 136–158.

Bailey, T. L., and Elkan, C. (1994). Fitting a mixture model by expectation maximization to discover motifs in biopolymers. *Proc. Int. Conf. Intell. Syst. Mol. Biol.* **2**, 28–36.

Bar-Sinai, A., Bassa, N., Fischette, M., Gottesman, M. M., Love, D. C., Hanover, J. A., and Hochman, J. (2005). Mouse mammary tumor virus Env-derived peptide associates with nucleolar targets in lymphoma, mammary carcinoma, and human breast cancer. *Cancer Res.* **65**, 7223–7230.

Bartel, D., Zapp, M., Green, M., and Szostak, J. (1991). HIV-1 Rev regulation involves recognition of non-Watson-Crick base pairs in viral RNA. *Cell* 67, 529–536.

Bear, J., Tan, W., Zolotukhin, A. S., Tabernero, C., Hudson, E. A., and Felber, B. K. (1999). Identification of novel import and export signals of human TAP, the protein that binds to the constitutive transport element of the type D retrovirus mRNAs. *Mol. Cell. Biol.* 19, 6306–6317.

Benko, D. M., Schwartz, S., Pavlakis, G. N., and Felber, B. K. (1990). A novel human immunodeficiency virus type 1 protein, *tev*, shares sequences with *tat*, *env*, and *rev* proteins. *J. Virol.* 64, 2505–2518.

Berthold, E., and Maldarelli, F. (1996). cis-acting elements in human immunodeficiency virus type 1 RNAs direct viral transcripts to distinct intranuclear locations. *J. Virol.* 70, 4667–4682.

Bevec, D., and Hauber, J. (1997). Eukaryotic initiation factor 5A activity and HIV-1 Rev function. *Biol. Signals* 6, 124–133.

Black, A. C., Luo, J., Watanabe, C., Chun, S., Bakker, A., Fraser, J. K., Morgan, J. P., and Rosenblatt, J. D. (1995). Polypyrimidine tract-binding protein and heterogeneous nuclear ribonucleoprotein A1 bind to human T-cell leukemia virus type 2 RNA regulatory elements. *J. Virol.* 69, 6852–6858.

Black, A. C., Luo, J., Chun, S., Bakker, A., Fraser, J. K., and Rosenblatt, J. D. (1996). Specific binding of polypyrimidine tract binding protein and hnRNP A1 to HIV-1 CRS elements. *Virus Genes* 12, 275–285.

Black, B. E., Holaska, J. M., Levesque, L., Ossareh-Nazari, B., Gwizdek, C., Dargemont, C., and Paschal, B. M. (2001). NXT1 is necessary for the terminal step of Crm1-mediated nuclear export. *J. Cell Biol.* 152, 141–155.

Bogerd, H. P., Huckaby, G. L., Ahmed, Y. F., Hanly, S. M., and Greene, W. C. (1991). The type I human T-cell leukemia virus (HTLV-I) Rex trans-activator binds directly to the HTLV-I Rex and the type 1 human immunodeficiency virus Rev RNA responsive element. *Proc. Natl. Acad. Sci. USA* 88, 5704–5708.

Bogerd, H. P., Wiegand, H. L., Yang, J., and Cullen, B. R. (2000). Mutational definition of functional domains within the Rev homolog encoded by human endogenous retrovirus K. *J. Virol.* 74, 9353–9361.

Boris-Lawrie, K., Roberts, T. M., and Hull, S. (2001). Retroviral RNA elements integrate components of post-transcriptional gene expression. *Life Sci.* 69, 2697–2709.

Braun, I., Rohrbach, E., Schmitt, C., and Izaurralde, E. (1999). TAP binds to the constitutive transport element through a novel RNA-binding motif that is sufficient to promote CTE-dependent RNA export from the nucleus. *EMBO J.* 18, 1953–1965.

Bray, M., Prasad, S., Dubay, J. W., Hunter, E., Jeang, K. T., Rekosh, D., and Hammarskjold, M. L. (1994). A small element from the Mason-Pfizer monkey virus genome makes human immunodeficiency virus type 1 expression and replication Rev-independent. *Proc. Natl. Acad. Sci. USA* 91, 1256–1260.

Chakrabarti, S., Robert-Guroff, M., Wong-Staal, F., Gallo, R. C., and Moss, B. (1986). Expression of the HTLV-III envelope gene by a recombinant vaccinia virus. *Nature* 320, 535–537.

Chang, D. D., and Sharp, P. A. (1989). Regulation by HIV Rev depends upon recognition of splice sites. *Cell* 59, 789–795.

Chen, C. Y., and Shyu, A. B. (1995). AU-rich elements: Characterization and importance in mRNA degradation. *Trends Biochem. Sci.* 20, 465–470.

Coburn, G. A., and Cullen, B. R. (2002). Potent and specific inhibition of human immunodeficiency virus type 1 replication by RNA interference. *J. Virol.* 76, 9225–9231.

Cochrane, A. (2004). Controlling HIV-1 Rev function. *Curr. Drug Targets Immune Endocr. Metabol. Disord.* 4, 287–295.

Cochrane, A. W., Chen, C.-H., and Rosen, C. A. (1990a). Specific interaction of the human immunodeficiency virus Rev protein with a structured region in the env mRNA. *Proc. Natl. Acad. Sci. USA* **87**, 1198–1202.

Cochrane, A. W., Perkins, A., and Rosen, C. A. (1990b). Identification of sequences important in the nucleolar localization of human immunodeficiency virus Rev: Relevance of nucleolar localization to function. *J. Virol.* **64**, 881–885.

Cochrane, A. W., Jones, K. S., Beidas, S., Dillon, P. J., Skalka, A. M., and Rosen, C. A. (1991). Identification and characterization of intragenic sequences which repress human immunodeficiency virus structural gene expression. *J. Virol.* **65**, 5305–5313.

Cochrane, A. W., McNally, M. T., and Mouland, A. J. (2006). The retrovirus RNA trafficking granule: From birth to maturity. *Retrovirology* **3**, 18–34.

Cole, C. N., and Scarcelli, J. J. (2006). Unravelling mRNA export. *Nat. Cell Biol.* **8**, 645–647.

Cole, J. L., Gehman, J. D., Shafer, J. A., and Kuo, L. C. (1993). Solution oligomerization of the rev protein of HIV-1: Implications for function. *Biochemistry* **32**, 11769–11775.

Cook, K. S., Fisk, G. J., Hauber, J., Usman, N., Daly, T. J., and Rusche, J. R. (1991). Characterization of HIV-1 REV protein: Binding stoichiometry and minimal RNA substrate. *Nucleic Acids Res.* **19**, 1577–1583.

Cullen, B. R. (2003). Nuclear mRNA export: Insights from virology. *Trends Biochem. Sci.* **28**, 419–424.

Cullen, B. R., Hauber, J., Campbell, K., Sodroski, J. G., Haseltine, W. A., and Rosen, C. A. (1988). Subcellular localization of the human immunodeficiency virus trans-acting art gene product. *J. Virol.* **62**, 2498–2501.

D'Agostino, D. M., Felber, B. K., Harrison, J. E., and Pavlakis, G. N. (1992). The Rev protein of human immunodeficiency virus type 1 promotes polysomal association and translation of *gag/pol* and *vpu/env* mRNA. *Mol. Cell. Biol.* **12**, 1375–1386.

D'Agostino, D. M., Ciminale, V., Pavlakis, G. P., and Chieco-Bianchi, L. (1995). Intracellular trafficking of the human immunodeficiency virus type 1 Rev protein: Involvement of continued rRNA synthesis in nuclear retention. *AIDS Res. Hum. Retroviruses* **11**, 1063–1072.

Daelemans, D., Costes, S. V., Cho, E. H., Erwin-Cohen, R. A., Lockett, S., and Pavlakis, G. N. (2004). *In vivo* HIV-1 Rev multimerization in the nucleolus and cytoplasm identified by fluorescence resonance energy transfer. *J. Biol. Chem.* **279**, 50167–50175.

Daelemans, D., Costes, S. V., Lockett, S., and Pavlakis, G. N. (2005a). Kinetic and molecular analysis of nuclear export factor CRM1 association with its cargo *in vivo*. *Mol. Cell. Biol.* **25**, 728–739.

Daelemans, D., Pannecouque, C., Pavlakis, G. N., Tabarrini, O., and De Clercq, E. (2005b). A novel and efficient approach to discriminate between pre- and post-transcription HIV inhibitors. *Mol. Pharmacol.* **67**, 1574–1580.

Daly, T. J., Cook, K. S., Gray, G. S., Maione, T. E., and Rusche, J. R. (1989). Specific binding of HIV-1 recombinant Rev protein to the Rev-responsive element *in vitro*. *Nature* **342**, 816–819.

Daly, T. J., Rennert, P., Lynch, P., Barry, J. K., Dundas, M., Rusche, J. R., Doten, R. C., Auer, M., and Farrington, C. K. (1993a). Perturbation of the carboxy terminus of HIV-1 Rev affects multimerization on the Rev responsive element. *Biochemistry* **32**, 8945–8954.

Daly, T. J., Rennert, P., Lynch, P., Barry, J. K., Dundas, M., Rusche, J. R., Doten, R. C., Auer, M., and Farrington, G. K. (1993b). Perturbation of the carboxy terminus of HIV-1 Rev affects multimerization on the Rev responsive element. *Biochemistry* **32**, 8945–8954.

Damgaard, C. K., Tange, T. O., and Kjems, J. (2002). hnRNP A1 controls HIV-1 mRNA splicing through cooperative binding to intron and exon splicing silencers in the context of a conserved secondary structure. *RNA* **8**, 1401–1415.

Dangerfield, J. A., Hohenadl, C., Egerbacher, M., Kodajova, P., Salmons, B., and Gunzburg, W. H. (2005). HIV-1 Rev can specifically interact with MMTV RNA and upregulate gene expression. *Gene* 358, 17–30.

Dayton, A. I., Terwilliger, E. F., Potz, J., Kowalski, M., Sodroski, J. G., and Haseltine, W. A. (1988). Cis-acting sequences responsive to the *rev* gene product of the human immunodeficiency virus. *J. Acquir. Immune Defic. Syndr.* 1, 441–452.

Dewannieux, M., Dupressoir, A., Harper, F., Pierron, G., and Heidmann, T. (2004). Identification of autonomous IAP LTR retrotransposons mobile in mammalian cells. *Nat. Genet.* 36, 534–539.

Dreyfuss, G., Matunis, M. J., Pinol-Roma, S., and Burd, C. G. (1993). hnRNP proteins and the biogenesis of mRNA. *Annu. Rev. Biochem.* 62, 289–321.

Dye, B. T., and Patton, J. G. (2001). An RNA recognition motif (RRM) is required for the localization of PTB-associated splicing factor (PSF) to subnuclear speckles. *Exp. Cell. Res.* 263, 131–144.

Elfgang, C., Rosorius, O., Hofer, L., Jaksche, H., Hauber, J., and Bevec, D. (1999). Evidence for specific nucleocytoplasmic transport pathways used by leucine-rich nuclear export signals. *Proc. Natl. Acad. Sci. USA* 96, 6229–6234.

Emerman, M., Vazeux, R., and Peden, K. (1989). The rev gene product of the human immunodeficiency virus affects envelope-specific RNA localization. *Cell* 57, 1155–1165.

Englmeier, L., Fornerod, M., Bischoff, F. R., Petosa, C., Mattaj, I. W., and Kutay, U. (2001). RanBP3 influences interactions between CRM1 and its nuclear protein export substrates. *EMBO Rep.* 2, 926–932.

Erkmann, J. A., and Kutay, U. (2004). Nuclear export of mRNA: From the site of transcription to the cytoplasm. *Exp. Cell Res.* 296, 12–20.

Ernst, R. K., Bray, M., Rekosh, D., and Hammarskjold, M.-L. (1997). Secondary structure and mutational analysis of the Mason-Pfizer monkey virus RNA constitutive transport element. *RNA* 3, 210–222.

Fang, J., Kubota, S., Yang, B., Zhou, N., Zhang, H., Godbout, R., and Pomerantz, R. J. (2004). A DEAD box protein facilitates HIV-1 replication as a cellular co-factor of Rev. *Virology* 330, 471–480.

Fang, J., Acheampong, E., Dave, R., Wang, F., Mukhtar, M., and Pomerantz, R. J. (2005). The RNA helicase DDX1 is involved in restricted HIV-1 Rev function in human astrocytes. *Virology* 336, 299–307.

Farjot, G., Sergeant, A., and Mikaelian, I. (1999). A new nucleoporin-like protein interacts with both HIV-1 Rev nuclear export signal and CRM-1. *J. Biol. Chem.* 274, 17309–17317.

Feinberg, M. B., Jarrett, R. F., Aldovini, A., Gallo, R. C., and Wong-Staal, F. (1986). HTLV-III expression and production involve complex regulation at the levels of splicing and translation of viral RNA. *Cell* 46, 807–817.

Felber, B. K., and Pavlakis, G. N. (1993). Molecular biology of HIV-1: Positive and negative regulatory elements important for virus expression. *AIDS* 7(Suppl. 1), S51–S62.

Felber, B. K., Derse, D., Athanassopoulos, A., Campbell, M., and Pavlakis, G. N. (1989a). Cross-activation of the Rex proteins of HTLV-1 and BLV and of the Rev protein of HIV-1 and nonreciprocal interactions with their RNA responsive elements. *New Biol.* 1, 318–330.

Felber, B. K., Hadzopoulou-Cladaras, M., Cladaras, C., Copeland, T., and Pavlakis, G. N. (1989b). rev protein of human immunodeficiency virus type 1 affects the stability and transport of the viral mRNA. *Proc. Natl. Acad. Sci. USA* 86, 1495–1499.

Felber, B. K., Drysdale, C. M., and Pavlakis, G. N. (1990). Feedback regulation of human immunodeficiency virus type 1 expression by the Rev protein. *J. Virol.* 64, 3734–3741.

Fischer, U., Huber, J., Boelens, W. C., Mattaj, I. W., and Luhrmann, R. (1995). The HIV-1 Rev activation domain is a nuclear export signal that accesses an export pathway used by specific cellular RNAs. *Cell* 82, 475–483.

Fornerod, M., and Ohno, M. (2002). Exportin-mediated nuclear export of proteins and ribonucleoproteins. *Results Probl. Cell Differ.* **35**, 67–91.

Fornerod, M., Ohno, M., Yoshida, M., and Mattaj, I. W. (1997). CRM1 is an export receptor for leucine-rich nuclear export signals. *Cell* **90**, 1051–1060.

Fox, A. H., Lam, Y. W., Leung, A. K., Lyon, C. E., Andersen, J., Mann, M., and Lamond, A. I. (2002). Paraspeckles: A novel nuclear domain. *Curr. Biol.* **12**, 13–25.

Fox, A. H., Bond, C. S., and Lamond, A. I. (2005). P54nrb forms a heterodimer with PSP1 that localizes to paraspeckles in a RNA-dependent manner. *Mol. Biol. Cell* **16**, 5305–5315.

Franchini, G., Gurunathan, S., Baglyos, L., Plotkin, S., and Tartaglia, J. (2004). Poxvirus-based vaccine candidates for HIV: Two decades of experience with special emphasis on canarypox vectors. *Expert Rev. Vaccines* **3**, S75–S88.

Fribourg, S., Braun, I. C., Izaurralde, E., and Conti, E. (2001). Structural basis for the recognition of a nucleoporin FG repeat by the NTF2-like domain of the TAP/p15 mRNA nuclear export factor. *Mol. Cell* **8**, 645–656.

Fried, H., and Kutay, U. (2003). Nucleocytoplasmic transport: Taking an inventory. *Cell. Mol. Life Sci.* **60**, 1659–1688.

Fritz, C. C., and Green, M. R. (1996). HIV Rev uses a conserved cellular protein export pathway for the nucleocytoplasmic transport of viral RNAs. *Curr. Biol.* **6**, 848–854.

Fritz, C. C., Zapp, M. L., and Green, M. R. (1995). A human nucleoporin-like protein that specifically interacts with HIV Rev. *Nature* **376**, 530–533.

Fukuda, M., Asano, S., Nakamura, T., Adachi, M., Yoshida, M., Yanagida, M., and Nishida, E. (1997). CRM1 is responsible for intracellular transport mediated by the nuclear export signal. *Nature* **390**, 308–311.

Graf, M., Bojak, A., Deml, L., Bieler, K., Wolf, H., and Wagner, R. (2000). Concerted action of multiple cis-acting sequences is required for Rev dependence of late human immunodeficiency virus type 1 gene expression. *J. Virol.* **74**, 10822–10826.

Graf, M., Ludwig, C., Kehlenbeck, S., Jungert, K., and Wagner, R. (2006). A quasi-lentiviral green fluorescent protein reporter exhibits nuclear export features of late human immunodeficiency virus type 1 transcripts. *Virology* **352**, 295–305.

Grantham, R., Gautier, C., and Gouy, M. (1980). Codon frequencies in 119 individual genes confirm consistent choices of degenerate bases according to genome type. *Nucleic Acids Res.* **8**, 1893–1912.

Grüter, P., Tabernero, C., von Kobbe, C., Schmitt, C., Saavedra, C., Bachi, A., Wilm, M., Felber, B. K., and Izaurralde, E. (1998). TAP, the human homolog of Mex67p, mediates CTE-dependent RNA export from the nucleus. *Mol. Cell* **1**, 649–659.

Guzik, B. W., Levesque, L., Prasad, S., Bor, Y. C., Black, B. E., Paschal, B. M., Rekosh, D., and Hammarskjold, M. L. (2001). NXT1 (p15) is a crucial cellular cofactor in TAP-dependent export of intron-containing RNA in mammalian cells. *Mol. Cell. Biol.* **21**, 2545–2554.

Haas, J., Park, E. C., and Seed, B. (1996). Codon usage limitation in the expression of HIV-1 envelope glycoprotein. *Curr. Biol.* **6**, 315–324.

Hadzopoulou-Cladaras, M., Felber, B. K., Cladaras, C., Athanassopoulos, A., Tse, A., and Pavlakis, G. N. (1989). The *rev* (*trs/art*) protein of human immunodeficiency virus type 1 affects viral mRNA and protein expression via a *cis*-acting sequence in the *env* region. *J. Virol.* **63**, 1265–1274.

Hammarskjöld, M. L., Heimer, J., Hammarskjöld, B., Sangwan, I., Albert, L., and Rekosh, D. (1989). Regulation of human immunodeficiency virus *env* expression by the *rev* gene product. *J. Virol.* **63**, 1959–1966.

Hanly, S. M., Rimsky, L. T., Malim, M. H., Kim, J. H., Hauber, J., Duc Dodon, M., Le, S.-Y., Maizel, J. V., Cullen, B. R., and Greene, W. C. (1989). Comparative analysis of the HTLV-1 Rex and HIV-1 Rev trans-regulatory proteins and their RNA response elements. *Genes Dev.* **3**, 1534–1544.

Heaphy, S., Dingwall, C., Ernberg, I., Gait, M. J., Green, S. M., Karn, J., Lowe, A. D., Singh, M., and Skinner, M. A. (1990). HIV-1 regulator of virion expression (Rev) protein binds to an RNA stem-loop structure located within the Rev response element region. *Cell* 60, 685–693.

Henderson, B. R., and Eleftheriou, A. (2000). A comparison of the activity, sequence specificity, and CRM1-dependence of different nuclear export signals. *Exp. Cell Res.* 256, 213–224.

Herold, A., Suyama, M., Rodrigues, J. P., Braun, I. C., Kutay, U., Carmo-Fonseca, M., Bork, P., and Izaurralde, E. (2000). TAP (NXF1) belongs to a multigene family of putative RNA export factors with a conserved modular architecture. *Mol. Cell. Biol.* 20, 8996–9008.

Herold, A., Klymenko, T., and Izaurralde, E. (2001). NXF1/p15 heterodimers are essential for mRNA nuclear export in *Drosophila*. *RNA* 7, 1768–1780.

Herold, A., Teixeira, L., and Izaurralde, E. (2003). Genome-wide analysis of nuclear mRNA export pathways in *Drosophila*. *EMBO J.* 22, 2472–2483.

Hidaka, M., Inoue, J., Yoshida, M., and Seiki, M. (1988). Post-transcriptional regulator (rex) of HTLV-1 initiates expression of viral structural proteins but suppresses expression of regulatory proteins. *EMBO J.* 7, 519–523.

Hofmann, W., Reichart, B., Ewald, A., Muller, E., Schmitt, I., Stauber, R. H., Lottspeich, F., Jockusch, B. M., Scheer, U., Hauber, J., and Dabauvalle, M. C. (2001). Cofactor requirements for nuclear export of Rev response element (RRE)- and constitutive transport element (CTE)-containing retroviral RNAs. An unexpected role for actin. *J. Cell Biol.* 152, 895–910.

Holland, S. M., Ahmad, N., Maitra, R. K., Wingfield, P., and Venkatesan, S. (1990). Human immunodeficiency virus Rev protein recognizes a target sequence in Rev-responsive element RNA within the context of RNA secondary structure. *J. Virol.* 64, 5966–5975.

Holland, S. M., Chavez, M., Gerstberger, S., and Venkatesan, S. (1992). A specific sequence with a bulged guanosine residue(s) in a stem-bulge-stem structure of Rev-responsive element RNA is required for trans activation by human immunodeficiency virus type 1 Rev. *J. Virol.* 66, 3699–3706.

Hope, T. J. (1999). The ins and outs of HIV Rev. *Arch. Biochem. Biophys.* 365, 186–191.

Huang, Y., and Steitz, J. A. (2001). Splicing factors SRp20 and 9G8 promote the nucleocytoplasmic export of mRNA. *Mol. Cell* 7, 899–905.

Huang, Y., Gattoni, R., Stevenin, J., and Steitz, J. A. (2003). SR splicing factors serve as adapter proteins for TAP-dependent mRNA export. *Mol. Cell* 11, 837–843.

Huang, Y., Yario, T. A., and Steitz, J. A. (2004). A molecular link between SR protein dephosphorylation and mRNA export. *Proc. Natl. Acad. Sci. USA* 101, 9666–9670.

Indik, S., Gunzburg, W. H., Salmons, B., and Rouault, F. (2005). A novel, mouse mammary tumor virus encoded protein with Rev-like properties. *Virology* 337, 1–6.

Ingraham, H. A., Flynn, S. E., Voss, J. W., Albert, V. R., Kapiloff, M. S., Wilson, L., and Rosenfeld, M. G. (1990). The POU-specific domain of Pit-1 is esssential for sequence-specific, high affinity DNA binding and DNA-dependent Pit-1 Pit-1 interactions. *Cell* 61, 1021–1033.

Inoue, J., Seiki, M., and Yoshida, M. (1986). The second pX product p27 chi-III of HTLV-1 is required for gag gene expression. *FEBS Lett.* 209, 187–190.

Inoue, J., Yoshida, M., and Seiki, M. (1987). Transcriptional (p40X) and post-transcriptional (p27X-III) regulators are required for the expression and replication of human T-cell leukemia virus type I genes. *Proc. Natl. Acad. Sci. USA* 84, 3653–3657.

Itoh, M., Inoue, J.-I., Toyoshima, H., Akizawa, T., Higashi, M., and Yoshida, M. (1989). HTLV-1 *rex* and HIV-1 *rev* act through similar mechanisms to relieve suppression of unspliced RNA expression. *Oncogene* 4, 1275–1279.

Izaurralde, E. (2002). Nuclear export of messenger RNA. *Results Probl. Cell Differ.* 35, 133–150.

Izaurralde, E. (2004). Directing mRNA export. *Nat. Struct. Mol. Biol.* **11**, 210–212.

Jain, C., and Belasco, J. G. (2001). Structural model for the cooperative assembly of HIV-1 Rev multimers on the RRE as deduced from analysis of assembly-defective mutants. *Mol. Cell* **7**, 603–614.

Jin, L., Guzik, B. W., Bor, Y. C., Rekosh, D., and Hammarskjold, M. L. (2003). Tap and NXT promote translation of unspliced mRNA. *Genes Dev.* **17**, 3075–3086.

Kalland, K. H., Szilvay, A. M., Brokstad, K. A., Sætrevik, W., and Haukenes, G. (1994). The human immunodeficiency virus type 1 Rev protein shuttles between the cytoplasm and nuclear compartments. *Mol. Cell. Biol.* **14**, 7436–7444.

Karacostas, V., Nagashima, K., Gonda, M. A., and Moss, B. (1989). Human immunodeficiency virus-like particles produced by a vaccinia virus expression vector. *Proc. Natl. Acad. Sci. USA* **86**, 8964–8967.

Katahira, J., Straesser, K., Saiwaki, T., Yoneda, Y., and Hurt, E. (2002). Complex formation between Tap and p15 affects binding to FG-repeat nucleoporins and nucleocytoplasmic shuttling. *J. Biol. Chem.* **277**, 9242–9246.

Kataoka, N., Yong, J., Kim, V. N., Velazquez, F., Perkinson, R. A., Wang, F., and Dreyfuss, G. (2000). Pre-mRNA splicing imprints mRNA in the nucleus with a novel RNA-binding protein that persists in the cytoplasm. *Mol. Cell* **6**, 673–682.

Kataoka, N., Diem, M. D., Kim, V. N., Yong, J., and Dreyfuss, G. (2001). Magoh, a human homolog of *Drosophila* mago nashi protein, is a component of the splicing-dependent exon-exon junction complex. *EMBO J.* **20**, 6424–6433.

Kimura, T., Hashimoto, I., Nagase, T., and Fujisawa, J. (2004). CRM1-dependent, but not ARE-mediated, nuclear export of IFN-alpha1 mRNA. *J. Cell Sci.* **117**, 2259–2270.

Kiss, A., Li, L., Gettemeier, T., and Venkatesh, L. K. (2003). Functional analysis of the interaction of the human immunodeficiency virus type 1 Rev nuclear export signal with its cofactors. *Virology* **314**, 591–600.

Kjems, J., Frankel, A. D., and Sharp, P. A. (1991). Specific regulation of mRNA splicing *in vitro* by a peptide from HIV-1 rev. *Cell* **67**, 169–178.

Kofman, A., Graf, M., Bojak, A., Deml, L., Bieler, K., Kharazova, A., Wolf, H., and Wagner, R. (2003). HIV-1 gag expression is quantitatively dependent on the ratio of native and optimized codons. *Tsitologiia* **45**, 86–93.

Kubota, S., Adachi, Y., Copeland, T. D., and Oroszlan, S. (1995). Binding of human prothymosin alpha to the leucine-motif/activation domains of HTLV-I Rex and HIV-1 Rev. *Eur. J. Biochem.* **233**, 48–54.

Kudo, N., Wolff, B., Sekimoto, T., Schreiner, E. P., Yoneda, Y., Yanagida, M., Horinouchi, S., and Yoshida, M. (1998). Leptomycin B inhibition of signal-mediated nuclear export by direct binding to CRM1. *Exp. Cell Res.* **242**, 540–547.

Kudo, N., Matsumori, N., Taoka, H., Fujiwara, D., Schreiner, E. P., Wolff, B., Yoshida, M., and Horinouchi, S. (1999). Leptomycin B inactivates CRM1/exportin 1 by covalent modification at a cysteine residue in the central conserved region. *Proc. Natl. Acad. Sci. USA* **96**, 9112–9117.

Kuersten, S., Segal, S. P., Verheyden, J., LaMartina, S. M., and Goodwin, E. B. (2004). NXF-2, REF-1, and REF-2 affect the choice of nuclear export pathway for tra-2 mRNA in C. elegans. *Mol. Cell* **14**, 599–610.

Kumar, S., Yan, J., Muthumani, K., Ramanathan, M. P., Yoon, H., Pavlakis, G. N., Felber, B. K., Sidhu, M., Boyer, J. D., and Weiner, D. B. (2006). Immunogenicity testing of a novel engineered HIV-1 envelope gp140 DNA vaccine construct. *DNA Cell Biol.* **25**, 383–392.

Kutay, U., and Guttinger, S. (2005). Leucine-rich nuclear-export signals: Born to be weak. *Trends Cell Biol.* **15**, 121–124.

la Cour, T., Gupta, R., Rapacki, K., Skriver, K., Poulsen, F. M., and Brunak, S. (Cour 2003). NESbase version 1.0: A database of nuclear export signals. *Nucleic Acids Res.* **31**, 393–396.

Lai, M. C., and Tarn, W. Y. (2004). Hypophosphorylated ASF/SF2 binds TAP and is present in messenger ribonucleoproteins. *J. Biol. Chem.* **279**, 31745–31749.

Lassen, K. G., Ramyar, K. X., Bailey, J. R., Zhou, Y., and Siliciano, R. F. (2006). Nuclear retention of multiply spliced HIV-1 RNA in resting CD4+ T cells. *PLoS Pathog.* **2**, e68.

Lawrence, J. B., Cochrane, A. W., Johnson, C. V., Perkins, A., and Rosen, C. A. (1991). The HIV-1 Rev protein: A model system for coupled RNA transport and translation. *New Biol.* **3**, 1220–1232.

Lee, N. S., Dohjima, T., Bauer, G., Li, H., Li, M. J., Ehsani, A., Salvaterra, P., and Rossi, J. (2002). Expression of small interfering RNAs targeted against HIV-1 rev transcripts in human cells. *Nat. Biotechnol.* **20**, 500–505.

Levesque, L., Guzik, B., Guan, T., Coyle, J., Black, B. E., Rekosh, D., Hammarskjold, M. L., and Paschal, B. M. (2001). RNA export mediated by tap involves NXT1-dependent interactions with the nuclear pore complex. *J. Biol. Chem.* **276**, 44953–44962.

Levesque, L., Bor, Y. C., Matzat, L. H., Jin, L., Berberoglu, S., Rekosh, D., Hammarskjold, M. L., and Paschal, B. M. (2006). Mutations in tap uncouple RNA export activity from translocation through the nuclear pore complex. *Mol. Biol. Cell* **17**, 931–943.

Lewis, N., Williams, J., Rekosh, D., and Hammarskjold, M. L. (1990). Identification of a *cis*-acting element in human immunodeficiency virus type 2 (HIV-2) that is responsive to the HIV-1 *rev* and human T-cell leukemia virus types I and II *rex* proteins. *J. Virol.* **64**, 1690–1697.

Li, J., Tang, H., Mullen, T. M., Westberg, C., Reddy, T. R., Rose, D. W., and Wong-Staal, F. (1999). A role for RNA helicase A in post-transcriptional regulation of HIV type 1. *Proc. Natl. Acad. Sci. USA* **96**, 709–714.

Li, J., Liu, Y., Kim, B. O., and He, J. J. (2002). Direct participation of Sam68, the 68-kilodalton Src-associated protein in mitosis, in the CRM1-mediated Rev nuclear export pathway. *J. Virol.* **76**, 8374–8382.

Li, Y., Bor, Y. C., Misawa, Y., Xue, Y., Rekosh, D., and Hammarskjold, M. L. (2006). An intron with a constitutive transport element is retained in a Tap messenger RNA. *Nature* **443**, 234–237.

Liker, E., Fernandez, E., Izaurralde, E., and Conti, E. (2000). The structure of the mRNA export factor TAP reveals a cis arrangement of a non-canonical RNP domain and an LRR domain. *EMBO J.* **19**, 5587–5598.

Lindsay, M. E., Holaska, J. M., Welch, K., Paschal, B. M., and Macara, I. G. (2001). Ran-binding protein 3 is a cofactor for Crm1-mediated nuclear protein export. *J. Cell Biol.* **153**, 1391–1402.

Lindtner, S., Zolotukhin, A. S., Uranishi, H., Bear, J., Kulkarni, V., Smulevitch, S., Samiotaki, M., Panayotou, G., Pavlakis, G. N., and Felber, B. K. (2006). RNA-binding motif protein 15 binds to the RNA transport element RTE and provides a direct link to the NXF1 export pathway. *J. Biol. Chem.* **281**, 36915–36928.

Linial, M. L. (1999). Foamy viruses are unconventional retroviruses. *J. Virol.* **73**, 1747–1755.

Liu, Y. P., Nemeroff, M., Yan, Y. P., and Chen, K. Y. (1997). Interaction of eukaryotic initiation factor 5A with the human immunodeficiency virus type 1 Rev response element RNA and U6 snRNA requires deoxyhypusine or hypusine modification. *Biol. Signals* **6**, 166–174.

Lochelt, M. (2003). Foamy virus transactivation and gene expression. *Curr. Top. Microbiol. Immunol.* **277**, 27–61.

Love, D. C., Sweitzer, T. D., and Hanover, J. A. (1998). Reconstitution of HIV-1 rev nuclear export: Independent requirements for nuclear import and export. *Proc. Natl. Acad. Sci. USA* **95**, 10608–10613.

Lower, R., Tonjes, R. R., Korbmacher, C., Kurth, R., and Lower, J. (1995). Identification of a Rev-related protein by analysis of spliced transcripts of the human endogenous retroviruses HTDV/HERV-K. *J. Virol.* **69**, 141–149.

Lu, X., Heimer, J., Rekosh, D., and Hammarskjöld, M.-L. (1990). U1 small nuclear RNA plays a direct role in the formation of a rev-regulated human immunodeficiency virus env mRNA that remains unspliced. *Proc. Natl. Acad. Sci. USA* **87**, 7598–7602.

Lutzelberger, M., Reinert, L. S., Das, A. T., Berkhout, B., and Kjems, J. (2006). A novel splice donor site in the gag-pol gene is required for HIV-1 RNA stability. *J. Biol. Chem.* **281**, 18644–18651.

Madore, S. J., Tiley, L. S., Malim, M. H., and Cullen, B. R. (1994). Sequence requirements for Rev multimerization *in vivo*. *Virology* **202**, 186–194.

Magin, C., Lower, R., and Lower, J. (1999). cORF and RcRE, the Rev/Rex and RRE/RxRE homologues of the human endogenous retrovirus family HTDV/HERV-K. *J. Virol.* **73**, 9496–9507.

Magin, C., Hesse, J., Lower, J., and Lower, R. (2000). Corf, the Rev/Rex homologue of HTDV/HERV-K, encodes an arginine-rich nuclear localization signal that exerts a trans-dominant phenotype when mutated. *Virology* **274**, 11–16.

Malim, M. H., and Cullen, B. R. (1991). HIV-1 structural gene expression requires the binding of multiple Rev monomers to the viral RRE: Implications for HIV-1 latency. *Cell* **65**, 241–248.

Malim, M. H., Böhnlein, S., Hauber, J., and Cullen, B. R. (1989a). Functional dissection of the HIV-1 Rev *trans*-activator derivation of a *trans*-dominant repressor of Rev function. *Cell* **58**, 205–214.

Malim, M. H., Hauber, J., Le, S.-Y., Maizel, J. V., and Cullen, B. R. (1989b). The HIV-1 *rev* *trans*-activator acts through a structured target sequence to activate nuclear export of unspliced viral mRNA. *Nature* **338**, 254–257.

McLaren, M., Asai, K., and Cochrane, A. (2004). A novel function for Sam68: Enhancement of HIV-1 RNA 3′ end processing. *RNA* **10**, 1119–1129.

Mermer, B., Felber, B. K., Campbell, M., and Pavlakis, G. N. (1990). Identification of *trans*-dominant HIV-1 rev protein mutants by direct transfer of bacterially produced proteins into human cells. *Nucleic Acids Res.* **18**, 2037–2044.

Mertz, J. A., Simper, M. S., Lozano, M. M., Payne, S. M., and Dudley, J. P. (2005). Mouse mammary tumor virus encodes a self-regulatory RNA export protein and is a complex retrovirus. *J. Virol.* **79**, 14737–14747.

Meyer, B. E., and Malim, M. H. (1994). The HIV-1 Rev *trans*-activator shuttles between the nucleus and the cytoplasm. *Genes Dev.* **8**, 1538–1547.

Meyer, B. E., Meinkoth, J. L., and Malim, M. H. (1996). Nuclear transport of human immunodeficiency virus type 1, visna virus, and equine infectious anemia virus Rev proteins: Identification of a family of transferable nuclear export signals. *J. Virol.* **70**, 2350–2359.

Michienzi, A., Cagnon, L., Bahner, I., and Rossi, J. J. (2000). Ribozyme-mediated inhibition of HIV 1 suggests nucleolar trafficking of HIV-1 RNA. *Proc. Natl. Acad. Sci. USA* **97**, 8955–8960.

Michienzi, A., De Angelis, F. G., Bozzoni, I., and Rossi, J. J. (2006). A nucleolar localizing Rev binding element inhibits HIV replication. *AIDS Res. Ther.* **3**, 13.

Mikaelian, I., Krieg, M., Gait, M. J., and Karn, J. (1996). Interactions of INS (CRS) elements and the splicing machinery regulate the production of Rev-responsive mRNAs. *J. Mol. Biol.* **257**, 246–264.

Modem, S., Badri, K. R., Holland, T. C., and Reddy, T. R. (2005). Sam68 is absolutely required for Rev function and HIV-1 production. *Nucleic Acids Res.* **33**, 873–879.

Mosammaparast, N., and Pemberton, L. F. (2004). Karyopherins: From nuclear-transport mediators to nuclear-function regulators. *Trends Cell Biol.* **14**, 547–556.

Moss, B., Ahn, B. Y., Amegadzie, B., Gershon, P. D., and Keck, J. G. (1991). Cytoplasmic transcription system encoded by vaccinia virus. *J. Biol. Chem.* **266**, 1355–1358.

Najera, I., Krieg, M., and Karn, J. (1999). Synergistic stimulation of HIV-1 rev-dependent export of unspliced mRNA to the cytoplasm by hnRNP A1. *J. Mol. Biol.* **285**, 1951–1964.

Nappi, F., Schneider, R., Zolotukhin, A., Smulevitch, S., Michalowski, D., Bear, J., Felber, B., and Pavlakis, G. (2001). Identification of a novel posttranscriptional regulatory element using a rev and RRE mutated HIV-1 DNA proviral clone as a molecular trap. *J. Virol.* **75**, 4558–4569.

Nasioulas, G., Zolotukhin, A. S., Tabernero, C., Solomin, L., Cunningham, C. P., Pavlakis, G. N., and Felber, B. K. (1994). Elements distinct from human immunodeficiency virus type 1 splice sites are responsible for the Rev dependence of env mRNA. *J. Virol.* **68**, 2986–2993.

Neumann, M., Harrison, J., Saltarelli, M., Hadziyannis, E., Felber, B. K., and Pavlakis, G. N. (1994). Splicing variability in HIV-1 revealed by quantitative RNA-PCR. *AIDS Res. Hum. Retroviruses* **10**, 1527–1538.

Neumann, M., Felber, B. K., Kleinschmidt, A., Froese, B., Erfle, V., Pavlakis, G. N., and Brack-Werner, R. (1995). Restriction of human immunodeficiency virus type 1 production in a human astrocytoma cell line is associated with a cellular block in Rev function. *J. Virol.* **69**, 2159–2167.

Neumann, M., Afonina, E., Ceccherini-Silberstein, F., Schlicht, S., Erfle, V., Pavlakis, G. N., and Brack-Werner, R. (2001). Nucleocytoplasmic transport in human astrocytes: Decreased nuclear uptake of the HIV Rev shuttle protein. *J. Cell Sci.* **114**, 1717–1729.

Neville, M., Stutz, F., Lee, L., Davis, L. I., and Rosbash, M. (1997). The importin-beta family member Crm1p bridges the interaction between Rev and the nuclear pore complex during nuclear export. *Curr. Biol.* **7**, 767–775.

Ogert, R. A., and Beemon, K. L. (1998). Mutational analysis of the rous sarcoma virus DR posttranscriptional control element. *J. Virol.* **72**, 3407–3411.

Ogert, R. A., Lee, L. H., and Beemon, K. L. (1996). Avian retroviral RNA element promotes unspliced RNA accumulation in the cytoplasm. *J. Virol.* **70**, 3834–3843.

Olsen, H. S., Beidas, S., Dillon, P., Rosen, C. A., and Cochrane, A. W. (1991). Mutational analysis of the HIV-1 Rev protein and its target sequence, the Rev responsive element. *J. Acquir. Immune Defic. Syndr.* **4**, 558–567.

Olsen, H. S., Cochrane, A. W., and Rosen, C. (1992). Interaction of cellular factors with intragenic cis-acting repressive sequences within the HIV genome. *Virology* **191**, 709–715.

Opi, S., Peloponese, J. M., Jr., Esquieu, D., Watkins, J., Campbell, G., De Mareuil, J., Jeang, K. T., Yirrell, D. L., Kaleebu, P., and Loret, E. P. (2004). Full-length HIV-1 Tat protein necessary for a vaccine. *Vaccine* **22**, 3105–3111.

Ossareh-Nazari, B., Maison, C., Black, B. E., Levesque, L., Paschal, B. M., and Dargemont, C. (2000). RanGTP-binding protein NXT1 facilitates nuclear export of different classes of RNA *in vitro*. *Mol. Cell. Biol.* **20**, 4562–4571.

Paca, R. E., Ogert, R. A., Hibbert, C. S., Izaurralde, E., and Beemon, K. L. (2000). Rous sarcoma virus DR posttranscriptional elements use a novel RNA export pathway. *J. Virol.* **74**, 9507–9514.

Paca-Uccaralertkun, S., Damgaard, C. K., Auewarakul, P., Thitithanyanont, A., Suphaphiphat, P., Essex, M., Kjems, J., and Lee, T. H. (2006). The Effect of a single nucleotide substitution in the splicing silencer in the tat/rev intron on HIV type 1 envelope expression. *AIDS Res. Hum. Retroviruses* **22**, 76–82.

Pavlakis, G. N., and Felber, B. K. (1990). Regulation of expression of human immunodeficiency virus. *New Biol.* **2**, 20–31.

Perkins, A., Cochrane, A. W., Ruben, S. M., and Rosen, C. A. (1989). Structural and functional characterization of the human immunodeficiency virus *rev* protein. *J. Acquir. Immune Defic. Syndr.* **2**, 256–263.

Petosa, C., Schoehn, G., Askjaer, P., Bauer, U., Moulin, M., Steuerwald, U., Soler-Lopez, M., Baudin, F., Mattaj, I. W., and Muller, C. W. (2004). Architecture of CRM1/Exportin1 suggests how cooperativity is achieved during formation of a nuclear export complex. *Mol. Cell* **16**, 761–775.

Pollard, V. W., and Malim, M. H. (1998). The HIV-1 Rev protein. *Annu. Rev. Microbiol.* **52**, 491–532.

Purcell, D. F. J., and Martin, M. A. (1993). Alternative splicing of human immunodeficiency virus type 1 mRNA modulates viral protein expression, replication, and infectivity. *J. Virol.* **67**, 6365–6378.

Reddy, T. R., Xu, W., Mau, J. K., Goodwin, C. D., Suhasini, M., Tang, H., Frimpong, K., Rose, D. W., and Wong-Staal, F. (1999). Inhibition of HIV replication by dominant negative mutants of Sam68, a functional homolog of HIV-1 Rev. *Nat. Med.* **5**, 635–642.

Reddy, T. R., Tang, H., Xu, W., and Wong-Staal, F. (2000a). Sam68, RNA helicase A and Tap cooperate in the post-transcriptional regulation of human immunodeficiency virus and type D retroviral mRNA. *Oncogene* **19**, 3570–3575.

Reddy, T. R., Xu, W. D., and Wong-Staal, F. (2000b). General effect of Sam68 on Rev/Rex regulated expression of complex retroviruses. *Oncogene* **19**, 4071–4074.

Reddy, T. R., Suhasini, M., Xu, W., Yeh, L. Y., Yang, J. P., Wu, J., Artzt, K., and Wong-Staal, F. (2002). A role for KH domain proteins (Sam68-like mammalian proteins and quaking proteins) in the post-transcriptional regulation of HIV replication. *J. Biol. Chem.* **277**, 5778–5784.

Rethwilm, A. (2003). The replication strategy of foamy viruses. *Curr. Top. Microbiol. Immunol.* **277**, 1–26.

Richard, N., Iacampo, S., and Cochrane, A. (1994). HIV-1 Rev is capable of shuttling between the nucleus and cytoplasm. *Virology* **204**, 123–131.

Rimsky, L., Hauber, J., Dukovich, M., Malim, M. H., Langlois, A., Cullen, B. R., and Greene, W. C. (1988). Functional replacement of the HIV-1 rev protein by the HTLV-1 rex protein. *Nature (London)* **335**, 738–740.

Romanov, V. I., Zolotukhin, A. S., Aleksandroff, N. N., Pinto da Silva, P., and Felber, B. K. (1997). Posttranscriptional regulation by Rev protein of human immunodeficiency virus type 1 results in non-random nuclear localization of *gag* mRNAs. *Virology* **228**, 360–370.

Rosati, M., von Gegerfelt, A., Roth, P., Alicea, C., Valentin, A., Robert-Guroff, M., Venzon, D., Montefiori, D. C., Markham, P., Felber, B. K., and Pavlakis, G. N. (2005). DNA vaccines expressing different forms of simian immunodeficiency virus antigens decrease viremia upon SIVmac251 challenge. *J. Virol.* **79**, 8480–8492.

Rosen, C. A. (1991). Tat and Rev: Positive modulators of human immunodeficiency virus gene expression. *Gene Expr.* **1**, 85–90.

Rosen, C. A., Terwilliger, E., Dayton, A., Sodroski, J. G., and Haseltine, W. A. (1988). Intragenic cis-acting *art* gene-responsive sequences of the human immunodeficiency virus. *Proc. Natl. Acad. Sci. USA* **85**, 2071–2075.

Rosorius, O., Reichart, B., Kratzer, F., Heger, P., Dabauvalle, M. C., and Hauber, J. (1999). Nuclear pore localization and nucleocytoplasmic transport of eIF-5A: Evidence for direct interaction with the export receptor CRM1. *J. Cell Sci.* **112**(Pt. 14), 2369–2380.

Ruhl, M., Himmelspach, M., Bahr, G. M., Hammerschmid, F., Jaksche, H., Wolff, B., Aschauer, H., Farrington, G. K., Probst, H., Bevec, D., and Hauber, J. (1993). Eukaryotic initiation factor 5A is a cellular target of the human immunodeficiency virus type 1 Rev activation domain mediating trans-activation. *J. Cell. Biol.* **123**, 1309–1320.

Salfeld, J., Gottlinger, H., Sia, R., Park, R., Sodroski, J., and Haseltine, W. (1990). A tripartite HIV-1 tat-env-rev fusion protein. *EMBO J.* **9**, 965–970.

Sanchez-Velar, N., Udofia, E. B., Yu, Z., and Zapp, M. L. (2004). hRIP, a cellular cofactor for Rev function, promotes release of HIV RNAs from the perinuclear region. *Genes Dev.* **18**, 23–34.

Schneider, R., Campbell, M., Nasioulas, G., Felber, B. K., and Pavlakis, G. N. (1997). Inactivation of the human immunodeficiency virus type 1 inhibitory elements allows Rev-independent expression of Gag and Gag/Protease and particle formation. *J. Virol.* **71**, 4892–4903.

Schneider, T. D., and Stephens, R. M. (1990). Sequence logos: A new way to display consensus sequences. *Nucleic Acids Res.* **18**, 6097–6100.

Schwartz, S., Felber, B. K., Benko, D. M., Fenyö, E. M., and Pavlakis, G. N. (1990a). Cloning and functional analysis of multiply spliced mRNA species of human immunodeficiency virus type 1. *J. Virol.* **64**, 2519–2529.

Schwartz, S., Felber, B. K., Fenyö, E. M., and Pavlakis, G. N. (1990b). Env and Vpu proteins of human immunodeficiency virus type 1 are produced from multiple bicistronic mRNAs. *J. Virol.* **64**, 5448–5456.

Schwartz, S., Felber, B. K., and Pavlakis, G. N. (1991). Expression of Human immunodeficiency virus type-1 vif and vpr mRNAs is Rev-dependent and regulated by splicing. *Virology* **183**, 677–686.

Schwartz, S., Campbell, M., Nasioulas, G., Harrison, J., Felber, B. K., and Pavlakis, G. N. (1992a). Mutational inactivation of an inhibitory sequence in human immunodeficiency virus type-1 results in Rev-independent *gag* expression. *J. Virol.* **66**, 7176–7182.

Schwartz, S., Felber, B. K., and Pavlakis, G. N. (1992b). Distinct RNA sequences in the *gag* region of human immunodeficiency virus type 1 decrease RNA stability and inhibit expression in the absence of Rev protein. *J. Virol.* **66**, 150–159.

Schwartz, S., Felber, B. K., and Pavlakis, G. N. (1992c). Mechanism of translation of monocistronic and multicistronic human immunodeficiency virus type 1 mRNAs. *Mol. Cell. Biol.* **12**, 207–219.

Segref, A., Sharma, K., Doye, V., Hellwig, A., Huber, J., Luhrmann, R., and Hurt, E. (1997). Mex67p, a novel factor for nuclear mRNA export, binds to both poly(A) + RNA and nuclear pores. *EMBO J.* **16**, 3256–3271.

Seiki, M., Inoue, J., Hidaka, M., and Yoshida, M. (1988). Two cis-acting elements responsible for posttranscriptional trans-regulation of gene expression of human T-cell leukemia virus type I. *Proc. Natl. Acad. Sci. USA* **85**, 7124–7128.

Shav-Tal, Y., and Zipori, D. (2002). PSF and p54(nrb)/NonO—multi-functional nuclear proteins. *FEBS Lett.* **531**, 109–114.

Shav-Tal, Y., Blechman, J., Darzacq, X., Montagna, C., Dye, B. T., Patton, J. G., Singer, R. H., and Zipori, D. (2005). Dynamic sorting of nuclear components into distinct nucleolar caps during transcriptional inhibition. *Mol. Biol. Cell* **16**, 2395–2413.

Shaw, G., and Kamen, R. (1986). A conserved AU sequence from the 3′ untranslated region of GM-CSF mRNA mediates selective mRNA degradation. *Cell* **46**, 659–667.

Shim, J., and Karin, M. (2002). The control of mRNA stability in response to extracellular stimuli. *Mol. Cell* **14**, 323–331.

Si, Z., Amendt, B. A., and Stoltzfus, C. M. (1997). Splicing efficiency of human immunodeficiency virus type 1 tat RNA is determined by both a suboptimal 3′ splice site and a 10 nucleotide exon splicing silencer element located within tat exon 2. *Nucleic Acids Res.* **25**, 861–867.

Smulevitch, S., Michalowski, D., Zolotukhin, A. S., Schneider, R., Bear, J., Roth, P., Pavlakis, G. N., and Felber, B. K. (2005). Structural and functional analysis of the RNA transport element, a member of an extensive family present in the mouse genome. *J. Virol.* **79**, 2356–2365.

Smulevitch, S., Bear, J., Alicea, C., Rosati, M., Jalah, R., Zolotukhin, A. S., von Gegerfelt, A. S., Michalowski, D., Moroni, C., Pavlakis, G. N., and Felber, B. K. (2006). RTE and CTE mRNA export elements synergistically increase expression of unstable, Rev-dependent HIV and SIV mRNAs. *Retrovirology* **3**, 6–14.

Sodroski, J., Goh, W. C., Rosen, C., Dayton, A., Terwilliger, E., and Haseltine, W. (1986). A second post-transcriptional trans-activator gene required for HTLV-III replication. *Nature* **321**, 412–417.

Spellman, R., Rideau, A., Matlin, A., Gooding, C., Robinson, F., McGlincy, N., Grellscheid, S. N., Southby, J., Wollerton, M., and Smith, C. W. (2005). Regulation of alternative splicing by PTB and associated factors. *Biochem. Soc. Trans.* **33**, 457–460.

Staffa, A., and Cochrane, A. (1994). The tat/rev intron of human immunodeficiency virus type 1 is inefficiently spliced because of suboptimal signals in the 3' splice site. *J. Virol.* **68**, 3071–3079.

Staffa, A., and Cochrane, A. (1995). Identification of positive and negative splicing regulation elements within the terminal tat-rev exon of human immunodeficiency virus type 1. *Mol. Cell. Biol.* **15**, 4597–4605.

Stauber, R., Gaitanaris, A. S., and Pavlakis, G. N. (1995). Analysis of trafficking of Rev and transdominant Rev proteins in living cells using green fluorescent protein fusions: Transdominant Rev blocks the export of Rev from the nucleus to the cytoplasm. *Virology* **213**, 439–454.

Stauber, R. H., Afonina, E., Gulnik, S., Erickson, J., and Pavlakis, G. N. (1998). Analysis of intracellular trafficking and interactions of cytoplasmic HIV-1 Rev mutants in living cells. *Virology* **251**, 38–48.

Stoltzfus, C. M., and Madsen, J. M. (2006). Role of viral splicing elements and cellular RNA binding proteins in regulation of HIV-1 alternative RNA splicing. *Curr. HIV Res.* **4**, 43–55.

Strasser, K., and Hurt, E. (2000). Yra1p, a conserved nuclear RNA-binding protein, interacts directly with Mex67p and is required for mRNA export. *EMBO J.* **19**, 410–420.

Stutz, F., Bachi, A., Doerks, T., Braun, I., Seraphin, B., Wilm, M., Bork, P., and Izaurralde, E. (2000). REF, an evolutionary conserved family of hnRNP-like proteins, interacts with TAP/Mex67p and participates in mRNA nuclear export. *RNA* **6**, 638–650.

Suyama, M., Doerks, T., Braun, I. C., Sattler, M., Izaurralde, E., and Bork, P. (2000). Prediction of structural domains of TAP reveals details of its interaction with p15 and nucleoporins. *EMBO Rep.* **1**, 53–58.

Szilvay, A. M., Brokstad, K. A., Kopperud, R., Haukenes, G., and Kalland, K.-H. (1995). Nuclear export of the human immunodeficiency virus type 1 nucleocytoplasmic shuttle protein Rev is mediated by its activation domain and is blocked by transdominant negative mutants. *J. Virol.* **69**, 3315–3323.

Tabernero, C., Zolotukhin, A. S., Valentin, A., Pavlakis, G. N., and Felber, B. K. (1996). The posttranscriptional control element of the simian retrovirus type 1 forms an extensive RNA secondary structure necessary for its function. *J. Virol.* **70**, 5998–6011.

Tabernero, C., Zolotukhin, A. S., Bear, J., Schneider, R., Karsenty, G., and Felber, B. K. (1997). Identification of an RNA sequence within an intracisternal-A particle element able to replace Rev-mediated posttranscriptional regulation of human immunodeficiency virus type 1. *J. Virol.* **71**, 95–101.

Tan, W., Zolotukhin, A. S., Bear, J., Patenaude, D. J., and Felber, B. K. (2000). The mRNA export in C. elegans is mediated by Ce-NXF-1, an ortholog of human TAP and S. cerevisiae Mex67p. *RNA* **6**, 1762–1772.

Tange, T. O., and Kjems, J. (2001). SF2/ASF binds to a splicing enhancer in the third HIV-1 tat exon and stimulates U2AF binding independently of the RS domain. *J. Mol. Biol.* **312**, 649–662.

Tange, T. O., Damgaard, C. K., Guth, S., Valcarcel, J., and Kjems, J. (2001). The hnRNP A1 protein regulates HIV-1 tat splicing via a novel intron silencer element. *EMBO J.* **20**, 5748–5758.

Thomas, S. L., Oft, M., Jaksche, H., Casari, G., Heger, P., Dobrovnik, M., Bevec, D., and Hauber, J. (1998). Functional analysis of the human immunodeficiency virus type 1 Rev protein oligomerization interface. *J. Virol.* **72**, 2935–2944.

Tretyakova, I., Zolotukhin, A. S., Tan, W., Bear, J., Propst, F., Ruthel, G., and Felber, B. K. (2005). Nuclear export factor family protein participates in cytoplasmic mRNA trafficking. *J. Biol. Chem.* **280**, 31981–31990.

Truant, R., Kang, Y., and Cullen, B. R. (1999). The human Tap nuclear RNA export factor contains a novel transportin-dependent nuclear localization signal that lacks nuclear export signal function. *J. Biol. Chem.* **274**, 32167–32171.

Valcarcel, J., and Gebauer, F. (1997). Post-transcriptional regulation: The dawn of PTB. *Curr. Biol.* **7**, R705–R708.

Valentin, A., Aldrovandi, G., Zolotukhin, A. S., Cole, S. W., Zack, J. A., Pavlakis, G. N., and Felber, B. K. (1997). Reduced viral load and lack of CD4 depletion in SCID-hu mice infected with Rev-independent clones of human immunodeficiency virus type 1. *J. Virol.* **71**, 9817–9822.

Venkatesh, L. K., and Chinnadurai, G. (1990). Mutants in a conserved region near the carboxy-terminus of HIV-1 Rev identify functionally important residues and exhibit a dominant negative phenotype. *Virology* **178**, 327–330.

Venkatesh, L. K., Mohammed, S., and Chinnadurai, G. (1990). Functional domains of the HIV-1 rev gene required for trans-regulation and subcellular localization. *Virology* **176**, 39–47.

Venkatesh, L. K., Gettemeier, T., and Chinnadurai, G. (2003). A nuclear kinesin-like protein interacts with and stimulates the activity of the leucine-rich nuclear export signal of the human immunodeficiency virus type 1 rev protein. *J. Virol.* **77**, 7236–7243.

Vinciguerra, P., and Stutz, F. (2004). mRNA export: An assembly line from genes to nuclear pores. *Curr. Opin. Cell Biol.* **16**, 285–292.

von Gegerfelt, A. S., and Felber, B. K. (1997). Replacement of posttranscriptional regulation in SIVmac239 generated a Rev-independent infectious virus able to propagate in rhesus peripheral blood mononuclear cells. *Virology* **232**, 291–299.

von Gegerfelt, A. S., Liska, V., Ray, N. B., McClure, H. M., Ruprecht, R. M., and Felber, B. K. (1999). Persistent infection of rhesus macaques by the rev-independent Nef(−) simian immunodeficiency virus SIVmac239: Replication kinetics and genomic stability. *J. Virol.* **73**, 6159–6165.

von Gegerfelt, A. S., Liska, V., Li, P. L., McClure, H. M., Horie, K., Nappi, F., Montefiori, D. C., Pavlakis, G. N., Marthas, M. L., Ruprecht, R. M., and Felber, B. K. (2002). Rev-independent simian immunodeficiency virus strains are nonpathogenic in neonatal macaques. *J. Virol.* **76**, 96–104.

von Gegerfelt, A. S., Alicea, C., Valentin, A., Morrow, M., van Rompay, K. K., Ayash-Rashkovsky, M., Markham, P., Else, J. G., Marthas, M. L., Pavlakis, G. N., Ruprecht, R. M., and Felber, B. K. (2006). Long lasting control and lack of pathogenicity of the attenuated Rev-independent SIV in rhesus macaques. *AIDS Res. Hum. Retroviruses* **22**, 516–528.

Weirich, C. S., Erzberger, J. P., Flick, J. S., Berger, J. M., Thorner, J., and Weis, K. (2006). Activation of the DExD/H-box protein Dbp5 by the nuclear-pore protein Gle1 and its coactivator InsP6 is required for mRNA export. *Nat. Cell Biol.* **8**, 668–676.

Wiegand, H. L., Coburn, G. A., Zeng, Y., Kang, Y., Bogerd, H. P., and Cullen, B. R. (2002). Formation of Tap/NXT1 heterodimers activates Tap-dependent nuclear mRNA export by enhancing recruitment to nuclear pore complexes. *Mol. Cell. Biol.* **22**, 245–256.

Wilkie, G. S., Zimyanin, V., Kirby, R., Korey, C., Francis-Lang, H., Van Vactor, D., and Davis, I. (2001). Small bristles, the Drosophila ortholog of NXF-1, is essential for mRNA export throughout development. *RNA* **7**, 1781–1792.

Wolff, B., Sanglier, J.-J., and Wang, Y. (1997). Leptomycin B is an inhibitor of nuclear export: Inhibition of nucleo-cytoplasmic translocation of the human immunodeficiency virus type 1 (HIV-1) Rev protein and Rev-dependent mRNA. *Chem. Biol.* **4**, 139–147.

Wolff, H., Hadian, K., Ziegler, M., Weierich, C., Kramer-Hammerle, S., Kleinschmidt, A., Erfle, V., and Brack-Werner, R. (2006). Analysis of the influence of subcellular localization of the HIV Rev protein on Rev-dependent gene expression by multi-fluorescence live-cell imaging. *Exp. Cell Res.* **312**, 443–456.

Yang, J., Bogerd, H. P., Peng, S., Wiegand, H., Truant, R., and Cullen, B. R. (1999). An ancient family of human endogenous retroviruses encodes a functional homolog of the HIV-1 Rev protein. *Proc. Natl. Acad. Sci. USA* **96**, 13404–13408.

Yang, J., Bogerd, H., Le, S. Y., and Cullen, B. R. (2000). The human endogenous retrovirus K Rev response element coincides with a predicted RNA folding region. *RNA* **6**, 1551–1564.

Yedavalli, V. S., Neuveut, C., Chi, Y. H., Kleiman, L., and Jeang, K. T. (2004). Requirement of DDX3 DEAD box RNA helicase for HIV-1 Rev-RRE export function. *Cell* **119**, 381–392.

Younis, I., and Green, P. L. (2005). The human T-cell leukemia virus Rex protein. *Front. Biosci.* **10**, 431–445.

Yu, Z., Sanchez-Velar, N., Catrina, I. E., Kittler, E. L., Udofia, E. B., and Zapp, M. L. (2005). The cellular HIV-1 Rev cofactor hRIP is required for viral replication. *Proc. Natl. Acad. Sci. USA* **102**, 4027–4032.

Zolotukhin, A. S., and Felber, B. K. (1999). Nucleoporins Nup98 and Nup214 participate in nuclear export of human immunodeficiency virus type 1 Rev. *J. Virol.* **73**, 120–127.

Zolotukhin, A. S., Valentin, A., Pavlakis, G. N., and Felber, B. K. (1994). Continuous propagation of RRE(-) and Rev(-)RRE(-) human immunodeficiency virus type 1 molecular clones containing a *cis*-acting element of simian retrovirus type 1 in human peripheral blood lymphocytes. *J. Virol.* **68**, 7944–7952.

Zolotukhin, A. S., Michalowski, D., Smulevitch, S., and Felber, B. K. (2001). Retroviral constitutive transport element evolved from cellular TAP(NXF1)-binding sequences. *J. Virol.* **75**, 5567–5575.

Zolotukhin, A. S., Tan, W., Bear, J., Smulevitch, S., and Felber, B. K. (2002). U2AF participates in the binding of TAP (NXF1) to mRNA. *J. Biol. Chem.* **277**, 3935–3942.

Zolotukhin, A. S., Michalowski, D., Bear, J., Smulevitch, S. V., Traish, A. M., Peng, R., Patton, J., Shatsky, I. N., and Felber, B. K. (2003). PSF acts through the human immunodeficiency virus type 1 mRNA instability elements to regulate virus expression. *Mol. Cell. Biol.* **23**, 6618–6630.

Klaus Strebel

Laboratory of Molecular Microbiology, National Institute of Allergy and Infectious
Diseases, National Institutes of Health, 4/312, Bethesda, Maryland 20892

HIV Accessory Genes Vif and Vpu

I. Chapter Overview

Primate immunodeficiency viruses, including HIV-1, are characterized
by the presence of a number of viral accessory genes that encompass *vif*, *vpr*,
vpx, *vpu*, and *nef* (Fig. 1). The *vif*, *vpr*, and *nef* genes are expressed in most
HIV-1, HIV-2, and SIV isolates (Huet *et al.*, 1990). In contrast, the *vpu* gene
is found only in HIV-1 and some SIV isolates. The *vpx* gene, on the other
hand, is not found in HIV-1 isolates but is common to HIV-2 and most SIV
isolates. Current knowledge indicates that none of the primate lentiviral
accessory proteins has enzymatic activity. Instead, it appears that these proteins serve primarily, if not exclusively, as adapter molecules to mediate the
physical interaction of other viral and/or host factors. This chapter attempts

Advances in Pharmacology, Volume 55   1054-3589/07 $35.00
                                        DOI: 10.1016/S1054-3589(07)55006-4

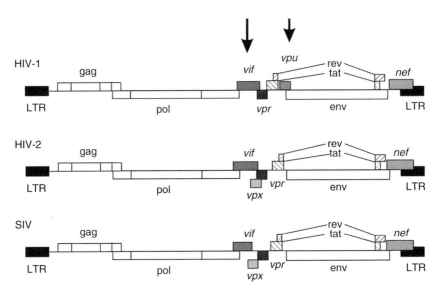

FIGURE I   Genome organization of primate lentiviruses. Map of prototypic HIV-1 and HIV-2/SIV proviruses showing the location of the *vif* and *vpu* gene.

to summarize our current knowledge of the function of the HIV accessory proteins Vif and Vpu.

II. Vif: A Potent Regulator of Viral Infectivity ——————

A. Introduction

Vif is encoded by all lentiviruses except *Equine infectious anemia virus* (Oberste and Gonda, 1992). Prior to the adoption of a standard nomenclature for HIV transcription units, Vif was known as sor, A, P′, or Q gene product (Gallo *et al.*, 1988). Its gene product is a 23-kDa basic protein, which is produced late in the infection cycle in a Rev-dependent manner (Garrett *et al.*, 1991; Schwartz *et al.*, 1991). Deletions in *vif* have been associated with a reduction or loss of viral infectivity (Fisher *et al.*, 1987; Kishi *et al.*, 1992; Strebel *et al.*, 1987), a phenomenon that is largely host cell dependent (Blanc *et al.*, 1993; Borman *et al.*, 1995; Fan and Peden, 1992; Gabuzda *et al.*, 1992; von Schwedler *et al.*, 1993; Sakai *et al.*, 1993) and can vary in its extent by several orders of magnitude (Fisher *et al.*, 1987; Kishi *et al.*, 1992; Strebel *et al.*, 1987). In permissive cell types, such as HeLa, COS, C8166, Jurkat, U937, or SupT1 (Fan and Peden, 1992; Gabuzda *et al.*, 1992; Sakai *et al.*, 1993), production of infectious particles does not require a functional *vif* gene product. In contrast, *vif*-deficient viruses produced from nonpermissive cells, such as H9, CEM, PBMC, or macrophages

(Borman *et al.*, 1995; Courcoul *et al.*, 1995; Fan and Peden, 1992; Gabuzda *et al.*, 1992, 1994; Sova and Volsky, 1993; von Schwedler *et al.*, 1993), are noninfectious regardless of the permissiveness of the target cells (Borman *et al.*, 1995; Gabuzda *et al.*, 1992; von Schwedler *et al.*, 1993). Of note, when permissive and nonpermissive cells were fused, the resulting heterokaryons exhibited a restrictive phenotype suggesting the presence of an inhibitory factor in nonpermissive cells (Madani and Kabat, 1998; Simon *et al.*, 1998a). It took almost 4 years after this discovery until the mysterious inhibitory factor was finally identified (Sheehy *et al.*, 2002). The identified protein whose expression in permissive cells rendered these cells nonpermissive for *vif*-deficient HIV-1 was initially referred to as CEM15 (Sheehy *et al.*, 2002). It quickly became clear that CEM15 belonged to a family of cytidine deaminases and was identical to APOBEC3G (apolipoprotein B mRNA-editing enzyme catalytic polypeptide-like 3G). The identification of CEM15 (APOBEC3G) in 2002 (Sheehy *et al.*, 2002) represented a milestone in Vif research as it brought to an end the long search for the elusive host factor targeted by Vif. It is interesting to note that CEM15 was not (despite many attempts) identified through yeast-two-hybrid screening using Vif as bait even though we now know that Vif and APOBEC3G closely interact. Instead, CEM15/APOBEC3G was identified through subtractive screening of cDNA libraries from the two closely related cell lines CEM and CEM-SS that exhibit permissive and nonpermissive phenotypes, respectively (Sheehy *et al.*, 2002).

B. Vif Function is Host Cell Specific

Several lines of evidence suggested early on that Vif exerts its function through interactions with species-specific host cell factor(s) (Simon *et al.*, 1995). For instance, HIV-1 Vif was able to regulate infectivity of HIV-1, HIV-2, and SIV_{agm} in human cells while SIV_{agm} Vif was inactive in human cells—even on SIV substrates—but was active in African green monkey (AGM) cells (Simon *et al.*, 1998c). Similarly, the identification of an HIV-2 isolate, HIV-2_{KR}, whose *vif*-defective variants exhibit cell type restrictions that are distinct from those observed for *vif*-deficient HIV-1, points to the involvement of cellular factor(s) for Vif function (Reddy *et al.*, 1995). Nevertheless, the observation that *vif* genes from HIV-1, HIV-2, and SIV are capable of functional complementation in appropriate cellular backgrounds (Reddy *et al.*, 1995; Simon *et al.*, 1995, 1998c) suggested a common mechanistic basis for Vif function.

Many models for Vif function have been proposed over the years. The observation that the defect in viruses produced in restrictive cells in the absence of Vif cannot be complemented by the presence of Vif in recipient cells (Borman *et al.*, 1995; von Schwedler *et al.*, 1993) suggested that Vif is required at the time of particle production in the host cell for regulating virus assembly or maturation (Blanc *et al.*, 1993; Borman *et al.*, 1995; Gabuzda *et al.*, 1992; von Schwedler *et al.*, 1993; Sakai *et al.*, 1993). This model is still valid today. It was further speculated that Vif might be involved in the posttranslational modification of one or several virion components. This model was based on the observation of morphological aberrancies in *vif*-defective virions from restrictive cells, which were not observed in wild-type virions or in *vif*-defective virions from permissive cells (Borman *et al.*, 1995; Hoglund *et al.*, 1994). More recently, the absence of Vif was associated with the formation of abnormal reverse transcription complexes in viruses derived from nonpermissive cells (Carr *et al.*, 2006). We know now that Vif-deficient viruses incorporate APOBEC3G and that virus-associated APOBEC3G is responsible for the loss of infectivity. Yet, only 20–50 copies of APOBEC3G are packaged in the absence of Vif into virus particles from nonpermissive H9 cells (K. S., unpublished data). Thus, the amount of virus-associated APOBEC3G is low when compared to the 4000–5000 copies of Gag present in a virion and it is not clear whether the presence of APOBEC3G can fully explain the above-noted morphological aberrancies.

C. Mechanisms of Vif Function

Introduction of CEM15/APOBEC3G into permissive 293T cells rendered these cells nonpermissive for *vif*-defective HIV-1 (Sheehy *et al.*, 2002). However, the antiviral activity of CEM15/APOBEC3G was severely inhibited in the presence of Vif. Thus, Vif has the intriguing ability to neutralize APOBEC3G. There is general agreement that the inhibition of APOBEC3G antiviral activity is mediated by a physical interaction with Vif and results in the exclusion of APOBEC3G from virions. The exact mechanism of Vif function is still under investigation. One of the unresolved issues concerns the domains in Vif and APOBEC3G that are involved in their interaction. The result from four independent studies published almost simultaneously points to a region in the N-terminal part of APOBEC3G (Bogerd *et al.*, 2004; Mangeat *et al.*, 2004; Schrofelbauer *et al.*, 2004; Xu *et al.*, 2004). All four groups found that a single amino acid change at position 128 in human APOBEC3G (D128K) was sufficient to change its sensitivity to Vif: normal human APOBEC3G was highly sensitive to HIV-1 Vif but insensitive to Vif from SIV_{agm}. In contrast, mutation of D128 to K rendered the resulting APOBEC3G protein insensitive to HIV-1 Vif but sensitive to SIV_{agm} Vif (Mangeat *et al.*, 2004; Schrofelbauer *et al.*, 2004; Xu *et al.*, 2004). In almost all of these studies, mutation at position 128 severely affected the binding of APOBEC3G to Vif (Bogerd *et al.*, 2004; Mangeat *et al.*, 2004; Schrofelbauer *et al.*, 2004). It is interesting to note that while the interaction of HIV-1 and SIV_{agm} Vif is limited to human and AGM APOBEC3G, respectively, Vif proteins encoded by HIV-2 and SIV_{mac} viruses can target both human and AGM APOBEC3G. These results suggest that residues other than amino acid 128 in APOBEC3G are important for the interaction with Vif. In this regard, it should be noted that Vif and APOBEC3G are both RNA-binding proteins, and it is possible that Vif–APOBEC3G interactions are mediated or facilitated by an RNA bridge even though one recent report found that the Vif–APOBEC3G interaction is insensitive to treatment with RNase (Kozak et al., 2006).

D. Degradation of APOBEC3G

Vif inhibits packaging of APOBEC3G into virus particles. The inhibition of APOBEC3G encapsidation by Vif is generally accompanied by a reduction of the intracellular expression level, which has been attributed to degradation by the cellular ubiquitin–dependent proteasome machinery (Conticello et al., 2003; Liddament et al., 2004; Marin et al., 2003; Mehle et al., 2004b; Sheehy et al., 2003; Stopak et al., 2003; Wiegand et al., 2004; Yu et al., 2003). Vif binds to APOBEC3G as well as to components of a cullin-ubiquitin ligase complex, including Cullin5 (Cul5), Elongin B, Elongin C, and the RING protein Rbx, and induces ubiquitination and subsequent degradation of APOBEC3G (Mehle et al., 2004b; Yu et al., 2003, 2004). A model for the proposed APOBEC3G ubiquitination complex is shown in Fig. 2. In this model, an Elongin B/C dimer interacts with a highly conserved SLQ motif in Vif also referred to as BC box motif (Mehle et al., 2004a; Yu et al., 2003; Fig. 2A). This is suggested by the fact that mutation or deletion of the SLQ motif reduces the affinity of Vif to Elongin B/C dimer, inhibits APOBEC3G ubiquitination, and results in the production of noninfectious virions (Mehle et al., 2004a; Yu et al., 2003). In addition to Elongin B and Elongin C, Vif also binds to Cul5. In this regard, a novel zinc-binding motif was recently identified in Vif, which is responsible for the binding of Vif to Cul5 and mediates cullin selection (Luo et al., 2005; Mehle et al., 2006). This novel HCCH motif is conserved in all primate lentiviral Vif proteins and has the consensus sequence $H\text{-}X_5\text{-}C\text{-}X_{17-18}\text{-}C\text{-}X_{3-5}\text{-}H$ (Fig. 2A). The HCCH motif represents a nonclassical zinc-binding motif, and mutation of any or all of the HCCH residues reduced zinc binding of Vif and significantly reduced the affinity of Vif to Cul5 (Mehle et al., 2006; Xiao et al., 2006). Interestingly, mutation of hydrophobic residues within the HCCH motif also reduced Cul5 binding without a simultaneous loss of Elongin B and Elongin C interaction with Vif (Xiao et al., 2006). On the basis of these results it was suggested that zinc coordination via the HCCH motif serves the purpose of properly positioning critical hydrophobic residues in Vif for interaction with Cul5 (Fig. 2A). The assembly on Vif of Cul5 and ElonginB/C together with Rbx and an E2 ubiquitin-conjugating enzyme into an active E3 ubiquitin ligase complex finally culminates in the ubiquitination and subsequent degradation of APOBEC3G (Fig. 2B).

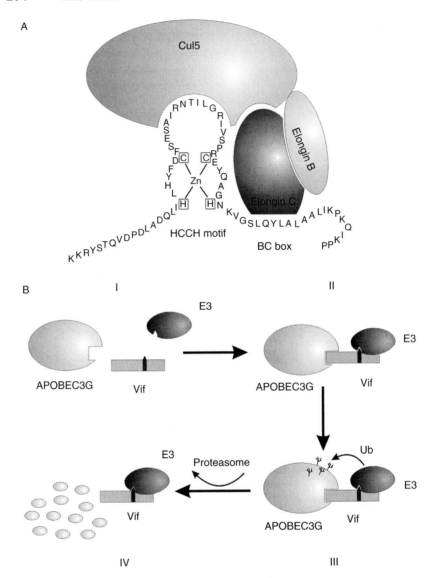

FIGURE 2 Vif induces proteasome-dependent degradation of APOBEC3G. (A) Two domains in Vif have been identified as crucial for the assembly of the Cul5-ubiquitin ligase complex. The BC box encompasses a highly conserved SLQ motif and constitutes a binding motif for the Elongin B/C heterodimer. A second conserved structure in Vif is the HCCH motif which confers zinc-binding property to Vif and is important for the association of Vif with Cul5. (B) Proposed model for the degradation of APOBEC3G by Vif. In this model, Vif functions as an adaptor molecule (I) to connect APOBEC3G to a Cul5-dependent E3 ubiquitin ligase complex (II). This results in the ubiquitination of APOBEC3G (III) and subsequent degradation of the ubiquitinated proteins by cytoplasmic proteasomes (IV).

As far as Vif is concerned it was observed that amino acid changes near the N-terminus (residues 14–17) affected the species-specific interaction with APOBEC3G (Schrofelbauer *et al.*, 2006). Consistent with this we found that deletions in that region of Vif reduced but did not abolish the interaction of Vif with APOBEC3G. The function of Vif as an adaptor between APOBEC3G and the Cul5 ubiquitination complex is reminiscent of the role of Vpu in the proteasome-mediated degradation of CD4, which will be discussed later in this chapter (Section III.C.1). It is interesting that thus far no dominant-negative mutants of Vif have been identified (Fujita *et al.*, 2002). Given the nature of the APOBEC3G–Vif–Cul5 complex, it should be possible to identify mutants of Vif that retain their ability to bind APOBEC3G but have lost their ability to connect to the Cul5 E3 ubiquitin ligase complex. Identification of such mutants could represent a promising step toward the development of novel Vif-based antivirals.

I. Does Vif Control APOBEC3G Through Multiple Mechanisms?

Degradation of APOBEC3G clearly contributes to the exclusion of APOBEC3G from viruses. However, there is increasing evidence that other mechanism(s) may come into play as well. For instance, it was noted that the reduction of virus-associated APOBEC3G was in some cases significantly more pronounced than the reduction of intracellular APOBEC3G levels (Kao *et al.*, 2003, 2004; Mariani *et al.*, 2003). Moreover, mutation of a serine residue at position 144 in Vif (S144A) did not affect its ability to induce APOBEC3G degradation yet severely impaired Vif's ability to govern the production of infectious viruses from APOBEC3G-expressing cells (Mehle *et al.*, 2004a). Finally, we recently identified an APOBEC3G variant that was stable in the presence of Vif and had antiviral activity but was excluded from virions in the presence of Vif (K. S., unpublished data). All of these data suggest that Vif is able to prevent the packaging of APOBEC3G through multiple mechanisms.

Additional evidence for degradation-independent effects of Vif on APO-BEC3G activity comes from a bacterial assay system that is based on the mutation of a rifampicin (Rif) test gene (Ramiro *et al.*, 2003). In this assay, deaminase activity is determined as the frequency of Rif-resistant colonies. HIV-1 Vif was found to inhibit enzymatic activity of both APOBEC3G and the B-cell-specific activation-induced deaminase (AID) (Santa-Marta *et al.*, 2005, 2007). Interestingly, inhibition by Vif was sensitive to mutation of residue D128 in APOBEC3G or the corresponding D118 in AID, which in other experiments was found to affect interaction of Vif and APOBEC3G (see Section II.C). Thus, interaction with Vif can affect the enzymatic activity of APOBEC3G in the absence of proteasomal protein degradation. It is unclear, how Vif in those examples inhibits deaminase activity. However, steric interference by mere binding of Vif to APOBEC3G seems unlikely since a Vif variant carrying a mutation in the HCCH box (C114F; Section II.D and Fig. 2A) was still capable of interacting with APOBEC3G but did not inhibit deaminase activity (Santa-Marta *et al.*, 2005, 2007).

2. APOBEC3G Complexes

APOBEC3G is enzymatically inactive when bound to RNA (Chiu *et al.*, 2005). In fact, in transcriptionally active cells, APOBEC3G copurifies with a large cytoplasmic ribonucleoprotein complex (Chiu *et al.*, 2005). Several studies employing affinity-tagged APOBEC3G proteins have identified RNA and protein components of this complex (Chiu *et al.*, 2006; Kozak *et al.*, 2006; Gallois-Montbrun *et al.*, 2007). The consensus seems to be that most of the APOBEC3G-associated proteins are RNA-binding proteins and that their interaction with APOBEC3G is sensitive to treatment with ribonuclease. The importance—if any—of the high-molecular-weight APOBEC3G ribonucleoprotein complexes for HIV-1 replication and/or Vif function remains unclear since at any given time there appear to be sufficient amounts of low-molecular-weight APOBEC3G in APOBEC3G-expressing cells to severely limit replication of Vif-defective HIV-1. The ability of APOBEC3G to form high-molecular-weight ribonucleoprotein complexes may reflect another function of APOBEC3G that aims at controlling intracellular events such as the retrotransposition of Alu retroelements, which is inhibited by APOBEC3G through sequestering Alu RNAs in cytoplasmic APOBEC3G ribonucleoprotein complexes away from the nuclear enzymatic retrotransposition machinery (Chiu *et al.*, 2006).

E. Vif is an RNA-Binding Protein

Fractionated extraction of Vif-transfected HeLa cells revealed that Vif partitions between soluble and detergent-insoluble fractions (Fujita *et al.*, 2004). Indeed, when cells were fractionated in the presence of RNase, Vif shifted almost entirely into the detergent-resistant fraction. This suggests that the soluble portion of Vif represents an RNA-bound form of Vif. Indeed, Vif was found to specifically associate with viral genomic RNA *in vitro* and was found to form a 40S mRNP complex in virus-producing cells (Dettenhofer *et al.*, 2000; Zhang *et al.*, 2000). Furthermore, Vif is packaged into virus particles through an association with viral genomic RNA (Khan *et al.*, 2001). *In vitro* studies revealed that Vif specifically binds to the 5' end of the viral genomic RNA (Henriet *et al.*, 2005) overlapping with a region required for the specific packaging of APOBEC3G (Khan *et al.*, 2005). Detergent-stripping of viruses demonstrated that Vif packaged together with viral genomic RNA is stably associated with the viral cores while Vif packaged in the absence of viral RNA can easily be separated from viral cores by mild detergent treatment (Khan *et al.*, 2001). Thus, Vif is an integral part of the viral reverse transcription complex.

Exactly how many copies of Vif are packaged into HIV-1 particles and its functional significance have been subject to debate. Estimates range from very low levels to more than 100 copies (Camaur and Trono, 1996; Dettenhofer and Yu, 1999; Gabuzda et al., 1992; Kao et al., 2003; Liu et al., 1995). However, it is clear that in acutely infected cultures the efficiency of Vif packaging was significantly higher than in chronically infected cultures (Kao et al., 2003).

F. Functional Domains in Vif

Vif tends to form nonspecific aggregates during purification and enrichment. This property has thus far precluded detailed structural analysis of Vif (Paul et al., 2006). All data regarding functional domains of Vif are therefore based on mutational analysis. With the exception of the BC box and HCCH motif (see Section II.D) functional domains including the APOBEC3G-binding region are poorly defined. Using a *Vaccinia virus*-based system for the expression of Vif in HeLa cells and supported by *in vitro* kinase assays on recombinant Vif, Yang et al. (1996) identified multiple phosphorylation sites in Vif, including Ser144, Thr155, and Thr188. In addition, Vif was found to be a substrate for mitogen-activated protein kinase (MAPK), which was reported to regulate phosphorylation of Vif at two additional sites, Thr96 and Ser165 (Yang and Gabuzda, 1998). Mutation of two of the phosphorylation sites (Thr96 and Ser144), which are highly conserved, abolished the ability of Vif to inhibit the APOBEC3G antiviral activity, suggesting that Vif phosphorylation may be important for its biological activity (Yang and Gabuzda, 1998; Yang et al., 1996). Other important sequences critical for Vif function include two conserved cysteine residues at positions 114 and 133 (Ma et al., 1994; Sova et al., 1997). Experimental evidence suggests that neither intracellular nor virus-associated Vif utilize Cys_{114} and Cys_{133} for the formation of sulfhydryl bonds (Sova et al., 1997). Nevertheless, the fact that mutation of either cysteine results in complete loss of Vif function (Ma et al., 1994; Simon et al., 1999) points to an important function of these residues. We now know that the conserved cysteine residues are part of an unusual zinc-coordination motif (see Section II.D) that is important for binding to Cul5 (Fig. 2A). In addition, a stretch of basic amino acids located near the C-terminus of Vif was found to be critical for interactions with cellular membranes (Goncalves et al., 1995) and the $Pr55^{Gag}$ precursor (see below). Membrane association of Vif was found to be sensitive to trypsin treatment, suggesting the involvement of a cellular protein whose identity, however, remains thus far unknown (Goncalves et al., 1995). Coimmunoprecipitation studies with differentially tagged Vif proteins demonstrated that Vif has the ability to form homomultimers (Yang et al., 2001). A proline-rich domain encompassed by residues 151–164 in Vif was found to be important for multimerization. However, other regions in Vif may contribute as well since deletion of residues 151–164 reduced the efficiency of Vif–Vif interaction only about threefold (Yang *et al.*, 2001).

Vif regulation of viral infectivity may be related to its ability to interact with the $Pr55^{Gag}$ precursor (Bouyac *et al.*, 1997). Vif–Gag interactions were abolished in a Vif mutant lacking the C-terminal 22 amino acids (Bouyac *et al.*, 1997), suggesting an involvement of this C-terminal basic domain in Vif, previously identified as a membrane-binding domain (Goncalves *et al.*, 1994, 1995). Using an insect cell system, Huvent *et al.* (1998) identified four discrete Gag-binding sites, which included residues T_{68}-L_{81} (site I) and W_{89}-P_{100} (site II) in the central domain, and residues P_{162}-R_{173} (III) and P_{177}-M_{189} (IV) at the C-terminus. Substitutions in site I and deletion of site IV were detrimental to Vif encapsidation, whereas substitution of basic residues for alanine in sites III and IV had a positive effect. The data suggest a direct intracellular Gag–Vif interaction and could point to a $Pr55^{Gag}$-mediated membrane-targeting pathway for Vif (Huvent *et al.*, 1998). The Vif-interacting domains in $Pr55^{Gag}$ were analyzed by screening of a phage-displayed library for Vif-interacting peptides (Huvent *et al.*, 1998). The Vif-binding domain in $Pr55^{Gag}$ identified with this technique spanned residues H_{421}-T_{470} and includes the C-terminal region of nucleocapsid (NC), including the second zinc finger, the intermediate spacer peptide sp2, and the N-terminal half of the p6 domain. Deletions in these Gag domains significantly decreased the Vif encapsidation efficiency, and complete deletion of NC or mutation of the cysteine residues in the zinc finger domain abolished Vif encapsidation (Huvent *et al.*, 1998; Khan *et al.*, 2001).

G. Vif Associates with the Cytoskeleton

Aside from its interaction with APOBEC3G and the proposed association of Vif with cellular membranes, the intracellular localization of Vif was found to be affected by the presence of the intermediate filament (IF) vimentin (Karczewski and Strebel, 1996). Fractionation of acutely infected T cells or transiently transfected HeLa cells revealed the existence of soluble, cytoskeletal, and detergent extractable forms of Vif. Confocal microscopic analysis of Vif-expressing HeLa cells suggests that Vif is predominantly present in the cytoplasm and closely colocalizes with the IF vimentin. The close association of Vif with vimentin is evidenced by the fact that treatment of cells with drugs affecting the structure of vimentin filaments similarly affected the localization of Vif (Karczewski and Strebel, 1996). The association of Vif with vimentin severely alters the structure of the IF network and can lead to its complete collapse in a perinuclear region (Karczewski and Strebel, 1996). This effect of Vif on vimentin was found to be reversible and depended on the microtubule network (K. S., unpublished data). Interestingly, the proper establishment of vimentin networks in normal fibroblasts was also found to require stable (detyrosinated) microtubules (Gurland and Gundersen, 1995). It is therefore possible that the observed effects of Vif on vimentin structure result from the disruption of such vimentin–microtubule interactions by Vif. Experimental evidence suggests that association of Vif with vimentin is cell cycle dependent (K. S., unpublished data). This could provide an explanation for the reported failure to detect vimentin association of Vif in syncytia of infected H9 cells (Simon *et al.*, 1997) and could further explain the reversible nature of the Vif-induced changes in the cytoskeletal structure.

H.   Vif as a Possible Regulator of Gag/Pol Polyprotein Processing

On the basis of its similarity to a family of cysteine proteases, Guy *et al.* (1991) initially proposed that Vif might act as a protease, targeting the cytoplasmic domain of the Env glycoprotein. However, even though Vif has been implicated in regulating incorporation of Env into virions (Borman *et al.*, 1995; Sakai *et al.*, 1993), a proteolytic activity of Vif has so far not been demonstrated and the processing of the C-terminal end of gp41 as suggested by Guy *et al.* (1991) could not be confirmed by others (Gabuzda *et al.*, 1992; von Schwedler *et al.*, 1993). In fact, a more recent model proposes that Vif acts as an inhibitor of the HIV protease and functions to prevent premature processing of the Gag/Pol polyprotein precursor (Baraz *et al.*, 1998; Friedler *et al.*, 1999a; Kotler *et al.*, 1997; Potash *et al.*, 1998). This proposed function of Vif is based on the observation that expression of Vif or an N-terminal Vif-derived peptide was able to inhibit autoprocessing of truncated Gag/Pol polyproteins in *Escherichia coli* and also inhibited processing of a synthetic model peptide *in vitro* (Kotler *et al.*, 1997). In addition, synthetic peptides corresponding to an N-terminal domain of Vif (residues 30–65 and 78–98) were found to inhibit HIV-1 replication in peripheral blood lymphocytes (Friedler *et al.*, 1999b; Potash *et al.*, 1998). Despite the obvious effect of Vif (or Vif-derived peptides) on Gag/Pol processing *in vitro*, the *in vivo* function of Vif, both with respect to the regulation of Gag processing and its site of action, remains controversial (Bouyac *et al.*, 1997; Fouchier *et al.*, 1996; Ochsenbauer *et al.*, 1997; Simm *et al.*, 1995; K. S., unpublished data).

I.   Virion-Associated Vif May Have a Crucial Role in Regulating Viral Infectivity

Aside from its proposed function in HIV-infected cells, Vif may also have a virion-associated activity. Like Vpr and Nef, Vif is packaged into virus particles (Borman *et al.*, 1995; Camaur and Trono, 1996; Karczewski and Strebel, 1996; Liu *et al.*, 1995). Unlike Vpr, which is packaged in significant quantities through specific interaction with the p6 domain in Gag (Kondo *et al.*, 1995; Lavallee *et al.*, 1994; Lu *et al.*, 1993, 1995; Paxton *et al.*, 1993; Selig *et al.*, 1999), Vif incorporation into virions was reported to be nonselective. While there is general agreement on the fact that Vif is packaged into virions, there is an ongoing discussion regarding the absolute amounts of Vif packaged. It is apparent that the amounts of Vif packaged into virions are low and vary depending on the intracellular expression levels of Vif (Camaur and Trono, 1996; Dettenhofer and Yu, 1999; Karczewski and Strebel, 1996; Liu *et al.*, 1995; Simon *et al.*, 1998b). Nevertheless, virion-associated Vif is found in tight association with the viral core (Karczewski and Strebel, 1996; Liu *et al.*, 1995) and consistently copurifies with viral reverse transcriptase, integrase, and unprocessed Pr55^{Gag} (K. S., unpublished data). It is thus likely that Vif is a component of the HIV nucleoprotein complex and as such could, despite its low abundance, perform a crucial function during the early phase of viral infection.

III. The HIV-1-Specific Vpu Protein

A. Introduction

Vpu is an 81 amino acid type 1 integral membrane protein composed of three discrete α-helices. (Cohen *et al.*, 1988; Strebel *et al.*, 1988). The N-terminal helix constitutes the transmembrane anchor and is followed by a cytoplasmic tail containing two amphipathic α-helices (Federau *et al.*, 1996; Willbold *et al.*, 1997). The Rev-dependent bicistronic mRNA that encodes Vpu also contains the downstream Env open reading frame (ORF) which is translated by leaky scanning of the Vpu initiation codon (Schwartz *et al.*, 1990). The *vpu* gene is not always functional due to the presence of mutated initiation codons or internal deletions suggesting a mechanism by which Vpu expression is regulated by the virus (Schubert *et al.*, 1999). Although the *vpu* gene is only found in HIV-1 strains, the envelope protein of certain isolates of HIV-2 have been shown to assume some of the functionality of the HIV-1 Vpu protein (Bour and Strebel, 1996; Bour *et al.*, 1996; Ritter *et al.*, 1996). The Vpu protein has two main roles in the viral life cycle: it promotes the efficient release of viral particles from the cell surface and it induces the degradation of CD4, and possibly other transmembrane proteins, in the endoplasmic reticulum (ER). Much progress has been made over the years to understand both functions of Vpu. However, there are a number of fundamental issues that remain to be addressed. This chapter aims at summarizing our current knowledge on Vpu.

B. Structure of the Vpu Protein

Vpu is an 81 amino acid type 1 integral membrane protein (Cohen *et al.*, 1988; Strebel *et al.*, 1988). Residues 1–27 constitute the N-terminal hydrophobic membrane anchor followed by 54 residues that protrude into the cytoplasm. A highly conserved region spanning residues 47–58 contains a pair of serine residues that are constitutively phosphorylated by casein kinase II (Schubert *et al.*, 1994). Initial attempts to resolve the structure of the Vpu protein were hampered by the presence of the N-terminal hydrophobic membrane anchor domain, which made the protein highly insoluble in aqueous solutions. Investigators therefore focused on partial structures using synthetic peptides corresponding to the hydrophilic region (residues 27–81) or fragments thereof. The inability to successfully crystallize Vpu made it necessary to use circular dichroism and proton NMR spectroscopy in solution to determine the structure of the Vpu cytoplasmic domain. Using synthetic peptides representing the Vpu cytoplasmic domain, such techniques detected two discrete α-helical structures encompassing amino acids 35–50 and 58–70, respectively separated by a flexible segment containing the two conserved phosphorylated serine residues (Federau *et al.*, 1996; Henklein *et al.*, 1993; Kochendoerfer *et al.*, 2004; Wray *et al.*, 1995; Zheng *et al.*, 2003). The Vpu helix 1 is amphipathic with hydrophobic, basic, and acidic residues clustered along the axis of the helix. The same is true for helix 2 albeit to a less striking degree. Using ^{15}N-labeled peptides encompassing residues 1–27, it was determined that the transmembrane domain forms a stable helical structure with a tilt angle of ~6° to 15° relative to the plane of the membrane (Kukol and Arkin, 1999; Park and Opella, 2005; Park *et al.*, 2003; Sharpe *et al.*, 2006). These data along with the extensive structure information available for the Vpu cytoplasmic tail in solution have led to a model of Vpu topology in a membrane environment as depicted in Fig. 3 (model I). In this model, the membrane-spanning N-terminal domain

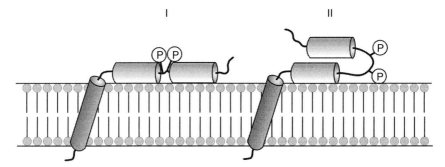

FIGURE 3 Model representation of the Vpu secondary structure as deducted from available NMR and modeling data. Two separate models are proposed. Model (I) is based on data presented by Park *et al.* (Park and Opella, 2005; Park *et al.*, 2003). Model II is based on data presented by Lemaitre *et al.* (2006). In both models the Vpu transmembrane helix is tilted. In model I, the two cytoplasmic helices are aligned with the lipid bilayer with the two phosphoserine residues protruding into the cytoplasm. Model II proposes that the two cytoplasmic helices are oriented almost parallel to each other with the two phosphoserine residues protruding from the connecting loop.

forms a stable a-helix connected to the soluble cytoplasmic tail by a short unstructured fragment. A string of positively charged residues within that flexible arm would allow interactions with the negatively charged lipid surface. The hydrophobic side of helix 1 in the cytoplasmic domain is partially buried in the lipid bilayer, exposing the hydrophilic (or charged) side to the cytoplasm. The flexible region joining the cytoplasmic helices 1 and 2 appears to form a loop pointing away from the membrane, mostly due to the acidic nature of the two conserved phosphorylated serine residues (Coadou *et al.*, 2002; Henklein *et al.*, 2000). In a second model (Fig. 3, model II), the two cytoplasmic helices of Vpu adopt a more compact structure where the two helices are oriented almost parallel to each other (Lemaitre *et al.*, 2006).

One of the limitations of all of these studies is that they are performed on highly purified Vpu protein. However, biochemical studies have revealed that in HIV-infected cells Vpu interacts with a number of host factors, including CD4 or βTrCP (see below). It is likely that the interaction of Vpu with such host factors affects its tertiary structure and in particular the orientation of the cytoplasmic helices. Also, homo-oligomerization of Vpu, which was first described by chemical cross-linking experiments (Maldarelli *et al.*, 1993) but which is not addressed in current structure models, may significantly affect on the overall conformation of Vpu in membranes. For a more comprehensive review of Vpu structure see Opella *et al.* (2005).

C. Biological Activities of the Vpu Protein

1. Vpu-Mediated Degradation of the CD4 Receptor

The gp160 envelope glycoprotein precursor (Env) and Vpu both significantly contribute to the viral effort to downregulate CD4. Gp160 is a major player in CD4 down-modulation that can, in most instances, quantitatively block the bulk of newly synthesized CD4 in the ER (Bour *et al.*, 1995; Crise *et al.*, 1990; Jabbar and Nayak, 1990). However, this strategy has two principal shortcomings. First, in contrast to Nef, Env is unable to remove preexisting CD4 molecules that have already reached the cell surface. Second, the formation of CD4-gp160 complexes in the ER blocks the transport and maturation of not only CD4 but of the Env protein itself (Bour *et al.*, 1991). In cases where equimolar amounts of CD4 and Env are synthesized, this could lead to the depletion of cell surface Env and thus the production of Env-deficient, noninfectious virions (Buonocore and Rose, 1990, 1993). An important function of Vpu is to induce the degradation of CD4 molecules trapped in intracellular complexes with Env thus allowing gp160 to resume transport toward the cell surface (Willey *et al.*, 1992a). In Vpu-expressing cells, CD4 is rapidly degraded in the ER and its half-life drops from 6 h to ~15 min (Willey *et al.*, 1992b). The importance of ER localization for CD4 susceptibility to Vpu-mediated degradation suggests that cellular factors essential for CD4 degradation are located in the ER and/or that the rate-limiting step of CD4 degradation is binding by Vpu (Chen *et al.*, 1993). In support of the latter option, coimmunoprecipitation experiments showed that CD4 and Vpu physically interact in the ER and that this interaction is essential for targeting CD4 to the degradation pathway (Bour *et al.*, 1995). The domains in Vpu required for CD4 binding are less well defined, suggesting that three-dimensional rather than linear structures are involved. While two conserved serine residues at positions 52 and 56 in the cytoplasmic domain of Vpu are critically important for CD4 degradation (Paul and Jabbar, 1997; Schubert and Strebel, 1994), they are not required for CD4 binding since phosphorylation-defective mutants of Vpu retained the capacity to interact with CD4 (Bour *et al.*, 1995). This finding led to the hypothesis that Vpu binding to CD4 was necessary but not sufficient to induce degradation (Bour *et al.*, 1995). The role of the Vpu phosphoserine residues in the induction of CD4 degradation was elucidated when yeast-two-hybrid assays as well as coimmunoprecipitation studies revealed an interaction of Vpu with the human beta *T*ransducin-*r*epeat Containing Protein (βTrCP; Margottin *et al.*, 1998). Interestingly, Vpu variants mutated at Ser52 and Ser56 were unable to interact with βTrCP, providing a mechanistic explanation for the requirement for Vpu phosphorylation and strongly suggesting that βTrCP was directly involved in the degradation of CD4 (Margottin *et al.*, 1998).

Structurally, βTrCP shows a modular organization. Similar to its *Xenopus laevis* homologue (Spevak *et al.*, 1993), human βTrCP contains seven C-terminal WD repeats, a structure known to mediate protein–protein interactions (Neer *et al.*, 1994). Accordingly, the WD repeats of human βTrCP were shown to mediate interactions with Vpu in a phosphoserine-dependent fashion (Margottin *et al.*, 1998). In addition to the WD repeats, βTrCP contains an F-box domain that functions as a connector between target proteins and the ubiquitin-dependent proteolytic machinery (Bai *et al.*, 1996). Although the molecular mechanisms, by which Vpu targets CD4 for degradation, are now reasonably well defined, it remains unclear how the membrane-anchored CD4 is ultimately brought into contact with cytoplasmic proteasome complexes. A number of proteasome degradation pathways involving βTrCP have recently been deciphered that resemble, at least in part, that of Vpu-mediated CD4 degradation. For example, ubiquitination and proteasome targeting of β-catenin or the NF-κB inhibitor IκBα was shown to involve the same TrCP-containing *S*kpI, Cullin, *F*-box protein (SCF^{TrCP}) E3 complex involved in CD4 degradation (Hatakeyama *et al.*, 1999; Spencer *et al.*, 1999; Winston *et al.*, 1999; Yaron *et al.*, 1998). Indeed, both β-catenin and IκB degradation are inhibited by Vpu (Besnard-Guerin *et al.*, 2004; Bour *et al.*, 2001).

Interestingly, the recognition motif on all known cellular substrates of βTrCP consists of a pair of conserved phosphoserine residues similar to those present in Vpu (Margottin *et al.*, 1998). These serine residues are arranged in a consensus motif present in all of these proteins ($DS^PG\Psi XS^P$, where S^P stands for phosphoserine, Ψ stands for a hydrophobic residue, and X stands for any residue). Serine-phosphorylation plays the major regulatory role in the stability of SCF target proteins. For example, activation of the IκB kinase complex (IKK) by external stimuli such as TNFα induces the serine-phosphorylation of IκBα followed by rapid TrCP-mediated proteasome degradation (Hochstrasser, 1996). Figure 4 summarizes our current understanding of Vpu-mediated degradation of CD4. According to this model, phosphorylated Vpu simultaneously binds to CD4 and TrCP and recruits the proteasome degradation machinery through SkpI, an F-box-binding protein that associates with TrCP (Margottin *et al.*, 1998). SkpI, in turn, interacts with Cul1, a Nedd8-modified entity that provides a docking site for the Cdc34 E2 ubiquitin conjugating enzyme. Cul1 also interacts with Rbx1, which can bind to both TrCP and Cdc34 and stabilize the E2-E3 complex (Skowyra *et al.*, 1999).

While the molecular machinery that assembles around CD4/Vpu complexes is now well defined, it is still not clear how CD4 goes from this targeted state to physical degradation in the cytosolic proteasome. There is only indirect evidence in mammalian assay systems that CD4 ubiquitination precedes its degradation by Vpu (Fujita *et al.*, 1997; Schubert *et al.*, 1998). In contrast, analysis of CD4 degradation in a yeast assay revealed ubiquitination of cytoplasmic but not luminal lysine residues on CD4 (Meusser and Sommer, 2004). It is not clear at present whether Vpu-induced degradation involves dislocation of CD4 from the ER membrane as shown for other

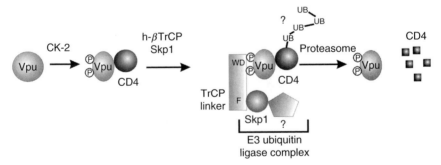

FIGURE 4   Model representation of the Vpu-mediated proteasome degradation of CD4. Vpu acts as an adaptor molecule to connect the CD4 cytoplasmic domain to an (SCF^{TrCP}) E3 complex. This results in the ubiquitination of lysine residues in the cytoplasmic tail of CD4 and subsequent degradation by proteasome complexes. Details of this model are described in the text.

membrane-bound proteasome substrates such as MHC class I heavy chains whose dislocation from the ER to the cytosol is catalyzed by the Human cytomegalovirus US11 gene product (Wiertz et al., 1996).

Vpu has one intriguing property that distinguishes it from all other known substrates of βTrCP: its resistance to proteasome degradation. Indeed, while the SCF^{TrCP} usually degrades the serine-phosphorylated protein directly bound to the TrCP WD domains (i.e., Vpu), CD4—bound to the Vpu cytoplasmic domain—is degraded instead. This phenomenon has serious implications for the regulation and availability of the SCF^{TrCP} in cells that express Vpu. Indeed, due to the fact that Vpu is constitutively phosphorylated (Schubert and Strebel, 1994), binds βTrCP with high affinity (Margottin et al., 1998), and is not released from the complex by degradation (Bour et al., 2001), Vpu expression in HIV-infected cells was likely to perturb the physiological function of the SCF^{TrCP} through competitive trapping of TrCP. Indeed, the dysregulation of IκB by Vpu was shown to lead to inhibition of both HIV- and TNF-α-induced activation of NF-κB (Bour et al., 2001). The dysregulation of NF-κB in Vpu expressing cells has far-reaching consequences since NF-κB is a central transcription factor that regulates the expression of key cellular genes involved in cell proliferation, cytokine production, and the induction of apoptosis (Barkett and Gilmore, 1999; Pahl, 1999). Inhibition of NF-κB activity by Vpu might therefore contribute to the induction of apoptosis in HIV-1-infected cells (Badley et al., 2000; Casella et al., 1999). This was confirmed experimentally by showing that in a population of Jurkat cells expressing wild-type HIV-1, twice as many cells underwent apoptosis than in cells infected with a Vpu-defective virus (Akari et al., 2001). Mechanistically, Vpu was shown to inhibit the NF-κB-dependent expression of antiapoptotic genes such as Bcl-2 family proteins, leading to enhanced intracellular levels of the apoptosis-promoting caspase-3 (Akari et al., 2001). Active caspase-3 then triggers a reaction that results in the cleavage of a number of target proteins including Bcl-2 family proteins and leads to cell death (Akari et al., 2001).

2. Vpu-Mediated Enhancement of Viral Particle Release

In addition to its destabilizing effect on CD4, Vpu mediates the efficient release of viral particles from HIV-1-infected cells (Klimkait et al., 1990; Strebel et al., 1989; Terwilliger et al., 1989). These two biological activities of Vpu appear to be mechanistically distinct and involve different structural domains in Vpu. For example, the particle release–enhancing activity of Vpu is independent of CD4 and does not require the envelope glycoprotein. Also, mutation of serine residues 52 and 56, which are crucial for CD4 degradation, only partially affect virus release (Friborg et al., 1995; Geraghty and Panganiban, 1993; Schubert et al., 1994; Yao et al., 1992). In addition, while the determinants for CD4 degradation are all contained in the cytoplasmic domain of Vpu, the transmembrane domain has been shown to play an essential role for the particle release activity (Paul *et al.*, 1998; Schubert *et al.*, 1996a). Early data suggested that Vpu regulates the detachment of otherwise functional virions from the cell surface (Klimkait *et al.*, 1990). In those experiments nearly 75% of cell-associated reverse transcriptase activity (i.e., virions) could be released by vortexing of the cells (Klimkait *et al.*, 1990). Similar results were obtained when cells producing Vpu-defective virus were treated with protease (Neil *et al.*, 2006). It is still debated whether Vpu enhances virus production through a global modification of the cellular environment or through discreet interactions with cellular or viral factors. The finding that Vpu forms ion-conductive channels at the cell surface (see below) argues in favor of the former possibility (Ewart *et al.*, 1996). Alternatively, it was suggested that interactions between Vpu and a novel cellular protein (Vpu-binding protein or UBP) may be involved in viral particle production (Callahan *et al.*, 1998). UBP is a 41-kDa protein that contains four copies of a so-called tetratricopeptide repeat (TPR), a degenerate 34-amino acid sequence involved in protein–protein interactions (Schatz *et al.*, 1998). Overexpression of UBP was found to abrogate the ability of Vpu to promote viral particle release, suggesting that UBP is a negative factor for virus assembly that needs to be displaced from Gag by Vpu (Callahan *et al.*, 1998). Examination of the subcellular location of Gag in the presence and absence of Vpu and/or UBP suggests that Vpu may enhance viral particle release either by promoting the transport of viral Gag precursors to the plasma membrane or by increasing the affinity of the N-terminal matrix domain for the plasma membrane lipids (Deora and Ratner, 2001; Handley *et al.*, 2001). More recent data suggest that Gag travels initially to the cell surface before accumulating in early and late endosomes (Harila *et al.*, 2006; Neil *et al.*, 2006). On the basis of these results it was proposed that Vpu inhibits nascent virion endocytosis. Interestingly, inhibition of clathrin-mediated endocytosis by expression of dominant-negative forms of dynamin or EPS-15 resulted in the accumulation of virions at the cell surface but did not increase virus release in the absence of Vpu. Instead, these virions were readily detachable by protease treatment (Neil *et al.*, 2006). These results are consistent with the results reported by Klimkait *et al.* (1990), which suggested that Vpu has no effect on virus assembly but regulates the detachment of virions from the cell surface. These results also suggest that Vpu acts at the cell surface. On the other hand, Varthakavi *et al.* (2006) demonstrated that Vpu traffics through the recycling endosome and that disruption of recycling endosome function led to an accumulation of Vpu in this compartment and abolished the enhancing effect of Vpu on virus release. Of note, disruption of endosome function also abolished the enhancing activity of HIV-2 Env, suggesting that Vpu and Env enhance virus release through a common mechanism (Varthakavi *et al.*, 2006). These results do not formally rule out that Vpu and HIV-2

Env regulate virus release per se from the cell surface; however, future studies will have to address that issue.

D. Ion Channel Activity

On the basis of the structural similarity of Vpu with the Influenza virus M2 ion channel protein, it was speculated that homo-oligomeric complexes of Vpu might possess pore-forming abilities (Maldarelli *et al.*, 1993). Indeed, Vpu ion channel activity was experimentally demonstrated in two independent studies by measuring current fluctuations across an artificial lipid bilayer containing either full-length recombinant Vpu protein or synthetic peptides corresponding to the cytoplasmic domain of Vpu (Ewart *et al.*, 1996). In addition, voltage clamp analysis on amphibian oocytes expressing full-length Vpu supports the notion that Vpu forms ion-conductive pores (Schubert *et al.*, 1996b). The Vpu channel appears to be selective for monovalent cations such as sodium and potassium. While some investigators argue that differences in membrane conductance in the presence of Vpu are not due to the opening of an ion channel but rather the result of alterations of the protein membrane composition by Vpu (Coady *et al.*, 1998), there is an intriguing correlation between the ability of Vpu to form ion-conductive channels and its ability to enhance viral particle release *in vivo*. Indeed, a Vpu mutant bearing a transmembrane domain with a scrambled amino acid sequence lacked ion channel activity and was unable to enhance virus particle release, yet retained full CD4 degradation activity (Schubert *et al.*, 1996a). Furthermore, scrambling the Vpu TM domain in the context of a SHIV virus (SHIV[TM]) significantly reduced viral pathogenicity (Hout *et al.*, 2005). Pig-tailed macaques infected with SHIV[TM] exhibited low viral load and did not show severe loss of CD4+ T cells (Hout *et al.*, 2005). Nevertheless, how an ion channel activity of Vpu could lead to enhanced viral particle production is still unclear. It is conceivable that the channel activity of Vpu locally modifies the electric potential at the plasma membrane, leading to facilitated formation and release of membrane budding structures. Alternatively, the action of the Vpu channel could induce cellular factors involved in the late stages of virus formation or exclude cellular factors inhibitory to the viral budding process. So far no inhibitors of Vpu channel activity or Vpu function have been identified. More recently, however, Hout *et al.* (2006b) demonstrated that substitution of the TM domain of Vpu in an SIV/HIV chimeric virus (SHIV(KU1bMC33)) with that of the Influenza virus M2 protein conferred sensitivity to rimantadine, a known inhibitor of the M2 channel. Indeed, the same authors demonstrated that replacement of an alanine residue in the Vpu TM domain by histidine was sufficient to render the protein sensitive to rimantadine (Hout *et al.*, 2006a). While it remains to be shown whether these mutants exhibit similar sensitivity to rimantadine in the context of other Vpu isolates or in the context of HIV, these results strongly imply that Vpu has ion channel activity not only *in vitro* but *in vivo* as well. These findings further support the notion that Vpu ion channel activity is relevant for Vpu function.

A different model for Vpu function was proposed by a recent study suggesting that Vpu affects the activity of the mammalian background K(+) channel TASK-1 (Hsu *et al.*, 2004). The N-terminal domain of TASK-1 exhibits significant structural homology to Vpu. Indeed, Vpu was found to interact with TASK-1 and coexpression of Vpu inhibited the TASK-1 ion channel activity (Hsu *et al.*, 2004). Also, coexpression of TASK-1 with the N-terminal fragment exhibiting homology to Vpu (Ttm1) inhibited TASK-1 ion channel function. Interestingly, expression of Ttm1 increased release of Vpu-defective virus from HeLa cells to a similar extent than wild-type Vpu (Hsu *et al.*, 2004). Thus, it is conceivable that TASK-1 is a cellular inhibitor whose function has to be inactivated by Vpu. If this is true, one would predict that TASK-1 is expressed in nonpermissive cell types such as HeLa or Jurkat but is absent in permissive cells, for example Cos-7 or 293T. Indeed, fusion of permissive Cos-7 cells with nonpermissive HeLa cells produced heterokaryons that exhibited a nonpermissive phenotype (Varthakavi *et al.*, 2003). These results therefore suggest that Vpu counteracts a human host cell restriction factor that inhibits HIV-1 particle production (Varthakavi *et al.*, 2003). Comparative analysis of TASK-1 in permissive and nonpermissive cells should reveal whether TASK-1 is responsible for the effects observed by Varthakavi *et al.*

E. Evolution of Vpu Biological Activities

Although the *vpu* gene is unique to HIV-1, the activity Vpu provides for enhanced viral particle release is not. Indeed, the envelope proteins of several HIV-2 isolates, including ROD10 and ST2, were shown to promote viral particle release in a manner indistinguishable from that of HIV-1 Vpu (Bour and Strebel, 1996; Ritter *et al.*, 1996). Both Vpu and the ROD10 Env are functionally interchangeable and each augments the release of HIV-1, HIV-2, and *Simian immunodeficiency virus* (SIV) particles, suggesting a common mechanism of action for these two proteins (Bour and Strebel, 1996; Gottlinger *et al.*, 1993). Because of its innate tendency to form homo-oligomeric complexes, it seems possible that HIV-2 Env, in analogy to Vpu, mediates the release of viral particles through the formation of a membrane pore. This is supported by the fact that Vpu and the HIV-2 Env both require the presence of a functional transmembrane domain for their activity (Bour and Strebel, 1996; Schubert *et al.*, 1996a) and adopt an oligomeric structure favorable to the formation of a membrane pore (Maldarelli *et al.*, 1993). Mutagenesis studies have delineated the regions in the HIV-2 Env important for its particle release activity. One study proposed that the C-terminal part of the Env cytoplasmic domain is required for efficient particle release (Ritter *et al.*, 1996). However, such correlation between the length of the cytoplasmic tail and the presence of particle release–promoting activity could not be confirmed for the ROD10 isolate (Bour *et al.*, 1999). In addition, ROD14, a molecular clone of HIV-2 closely related to ROD10 that originated from the same patient (Clavel *et al.*, 1986), does not support viral particle release irrespective of the length of its cytoplasmic domain (Bour *et al.*, 1999). Instead, site-directed mutagenesis revealed that the ability of the HIV-2 ROD Env protein to enhance viral particle release is regulated by a single amino acid substitution (position 598) in the ectodomain of the gp36 TM subunit (Bour *et al.*, 2003). Substituting the threonine at that position in the inactive ROD14 Env by the alanine found at the same position in the active ROD10 Env restored full particle release activity to the ROD14 Env in transfected HeLa cells (Bour *et al.*, 2003). In addition to residue 598, Abada *et al.* (2005) have identified two separate functional domains in the HIV-2 Env, located in the ectodomain and the cytoplasmic domain. The cytoplasmic domain important for the enhancing effect of HIV-2 contains a glycine-tyrosine-x-x-hydrophobic (GYxxθ) motif that was previously shown to mediate interaction of HIV-1 Env with the AP-2 adapter complex (Boge *et al.*, 1998; Ohno *et al.*, 1997). Indeed, the GYxxθ motif in HIV-2 Env functions to recruit AP-2 in order to direct Env to an appropriate cellular location required for the enhancement of virus release (Abada *et al.*, 2005). How HIV-2 Env ultimately regulates virus release remains unknown.

Unlike Vpu, the HIV-2 Env protein is unable to induce CD4 degradation (Bour and Strebel, 1996). The absence of a degradative activity in the ROD10 Env suggests that this additional function may have evolved in Vpu from the ancestral particle release activity in response to increased affinity between the HIV-1 Env and CD4 (Bour and Strebel, 1996; Willey *et al.*, 1992a). Additional evidence in favor of this hypothesis comes from examining the sequence of SIV$_{cpz}$ isolates. The serine residues at positions 52 and 56 essential for interaction with TrCP are less conserved in SIV$_{cpz}$ than in the prototypical subtype C HIV-1 isolates (McCormick-Davis *et al.*, 2000). Interestingly, the ability of Vpu to induce CD4 degradation is conserved among highly divergent strains of SIV$_{cpz}$ despite the fact that several of the Vpu variants contain only one of the two phosphoserine residues required for interaction with βTrCP (Gomez *et al.*, 2005). A possible explanation for the dispensability of Ser56 in these isolates is the presence of a string of negatively charged residues downstream of Ser52 that may substitute for the missing phosphoserine (S_{56}). In support of this, substitution of one or more of the negatively charged amino acids by lysine abolished their ability to degrade CD4 (Gomez *et al.*, 2005).

F. Vpu Contributes to HIV-1 Pathogenesis by Raising Viral Loads

Vpu is one of the least antigenic proteins of HIV-1. Despite the delineation of two immunodominant B-cell epitopes in Vpu, only 20–30% of patients tested exhibit detectable immune response to Vpu (Kusk *et al.*, 1993; Schneider *et al.*, 1990a). Vpu also appears to be a poor target for cytotoxic T cells. Although a major cytotoxic T-lymphocyte (CTL) epitope was identified between residues 28 and 36, less than 3% of patients screened have detectable Vpu-specific CTL responses against this peptide (Addo *et al.*, 2002). There are conflicting reports on the possible link between the presence of Vpu-specific antibodies in patients and disease progression. One early study found no temporal relationship between the presence or absence of Vpu antibodies and the onset of HIV-1-related disease (Reiss and Hershko, 1990). In contrast, Kusk *et al.* (1993) found a statistically relevant correlation between the presence of antibodies against the immunodominant epitope 31–50 and a late disease stage characterized by CD4+ T cell counts of <400 cells/μl. However, the notion that antibodies against Vpu are a valid marker of disease progression is further challenged by the finding that in a cohort of 243 HIV-1-infected patients Vpu-specific antibodies against another immunodominant epitope (residues 64–81) were actually more prevalent in individuals in the early stages of disease (Schneider *et al.*, 1990b). Furthermore, Chen *et al.* (2003) reported an association of the presence of anti-Vpu antibodies with improved prognosis following HIV-1 infection in a cohort of 162 highly active antiretroviral therapy (HAART) patients. A possible explanation for these divergent sets of data may be that the Vpu sequence appears to be the most variable among all HIV-1 genes (Yusim *et al.*, 2002). Indeed, experimental methods employed to detect both humoral and CTL activities rely on reactions against synthetic peptides whose sequences are based on the consensus of cloned viruses. Given the rate of variability of the immunodominant epitopes in Vpu, it is entirely possible that such diagnostic assays give false-negative readouts when used against widely divergent Vpu sequences.

Stronger lines of evidence point to a role of Vpu in HIV pathogenesis. Studies in pig-tailed macaque using SIV/HIV chimeric viruses (SHIV) have shown that mutation of the *vpu* initiation codon rapidly reverts to give rise to a functional *vpu* ORF (Stephens *et al.*, 1997). Such reversion occurs as early as 16 weeks postinfection and correlates with a phase of profound loss of CD4+ cells (McCormick-Davis *et al.*, 1998). The rapid loss of CD4+ T cells was correlated with the phosphorylation of Vpu (Singh *et al.*, 2003). Animals infected with a SHIV variant carrying mutations in the phosphoserine sites developed no or only gradual CD4+ T-cell loss and maintained low viral burden (Singh *et al.*, 2003).

Similar results were obtained in cynomolgus monkeys where the presence of Vpu was correlated with a vast increase in the plasma viral RNA levels 2 weeks postinfection (Li *et al.*, 1995). The increased viral fitness and pathogenicity conferred by Vpu is bimodal. First, Vpu increases viral loads in the plasma, thereby contributing to viral spread. Second, the higher frequency of *de novo* infections that results from these higher viral loads leads to increased rates of mutations in the *env* gene (Li *et al.*, 1995; Mackay *et al.*, 2002). This in turn leads to more rapid and efficient escape from neutralizing antibodies and accelerated disease progression (Li *et al.*, 1995). In animals infected with viruses where *vpu* deletions were large enough to prevent reversions, investigators observed long-term nonprogressing infections characterized by a lack of circulating CD4+ T-cells loss (Stephens *et al.*, 2002). Finally, studies in pig-tailed macaques showed that in the presence of large deletions in *vpu*, additional mutations in the *env* gene were acquired that partially compensated for the lack of Vpu (McCormick-Davis *et al.*, 2000). Although the mechanism by which Env would recapitulate the activity of Vpu in these animals is unclear, it is tempting to speculate that Env might have acquired a particle release activity similar to that displayed by some HIV-1 macrophage tropic isolates (Schubert *et al.*, 1999) and some HIV-2 isolates (Bour *et al.*, 1996; Ritter *et al.*, 1996).

While Vpu might still be referred to as an accessory protein, there is clear evidence that its role in enhancing viral particle production, downregulating cell surface CD4, and raising viral loads *in vivo* is key to the fitness and pathogenesis of HIV-1. It may be too early to call Vpu a viral pathogenesis factor but it is interesting to note that closely related retroviruses such as HIV-2 and SIV with less severe pathogenesis and disease outcome all lack expression of the Vpu protein.

References

Abada, P., Noble, B., and Cannon, P. M. (2005). Functional domains within the human immunodeficiency virus type 2 envelope protein required to enhance virus production. *J. Virol.* **79**, 3627–3638.

Addo, M. M., Altfeld, M., Rathod, A., Yu, M., Yu, X. G., Goulder, P. J., Rosenberg, E. S., and Walker, B. D. (2002). HIV-1 Vpu represents a minor target for cytotoxic T lymphocytes in HIV-1-infection. *AIDS* **16**, 1071–1073.

Akari, H., Bour, S., Kao, S., Adachi, A., and Strebel, K. (2001). The human immunodeficiency virus type 1 accessory protein Vpu induces apoptosis by suppressing the nuclear factor kappaB-dependent expression of antiapoptotic factors. *J. Exp. Med.* **194**, 1299–1311.

Badley, A. D., Pilon, A. A., Landay, A., and Lynch, D. H. (2000). Mechanisms of HIV-associated lymphocyte apoptosis. *Blood* **96**, 2951–2964.

Bai, C., Sen, P., Hofmann, K., Ma, L., Goebl, M., Harper, J. W., and Elledge, S. J. (1996). SKP1 connects cell cycle regulators to the ubiquitin proteolysis machinery through a novel motif, the F-box. *Cell* **86**, 263–274.

Baraz, L., Friedler, A., Blumenzweig, I., Nussinuv, O., Chen, N., Steinitz, M., Gilon, C., and Kotler, M. (1998). Human immunodeficiency virus type 1 Vif-derived peptides inhibit the viral protease and arrest virus production. *FEBS Lett.* **441**, 419–426.

Barkett, M., and Gilmore, T. D. (1999). Control of apoptosis by Rel/NF-kappaB transcription factors. *Oncogene* **18**, 6910–6924.

Besnard-Guerin, C., Belaidouni, N., Lassot, I., Segeral, E., Jobart, A., Marchal, C., and Benarous, R. (2004). HIV-1 Vpu sequesters {beta}-transducin repeat-containing protein ({beta}TrCP) in the cytoplasm and provokes the accumulation of {beta}-catenin and other SCF{beta}TrCP substrates. *J. Biol. Chem.* **279**, 788–795.

Blanc, D., Patience, C., Schulz, T. F., Weiss, R., and Spire, B. (1993). Transcomplementation of VIF- HIV-1 mutants in CEM cells suggests that VIF affects late steps of the viral life cycle. *Virology* **193**, 186–192.

Boge, M., Wyss, S., Bonifacino, J. S., and Thali, M. (1998). A membrane-proximal tyrosine-based signal mediates internalization of the HIV-1 envelope glycoprotein via interaction with the AP-2 clathrin adaptor. *J. Biol. Chem.* **273**, 15773–15778.

Bogerd, H. P., Doehle, B. P., Wiegand, H. L., and Cullen, B. R. (2004). A single amino acid difference in the host APOBEC3G protein controls the primate species specificity of HIV type 1 virion infectivity factor. *Proc. Natl. Acad. Sci. USA* **101**, 3770–3774.

Borman, A. M., Quillent, C., Charneau, P., Dauguet, C., and Clavel, F. (1995). Human immunodeficiency virus type 1 Vif-mutant particles from restrictive cells: Role of Vif in correct particle assembly and infectivity. *J. Virol.* **69**, 2058–2067.

Bour, S., and Strebel, K. (1996). The human immunodeficiency virus (HIV) type 2 envelope protein is a functional complement to HIV type 1 Vpu that enhances particle release of heterologous retroviruses. *J. Virol.* **70**, 8285–8300.

Bour, S., Boulerice, F., and Wainberg, M. A. (1991). Inhibition of gp160 and CD4 maturation in U937 cells after both defective and productive infections by human immunodeficiency virus type 1. *J. Virol.* **65**, 6387–6396.

Bour, S., Schubert, U., and Strebel, K. (1995). The human immunodeficiency virus type 1 Vpu protein specifically binds to the cytoplasmic domain of CD4: Implications for the mechanism of degradation. *J. Virol.* **69**, 1510–1520.

Bour, S., Schubert, U., Peden, K., and Strebel, K. (1996). The envelope glycoprotein of human immunodeficiency virus type 2 enhances viral particle release: A Vpu-like factor? *J. Virol.* **70**, 820–829.

Bour, S., Perrin, C., Akari, H., and Strebel, K. (2001). The Human immunodeficiency virus type 1 Vpu protein inhibits NF-kappa B activation by interfering with beta TrCP-mediated degradation of Ikappa B. *J. Biol. Chem.* **276**, 15920–15928.

Bour, S., Akari, H., Miyagi, E., and Strebel, K. (2003). Naturally occurring amino acid substitutions in the HIV-2 ROD envelope glycoprotein regulate its ability to augment viral particle release. *Virology* **309**, 85–98.

Bour, S. P., Aberham, C., Perrin, C., and Strebel, K. (1999). Lack of effect of cytoplasmic tail truncations on human immunodeficiency virus type 2 ROD env particle release activity. *J. Virol.* **73**, 778–782.

Bouyac, M., Courcoul, M., Bertoia, G., Baudat, Y., Gabuzda, D., Blanc, D., Chazal, N., Boulanger, P., Sire, J., Vigne, R., and Spire, B. (1997). Human immunodeficiency virus type 1 Vif protein binds to the Pr55Gag precursor. *J. Virol.* **71**, 9358–9365.

Buonocore, L., and Rose, J. K. (1990). Prevention of HIV-1 glycoprotein transport by soluble CD4 retained in the endoplasmic reticulum. *Nature* **345**, 625–628.

Buonocore, L., and Rose, J. K. (1993). Blockade of human immunodeficiency virus type 1 production in CD4+ T cells by an intracellular CD4 expressed under control of the viral long terminal repeat. *Proc. Natl. Acad. Sci. USA* **90**, 2695–2699.

Callahan, M. A., Handley, M. A., Lee, Y. H., Talbot, K. J., Harper, J. W., and Panganiban, A. T. (1998). Functional interaction of human immunodeficiency virus type 1 Vpu and Gag with a novel member of the tetratricopeptide repeat protein family. *J. Virol.* **72**, 5189–5197.

Camaur, D., and Trono, D. (1996). Characterization of human immunodeficiency virus type 1 Vif particle incorporation. *J. Virol.* **70**, 6106–6111.

Carr, J. M., Davis, A. J., Coolen, C., Cheney, K., Burrell, C. J., and Li, P. (2006). Vif-deficient HIV reverse transcription complexes (RTCs) are subject to structural changes and mutation of RTC-associated reverse transcription products. *Virology* **351**, 80–91.

Casella, C. R., Rapaport, E. L., and Finkel, T. H. (1999). Vpu increases susceptibility of human immunodeficiency virus type 1-infected cells to fas killing. *J. Virol.* **73**, 92–100.

Chen, M. Y., Maldarelli, F., Karczewski, M. K., Willey, R. L., and Strebel, K. (1993). Human immunodeficiency virus type 1 Vpu protein induces degradation of CD4 *in vitro*: The cytoplasmic domain of CD4 contributes to Vpu sensitivity. *J. Virol.* **67**, 3877–3884.

Chen, Y. M., Rey, W. Y., Lan, Y. C., Lai, S. F., Huang, Y. C., Wu, S. I., Liu, T. T., and Hsiao, K. J. (2003). Antibody reactivity to HIV-1 Vpu in HIV-1/AIDS patients on highly active antiretroviral therapy. *J. Biomed. Sci.* **10**, 266–275.

Chiu, Y. L., Soros, V. B., Kreisberg, J. F., Stopak, K., Yonemoto, W., and Greene, W. C. (2005). Cellular APOBEC3G restricts HIV-1 infection in resting CD4+ T cells. *Nature* **435**, 108–114.

Chiu, Y. L., Witkowska, H. E., Hall, S. C., Santiago, M., Soros, V. B., Esnault, C., Heidmann, T., and Greene, W. C. (2006). High-molecular-mass APOBEC3G complexes restrict alu retrotransposition. *Proc. Natl. Acad. Sci. USA* **103**(42), 15588–15593.

Clavel, F., Guyader, M., Guetard, D., Salle, M., Montagnier, L., and Alizon, M. (1986). Molecular cloning and polymorphism of the human immunodeficiency virus type 2. *Nature* **324**, 691–695.

Coadou, G., Evrard-Todeschi, N., Gharbi-Benarous, J., Benarous, R., and Girault, J. P. (2002). HIV-1 encoded virus protein U (Vpu) solution structure of the 41–62 hydrophilic region containing the phosphorylated sites Ser52 and Ser56. *Int. J. Biol. Macromol.* **30**, 23–40.

Coady, M. J., Daniel, N. G., Tiganos, E., Allain, B., Friborg, J., Lapointe, J. Y., and Cohen, E. A. (1998). Effects of Vpu expression on Xenopus oocyte membrane conductance. *Virology* **244**, 39–49.

Cohen, E. A., Terwilliger, E. F., Sodroski, J. G., and Haseltine, W. A. (1988). Identification of a protein encoded by the vpu gene of HIV-1. *Nature* **334**, 532–534.

Conticello, S. G., Harris, R. S., and Neuberger, M. S. (2003). The Vif protein of HIV triggers degradation of the human antiretroviral DNA deaminase APOBEC3G. *Curr. Biol.* **13**, 2009–2013.

Courcoul, M., Patience, C., Rey, F., Blanc, D., Harmache, A., Sire, J., Vigne, R., and Spire, B. (1995). Peripheral blood mononuclear cells produce normal amounts of defective Vif- human immunodeficiency virus type 1 particles which are restricted for the preretrotranscription steps. *J. Virol.* **69**, 2068–2074.

Crise, B., Buonocore, L., and Rose, J. K. (1990). CD4 is retained in the endoplasmic reticulum by the human immunodeficiency virus type 1 glycoprotein precursor. *J. Virol.* **64**, 5585–5593.

Deora, A., and Ratner, L. (2001). Viral protein U (Vpu)-mediated enhancement of human immunodeficiency virus type 1 particle release depends on the rate of cellular proliferation. *J. Virol.* **75**, 6714–6718.

Dettenhofer, M., and Yu, X. F. (1999). Highly purified human immunodeficiency virus type 1 reveals a virtual absence of Vif in virions. *J. Virol.* **73**, 1460–1467.

Dettenhofer, M., Cen, S., Carlson, B. A., Kleiman, L., and Yu, X. F. (2000). Association of human immunodeficiency virus type 1 Vif with RNA and its role in reverse transcription. *J. Virol.* **74**, 8938–8945.

Ewart, G. D., Sutherland, T., Gage, P. W., and Cox, G. B. (1996). The Vpu protein of human immunodeficiency virus type 1 forms cation-selective ion channels. *J. Virol.* **70**, 7108–7115.

Fan, L., and Peden, K. (1992). Cell-free transmission of Vif mutants of HIV-1. *Virology* **190**, 19–29.

Federau, T., Schubert, U., Flossdorf, J., Henklein, P., Schomburg, D., and Wray, V. (1996). Solution structure of the cytoplasmic domain of the human immunoodeficiency virus type 1 encoded virus protein U (Vpu). *Int. J. Peptide Res.* **47**, 297–310.

Fisher, A. G., Ensoli, B., Ivanoff, L., Chamberlain, M., Petteway, S., Ratner, L., Gallo, R. C., and Wong-Staal, F. (1987). The *sor* gene of HIV-1 is required for efficient virus transmission *in vitro*. *Science* **237**, 888–893.

Fouchier, R. A., Simon, J. H., Jaffe, A. B., and Malim, M. H. (1996). Human immunodeficiency virus type 1 Vif does not influence expression or virion incorporation of gag-, pol-, and env-encoded proteins. *J. Virol.* **70**, 8263–8269.

Friborg, J., Ladha, A., Goettlinger, H., Haseltine, W. A., and Cohen, E. A. (1995). Functional analysis of the phosphorylation sites on the human immunodeficiency virus type 1 Vpu protein. *J. Acquired Immune Def. Syndr. Hum Retrovir.* **8**, 10–22.

Friedler, A., Blumenzweig, I., Baraz, L., Steinitz, M., Kotler, M., and Gilon, C. (1999a). Peptides derived from HIV-1 Vif: A non-substrate based novel type of HIV-1 protease inhibitors. *J. Mol. Biol.* **287**, 93–101.

Friedler, A., Zakai, N., Karni, O., Friedler, D., Gilon, C., and Loyter, A. (1999b). Identification of a nuclear transport inhibitory signal (NTIS) in the basic domain of HIV-1 Vif protein. *J. Mol. Biol.* **289**, 431–437.

Fujita, K., Omura, S., and Silver, J. (1997). Rapid degradation of CD4 in cells expressing HIV-1 Env and Vpu is blocked by proteasome inhibitors. *J. Gen. Virol.* **78**, 619–625.

Fujita, M., Matsumoto, S., Sakurai, A., Doi, N., Miyaura, M., Yoshida, A., and Adachi, A. (2002). Apparent lack of trans-dominant negative effects of various vif mutants on the replication of HIV-1. *Microbes Infect.* **4**, 1203–1207.

Fujita, M., Akari, H., Sakurai, A., Yoshida, A., Chiba, T., Tanaka, K., Strebel, K., and Adachi, A. (2004). Expression of HIV-1 accessory protein Vif is controlled uniquely to be low and optimal by proteasome degradation. *Microbes Infect.* **6**, 791–798.

Gabuzda, D. H., Lawrence, K., Langhoff, E., Terwilliger, E., Dorfman, T., Haseltine, W. A., and Sodroski, J. (1992). Role of vif in replication of human immunodeficiency virus type 1 in CD4+ T lymphocytes. *J. Virol.* **66**, 6489–6495.

Gabuzda, D. H., Li, H., Lawrence, K., Vasir, B. S., Crawford, K., and Langhoff, E. (1994). Essential role of vif in establishing productive HIV-1 infection in peripheral blood T lymphocytes and monocyte/macrophages. *J. Acq. Immune Def. Syndr.* **7**, 908–915.

Gallo, R., Wong-Staal, F., Montagnier, L., Haseltine, W. A., and Yoshida, M. (1988). HIV/HTLV gene nomenclature. *Nature* **333**, 514.

Gallois-Montbrun, S., Kramer, B., Swanson, C. M., Byers, H., Lynham, S., Ward, M., and Malim, M. H. (2007). Antiviral protein APOBEC3G localizes to ribonucleoprotein complexes found in P bodies and stress granules. *J. Virol.* **81**, 2165–2178.

Garrett, E. D., Tiley, L. S., and Cullen, B. R. (1991). Rev activates expression of the human immunodeficiency virus type 1 vif and vpr gene products. *J. Virol.* **65**, 1653–1657.

Geraghty, R. J., and Panganiban, A. T. (1993). Human immunodeficiency virus type 1 Vpu has a CD4− and an envelope glycoprotein-independent function. *J. Virol.* **67**, 4190–4194.

Gomez, L. M., Pacyniak, E., Flick, M., Hout, D. R., Gomez, M. L., Nerrienet, E., Ayouba, A., Santiago, M. L., Hahn, B. H., and Stephens, E. B. (2005). Vpu-mediated CD4 down-regulation and degradation is conserved among highly divergent SIV(cpz) strains. *Virology* **335**, 46–60.

Goncalves, J., Jallepalli, P., and Gabuzda, D. H. (1994). Subcellular localization of the Vif protein of human immunodeficiency virus type 1. *J. Virol.* **68**, 704–712.

Goncalves, J., Shi, B., Yang, X., and Gabuzda, D. (1995). Biological activity of human immunodeficiency virus type 1 Vif requires membrane targeting by C-terminal basic domains. *J. Virol.* **69**, 7196–7204.

Gottlinger, H. G., Dorfman, T., Cohen, E. A., and Haseltine, W. A. (1993). Vpu protein of human immunodeficiency virus type 1 enhances the release of capsids produced by gag gene constructs of widely divergent retroviruses. *Proc. Natl. Acad. Sci. USA* **90**, 7381–7385.

Gurland, G., and Gundersen, G. G. (1995). Stable, detyrosinated microtubules function to localize vimentin intermediate filaments in fibroblasts. *J. Cell Biol.* **131**, 1275–1290.

Guy, B., Geist, M., Dott, K., Spehner, D., Kieny, M. P., and Lecocq, J. P. (1991). A specific inhibitor of cysteine proteases impairs a vif-dependent modification of human immunodeficiency virus type 1 env protein. *J. Virol.* **65**, 1325–1331.

Handley, M. A., Paddock, S., Dall, A., and Panganiban, A. T. (2001). Association of Vpu-binding protein with microtubules and Vpu-dependent redistribution of HIV-1 Gag protein. *Virology* **291**, 198–207.

Harila, K., Prior, I., Sjoberg, M., Salminen, A., Hinkula, J., and Suomalainen, M. (2006). Vpu and Tsg101 regulate intracellular targeting of the human immunodeficiency virus type 1 core protein precursor Pr55gag. *J. Virol.* **80**, 3765–3772.

Hatakeyama, S., Kitagawa, M., Nakayama, K., Shirane, M., Matsumoto, M., Hattori, K., Higashi, H., Nakano, H., Okumura, K., Onoe, K., Good, R. A., and Nakayama, K. I. (1999). Ubiquitin-dependent degradation of IkappaBalpha is mediated by aubiquitin ligase Skp1/Cul 1/F-box protein FWD1. *Proc. Natl. Acad. Sci. USA* **96**, 3859–3863.

Henklein, P., Schubert, U., Kunert, O., Klabunde, S., Wray, V., Kloeppel, K. D., Kiess, M., Porstmann, T., and Schomburg, D. (1993). Synthesis and characterization of the hydrophilic C-terminal domain of the human immunodeficiency virus type 1-encoded virus protein U (Vpu). *Pept. Res.* **6**, 79–87.

Henklein, P., Kinder, R., Schubert, U., and Bechinger, B. (2000). Membrane interactions and alignment of structures within the HIV-1 Vpu cytoplasmic domain: Effect of phosphorylation of serines 52 and 56. *FEBS Lett.* **482**, 220–224.

Henriet, S., Richer, D., Bernacchi, S., Decroly, E., Vigne, R., Ehresmann, B., Ehresmann, C., Paillart, J. C., and Marquet, R. (2005). Cooperative and specific binding of Vif to the 5′ region of HIV-1 genomic RNA. *J. Mol. Biol.* **354**, 55–72.

Hochstrasser, M. (1996). Protein degradation or regulation: Ub the judge. *Cell* **84**, 813–815.

Hoglund, S., Ohagen, A., Lawrence, K., and Gabuzda, D. (1994). Role of vif during packing of the core of HIV-1. *Virology* **201**, 349–355.

Hout, D. R., Gomez, M. L., Pacyniak, E., Gomez, L. M., Inbody, S. H., Mulcahy, E. R., Culley, N., Pinson, D. M., Powers, M. F., Wong, S. W., and Stephens, E. B. (2005). Scrambling of the amino acids within the transmembrane domain of Vpu results in a simian-human immunodeficiency virus (SHIV(TM)) that is less pathogenic for pig-tailed macaques. *Virology* **339**, 56–69.

Hout, D. R., Gomez, L. M., Pacyniak, E., Miller, J. M., Hill, M. S., and Stephens, E. B. (2006a). A single amino acid substitution within the transmembrane domain of the human immunodeficiency virus type 1 Vpu protein renders simian-human immunodeficiency virus (SHIV(KU-1bMC33)) susceptible to rimantadine. *Virology* **348**, 449–461.

Hout, D. R., Gomez, M. L., Pacyniak, E., Gomez, L. M., Fegley, B., Mulcahy, E. R., Hill, M. S., Culley, N., Pinson, D. M., Nothnick, W., Powers, M. F., Wong, S. W., *et al.* (2006b). Substitution of the transmembrane domain of Vpu in simian-human immunodeficiency virus (SHIV(KU1bMC33)) with that of M2 of influenza A results in a virus that is sensitive to inhibitors of the M2 ion channel and is pathogenic for pig-tailed macaques. *Virology* **344**, 541–559.

Hsu, K., Seharaseyon, J., Dong, P., Bour, S., and Marban, E. (2004). Mutual functional destruction of HIV-1 Vpu and host TASK-1 channel. *Mol. Cell.* **14**, 259–267.

Huet, T., Cheynier, R., Meyerhans, A., Roelants, G., and Wain-Hobson, S. (1990). Genetic organization of a chimpanzee lentivirus related to HIV-1. *Nature* **345**, 356–359.

Huvent, I., Hong, S. S., Fournier, C., Gay, B., Tournier, J., Carriere, C., Courcoul, M., Vigne, R., Spire, B., and Boulanger, P. (1998). Interaction and co-encapsidation of human immunodeficiency virus type 1 Gag and Vif recombinant proteins. *J. Gen. Virol.* **79**(Pt. 5), 1069–1081.

Jabbar, M. A., and Nayak, D. P. (1990). Intracellular interaction of human immunodeficiency virus type 1 (ARV-2) envelope glycoprotein gp160 with CD4 blocks the movement and maturation of CD4 to the plasma membrane. *J. Virol.* **64**, 6297–6304.

Kao, S., Akari, H., Khan, M. A., Dettenhofer, M., Yu, X. F., and Strebel, K. (2003). Human immunodeficiency virus type 1 Vif is efficiently packaged into virions during productive but not chronic infection. *J. Virol.* **77**, 1131–1140.

Kao, S., Miyagi, E., Khan, M. A., Takeuchi, H., Opi, S., Goila-Gaur, R., and Strebel, K. (2004). Production of infectious human immunodeficiency virus type 1 does not require depletion of APOBEC3G from virus-producing cells. *Retrovirology* **1**, 27.

Karczewski, M. K., and Strebel, K. (1996). Cytoskeleton association and virion incorporation of the human immunodeficiency virus type 1 Vif protein. *J. Virol.* **70**, 494–507.

Khan, M. A., Aberham, C., Kao, S., Akari, H., Gorelick, R., Bour, S., and Strebel, K. (2001). Human immunodeficiency virus type 1 Vif protein is packaged into the nucleoprotein complex through an interaction with viral genomic RNA. *J. Virol.* **75**, 7252–7265.

Khan, M. A., Kao, S., Miyagi, E., Takeuchi, H., Goila-Gaur, R., Opi, S., Gipson, C. L., Parslow, T. G., Ly, H., and Strebel, K. (2005). Viral RNA is required for the association of APOBEC3G with human immunodeficiency virus type 1 nucleoprotein complexes. *J. Virol.* **79**, 5870–5874.

Kishi, M., Nishino, Y., Sumiya, M., Ohki, K., Kimura, T., Goto, T., Nakai, M., Kakinuma, M., and Ikuta, K. (1992). Cells surviving infection by human immunodeficiency virus type 1: Vif or vpu mutants produce non-infectious or markedly less cytopathic viruses. *J. Gen. Virol.* **73**(Pt. 1), 77–87.

Klimkait, T., Strebel, K., Hoggan, M. D., Martin, M. A., and Orenstein, J. M. (1990). The human immunodeficiency virus type 1-specific protein vpu is required for efficient virus maturation and release. *J. Virol.* **64**, 621–629.

Kochendoerfer, G. G., Jones, D. H., Lee, S., Oblatt-Montal, M., Opella, S. J., and Montal, M. (2004). Functional characterization and NMR spectroscopy on full-length Vpu from HIV-1 prepared by total chemical synthesis. *J. Am. Chem. Soc.* **126**, 2439–2446.

Kondo, E., Mammano, F., Cohen, E. A., and Gottlinger, H. G. (1995). The p6gag domain of human immunodeficiency virus type 1 is sufficient for the incorporation of Vpr into heterologous viral particles. *J. Virol.* **69**, 2759–2764.

Kotler, M., Simm, M., Zhao, Y. S., Sova, P., Chao, W., Ohnona, S. F., Roller, R., Krachmarov, C., Potash, M. J., and Volsky, D. J. (1997). Human immunodeficiency virus Type 1 (HIV-1) protein Vif inhibits the activity of HIV-1 protease in bacteria and *in vitro*. *J. Virol.* **71**, 5774–5781.

Kozak, S. L., Marin, M., Rose, K. M., Bystrom, C., and Kabat, D. (2006). The anti-HIV-1 editing enzyme APOBEC3G binds HIV-1 RNA and messenger RNAs that shuttle between polysomes and stress granules. *J. Biol. Chem.* **281**(39), 29105–29119.

Kukol, A., and Arkin, I. T. (1999). vpu transmembrane peptide structure obtained by site-specific fourier transform infrared dichroism and global molecular dynamics searching. *Biophys. J.* **77**, 1594–1601.

Kusk, P., Lindhardt, B. O., Bugge, T. H., Holmback, K., and Hulgaard, E. F. (1993). Mapping of a new immunodominant human linear B-cell epitope on the vpu protein of the human immunodeficiency virus type 1. *J. Acquir. Immune Defic. Syndr.* **6**, 334–338.

Lavallee, C., Yao, X. J., Ladha, A., Gottlinger, H., Haseltine, W. A., and Cohen, E. A. (1994). Requirement of the Pr55gag precursor for incorporation of the Vpr product into human immunodeficiency virus type 1 viral particles. *J. Virol.* **68**, 1926–1934.

Lemaitre, V., Willbold, D., Watts, A., and Fischer, W. B. (2006). Full length Vpu from HIV-1: Combining molecular dynamics simulations with NMR Spectroscopy. *J. Biomol. Struct. Dyn.* **23**, 485–496.

Li, J. T., Halloran, M., Lord, C. I., Watson, A., Ranchalis, J., Fung, M., Letvin, N. L., and Sodroski, J. G. (1995). Persistent infection of macaques with simian-human immunodeficiency viruses. *J. Virol.* **69**, 7061–7067.

Liddament, M. T., Brown, W. L., Schumacher, A. J., and Harris, R. S. (2004). APOBEC3F properties and hypermutation preferences indicate activity against HIV-1 *in vivo*. *Curr. Biol.* **14**, 1385–1391.

Liu, H., Wu, X., Newman, M., Shaw, G. M., Hahn, B. H., and Kappes, J. C. (1995). The Vif protein of human and simian immunodeficiency viruses is packaged into virions and associates with viral core structures. *J. Virol.* **69**, 7630–7638.

Lu, Y. L., Spearman, P., and Ratner, L. (1993). Human immunodeficiency virus type 1 viral protein R localization in infected cells and virions. *J. Virol.* **67**, 6542–6550.

Lu, Y. L., Bennett, R. P., Wills, J. W., Gorelick, R., and Ratner, L. (1995). A leucine triplet repeat sequence (LXX)4 in p6gag is important for Vpr incorporation into human immunodeficiency virus type 1 particles. *J. Virol.* **69**, 6873–6879.

Luo, K., Xiao, Z., Ehrlich, E., Yu, Y., Liu, B., Zheng, S., and Yu, X. F. (2005). Primate lentiviral virion infectivity factors are substrate receptors that assemble with cullin 5-E3 ligase through a HCCH motif to suppress APOBEC3G. *Proc. Natl. Acad. Sci. USA* **102**, 11444–11449.

Ma, X. Y., Sova, P., Chao, W., and Volsky, D. J. (1994). Cysteine residues in the Vif protein of human immunodeficiency virus type 1 are essential for viral infectivity. *J. Virol.* **68**, 1714–1720.

Mackay, G. A., Niu, Y., Liu, Z. Q., Mukherjee, S., Li, Z., Adany, I., Buch, S., Zhuge, W., McClure, H. M., Narayan, O., and Smith, M. S. (2002). Presence of Intact vpu and nef genes in nonpathogenic SHIV is essential for acquisition of pathogenicity of this virus by serial passage in macaques. *Virology* **295**, 133–146.

Madani, N., and Kabat, D. (1998). An endogenous inhibitor of human immunodeficiency virus in human lymphocytes is overcome by the viral Vif protein. *J. Virol.* **72**, 10251–10255.

Maldarelli, F., Chen, M. Y., Willey, R. L., and Strebel, K. (1993). Human immunodeficiency virus type 1 Vpu protein is an oligomeric type I integral membrane protein. *J. Virol.* **67**, 5056–5061.

Mangeat, B., Turelli, P., Liao, S., and Trono, D. (2004). A single amino acid determinant governs the species-specific sensitivity of APOBEC3G to Vif action. *J. Biol. Chem.* **279**, 14481–14483.

Margottin, F., Bour, S. P., Durand, H., Selig, L., Benichou, S., Richard, V., Thomas, D., Strebel, K., and Benarous, R. (1998). A novel human WD protein, h-beta TrCp, that interacts with HIV-1 Vpu connects CD4 to the ER degradation pathway through an F-box motif. *Mol. Cell.* **1**, 565–574.

Mariani, R., Chen, D., Schrofelbauer, B., Navarro, F., Konig, R., Bollman, B., Munk, C., Nymark-McMahon, H., and Landau, N. R. (2003). Species-specific exclusion of APOBEC3G from HIV-1 virions by Vif. *Cell* **114**, 21–31.

Marin, M., Rose, K. M., Kozak, S. L., and Kabat, D. (2003). HIV-1 Vif protein binds the editing enzyme APOBEC3G and induces its degradation. *Nat. Med.* **9**, 1398–1403.

McCormick-Davis, C., Zhao, L. J., Mukherjee, S., Leung, K., Sheffer, D., Joag, S. V., Narayan, O., and Stephens, E. B. (1998). Chronology of genetic changes in the vpu, env, and nef genes of chimeric simian-human immunodeficiency virus (strain HXB2) during acquisition of virulence for pig-tailed macaques. *Virology* **248**, 275–283.

McCormick-Davis, C., Dalton, S. B., Hout, D. R., Singh, D. K., Berman, N. E., Yong, C., Pinson, D. M., Foresman, L., and Stephens, E. B. (2000). A molecular clone of simian-human immunodeficiency virus (DeltavpuSHIV(KU-1bMC33)) with a truncated, non-membrane-bound vpu results in rapid CD4(+) T cell loss and neuro-AIDS in pig-tailed macaques. *Virology* **272**, 112–126.

Mehle, A., Goncalves, J., Santa-Marta, M., McPike, M., and Gabuzda, D. (2004a). Phosphorylation of a novel SOCS-box regulates assembly of the HIV-1 Vif-Cul5 complex that promotes APOBEC3G degradation. *Genes Dev.* **18**, 2861–2866.

Mehle, A., Strack, B., Ancuta, P., Zhang, C., McPike, M., and Gabuzda, D. (2004b). Vif overcomes the innate antiviral activity of APOBEC3G by promoting its degradation in the ubiquitin-proteasome pathway. *J. Biol. Chem.* **279**, 7792–7798.

Mehle, A., Thomas, E. R., Rajendran, K. S., and Gabuzda, D. (2006). A zinc-binding region in Vif binds Cul5 and determines cullin selection. *J. Biol. Chem.* **281**, 17259–17265.

Meusser, B., and Sommer, T. (2004). Vpu-mediated degradation of CD4 reconstituted in yeast reveals mechanistic differences to cellular ER-associated protein degradation. *Mol. Cell.* **14**, 247–258.

Neer, E. J., Schmidt, C. J., Nambudripad, R., and Smith, T. F. (1994). The ancient regulatory-protein family of WD-repeat proteins. *Nature* **371**, 297–300.

Neil, S. J., Eastman, S. W., Jouvenet, N., and Bieniasz, P. D. (2006). HIV-1 Vpu promotes release and prevents endocytosis of nascent retrovirus particles from the plasma membrane. *PLoS Pathog.* **2**, e39.

Oberste, M. S., and Gonda, M. A. (1992). Conservation of amino-acid sequence motifs in lentivirus Vif proteins. *Virus Genes* **6**, 95–102.

Ochsenbauer, C., Wilk, T., and Bosch, V. (1997). Analysis of vif-defective human immunodeficiency virus type 1 (HIV-1) virions synthesized in 'non-permissive' T lymphoid cells stably infected with selectable HIV-1. *J. Gen. Virol.* **78**(Pt. 3), 627–635.

Ohno, H., Aguilar, R. C., Fournier, M. C., Hennecke, S., Cosson, P., and Bonifacino, J. S. (1997). Interaction of endocytic signals from the HIV-1 envelope glycoprotein complex with members of the adaptor medium chain family. *Virology* **238**, 305–315.

Opella, S. J., Park, S., Lee, S., Jones, D., Nevzorov, A., Meslet, M., Mrse, A., Marassi, F. M., Oblatt-Montal, M., Montal, M., Strebel, K., and Bour, S. (2005). Structure and function of Vpu from HIV-1. *In* "Viral Membrane Proteins: Structure, Function, and Drug Design" (W. Fischer, Ed.), pp. 147–163. Kluwer Academic, New York.

Pahl, H. L. (1999). Activators and target genes of Rel/NF-kappaB transcription factors. *Oncogene* **18**, 6853–6866.

Park, S. H., and Opella, S. J. (2005). Tilt angle of a trans-membrane helix is determined by hydrophobic mismatch. *J. Mol. Biol.* **350**, 310–318.

Park, S. H., Mrse, A. A., Nevzorov, A. A., Mesleh, M. F., Oblatt-Montal, M., Montal, M., and Opella, S. J. (2003). Three-dimensional structure of the channel-forming trans-membrane domain of virus protein "U" (Vpu) from HIV-1. *J. Mol. Biol.* **333**, 409–424.

Paul, I., Cui, J., and Maynard, E. L. (2006). Zinc binding to the HCCH motif of HIV-1 Virion infectivity factor induces a conformational change that mediates protein-protein interactions. *Proc. Natl. Acad. Sci. USA* **103**, 18475–18480.

Paul, M., and Jabbar, M. A. (1997). Phosphorylation of both phosphoacceptor sites in the HIV-1 Vpu cytoplasmic domain is essential for Vpu-mediated ER degradation of CD4. *Virology* **232**, 207–216.

Paul, M., Mazumder, S., Raja, N., and Jabbar, M. A. (1998). Mutational analysis of the human immunodeficiency virus type 1 Vpu transmembrane domain that promotes the enhanced release of virus-like particles from the plasma membrane of mammalian cells. *J. Virol.* **72**, 1270–1279.

Paxton, W., Connor, R. I., and Landau, N. R. (1993). Incorporation of Vpr into human immunodeficiency virus type 1 virions: Requirement for the p6 region of gag and mutational analysis. *J. Virol.* **67**, 7229–7237.

Potash, M. J., Bentsman, G., Muir, T., Krachmarov, C., Sova, P., and Volsky, D. J. (1998). Peptide inhibitors of HIV-1 protease and viral infection of peripheral blood lymphocytes based on HIV-1 Vif. *Proc. Natl. Acad. Sci. USA* **95**, 13865–13868.

Ramiro, A. R., Stavropoulos, P., Jankovic, M., and Nussenzweig, M. C. (2003). Transcription enhances AID-mediated cytidine deamination by exposing single-stranded DNA on the nontemplate strand. *Nat. Immunol.* **4**, 452–456.

Reddy, T. R., Kraus, G., Yamada, O., Looney, D. J., Suhasini, M., and Wong-Staal, F. (1995). Comparative analyses of human immunodeficiency virus type 1 (HIV-1) and HIV-2 Vif mutants. *J. Virol.* **69**, 3549–3553.

Reiss, Y., and Hershko, A. (1990). Affinity purification of ubiquitin-protein ligase on immobilized protein substrates. *J. Biol. Chem.* **265**, 3685–3690.

Ritter, G. D., Yamshchikov, G., Cohen, S. J., and Mulligan, M. J. (1996). Human immunodeficiency virus type 2 glycoprotein enhancement of particle budding: Role of the cytoplasmic domain. *J. Virol.* **70**, 2669–2673.

Sakai, H., Shibata, R., Sakuragi, J., Sakuragi, S., Kawamura, M., and Adachi, A. (1993). Cell-dependent requirement of human immunodeficiency virus type 1 Vif protein for maturation of virus particles. *J. Virol.* **67**, 1663–1666.

Santa-Marta, M., da Silva, F. A., Fonseca, A. M., and Goncalves, J. (2005). HIV-1 Vif can directly inhibit apolipoprotein B mRNA-editing enzyme catalytic polypeptide-like 3G-mediated cytidine deamination by using a single amino acid interaction and without protein degradation. *J. Biol. Chem.* **280**, 8765–8775.

Santa-Marta, M., Aires da Silva, F., Fonseca, A. M., Rato, S., and Goncalves, J. (2007). HIV-1 Vif protein blocks the cytidine deaminase activity of B-cell specific AID in *E. coli* by a similar mechanism of action. *Mol. Immunol.* **44**, 583–590.

Schatz, O., Oft, M., Dascher, C., Schebesta, M., Rosorius, O., Jaksche, H., Dobrovnik, M., Bevec, D., and Hauber, J. (1998). Interaction of the HIV-1 rev cofactor eukaryotic initiation factor 5A with ribosomal protein L5. *Proc. Natl. Acad. Sci. USA* **95**, 1607–1612.

Schneider, J., Lüke, W., Kirchhoff, F., Jung, R., Jurkewicz, E., Stahl-Henning, C., Nick, S., Klemm, E., Jentsch, K. D., and Hunsmann, G. (1990a). Isolation and characterization of HIV-2ben obtained from a patient with predominantly neurological defects. *Aids* **4**, 455–457.

Schneider, T., Hildebrandt, P., Rönspeck, W., Weigelt, W., and Pauli, G. (1990b). The antibody response to the HIV-1 specific "out" (vpu) protein: Identification of an immunodominant epitope and correlation of antibody detectability to clinical stages. *AIDS Res. Hum. Retrovir.* **6**, 943–950.

Schrofelbauer, B., Chen, D., and Landau, N. R. (2004). A single amino acid of APOBEC3G controls its species-specific interaction with virion infectivity factor (Vif). *Proc. Natl. Acad. Sci. USA* **101**, 3927–3932.

Schrofelbauer, B., Senger, T., Manning, G., and Landau, N. R. (2006). Mutational alteration of human immunodeficiency virus type 1 Vif allows for functional interaction with nonhuman primate APOBEC3G. *J. Virol.* **80**, 5984–5991.

Schubert, U., and Strebel, K. (1994). Differential activities of the human immunodeficiency virus type 1-encoded Vpu protein are regulated by phosphorylation and occur in different cellular compartments. *J. Virol.* **68**, 2260–2271.

Schubert, U., Henklein, P., Boldyreff, B., Wingender, E., Strebel, K., and Porstmann, T. (1994). The human immunodeficiency virus type 1 encoded Vpu protein is phosphorylated by casein kinase-2 (CK-2) at positions Ser52 and Ser56 within a predicted alpha-helix-turn-alpha-helix-motif. *J. Mol. Biol.* **236**, 16–25.

Schubert, U., Bour, S., Ferrer-Montiel, A. V., Montal, M., Maldarell, F., and Strebel, K. (1996a). The two biological activities of human immunodeficiency virus type 1 Vpu protein involve two separable structural domains. *J. Virol.* **70**, 809–819.

Schubert, U., Ferrer-Montiel, A. V., Oblatt-Montal, M., Henklein, P., Strebel, K., and Montal, M. (1996b). Identification of an ion channel activity of the Vpu transmembrane domain and its involvement in the regulation of virus release from HIV-1-infected cells. *FEBS Lett.* **398**, 12–18.

Schubert, U., Anton, L. C., Bacik, I., Cox, J. H., Bour, S., Bennink, J. R., Orlowski, M., Strebel, K., and Yewdell, J. W. (1998). CD4 glycoprotein degradation induced by human immunodeficiency virus type 1 Vpu protein requires the function of proteasomes and the ubiquitin-conjugating pathway. *J. Virol.* **72**, 2280–2288.

Schubert, U., Bour, S., Willey, R. L., and Strebel, K. (1999). Regulation of virus release by the macrophage-tropic human immunodeficiency virus type 1 AD8 isolate is redundant and can be controlled by either Vpu or Env. *J. Virol.* **73**, 887–896.

Schwartz, S., Felber, B. K., Fenyö, E. M., and Pavlakis, G. N. (1990). Env and vpu proteins of human immunodeficiency virus type-1 are produced from multiple bicistronic mRNAs. *J. Virol.* **64**, 5448–5456.

Schwartz, S., Felber, B. K., and Pavlakis, G. N. (1991). Expression of human immunodeficiency virus type 1 vif and vpr mRNAs is Rev-dependent and regulated by splicing. *Virology* **183**, 677–686.

Selig, L., Pages, J. C., Tanchou, V., Preveral, S., Berlioz-Torrent, C., Liu, L. X., Erdtmann, L., Darlix, J., Benarous, R., and Benichou, S. (1999). Interaction with the p6 domain of the gag precursor mediates incorporation into virions of Vpr and Vpx proteins from primate lentiviruses. *J. Virol.* **73**, 592–600.

Sharpe, S., Yau, W. M., and Tycko, R. (2006). Structure and dynamics of the HIV-1 Vpu transmembrane domain revealed by solid-state NMR with magic-angle spinning. *Biochemistry* **45**, 918–933.

Sheehy, A. M., Gaddis, N. C., Choi, J. D., and Malim, M. H. (2002). Isolation of a human gene that inhibits HIV-1 infection and is suppressed by the viral Vif protein. *Nature* **418**, 646–650.

Sheehy, A. M., Gaddis, N. C., and Malim, M. H. (2003). The antiretroviral enzyme APOBEC3G is degraded by the proteasome in response to HIV-1 Vif. *Nat. Med.* **9**, 1404–1407.

Simm, M., Shahabuddin, M., Chao, W., Allan, J. S., and Volsky, D. J. (1995). Aberrant Gag protein composition of a human immunodeficiency virus type 1 vif mutant produced in primary lymphocytes. *J. Virol.* **69**, 4582–4586.

Simon, J. H., Southerling, T. E., Peterson, J. C., Meyer, B. E., and Malim, M. H. (1995). Complementation of vif-defective human immunodeficiency virus type 1 by primate, but not nonprimate, lentivirus vif genes. *J. Virol.* **69**, 4166–4172.

Simon, J. H., Fouchier, R. A., Southerling, T. E., Guerra, C. B., Grant, C. K., and Malim, M. H. (1997). The Vif and Gag proteins of human immunodeficiency virus type 1 colocalize in infected human T cells. *J. Virol.* **71**, 5259–5267.

Simon, J. H., Gaddis, N. C., Fouchier, R. A., and Malim, M. H. (1998a). Evidence for a newly discovered cellular anti-HIV-1 phenotype. *Nat. Med.* **4**, 1397–1400.

Simon, J. H., Miller, D. L., Fouchier, R. A., and Malim, M. H. (1998b). Virion incorporation of human immunodeficiency virus type-1 Vif is determined by intracellular expression level and may not be necessary for function. *Virology* **248**, 182–187.

Simon, J. H., Miller, D. L., Fouchier, R. A., Soares, M. A., Peden, K. W., and Malim, M. H. (1998c). The regulation of primate immunodeficiency virus infectivity by Vif is cell species restricted: A role for Vif in determining virus host range and cross-species transmission. *EMBO J.* **17**, 1259–1267.

Simon, J. H., Sheehy, A. M., Carpenter, E. A., Fouchier, R. A., and Malim, M. H. (1999). Mutational analysis of the human immunodeficiency virus type 1 Vif protein. *J. Virol.* **73**, 2675–2681.

Singh, D. K., Griffin, D. M., Pacyniak, E., Jackson, M., Werle, M. J., Wisdom, B., Sun, F., Hout, D. R., Pinson, D. M., Gunderson, R. S., Powers, M. F., Wong, S. W., *et al.* (2003). The presence of the casein kinase II phosphorylation sites of Vpu enhances the CD4(+) T cell loss caused by the simian-human immunodeficiency virus SHIV(KU-lbMC33) in pig-tailed macaques. *Virology* **313**, 435–451.

Skowyra, D., Koepp, D. M., Kamura, T., Conrad, M. N., Conaway, R. C., Conaway, J. W., Elledge, S. J., and Harper, J. W. (1999). Reconstitution of G1 cyclin ubiquitination with complexes containing SCFGrr1 and Rbx1. *Science* **284**, 662–665.

Sova, P., and Volsky, D. J. (1993). Efficiency of viral DNA synthesis during infection of permissive and nonpermissive cells with vif-negative human immunodeficiency virus type 1. *J. Virol.* **67**, 6322–6326.

Sova, P., Chao, W., and Volsky, D. J. (1997). The redox state of cysteines in human immunodeficiency virus type 1 Vif in infected cells and in virions. *Biochem. Biophys. Res. Commun.* **240**, 257–260.

Spencer, E., Jiang, J., and Chen, Z. J. (1999). Signal-induced ubiquitination of IkappaBalpha by the F-box protein Slimb/beta-TrCP. *Genes Dev.* **13**, 284–294.

Spevak, W., Keiper, B. D., Stratowa, C., and Castanon, M. J. (1993). *Saccharomyces cerevisiae* cdc15 mutants arrested at a late stage in anaphase are rescued by xenopus cDNAs encoding N-ras or a protein with beta-transducin repeats. *Mol. Cell. Biol.* **13**, 4953–4966.

Stephens, E. B., Mukherjee, S., Sahni, M., Zhuge, W., Raghavan, R., Singh, D. K., Leung, K., Atkinson, B., Li, Z., Joag, S. V., Liu, Z. Q., and Narayan, O. (1997). A cell-free stock of simian-human immunodeficiency virus that causes AIDS in pig-tailed macaques has a limited number of amino acid substitutions in both SIVmac and HIV-1 regions of the genome and has offered cytotropism. *Virology* **231**, 313–321.

Stephens, E. B., McCormick, C., Pacyniak, E., Griffin, D., Pinson, D. M., Sun, F., Nothnick, W., Wong, S. W., Gunderson, R., Berman, N. E., and Singh, D. K. (2002). Deletion of the vpu sequences prior to the env in a Simian–Human immunodeficiency virus results in enhanced env precursor synthesis but is less pathogenic for pig-tailed macaques. *Virology* **293**, 252–261.

Stopak, K., de Noronha, C., Yonemoto, W., and Greene, W. C. (2003). HIV-1 Vif blocks the antiviral activity of APOBEC3G by impairing both its translation and intracellular stability. *Mol. Cell.* **12**, 591–601.

Strebel, K., Daugherty, D., Clouse, K., Cohen, D., Folks, T., and Martin, M. A. (1987). The HIV 'A' (sor) gene product is essential for virus infectivity. *Nature* **328**, 728–730.

Strebel, K., Klimkait, T., and Martin, M. A. (1988). A novel gene of HIV-1, vpu, and its 16-kilodalton product. *Science* **241**, 1221–1223.

Strebel, K., Klimkait, T., Maldarelli, F., and Martin, M. A. (1989). Molecular and biochemical analyses of human immunodeficiency virus type 1 vpu protein. *J. Virol.* **63**, 3784–3791.

Terwilliger, E. F., Cohen, E. A., Lu, Y., Sodroski, J. G., and Haseltine, W. A. (1989). Functional role of human immunodeficiency virus type 1 vpu. *Proc. Natl. Acad. Sci. USA* **86**, 5163–5167.

Varthakavi, V., Smith, R. M., Bour, S. P., Strebel, K., and Spearman, P. (2003). Viral protein U counteracts a human host cell restriction that inhibits HIV-1 particle production. *Proc. Natl. Acad. Sci. USA* **100**, 15154–15159.

Varthakavi, V., Smith, R. M., Martin, K. L., Derdowski, A., Lapierre, L. A., Goldenring, J. R., and Spearman, P. (2006). The pericentriolar recycling endosome plays a key role in Vpu-mediated enhancement of HIV-1 particle release. *Traffic* **7**, 298–307.

von Schwedler, U., Song, J., Aiken, C., and Trono, D. (Schwedler 1993). Vif is crucial for human immunodeficiency virus type 1 proviral DNA synthesis in infected cells. *J. Virol.* **67**, 4945–4955.

Wiegand, H. L., Doehle, B. P., Bogerd, H. P., and Cullen, B. R. (2004). A second human antiretroviral factor, APOBEC3F, is suppressed by the HIV-1 and HIV-2 Vif proteins. *EMBO J.* **23**, 2451–2458.

Wiertz, E. J., Jones, T. R., Sun, L., Bogyo, M., Geuze, H. J., and Ploegh, H. L. (1996). The human cytomegalovirus US11 gene product dislocates MHC class I heavy chains from the endoplasmic reticulum to the cytosol. *Cell* **84**, 769–779.

Willbold, D., Hoffmann, S., and Roesch, P. (1997). Secondary structure and tertiary fold of the human immunodeficiency virus protein U (Vpu) cytoplasmic domain in solution. *Eur. J. Biochem.* **245**, 581–588.

Willey, R. L., Maldarelli, F., Martin, M. A., and Strebel, K. (1992a). Human immunodeficiency virus type 1 Vpu protein regulates the formation of intracellular gp160-CD4 complexes. *J. Virol.* **66**, 226–234.

Willey, R. L., Maldarelli, F., Martin, M. A., and Strebel, K. (1992b). Human immunodeficiency virus type 1 Vpu protein induces rapid degradation of CD4. *J. Virol.* **66**, 7193–7200.

Winston, J. T., Strack, P., Beer-Romero, P., Chu, C. Y., Elledge, S. J., and Harper, J. W. (1999). The SCFbeta-TRCP-ubiquitin ligase complex associates specifically with phosphorylated destruction motifs in IkappaBalpha and beta-catenin and stimulates IkappaBalpha ubiquitination *in vitro*. *Genes Dev.* **13**, 270–283.

Wray, V., Federau, T., Henklein, P., Klabunde, S., Kunert, O., Schomburg, D., and Schubert, U. (1995). Solution structure of the hydrophilic region of HIV-1 encoded virus protein U (Vpu) by CD and 1H NMR spectroscopy. *Int. J. Peptide Protein Res.* **45**, 35–43.

Xiao, Z., Ehrlich, E., Yu, Y., Luo, K., Wang, T., Tian, C., and Yu, X. F. (2006). Assembly of HIV-1 Vif-Cul5 E3 ubiquitin ligase through a novel zinc-binding domain-stabilized hydrophobic interface in Vif. *Virology* **349**, 290–299.

Xu, H., Svarovskaia, E. S., Barr, R., Zhang, Y., Khan, M. A., Strebel, K., and Pathak, V. K. (2004). A single amino acid substitution in human APOBEC3G antiretroviral enzyme confers resistance to HIV-1 virion infectivity factor-induced depletion. *Proc. Natl. Acad. Sci. USA* **101**, 5652–5657.

Yang, S., Sun, Y., and Zhang, H. (2001). The multimerization of human immunodeficiency virus type I Vif protein: A requirement for Vif function in the viral life cycle. *J. Biol. Chem.* **276**, 4889–4893.

Yang, X., and Gabuzda, D. (1998). Mitogen-activated protein kinase phosphorylates and regulates the HIV-1 Vif protein. *J. Biol. Chem.* **273**, 29879–29887.

Yang, X., Goncalves, J., and Gabuzda, D. (1996). Phosphorylation of Vif and its role in HIV-1 replication. *J. Biol. Chem.* **271**, 10121–10129.

Yao, X. J. Y., Goettlinger, H., Haseltine, W. A., and Cohen, E. A. (1992). Envelope glycoprotein and CD4 independence of Vpu-facilitated human immunodeficiency virus type 1 capsid export. *J. Virol.* **66**, 5119–5126.

Yaron, A., Hatzubai, A., Davis, M., Lavon, I., Amit, S., Manning, A. M., Andersen, J. S., Mann, M., Mercurio, F., and Ben-Neriah, Y. (1998). Identification of the receptor component of the IkappaBalpha-ubiquitin ligase. *Nature* **396**, 590–594.

Yu, X., Yu, Y., Liu, B., Luo, K., Kong, W., Mao, P., and Yu, X. F. (2003). Induction of APOBEC3G ubiquitination and degradation by an HIV-1 Vif-Cul5-SCF complex. *Science* **302**, 1056–1060.

Yu, Y., Xiao, Z., Ehrlich, E. S., Yu, X., and Yu, X. F. (2004). Selective assembly of HIV-1 Vif-Cul5-ElonginB-ElonginC E3 ubiquitin ligase complex through a novel SOCS box and upstream cysteines. *Genes Dev.* **18**, 2867–2872.

Yusim, K., Kesmir, C., Gaschen, B., Addo, M. M., Altfeld, M., Brunak, S., Chigaev, A., Detours, V., and Korber, B. T. (2002). Clustering patterns of cytotoxic T-lymphocyte epitopes in human immunodeficiency virus type 1 (HIV-1) proteins reveal imprints of immune evasion on HIV-1 global variation. *J. Virol.* **76**, 8757–8768.

Zhang, H., Pomerantz, R. J., Dornadula, G., and Sun, Y. (2000). Human immunodeficiency virus type 1 vif protein is an integral component of an mRNP complex of viral RNA and could be involved in the viral RNA folding and packaging process. *J. Virol.* **74**, 8252–8261.

Zheng, S., Strzalka, J., Jones, D. H., Opella, S. J., and Blasie, J. K. (2003). Comparative structural studies of Vpu peptides in phospholipid monolayers by X-ray scattering. *Biophys. J.* **84**, 2393–2415.

Richard Y. Zhao[*,†,‡],
Robert T. Elder[‡], and Michael Bukrinsky[§]

[*]Department of Pathology, University of Maryland School of Medicine
Baltimore, Maryland 21201

[†]Department of Microbiology-Immunology, University of Maryland School of Medicine
Baltimore, Maryland 21201

[‡]Department of Pediatrics and Children's Memorial Research Center, Northwestern
University Feinberg School of Medicine, Chicago, Illinois 60614

[§]Department of Microbiology, Immunology, and Tropical Medicine, The George
Washington University, Washington, District of Columbia 20037

Interactions of HIV-1 Viral Protein R with Host Cell Proteins

I. Chapter Overview

Active host–pathogen interactions take place during *human immuno-deficiency virus type 1* (HIV-1) infection of host cells. HIV-infected cells respond to viral invasion with various antiviral strategies, such as innate, cellular, and humoral immune antiviral defense mechanisms, and the virus has developed tactics to suppress these host responses to infection. The final balance between these interactions determines the efficiency of the viral infection and subsequent disease progression. In this chapter, we will review the virus-host interactions taking place with the HIV viral protein R (Vpr). Recent findings suggest that Vpr interacts with some of the host innate

Advances in Pharmacology, Volume 55
1054-3589/07 $35.00
DOI: 10.1016/S1054-3589(07)55007-6

antiviral responses, such as heat stress responses, and plays an active role as a viral pathogenic factor; cellular heat stress response factors counteract such Vpr activities as nuclear import, induction of cell cycle G2/M arrest, and apoptosis of the host cells, and also inhibit HIV replication. Other Vpr-interacting proteins and their potential roles in HIV replication, as well as strategies for the development of future antiviral therapies directed at suppressing Vpr activities, are also discussed.

II. Introduction

On infection by HIV-1, host reacts with various innate, cellular, and humoral immune responses to counteract the viral invasion. Limited and transient restriction of viral infection is normally achieved. However, HIV ultimately overcomes these antiviral responses resulting in successful viral replication. Expression of several HIV-1 regulatory and accessory genes such as *tat, nef, vif,* and *vpu* is known to regulate some of these immune responses to maximize viral replication. For example, Nef suppresses adaptive antiviral immunity by downregulating several cellular molecules critical for antigen presentation and interaction between the immune cells such as class I MHC, CD28, and CD4 (reviewed in Wei *et al.*, 2003). Another HIV protein, Tat, was shown to abrogate one of innate immunity mechanisms working at the cellular level, the cell's RNA-silencing defense (Bennasser *et al.*, 2005). The innate antiviral responses operating at the cellular level, also called intrinsic immunity, are targeted by several other HIV-1 accessory proteins, including Vif, which inactivates a cellular deaminase APOBEC3G that affects HIV reverse transcription (Bishop *et al.*, 2006), and Vpu, which inactivates acid-sensitive K^+ channel TASK-1 whose expression inhibits HIV virus release from infected cells (Hsu *et al.*, 2004).

HIV-1 Vpr is a virion-associated accessory protein with an average length of 96 amino acids and a calculated molecular weight of 12.7 kDa. Vpr is highly conserved among HIV, simian immunodeficiency viruses (SIV), and other lentiviruses (Tristem *et al.*, 1992, 1998). Besides lentiviruses, the Vpr protein sequence shares no strong homology with any other known protein. A tertiary structure of Vpr proposed on the basis of NMR analysis consists of an α-helix-turn-α-helix domain in the N-terminal half from amino acids 17 to 46 and a long α-helix from amino acids 53 to 78 in the C-terminal half (Schuler *et al.*, 1999; Wecker and Roques, 1999). These three α-helices are folded around a hydrophobic core in a structure which allows interaction of Vpr with different cellular proteins (Morellet *et al.*, 2003). These interactions underlie the role of Vpr as a pathogenic factor.

Vpr displays several distinct activities in host cells. These include cytoplasmic-nuclear shuttling (Heinzinger *et al.*, 1994), induction of cell cycle G2 arrest (He *et al.*, 1995), and cell killing (Stewart *et al.*, 1997).

These three Vpr-specific activities were shown to be functionally independent of each other (Chen *et al.*, 1999; Elder *et al.*, 2000; Subbramanian *et al.*, 1998; Vodicka *et al.*, 1998) and have been demonstrated in a wide variety of eukaryotic cells ranging from yeast to humans, indicating that Vpr most likely affects highly conserved cellular processes.

In this chapter, we describe our current understanding of the host–Vpr interactions and the potential roles of Vpr activities in viral pathogenesis.

III. Effects of HIV-1 Vpr on Host Cellular Activities _____

A. Induction of Cell Cycle G2/M Arrest

To ensure accurate transmission of the genetic information, eukaryotic cells have developed an elaborate network of checkpoints to monitor the successful completion of every cell cycle step and to respond to certain abnormalities, such as DNA damage or replication inhibition, as they arise during cell proliferation. Two of the best-characterized G2/M checkpoints, DNA damage and DNA replication (for reviews, see Boddy *et al.*, 1998; Caspari and Carr, 1999; Elledge, 1996; Rhind and Russell, 1998a), were first characterized in detail by genetic analysis in fission yeast (Fig. 1A). The G2 to M transition is controlled in fission yeast by the phosphorylation status of Tyr15 on Cdc2, the cyclin-dependent kinase which regulates the cell cycle in all eukaryotic cells (Morgan, 1995). Tyr15 is phosphorylated by the Wee1 and Mik1 kinases to hold the cell in G2, and rapid dephosphorylation by the Cdc25 phosphatase triggers the G2 to M transition (Gould and Nurse, 1989; Krek and Nigg, 1991; Morgan, 1995; Norbury *et al.*, 1991).

The DNA damage checkpoint is activated by ionizing radiation or ultraviolet light, and activation of this checkpoint leads to inhibitory phosphorylation of Cdc2 at Tyr15 by a multistep pathway (Nurse, 1997; Rhind and Russell, 1998b). The early genes in the pathway, which include Rad1, Rad3, Rad9, Rad17, Rad26, and Hus1, are thought to sense the DNA damage and lead to phosphorylation of the Chk1 protein by the activated Rad3 kinase (Walworth and Bernards, 1996). For example, in response to double strand DNA breaks induced by ionizing radiation, Rad17 acts as a checkpoint-specific loading factor (CCL), which responds to the DNA damage by loading a 9-1-1 protein complex onto the sites where DNA is damaged (Burtelow *et al.*, 2001; Carr, 2002). The 9-1-1 protein complex, also known as the checkpoint clamp complex (CCC), is composed of Rad1, Rad9, and Hus1 (Carr, 2002). The Rad3-Rad26 protein complex also binds to sites of DNA damage independently of the 9-1-1 protein complex. The independent binding of these two protein complexes to DNA damage, which is believed to protect the cell against inappropriate checkpoint activation, initiates the DNA structure checkpoint (Carr, 2002; Caspari and Carr, 1999, 2002).

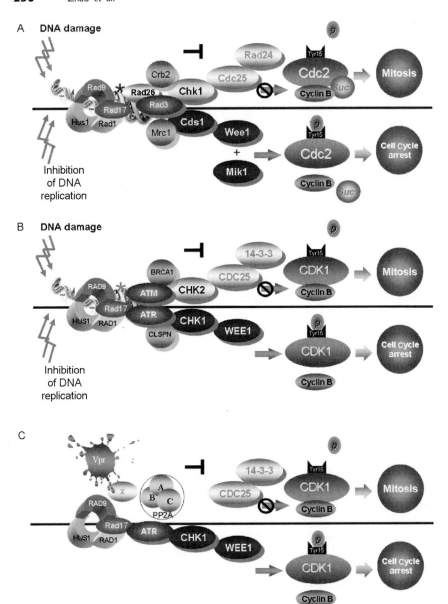

FIGURE 1 Comparison of cell cycle arrest induced by cellular DNA damage and DNA replication checkpoints with that induced by HIV-1 Vpr. The figure denotes cell cycle G2/M regulation in fission yeast (*Schizosaccharomyces pombe*) (A), in mammalian cells (B), and putative regulation by HIV-1 Vpr (C). Asterisks on the double-stranded DNA in (A) and (B) represent DNA damage or modification. The X in (C) indicates that Vpr may bind to another protein(s) before the resulting complex binds to and regulates the PP2A holoenzyme. →, activation; ⊣, inhibition.

Activation of Chk1, a downstream kinase activated by Rad3, is mediated by an adaptor protein Crb2, which bridges Rad3-Rad26 and Chk1 (Du et al., 2003; Esashi et al., 2000; Francesconi et al., 2002; Saka et al., 1997). The activated Chk1 kinase then directly phosphorylates the Cdc25 phosphatase (Furnari et al., 1997). The phosphorylated Cdc25 binds Rad24/Rad25 protein, and this complex is transported out of the nucleus to render Cdc25 inactive (Lopez-Girona et al., 1999). The activated Chk1 also regulates the Mik1 kinase to inhibit Cdc2 (Baber-Furnari et al., 2000). DNA damage thus initiates a Chk1-mediated protein phosphorylation cascade ending in the inactivation of Cdc25 phosphorylase and activation of Mik1 kinase to increase inhibitory phosphorylation of Tyr15 on Cdc2 (Fig. 1A).

The DNA replication checkpoint is activated by treatment with hydroxyurea, which inhibits DNA replication, and this checkpoint also controls the G2 to M transition through inhibitory phosphorylation of Cdc2 (Rhind and Russell, 1998b). Parts of this DNA replication checkpoint are shared with the DNA damage checkpoint as Rad1, Rad3, Rad9, Rad17, Rad26, and Hus1 are required for both checkpoints in fission yeast (al-Khodairy and Carr, 1992). The same 9-1-1 and Rad3-Rad26 checkpoint protein complexes may associate with the DNA replication complex (Carr, 2002). However, the DNA replication checkpoint acts primarily through phosphorylation of Cds1 kinase, which is mediated by another protein Mrc1 (Alcasabas et al., 2001; Tanaka and Russell, 2001; Zhao and Russell, 2004). Mrc1 is a replication checkpoint adaptor protein that allows the sensor kinase Rad3-Rad26 to activate the effector kinase Cds1. There is a minor contribution from the Chk1 kinase, and either kinase is sufficient by itself to accomplish the cell cycle arrest when DNA synthesis is inhibited (Zeng et al., 1998). Activated Cds1 kinase inactivates Cdc25 through the same mechanism as Chk1 and may also activate the Wee1 and Mik1 kinases, which phosphorylate Tyr15 of Cdc2 (Boddy et al., 1998; Zeng et al., 1998).

The cell cycle G2/M control mechanisms, which were initially defined in fission yeast, are highly conserved, and most of the genes required for the checkpoints have human homologues (Table I). In general, these homologues have similar, although not always identical, roles in the control of the human cell cycle (Fig. 1B). One example of a similar but not identical role is the Chk1 protein in fission yeast which is the effector kinase for the DNA damage checkpoint while Chk1 in human cells is the effector kinase for the DNA replication checkpoint (Carr, 2002). In a second example, Claspin (CLSPN) is a homologue of Mrc1, a checkpoint protein required for the DNA replication checkpoint in yeast (Lin et al., 2004). However, Claspin is required for cellular checkpoint responses to both DNA damage, such as by UV or ionizing radiation, and inhibition of DNA replication by hydroxyurea. On DNA damage or replication stress, ATR activates Claspin by phosphorylation, which in turn recruits and phosphorylates BRCA1.

TABLE I   Human and Fission Yeast Equivalent Proteins That Are Involved in Cell Cycle G2/M Regulation and Vpr Interactions

Fission yeast	Human	Putative activity	References[a]
Mitotic regulators			
Cdc2	CDK1	Cyclin B-dependent kinase	(Lee and Nurse, 1987)
Cdc13	Cyclin B	B-type cyclin	(Ozon, 1991)
Wee1	WEE1	Mitotic inhibitor kinase	(Igarashi *et al.*, 1991)
Mik1	---	Mitotic inhibitor kinase	
Cdc25	CDC25A/B/C	Mitotic-promoting phosphatase	(Sadhu *et al.*, 1990) (Nagata *et al.*, 1991)
Suc1	---	Cdc2 regulatory subunit	
DNA damage and replication checkpoints			
Rad1	RAD1	Part of 9-1-1 complex	(Marathi *et al.*, 1998)
Rad3	ATM/ATR	Protein kinase	(Bentley *et al.*, 1996)
Rad9	RAD9	Part of 9-1-1 complex	(Lieberman *et al.*, 1996)
Rad17	RAD17	RFC-related protein	(Parker *et al.*, 1998)
Rad24/25	14-3-3	Binds to phosphorylated Ser	(Ford *et al.*, 1994)
Rad26	ATRIP	ATR regulatory subunit	(McGowan and Russell, 2004)
Hus1	HUS1	Part of 9-1-1 complex	(Volkmer and Karnitz, 1999)
Chk1	CHK1	Serine/threonine kinase	(Furnari *et al.*, 1997)
Cds1	CHK2	Serine/threonine kinase	(Matsuoka *et al.*, 1998)
Crb2	BRCA1	Adaptor protein linking Rad3-Rad26 and Chk1	(Du *et al.*, 2003)
Mrc1	CLSPN	Adaptor protein linking Rad3-Rad26 and Cds1	(Zhao and Russell, 2004)
Cellular proteins involved in Vpr-induced G2 arrest			
PP2A	PP2A	Protein phosphatase 2A	(Kinoshita *et al.*, 1990)
Paa1	A	A regulatory subunit	
Pab1	B	B regulatory subunit	
Ppa2	C	Major C catalytic subunit	
Ppa1	C	Minor C catalytic subunit	
Wos2	P23	Wee1 inhibitor	(Munoz *et al.*, 1999)
Sum1	TRIP-1	Cdc25 inhibitor	(Humphrey and Enoch, 1998)
Vpr-binding proteins			
Rhp23	HHR23A/B	Excision DNA repair enzyme	(Elder *et al.*, 2002)
Ung1	UNG1/2	Uracil-N-glycosylase	(Elder *et al.*, 2003)

[a]Only references that report mammalian homologues are listed.
Note: "---," not found; RFC, replication factor C.

Claspin and BRCA1 work in concert to activate CHK1 for initiation of cell cycle arrest. Thus, activation of Claspin is a clear indication of checkpoint activation. There is also a tendency for multiple, partially redundant checkpoints in human cells compared to simpler checkpoints in yeast, probably reflecting the more complex requirements for cell cycle control in multicellular eukaryotes. For example, the single *rad3* gene in fission yeast is required for both the DNA damage and replication checkpoints and activation of the *chk1* and *cds1* checkpoint kinases (Carr, 2002; Caspari and Carr, 1999, 2002). In human cells, there are two homologues of *rad3*, *ATM* and *ATR*. The primary role of *ATM* is in the DNA damage checkpoint initiated by double strand breaks and activation of *CHK2*, the human homologue of *cds1*, whereas the primary role of the essential *ATR* gene is in the DNA replication checkpoint or responses to many forms of DNA damage and activation of *CHK1* (Abraham, 2001; Shiloh, 2001). Similarly, there is only one tyrosine phosphatase Cdc25 that dephosphorylates Cdc2 in fission yeast, whereas in human cells, there are three CDC25 homologues, CDC25A, CDC25B, and CDC25C, and each of them can be phosphorylated by CHK1 (Sanchez *et al.*, 1997). All three of these phosphatases have been shown to be involved in the control of the G2 to M transition, although their specific roles in this process have not yet been well characterized (Cans *et al.*, 1999; Lammer *et al.*, 1998; Mils *et al.*, 2000). The conservation of checkpoints even extends to the regulatory mechanisms, as illustrated by the negative regulation of CDC25 by relocation to the cytoplasm from the nucleus in both fission yeast and human cells. This relocation in both organisms is dependent on 14-3-3 proteins (Graves *et al.*, 2001; Lopez-Girona *et al.*, 1999).

The HIV-1 Vpr protein induces cell cycle G2 arrest through inhibitory phosphorylation of Cdc2 in both fission yeast and human cells, suggesting that Vpr affects a conserved cellular process (Fig. 1C). Specifically, Vpr induces hyperphosphorylation of fission yeast Cdc2 or human CDK1, the human homologue of Cdc2 (He *et al.*, 1995; Re *et al.*, 1995; Zhao *et al.*, 1996). It exerts its inhibitory effect through T14 and Y15 of CDK1 and Y15 of Cdc2, as expression of nonphosphorylated mutants, T14A Y15F of CDK1 or Y15F of Cdc2 prevents Vpr-induced G2 arrest (Elder *et al.*, 2000; He *et al.*, 1995). Furthermore, Vpr inhibits the Cdc25 phosphatase (Bartz *et al.*, 1996; Elder *et al.*, 2001) and activates Wee1 kinase (Elder *et al.*, 2001; Yuan *et al.*, 2004) to promote phosphorylation of Cdc2/CDK1 during induction of G2 arrest. Consistent with the roles of Wee1 and Cdc25 in Vpr-induced G2 arrest, proteins that are involved in regulation of Cdc25 or Wee1 have also been identified to either enhance or inhibit Vpr-induced G2 arrest. Fission yeast Wos2, which is a human p23 homologue and a Wee1 inhibitor (Munoz *et al.*, 1999), has been shown to be a multicopy Vpr suppressor (Elder *et al.*, 2001; Matsuda *et al.*, 2006). A Cdc25 inhibitor *rad25* (Lopez-Girona *et al.*, 1999), which is the human 14-3-3 homologue, enhances Vpr-induced G2 arrest when overproduced in fission yeast (Elder *et al.*, 2001). Recent studies demonstrated that Vpr binds to Cdc25C and 14-3-3 in human cells (Goh *et al.*, 2004; Kino and Pavlakis, 2004), providing a possible mechanistic basis for Vpr's effect on the cell cycle.

Given that the DNA checkpoints and Vpr both induce G2 arrest through inhibitory phosphorylation of Cdc2, Vpr might induce G2 arrest through a checkpoint pathway. This possibility has been evaluated in fission yeast by expressing *vpr* in mutant fission yeast strains defective in early and late steps of the checkpoint pathways. None of the early checkpoint-specific mutants (*rad1, rad3, rad9,* and *rad17*) showed a significant effect on the induction of G2 arrest by Vpr (Elder *et al.*, 2000, 2001; Masuda *et al.*, 2000). Furthermore, mutations in both *chk1* and *cds1*, which are thought to be the last steps specific for the checkpoint (Boddy *et al.*, 1998; Furnari *et al.*, 1997; Zeng *et al.*, 1998), also did not block Vpr-induced G2 arrest (Elder *et al.*, 2001; Masuda *et al.*, 2000). Therefore, Vpr does not appear to use the DNA-damage or DNA-replication checkpoint pathways to induce G2 arrest in fission yeast.

Early data in human cells tended to support the conclusion that Vpr does not induce G2 arrest through the DNA damage checkpoint pathways. Vpr still induced G2 arrest in cells from patients with ataxia telangiectasia (AT) (Bartz *et al.*, 1996). The AT cells are mutant for the ATM gene, which is a human homologue of fission yeast Rad3, and they do not arrest in G2 in response to DNA damage (Bentley *et al.*, 1996; Matsuoka *et al.*, 1998; Savitsky *et al.*, 1995). However, recent reports showed that Vpr activates ATR and CHK1, as well as other steps in this checkpoint pathway dependent on such proteins as Rad17, Hus1, BRCA1, and γ-H2AX (Zhu *et al.*, 2003; Zimmerman *et al.*, 2004). Considering that G2/M DNA checkpoints are highly conserved between mammalian and fission yeast cells (Table I), it is unclear at the moment why, given that activation of human ATR and CHK1 by Vpr is necessary for G2 arrest, deletion of *rad3* (the fission yeast homologue of ATR/ATM) or *chk1/cds1* (homologues of CHK1/CHK2) does not block Vpr-induced G2 arrest in fission yeast (Elder *et al.*, 2000, 2001). One possibility is that, unlike fission yeast Rad3, activation of mammalian ATR might not necessarily be an indication of only the classic checkpoint responses. Rather ATR may also be activated through other cellular stresses. This possibility is certainly supported by our recent observation showing that Vpr-induced cell cycle arrest does not require Claspin (RYZ, Unpublished data), which is typically needed for the checkpoints activation (Chini and Chen, 2003, 2004). Interestingly, Roshal *et al.* (2003) showed that treatment of Vpr-producing mammalian cells with caffeine completely blocked Vpr-induced G2 arrest. Caffeine is part of the methylxanthine family, and, similar to the caffeine effect, another methylxanthine, pentoxifylline (PTX), also inhibited Vpr-induced G2 arrest in mammalian cells (Poon *et al.*, 1998). Similarly, both PTX and caffeine suppress Vpr-induced G2 arrest in fission yeast (Elder *et al.*, 2001; Zhao *et al.*, 1998). Since PTX and caffeine inhibit Vpr-induced G2 arrest in fission yeast where the classic DNA checkpoints apparently play no role, these observations suggest that molecular mechanisms other than the classic DNA checkpoints may be involved in the activation of ATR and regulation of CDC25 and WEE1.

These additional mechanisms might involve protein phosphatase 2A (PP2A). Although this protein phosphatase has no known role in the activation of ATR-dependent checkpoints, it has an important role in Vpr-induced G2 arrest. Okadaic acid, a specific inhibitor of PP2A, was shown to inhibit Vpr-induced G2 arrest both in human (Li *et al.*, 2007; Re *et al.*, 1995) and fission yeast cells (Zhao *et al.*, 1996). Further evidence for an important role of PP2A comes from PP2A mutant strains. PP2A is composed of three subunits, one catalytic (C) and two regulatory (A and B). When *vpr* was expressed in a strain with a deletion for a catalytic subunit (*ppa2*) or a regulatory subunit (*pab1*) of PP2A, Vpr-induced G2 arrest was reduced (Elder *et al.*, 2001; Masuda *et al.*, 2000). Recent siRNA studies have directly shown that PP2A has an essential role in the G2 arrest induced by Vpr in human cells (Li *et al.* 2007). PP2A appears to be a common viral target since other viruses, such as *Simian virus 40* (SV40), *Polyomavirus*, human T lymphotropic retrovirus, and adenovirus, affect the enzymatic activity of at least a subset of PP2A proteins (see review Janssens and Goris, 2001). Even though these viruses are not otherwise related, they all seem to have adapted a similar strategy to affect cellular processes by directly interacting with PP2A. Similar to the Vpr effects, adenoviral E4orf4 (Kornitzer *et al.*, 2001; Roopchand *et al.*, 2001; Shtrichman *et al.*, 1999) and HTLV-1 Tax protein induce cell cycle G2 arrest (Haoudi *et al.*, 2003). These two viral proteins both bind to PP2A and affect its enzymatic activity (Fu *et al.*, 2003; Kornitzer *et al.*, 2001). Interestingly, the effect of E4orf4 on PP2A is independent of cellular checkpoint (O'Shea *et al.*, 2005); similar to Vpr, Tax-induced G2 arrest is reversible by caffeine (Haoudi *et al.*, 2003). Further examinations indicated that Tax binds to CHK2 in Jurkat T cells (Haoudi *et al.*, 2003) but it complexes with CHK1 in other T cells (Park *et al.*, 2004). With regard to Vpr, it is possible that a concerted cellular mechanism interlinks PP2A and ATR/CHK1 in the cellular response to *vpr* gene expression during the induction of G2 arrest (Fig. 1C).

The cellular target to which Vpr binds directly to induce cell cycle arrest has not been clearly defined. A recent report showed that Vpr induces G2 arrest by binding to the CUS1 domain of SAP145 and interfering with the functions of the SAP145 and SAP49 proteins, two subunits of the multimeric splicing factor 3b (Terada and Yasuda, 2006). Depletion of either SAP145 or SAP49 led to cell cycle G2 arrest suggesting that Vpr inhibits the formation of SAP145–SAP49 complex. This finding is interesting as SAP145 has not been implicated in cellular checkpoints previously. The fact that Vpr inhibits SAP145 suggests that the G2 arrest is the result of active and unique action of Vpr rather than a passive activation of cellular checkpoints seen after DNA damage.

Based on our current knowledge about the effect of Vpr on cell cycle G2/M regulation, we propose a new working model for the cell cycle regulation by HIV-1 Vpr (Fig. 1C). This model integrates the classic G2/M checkpoint pathways (Fig. 1B) with a PP2A-dependent pathway for G2/M control by Vpr. We hypothesize that Vpr induces G2 arrest at least in part by stimulating PP2A activity either by direct association with the PP2A enzyme complex or by association with an intermediate protein(s). In addition, it is also possible that there might be a concerted cellular mechanism inter-linking PP2A and ATR/CHK1 in the cellular response to *vpr* gene expression. A protein phosphorylation cascade including PP2A is probably in part responsible for activation of ATR, which in turn activates CHK1 and inhibits CDK1 by Tyr15 phosphorylation. While WEE1 plays the major role in the induction of G2 arrest by Vpr, CDC25 appears to play only a minor role and to be partially inhibited by this proposed regulatory pathway. On the basis of the fact that DNA damage and replication checkpoints are not involved in Vpr-induced G2 arrest in fission yeast and Claspin may not be required for the induction of G2 in mammalian cells, we further propose that Vpr induces G2 arrest through an active and unique mechanism that is distinguishable from the classic cellular checkpoints responses.

B. Nuclear Transport of HIV-1 Preintegration Complex

The ability to replicate in nondividing cells (terminally differentiated macrophages and incompletely activated CD4+ T lymphocytes) is the characteristic feature of HIV-1 which determines to a large extent its high replicative capacity and pathogenesis. To infect nondividing cells, HIV-1 needs to transport its genomic DNA [in the context of the viral preintegration complex (PIC)] from the cytoplasm into the nucleus of a target cell. Vpr is believed to be among the main regulators of HIV-1 nuclear import (Connor *et al.*, 1995; Heinzinger *et al.*, 1994). Interestingly, a small fraction of Vpr is phosphorylated (Muller *et al.*, 2000), and phosphorylation on Ser79 is critical for Vpr activity in HIV nuclear import (Agostini *et al.*, 2002).

Proteins engaged in nuclear transport typically contain a classical nuclear localization sequence (NLS) (Nakielny and Dreyfuss, 1999; Wente, 2000), which is a short region rich in basic amino acids (lysines and arginines) that binds to the adaptor protein importin α. The complex of NLS-importin α then binds to the receptor importin β through the importin β-binding domain (IBB) on importin α. Importin β interacts with components of the nuclear pore complex (NPC) as an essential part of the nuclear translocation process. The NPC is a large structure composed of 50–100 proteins called nucleoporins and containing a central 10-nm aqueous channel through which proteins are actively transported. Directionality of this translocation process is ensured by Ran. A high concentration of Ran-GTP inside the nucleus stimulates binding of Ran-GTP to NLS-importin α–importin β complex and disassembles it to release the protein carrying the NLS into the nucleoplasm. Importin α and importin β are then exported out of the nucleus to be reused in another round of nuclear transport. This model for NLS translocation is partially based on work done in budding yeast, and the high degree of conservation is demonstrated by functional complementation of many budding yeast mutants in nuclear transport proteins by human homologues (Corbett and Silver, 1997).

It is well established that Vpr expressed without other viral proteins localizes predominantly to the nuclear envelope in human, fission yeast, and budding yeast cells (Chen *et al.*, 1999; Lu *et al.*, 1993; Vodicka *et al.*, 1998). Two hypotheses (not necessarily mutually exclusive) for the mode of action of Vpr in HIV-1 nuclear import have been proposed (Fig. 2): (1) Vpr targets the HIV-1 PIC to the nucleus via a distinct, importin-independent pathway (Gallay *et al.*, 1996; Jenkins *et al.*, 1998) or (2) Vpr modifies cellular importin-dependent import machinery (Popov *et al.*, 1998a,b). The first model was based on the observation that in the *in vitro* nuclear import assay Vpr can enter nuclei in the absence of soluble import factors (Jenkins *et al.*, 1998). Consistent with this concept, Vpr was shown to induce dynamic disruptions in the nuclear envelope (de Noronha *et al.*, 2001) which may serve as entry points for isolated Vpr and for the PICs. HIV-1 Vpr has been shown to coprecipitate with fission yeast nucleoporin Nup124p and its human homologue, Nup153, and nuclear import of Vpr was impaired in nup124 null mutant strain (Varadarajan *et al.*, 2005). Vpr also interacts

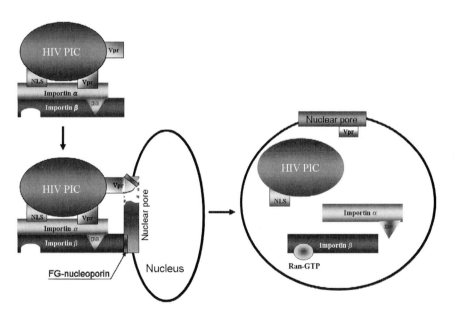

FIGURE 2   Vpr and PIC nuclear import. Proposed mechanisms of Vpr-mediated nuclear import of HIV-1 PIC are denoted. Vpr binds importin α and enhances its interaction with NLS-containing PIC proteins, thus stimulating HIV nuclear import via a classical importin α/β-dependent pathway. Other Vpr molecules in the PIC may directly interact with FG repeat–containing nucleoporins and also cause dynamic disruptions of the nuclear envelope (it is unclear whether nuclear envelope disruption is related to nucleoporin binding), which may serve as entry sites for PIC. Inside the nucleus, the importin complex dissociates after binding of Ran-GTP, thus releasing the PIC. Nucleoporin-bound Vpr likely stays at the nuclear membrane. Details are in the text. Not drawn to scale.

with human nucleoporin CG1, which contributes to Vpr docking to the nuclear envelope (Le Rouzic et al., 2002). Therefore, Vpr may function as a substitute for importin β, which also interacts with nucleoporins to mediate nuclear translocation of its cargo (Pemberton and Paschal, 2005). Consistent with this notion, Vpr was shown to interact specifically with nucleoporin phenylalanine-glycine (FG)-repeat regions, critical for importin-mediated nuclear import (Fouchier et al., 1998).

Another hypothesis postulates that Vpr uses a modification of the importin α-dependent pathway to enter the nucleus (Bukrinsky, 2004). Vpr was shown to bind to importin α both from human and budding yeast cells, but the binding site is different from the binding site for NLS (Agostini et al., 2000; Popov et al., 1998a,b; Vodicka et al., 1998). This binding of Vpr to importin α appears to stimulate subsequent nuclear import of the cargo (Popov et al., 1998b), likely by increasing the affinity of NLS–importin α interaction (Agostini et al., 2000). The effect of Ran-GTP binding to importin β on the Vpr ternary complex has not been reported and it is not understood why Vpr is frequently observed to localize at the nuclear envelope, although this may be related to the binding of Vpr to nucleoporins described above. One study found Vpr to be at the inside of the nuclear envelope (Vodicka et al., 1998) suggesting that Vpr is transported through the pore but is not released into the nucleoplasm.

One interesting implication of a conserved Vpr-binding site present both on human and budding yeast importin α is that this binding site might have some important cellular function in nuclear transport and that a cellular protein might bind to this site. Agostini et al. (2000) have identified this cellular protein as HSP70, a highly conserved heat shock protein (HSP), which competes with Vpr for binding to importin α. HSP70 can in fact replace Vpr in the nuclear transport of PIC and, similar to Vpr, also strengthens the binding of MA NLS to importin α (Agostini et al., 2000). One cellular role of this binding thus appears to be strengthening the interaction of a weak NLS with importin α. Therefore, one possible function for HSP70 may be to stimulate efficient translocation of large cargo complexes through the nuclear pore, similar to the role of Vpr in the nuclear import of the HIV-1 PIC. Interestingly, while HSP70 stimulates nuclear import and replication in macrophages of Vpr-deficient virus, it inhibits replication of a Vpr-positive HIV-1 (Iordanskiy et al., 2004a). The mechanism of this effect is unclear yet. Together with inhibition of other Vpr activities by HSP70 (Iordanskiy et al., 2004b), these results suggest that HSP70 might function as an innate antiviral factor.

C. Induction of Apoptosis

A major pathway for the induction of apoptosis by Vpr is through the mitochondria. This intrinsic pathway for apoptosis is initiated by mitochondrial membrane permeabilization (MMP; Green and Kroemer, 2004).

The release of proteins from the space between the inner and outer mitochondrial membranes ultimately leads to apoptosis. Cytochrome c is particularly important in this process since it cooperates in the cytoplasm with Apaf-1 to activate procaspase-9, the initiating caspase for the intrinsic pathway. Activated caspase-9 in turn activates the downstream caspases, such as caspase-3, which carry out many of the apoptotic events (Green and Kroemer, 2004).

Vpr is thought to lead to MMP by virtue of binding to ANT (adenine nucleotide translocator) protein of the inner mitochondrial membrane (Brenner and Kroemer, 2003; Jacotot et al., 2000, 2001). This binding occurs after Vpr crossing of the outer mitochondrial membrane, possibly through VDA (voltage dependent anion) channel, and leads to depolarization of the inner mitochondrial membrane, swelling of the inner mitochondria and ultimately to MMP with release of the apoptosis factors. Among the considerable evidence supporting this model are depolarization of the inner mitochondrial membrane by Vpr in intact cells, depolarization of isolated mitochondria by purified Vpr, strong binding between Vpr and ANT shown by several methods, reduced cell killing when ANT levels are decreased (Brenner and Kroemer, 2003; Jacotot et al., 2000, 2001), and activation of caspase-9 and caspase-3 by Vpr (Muthumani et al., 2002a,b; Zelivianski et al., 2006).

A potential problem with ANT as a mediator of Vpr-induced apoptosis is localization of ANT at the mitochondrial inner membrane (Klingenberg and Rottenberg, 1977), making it unclear how an interaction or disturbance at the inner mitochondrial membrane can provoke perforation of the outer membrane leading to the release of apoptogenic factors normally resident in the intermembranous space. A recent demonstration that Vpr also targets an outer membrane factor, HAX-1, provides an insight into possible mechanisms of MMP (Yedavalli et al., 2005). HAX-1 is an antiapoptotic factor that can bind directly to Bcl2 (Matsuda et al., 2003). Vpr–HAX-1 interaction was localized to the C-terminal portion of Vpr and the region between amino acids 118 and 141 of HAX-1, and this interaction correlated with Vpr-induced apoptosis (Yedavalli et al., 2005). Therefore, Vpr appears to sequester and dislocate mitochondrion-protective HAX-1. Consistent with this model, overexpression of Vpr-binding HAX-1 mutants protected cells from Vpr-induced apoptosis (Yedavalli et al., 2005).

While there is ample support for involvement of MMP in Vpr-induced apoptosis, there are some reports that do not readily fit into this model and which raise the possibility that Vpr may kill cells through other pathways. The localization of Vpr raises one question about the MMP model since Vpr has been consistently reported to be in the nucleus or at the nuclear membrane (Chen et al., 1999; Di Marzio et al., 1995; Lu et al., 1993; Mahalingam et al., 1995; Vodicka et al., 1998; Waldhuber et al., 2003) rather than in the mitochondria (Jacotot et al., 2000). It may be that only a small fraction of Vpr molecules localizes to the mitochondria, which is sufficient to induce apoptosis, and methods used to visualize Vpr may have overlooked this small amount. However, the predominant nuclear localization of Vpr and the association of nuclear localization with cell killing in Vpr mutants (Chen et al., 1999; Waldhuber et al., 2003) suggest that Vpr located in the nucleus may have some role in initiating cell killing. Consistent with this idea, Anderson et al. (2005) have recently presented evidence that ATR is not only responsible for the G2 arrest but has an essential role in Vpr-induced apoptosis of human cells as well.

Other observations seemingly inconsistent with the MMP model concern the activation of caspases by Vpr. While activation of caspase-9 with no activation of caspase-8 supports the role of MMP in the induction of apoptosis by Vpr (Muthumani et al., 2002a), there have been other conflicting reports that Vpr does activate caspase-8 (Lum et al., 2003; Patel et al., 2000). Caspase-8 activation is thought to be a hallmark of the extrinsic pathway for apoptosis induction by death receptors such as FAS and TNFR1 (Barnhart and Peter, 2003). It has also been reported that a fragment of Vpr is able to induce cell death without caspase activation (Roumier et al., 2002), and even that Vpr induces a necrotic type of cell death in neurons (Huang et al., 2000). The observation that Vpr is able to kill fission yeast cells (Zhao et al., 1998), where caspases play at most a minor role in cell death (Madeo et al., 2002), also suggests that there may be a caspase- and mitochondria-independent pathways for cell killing by Vpr.

D. Interaction of Vpr with Other Cellular Proteins

Some interactions between Vpr and cellular proteins have not yet been linked to a defined effect on viral replication or HIV pathogenesis. For example, Vpr interacts with a human HHR23A, which is a homologue of the well-characterized budding yeast Rad23 (Gragerov et al., 1998; Withers-Ward et al., 1997) and fission yeast Rhp23 (Elder et al., 2002). Vpr binds to HHR23A through its C-terminal ubiquitin-associated (UBA) domain (Dieckmann et al., 1998), which is a binding site for ubiquitin (Bertolaet et al., 2001; Chen et al., 2001; Elder et al., 2002). Rad23 and its homologues interact with the proteasome via the UbL domain (Hiyama et al., 1999; Schauber et al., 1998; Wilkinson et al., 2001). Specifically, both HHR23A and Rad23 bind via UbL directly to S5a, a protein which is part of the 19S regulatory subunit of the proteasome (Hiyama et al., 1999; Lambertson, 1999; Layfield et al., 2001). Deletion of S5a or HHR23A homologues in budding and fission yeast induced accumulation of polyubiquitinated proteins and prevented the degradation of a proteasome-specific substrate such as Ub-Pro-βgal (Lambertson, 1999; van Nocker et al., 1996; Wilkinson et al., 2001). Similarly, HHR23A also inhibited the degradation of iodinated lysozyme by the proteasome in the rabbit reticulocyte lysate (Hiyama et al., 1999). These results indicating that Vpr interacts with a ubiquitin binding site on proteins with essential roles in proteasome function suggest a potential effect of Vpr on cellular proteasomes. In fact, there have been two reports that Vpr can target a protein to the proteasome (Schrofelbauer *et al.*, 2005; Zhao *et al.*, 2004), indicating that the possible interactions between Vpr and the proteasome merit further exploration.

Vpr also binds to uracil-DNA glycosylase (UNG) (Bouhamdan *et al.*, 1996), which removes the uracil base from DNA. This reaction initiates the base excision repair pathway for removal from DNA of deoxyuracil resulting from spontaneous deamination of cytosine or misincorporation of dUMP during DNA synthesis (Kubota *et al.*, 1996; Parikh *et al.*, 2000; Wang *et al.*, 1997). UNG is highly conserved among species and is present in evolutionarily distant organisms ranging from bacteria and animal viruses to plants and mammals (Krokan *et al.*, 1997, 2000; Olsen *et al.*, 1991; Percival *et al.*, 1989; Varshney *et al.*, 1988). In human cells, there are two isoforms of UNG, which are encoded by the same gene (Slupphaug *et al.*, 1993) and produced by alternative splicing (Nilsen *et al.*, 1997). The UNG1 predominantly localizes to mitochondria while UNG2 is found mostly in the nucleus. The subcellular distribution of these two UNG isoforms is determined by different N-terminal presequence, whereas the rest of the protein sequence is identical (Slupphaug *et al.*, 1993).

Interestingly, primate lentiviruses do not produce UNG, whereas all known nonprimate lentiviruses encode a similar enzyme, dUTPase. The dUTPase enzyme, like UNG, minimizes the misincorporation of uracil into the viral DNA and plays an important role during viral replication in primary nondividing macrophages (Turelli *et al.*, 1997). Therefore, one possibility is that Vpr attracts UNG to proofread the viral reverse transcription. Indeed, interaction of Vpr with UNG was shown to decrease the mutation rate of HIV-1 *in vivo* (Chen *et al.*, 2004; Mansky *et al.*, 2000). However, this model was questioned in a recent report (Schrofelbauer *et al.*, 2005), which demonstrated that the binding of Vpr to UNG and to the related enzyme SMUG induces their proteasomal degradation and prevents their incorporation into nascent virions. These authors suggested that Vpr-assisted UNG degradation helps the virus to reduce the frequency of abasic sites in viral reverse transcripts at uracil residues caused by APOBEC3-catalyzed deamination of cytosine residues (Schrofelbauer *et al.*, 2005). This idea seems to contradict a report by Priet *et al.* (2005) who demonstrated that UNG2, recruited into viral particles by the HIV-1-encoded integrase domain, functions to excise uracils from the viral cDNA in a repair process which is required to produce infectious virus. This controversy regarding the role of UNG and Vpr–UNG interaction in the HIV life cycle awaits resolution.

Vpr also binds to p300/CBP transcriptional coactivators (Kino *et al.*, 2002). This binding, as well as previously described interaction with cellular transcription factor Sp1 (Wang *et al.*, 1995), may account for transactivating activity of Vpr on HIV promoter (Forget et al., 1998; Thotala et al., 2004). Also relevant to the transactivating effect of Vpr may be its interaction with the glucocorticoid receptor (GR) (Muthumani et al., 2006), as complex of Vpr and GR may transactivate HIV-1 transcription through glucocorticoid response element (GRE) in the LTR (Schafer et al., 2006).

Vpr was also reported to interact with Lys-tRNA synthetase (LysRS) (Stark and Hay, 1998). In the presence of Vpr, LysRS-mediated aminoacylation of tRNA(Lys) was inhibited. Since tRNA(Lys) is the primer for reverse transcription of the HIV-1 genome, this result suggests that the interaction between Vpr and LysRS may influence the initiation of HIV-1 reverse transcription.

IV. Activation and Counteraction of Host Immune Responses by Vpr

All regulatory and accessory HIV-1 proteins are targeted by HIV-1-specific CD8+ cytotoxic T-lymphocytes (CTLs) (Addo et al., 2002). However, Vpr is preferentially targeted by the CTL response in comparison to other viral proteins, at least during the acute phase of infection (Altfeld et al., 2001; Mothe et al., 2002), suggesting an important role for Vpr during the early phase of infection. Vpr suppresses antigen-specific CD8-mediated CTL and Th1 immune responses (Ayyavoo et al., 2002). Consistent with idea that Vpr suppresses the immune response, rhesus macaques infected with HIV-2 lacking the vpr gene had increased antibody titers compared to monkeys infected with the wild-type virus (Abimiku et al., 1995). Although the molecular mechanisms underlying the suppression of CTL and antibody production by Vpr are presently unknown, one possibility is that Vpr inhibits T-helper activity by suppressing T-cell proliferation and inducing cell cycle G2/M arrest (Poon et al., 1998).

Evidence also suggests that Vpr may suppress host inflammatory responses, which present another level of the host immune responses to viral infections (for review, see Muthumani et al., 2004). Vpr inhibits host inflammatory responses by downregulating proinflammatory cytokines (TNF-α and IL-12) and chemokines (RANTES, MIP-1α, and MIP-1β) in a manner similar to glucocorticoids (Ayyavoo et al., 1997; Refaeli et al., 1995); Vpr additionally suppresses host inflammatory response by inhibiting NF-κB activity through the induction of IκB (Ayyavoo et al., 1997).

In addition, Vpr induces expression of HSPs (Liang et al., 2007), indicating initiation of the heat stress response to Vpr. For example, HSP27 and HSP70 mRNA transcription appeared as early as 3–8 h following HIV infection. We now know that some of the HSPs, such as HSP27 or HSP70, have a protective effect against some or all of the Vpr activities (Iordanskiy et al., 2004a,b; Liang et al., 2007), suggesting that the heat stress response is part of the anti-HIV intrinsic immunity mechanism. Interestingly, the fission yeast heat shock protein Hsp16 also showed similar protective effect against Vpr activities suggesting a highly conserved nature of Vpr-induced stress response (Benko *et al.*, 2004, 2007). However, the elevation of HSPs in response to HIV-1 infection is transient as the *HSP27* and *HSP70* mRNA transcripts are significantly downregulated by 24 h after viral infection, concomitant with the first appearance of the full-length genomic HIV-1 mRNA (Wainberg *et al.*, 1997). This observation implies an active interplay between HIV viral proteins, and in particular Vpr, and HSP27 or HSP70. Consistent with this notion, an active and antagonistic interaction was seen between Vpr and a yeast homologue of HSP27, Hsp16 (Benko *et al.*, 2007).

Therefore, there appears to be at least two levels of host responses to *vpr* gene expression: one is the cellular immune response mediated by CD8+ CTLs, and the other is an innate immune response involving some of the cellular chaperone proteins. Vpr counteracts both these host responses: it prevents T-cell proliferation, suppresses host inflammatory responses including production of cytokines and chemokines, and downregulates production of HSPs, which have specific suppressive activities against Vpr. These specific host responses to Vpr and the counteracting effect by Vpr strongly suggest a very dynamic interaction between *vpr* gene expression and the host. Future studies should reveal to what extent these interactions contribute to the success of viral infection and will determine the best way to exploit the specific host responses to optimize strategies aimed at suppressing Vpr.

V. Development of Anti-Vpr Therapies

The results described in this chapter suggest that Vpr plays a pivotal role in viral pathogenesis. Specifically, Vpr activities are linked to promotion of viral infection in nondividing macrophages and monocytes, prevention of T-cell clonal expansion, and depletion of CD4 T-lymphocytes. Therefore, strategies to inhibit these adverse Vpr effects could potentially alleviate the impact of the virus and benefit infected patients. Thus, it is desirable to identify Vpr-specific inhibitors as a basis for the design of future anti-HIV regimens. Simple model systems have thus far been useful in identifying Vpr-specific inhibitors. For example, the translational elongation factor 2 (EF2) isolated from both fission yeast and mammalian cells specifically suppresses Vpr-induced apoptosis (Zelivianski *et al.*, 2006). A number of hexameric peptides with a ditryptophan motif were found by genetic selection in budding yeast to suppress Vpr-induced G2 arrest and apoptosis in T cells (Benko *et al.*, 2007; Yao *et al.*, 2002). A fission yeast small heat shock protein 16 (Hsp16) has been shown to specifically block all pathogenic

Vpr activities (Benko *et al.*, 2004, 2007). These Vpr-specific inhibitors and others being identified provide leads for the development of anti-HIV therapies with the potential to benefit HIV-infected patients in the future.

Acknowledgment

The work was supported in part by grants from the National Institute of Health AI40891 and GM63080 (R.Y.Z.) and AI33776 (M.B.).

References

Abimiku, A. G., Franchini, G., Aldrich, K., Myagkikh, M., Markham, P., Gard, E., Gallo, R. C., and Robert-Guroff, M. (1995). Humoral and cellular immune responses in rhesus macaques infected with human immunodeficiency virus type 2. *AIDS Res. Hum. Retroviruses* **11**(3), 383–393.

Abraham, R. T. (2001). Cell cycle checkpoint signaling through the ATM and ATR kinases. *Genes Dev.* **15**(17), 2177–2196.

Addo, M. M., Yu, X. G., Rosenberg, E. S., Walker, B. D., and Altfeld, M. (2002). Cytotoxic T-lymphocyte (CTL) responses directed against regulatory and accessory proteins in HIV-1 infection. *DNA Cell Biol.* **21**(9), 671–678.

Agostini, I., Popov, S., Li, J., Dubrovsky, L., Hao, T., and Bukrinsky, M. (2000). Heat-shock protein 70 can replace viral protein R of HIV-1 during nuclear import of the viral preintegration complex. *Exp. Cell Res.* **259**(2), 398–403.

Agostini, I., Popov, S., Hao, T., Li, J. H., Dubrovsky, L., Chaika, O., Chaika, N., Lewis, R., and Bukrinsky, M. (2002). Phosphorylation of Vpr regulates HIV type 1 nuclear import and macrophage infection. *AIDS Res. Hum. Retroviruses* **18**(4), 283–288.

al-Khodairy, F., and Carr, A. M. (1992). DNA repair mutants defining G2 checkpoint pathways in Schizosaccharomyces pombe. *EMBO J.* **11**(4), 1343–1350.

Alcasabas, A. A., Osborn, A. J., Bachant, J., Hu, F., Werler, P. J., Bousset, K., Furuya, K., Diffley, J. F., Carr, A. M., and Elledge, S. J. (2001). Mrc1 transduces signals of DNA replication stress to activate Rad53. *Nat. Cell Biol.* **3**(11), 958–965.

Altfeld, M., Addo, M. M., Eldridge, R. L., Yu, X. G., Thomas, S., Khatri, A., Strick, D., Phillips, M. N., Cohen, G. B., Islam, S. A., Kalams, S. A., Brander, C., *et al.* (2001). Vpr is preferentially targeted by CTL during HIV-1 infection. *J. Immunol.* **167**(5), 2743–2752.

Andersen, J. L., Zimmerman, E. S., DeHart, J. L., Murala, S., Ardon, O., Blackett, J., Chen, J., and Planelles, V. (2001). ATR and GADD45alpha mediate HIV-1 Vpr included apoptosis. Cell Death Differ **12**(4), 326–334.

Ayyavoo, V., Mahboubi, A., Mahalingam, S., Ramalingam, R., Kudchodkar, S., Williams, W. V., Green, D. R., and Weiner, D. B. (1997). HIV-1 Vpr suppresses immune activation and apoptosis through regulation of nuclear factor kappa B. *Nat. Med.* **3**(10), 1117–1123.

Ayyavoo, V., Muthumani, K., Kudchodkar, S., Zhang, D., Ramanathan, P., Dayes, N. S., Kim, J. J., Sin, J. I., Montaner, L. J., and Weiner, D. B. (2002). HIV-1 viral protein R compromises cellular immune function *in vivo*. *Int. Immunol.* **14**(1), 13–22.

Baber-Furnari, B. A., Rhind, N., Boddy, M. N., Shanahan, P., Lopez-Girona, A., and Russell, P. (2000). Regulation of mitotic inhibitor Mik1 helps to enforce the DNA damage checkpoint. *Mol. Biol. Cell* **11**(1), 1–11.

Barnhart, B. C., and Peter, M. E. (2003). The TNF receptor 1: A split personality complex. *Cell* **114**(2), 148–150.

Bartz, S. R., Rogel, M. E., and Emerman, M. (1996). Human immunodeficiency virus type 1 cell cycle control: Vpr is cytostatic and mediates G2 accumulation by a mechanism which differs from DNA damage checkpoint control. *J. Virol.* **70**(4), 2324–2331.

Benko, Z., Liang, D., Agbottah, E., Hou, J., Chiu, K., Yu, M., Innis, S., Reed, P., Kabat, W., Elder, R. T., Di Marzio, P., Taricani, L., *et al.* (2004). Anti-Vpr activity of a yeast chaperone protein. *J. Virol.* **78**(20), 11016–11029.

Benko, Z., Liang, D., Agbottah, E., Hou, J., Taricani, L., Young, P. G., Bukrinsky, M., and Zhao, R. Y. (2007). Antagonistic interaction of HIV-1 Vpr with Hsf-mediated cellular heat shock response and Hsp16 in fission yeast (*Schizosaccharomyces pombe*). *Retrovirology* **4**, 16.

Bennasser, Y., Le, S. Y., Benkirane, M., and Jeang, K. T. (2005). Evidence that HIV-1 encodes an siRNA and a suppressor of RNA silencing. *Immunity* **22**(5), 607–619.

Bentley, N. J., Holtzman, D. A., Flaggs, G., Keegan, K. S., DeMaggio, A., Ford, J. C., Hoekstra, M., and Carr, A. M. (1996). The *Schizosaccharomyces pombe rad3* checkpoint gene. *EMBO J.* **15**(23), 6641–6651.

Bertolaet, B. L., Clarke, D. J., Wolff, M., Watson, M. H., Henze, M., Divita, G., and Reed, S. I. (2001). UBA domains of DNA damage-inducible proteins interact with ubiquitin. *Nat. Struct. Biol.* **8**(5), 417–422.

Bishop, K. N., Holmes, R. K., and Malim, M. H. (2006). Antiviral potency of APOBEC proteins does not correlate with cytidine deamination. *J. Virol.* **80**(17), 8450–8458.

Boddy, M., Furnari, B., Mondesert, O., and Russell, P. (1998). Replication checkpoint enforced by kinases Cds1 and Chk1. *Science* **280**, 909–912.

Bouhamdan, M., Benichou, S., Rey, F., Navarro, J. M., Agostini, I., Spire, B., Camonis, J., Slupphaug, G., Vigne, R., Benarous, R., and Sire, J. (1996). Human immunodeficiency virus type 1 Vpr protein binds to the uracil DNA glycosylase DNA repair enzyme. *J. Virol.* **70**, 697–704.

Brenner, C., and Kroemer, G. (2003). The mitochondriotoxic domain of Vpr determines HIV-1 virulence. *J. Clin. Invest.* **111**(10), 1455–1457.

Bukrinsky, M. (2004). A hard way to the nucleus. *Mol. Med.* **10**(1–6), 1–5.

Burtelow, M. A., Roos-Mattjus, P. M., Rauen, M., Babendure, J. R., and Karnitz, L. M. (2001). Reconstitution and molecular analysis of the hRad9-hHus1-hRad1 (9–1–1) DNA damage responsive checkpoint complex. *J. Biol. Chem.* **276**(28), 25903–25909.

Cans, C., Ducommun, B., and Baldin, V. (1999). Proteasome-dependent degradation of human CDC25B phosphatase. *Mol. Biol. Rep.* **26**(1–2), 53–57.

Carr, A. M. (2002). DNA structure dependent checkpoints as regulators of DNA repair. *DNA Repair (Amst.)* **1**(12), 983–994.

Caspari, T., and Carr, A. M. (1999). DNA structure checkpoint pathways in Schizosaccharomyces pombe. *Biochimie* **81**(1–2), 173–181.

Caspari, T., and Carr, A. M. (2002). Checkpoints: How to flag up double-strand breaks. *Curr. Biol.* **12**(3), R105–R107.

Chen, L., Shinde, U., Ortolan, T. G., and Madura, K. (2001). Ubiquitin-associated (UBA) domains in Rad23 bind ubiquitin and promote inhibition of multi-ubiquitin chain assembly. *EMBO Rep.* **2**(10), 933–938.

Chen, M., Elder, R. T., Yu, M., O'Gorman, M. G., Selig, L., Benarous, R., Yamamoto, A., and Zhao, Y. (1999). Mutational analysis of Vpr-induced G2 arrest, nuclear localization, and cell death in fission yeast. *J. Virol.* **73**(4), 3236–3245.

Chen, R., Le Rouzic, E., Kearney, J. A., Mansky, L. M., and Benichou, S. (2004). Vpr-mediated incorporation of UNG2 into HIV-1 particles is required to modulate the virus mutation rate and for replication in macrophages. *J. Biol. Chem.* **279**(27), 28419–28425.

Chini, C. C., and Chen, J. (2003). Human claspin is required for replication checkpoint control. *J. Biol. Chem.* **278**(32), 30057–30062.

Chini, C. C., and Chen, J. (2004). Claspin, a regulator of Chk1 in DNA replication stress pathway. *DNA Repair (Amst.)* **3**(8–9), 1033–1037.

Connor, R. I., Chen, B. K., Choe, S., and Landau, N. R. (1995). Vpr is required for efficient replication of human immunodeficiency virus type-1 in mononuclear phagocytes. *Virology* **206**(2), 935–944.

Corbett, A. H., and Silver, P. A. (1997). Nucleocytoplasmic transport of macromolecules. *Microbiol. Mol. Biol. Rev.* **61**(2), 193–211.

de Noronha, C. M., Sherman, M. P., Lin, H. W., Cavrois, M. V., Moir, R. D., Goldman, R. D., and Greene, W. C. (2001). Dynamic disruptions in nuclear envelope architecture and integrity induced by HIV-1 Vpr. *Science* **294**(5544), 1105–1108.

Dieckmann, T., Withers-Ward, E. S., Jarosinski, M. A., Liu, C. F., Chen, I. S., and Feigon, J. (1998). Structure of a human DNA repair protein UBA domain that interacts with HIV-1 Vpr. *Nat. Struct. Biol.* **5**(12), 1042–1047.

Di Marzio, P., Choe, S., Ebright, M., Knoblauch, R., and Landau, N. R. (1995). Mutational analysis of cell cycle arrest, nuclear localization and virion packaging of human immunodeficiency virus type 1 Vpr. *J. Virol.* **69**(12), 7909–7916.

Du, L. L., Nakamura, T. M., Moser, B. A., and Russell, P. (2003). Retention but not recruitment of Crb2 at double-strand breaks requires Rad1 and Rad3 complexes. *Mol. Cell. Biol.* **23**(17), 6150–6158.

Elder, R. T., Yu, M., Chen, M., Edelson, S., and Zhao, Y. (2000). Cell cycle G2 arrest induced by HIV-1 Vpr in fission yeast (*Schizosaccharomyces pombe*) is independent of cell death and early genes in the DNA damage checkpoint. *Virus Res.* **68**, 161–173.

Elder, R. T., Yu, M.M, Chen, M., Zhu, X., Yanagida, M., and Zhao, Y (2001). HIV-1 Vpr induces cell cycle G2 arrest in fission yeast (*Schizosaccharomyces pombe*) through a pathway involving regulatory and catalytic subunits of PP2A and acting on both Wee1 and Cdc25. *Virology* **287**(2), 359–370.

Elder, R. T., Song, X. Q., Chen, M., Hopkins, K. M., Lieberman, H. B., and Zhao, Y. (2002). Involvement of rhp23, a Schizosaccharomyces pombe homolog of the human HHR23A and Saccharomyces cerevisiae RAD23 nucleotide excision repair genes, in cell cycle control and protein ubiquitination. *Nucleic Acids Res.* **30**(2), 581–591.

Elder, R. T., Zhu, X., Priet, S., Chen, M., Yu, M., Navarro, J. M., Sire, J., and Zhao, Y. (2003). A fission yeast homologue of the human uracil-DNA-glycosylase and their roles in causing DNA damage after overexpression. *Biochem. Biophys. Res. Commun.* **306**(3), 693–700.

Elledge, S. J. (1996). Cell cycle checkpoints: Preventing an identity crisis. *Science* **274**(5293), 1664–1672.

Esashi, F., Mochida, S., Matsusaka, T., Obara, T., Ogawa, A., Tamai, K., and Yanagida, M. (2000). Establishment of and recovery from damage checkpoint requires sequential interactions of Crb2 with protein kinases Rad3, Chk1, and Cdc2. *Cold Spring Harb. Symp. Quant. Biol.* **65**, 443–449.

Ford, J. C., al-Khodairy, F., Fotou, E., Sheldrick, K. S., Griffiths, D. J., and Carr, A. M. (1994). 14-3-3 protein homologs required for the DNA damage checkpoint in fission yeast. *Science* **265**(5171), 533–535.

Forget, J., Yao, X. J., Mercier, J., and Cohen, E. A. (1998). Human immunodeficiency virus type 1 Vpr protein transactivation function: Mechanism and identification of domains involved. *J. Mol. Biol.* **284**, 915–923.

Fouchier, R. A., Meyer, B. E., Simon, J. H., Fischer, U., Albright, A. V., Gonzalez-Scarano, F., and Malim, M. H. (1998). Interaction of the human immunodeficiency virus type 1 Vpr protein with the nuclear pore complex. *J. Virol.* **72**(7), 6004–6013.

Francesconi, S., Smeets, M., Grenon, M., Tillit, J., Blaisonneau, J., and Baldacci, G. (2002). Fission yeast chk1 mutants show distinct responses to different types of DNA damaging treatments. *Genes Cells* **7**(7), 663–673.

Fu, D. X., Kuo, Y. L., Liu, B. Y., Jeang, K. T., and Giam, C. Z. (2003). Human T-lymphotropic virus type I tax activates I-kappa B kinase by inhibiting I-kappa B kinase-associated serine/threonine protein phosphatase 2A. *J. Biol. Chem.* **278**(3), 1487–1493.

Furnari, B., Rhind, N., and Russell, P. (1997). Cdc25 mitotic inducer targeted by Chk1 DNA damage checkpoint kinase. *Science* 277(5331), 1495–1497.

Gallay, P., Stitt, V., Mundy, C., Oettinger, M., and Trono, D. (1996). Role of the karyopherin pathway in human immunodeficiency virus type 1 nuclear import. *J. Virol.* 70(2), 1027–1032.

Goh, W. C., Manel, N., and Emerman, M. (2004). The human immunodeficiency virus Vpr protein binds Cdc25C: Implications for G2 arrest. *Virology* 318(1), 337–349.

Gould, K. L., and Nurse, P. (1989). Tyrosine phosphorylation of the fission yeast *cdc2*⁺ protein kinase regulates entry into mitosis. *Nature* 342(6245), 39–45.

Gragerov, A., Kino, T., Ilyina-Gragerova, G., Chrousos, G. P., and Pavlakis, G. N. (1998). HHR23A, the human homologue of the yeast repair protein RAD23, interacts specifically with Vpr protein and prevents cell cycle arrest but not the transcriptional effects of Vpr. *Virol.* 245(2), 323–330.

Graves, P. R., Lovly, C. M., Uy, G. L., and Piwnica-Worms, H. (2001). Localization of human Cdc25C is regulated both by nuclear export and 14-3-3 protein binding. *Oncogene* 20(15), 1839–1851.

Green, D. R., and Kroemer, G. (2004). The pathophysiology of mitochondrial cell death. *Science* 305(5684), 626–629.

Haoudi, A., Daniels, R. C., Wong, E., Kupfer, G., and Semmes, O. J. (2003). Human T-cell leukemia virus-I tax oncoprotein functionally targets a subnuclear complex involved in cellular DNA damage-response. *J. Biol. Chem.* 278(39), 37736–37744.

He, J., Choe, S., Walker, R., Di Marzio, P., Morgan, D. O., and Landau, N. R. (1995). Human immunodeficiency virus type 1 viral protein R (Vpr) arrests cells in the G2 phase of the cell cycle by inhibiting p34cdc2 activity. *J. Virol.* 69(11), 6705–6711.

Heinzinger, N., Bukinsky, M., Haggerty, S., Ragland, A., Kewalramani, V., Lee, M., Gendelman, H., Ratner, L., Stevenson, M., and Emerman, M. (1994). The Vpr protein of human immunodeficiency virus type 1 influences nuclear localization of viral nucleic acids in nondividing host cells. *Proc. Natl. Acad. Sci. USA* 91(15), 7311–7315.

Hiyama, H., Yokoi, M., Masutani, C., Sugasawa, K., Maekawa, T., Tanaka, K., Hoeijmakers, J. H., and Hanaoka, F. (1999). Interaction of hHR23 with S5a. The ubiquitin-like domain of hhr23 mediates interaction with s5a subunit of 26 s proteasome. *J. Biol. Chem.* 274(39), 28019–28025.

Hsu, K., Seharaseyon, J., Dong, P., Bour, S., and Marban, E. (2004). Mutual functional destruction of HIV-1 Vpu and host TASK-1 channel. *Mol. Cell* 14(2), 259–267.

Huang, M. B., Weeks, O., Zhao, L. J., Saltarelli, M., and Bond, V. C. (2000). Effects of extracellular human immunodeficiency virus type 1 vpr protein in primary rat cortical cell cultures. *J. Neurovirol.* 6(3), 202–220.

Humphrey, T., and Enoch, T. (1998). Sum1, a highly conserved WD-repeat protein, suppresses S-M checkpoint mutants and inhibits the osmotic stress cell cycle response in fission yeast. *Genetics* 148(4), 1731–1742.

Igarashi, M., Nagata, A., Jinno, S., Suto, K., and Okayama, H. (1991). Wee1(+)-like gene in human cells. *Nature* 353(6339), 80–83.

Iordanskiy, S., Zhao, Y., DiMarzio, P., Agostini, I., Dubrovsky, L., and Bukrinsky, M. (2004a). Heat-shock protein 70 exerts opposing effects on Vpr-dependent and Vpr-independent HIV-1 replication in macrophages. *Blood* 104(6), 1867–1872.

Iordanskiy, S., Zhao, Y., Dubrovsky, L., Iordanskaya, T., Chen, M., Liang, D., and Bukrinsky, M. (2004b). Heat shock protein 70 protects cells from cell cycle arrest and apoptosis induced by human immunodeficiency virus type 1 viral protein R. *J. Virol.* 78(18), 9697–9704.

Jacotot, E., Ravagnan, L., Loeffler, M., Ferri, K. F., Vieira, H. L., Zamzami, N., Costantini, P., Druillennec, S., Hoebeke, J., Briand, J. P., Irinopoulou, T., Daugas, E., *et al.* (2000). The

HIV-1 viral protein R induces apoptosis via a direct effect on the mitochondrial permeability transition pore. *J. Exp. Med.* **191**(1), 33–46.

Jacotot, E., Ferri, K. F., El Hamel, C., Brenner, C., Druillennec, S., Hoebeke, J., Rustin, P., Metivier, D., Lenoir, C., Geuskens, M., Vieira, H. L., Loeffler, M., *et al.* (2001). Control of mitochondrial membrane permeabilization by adenine nucleotide translocator interacting with HIV-1 viral protein rR and Bcl-2. *J. Exp. Med.* **193**(4), 509–519.

Janssens, V., and Goris, J. (2001). Protein phosphatase 2A: A highly regulated family of serine/threonine phosphatases implicated in cell growth and signalling. *Biochem. J.* **353**(Pt. 3), 417–439.

Jenkins, Y., McEntee, M., Weis, K., and Greene, W. C. (1998). Characterization of HIV-1 vpr nuclear import: Analysis of signals and pathways. *J. Cell Biol.* **143**(4), 875–885.

Kino, T., and Pavlakis, G. N. (2004). Partner molecules of accessory protein Vpr of the human immunodeficiency virus type 1. *DNA Cell Biol.* **23**(4), 193–205.

Kino, T., Gragerov, A., Slobodskaya, O., Tsopanomichalou, M., Chrousos, G. P., and Pavlakis, G. N. (2002). Human immunodeficiency virus type 1 (HIV-1) accessory protein Vpr induces transcription of the HIV-1 and glucocorticoid-responsive promoters by binding directly to p300/CBP coactivators. *J. Virol.* **76**(19), 9724–9734.

Kinoshita, N., Ohkura, H., and Yanagida, M. (1990). Distinct, essential roles of type 1 and 2A protein phosphatases in the control of the fission yeast cell division cycle. *Cell* **63**(2), 405–415.

Klingenberg, M., and Rottenberg, H. (1977). Relation between the gradient of the ATP/ADP ratio and the membrane potential across the mitochondrial membrane. *Eur. J. Biochem.* **73**(1), 125–130.

Kornitzer, D., Sharf, R., and Kleinberger, T. (2001). Adenovirus E4orf4 protein induces PP2A-dependent growth arrest in Saccharomyces cerevisiae and interacts with the anaphase-promoting complex/cyclosome. *J. Cell Biol.* **154**(2), 331–344.

Krokan, H. E., Standal, R., and Slupphaug, G. (1997). DNA glycosylases in the base excision repair of DNA. *Biochem. J.* **325**(Pt 1), 1–16.

Krokan, H. E., Nilsen, H., Skorpen, F., Otterlei, M., and Slupphaug, G. (2000). Base excision repair of DNA in mammalian cells. *FEBS Lett.* **476**(1–2), 73–77.

Krek, W., and Nigg, E. A. (1991). Differential phosphorylation of vertebrate p34^{cdc2} kinase at the G1/S and G2/M transitions of the cell cycle: Identification of major phosphorylation sites. *EMBO J.* **10**(2), 305–316.

Kubota, Y., Nash, R. A., Klungland, A., Schar, P., Barnes, D. E., and Lindahl, T. (1996). Reconstitution of DNA base excision-repair with purified human proteins: Interaction between DNA polymerase beta and the XRCC1 protein. *EMBO J.* **15**(23), 6662–6670.

Lambertson, D., Chen, L., and Madura, K. (1999). Pleiotropic defects caused by loss of the proteasome-interacting factors rad23 and rpn10 of *saccharomyces cerevisiae*. *Genetics* **153**(1), 69–79.

Lammer, C., Wagerer, S., Saffrich, R., Mertens, D., Ansorge, W., and Hoffmann, I. (1998). The cdc25B phosphatase is essential for the G2/M phase transition in human cells. *J. Cell Sci.* **111**(Pt. 16), 2445–2453.

Layfield, R., Tooth, D., Landon, M., Dawson, S., Mayer, J., and Alban, A. (2001). Purification of poly-ubiquitinated proteins by S5a-affinity chromatography. *Proteomics* **1**(6), 773–777.

Le Rouzic, E., Mousnier, A., Rustum, C., Stutz, F., Hallberg, E., Dargemont, C., and Benichou, S. (2002). Docking of HIV-1 Vpr to the nuclear envelope is mediated by the interaction with the nucleoporin hCG1. *J. Biol. Chem.* **277**(47), 45091–45098.

Lee, M. G., and Nurse, P. (1987). Complementation used to clone a human homologue of the fission yeast cell cycle control gene cdc2. *Nature* **327**(6117), 31–35.

Li, G., Elder, R. T., Qin, K., Park, H. U., Liang, D., and Zhao, R. Y. (2007). Phosphatase type 2A-dependent and -independent pathways for ATR phosphorylation of Chk1. *J. Biol. Chem.* **282**(10), 7287–7298.

Liang, D., Benko, Z., Agbottah, E., Bukrinsky, M., and Zhao, R. Y. (2007). HSF27 as a Potential Intrinsic Anti-HIV Factor Targeting the HIV-1 Viral Protein R. *Mol. Med.* In press.

Lieberman, H. B., Hopkins, K. M., Nass, M., Demetrick, D., and Davey, S. (1996). A human homolog of the Schizosaccharomyces pombe rad9+ checkpoint control gene. *Proc. Natl. Acad. Sci. USA* **93**(24), 13890–13895.

Lin, S. Y., Li, K., Stewart, G. S., and Elledge, S. J. (2004). Human Claspin works with BRCA1 to both positively and negatively regulate cell proliferation. *Proc. Natl. Acad. Sci. USA* **101**(17), 6484–6489.

Lopez-Girona, A., Furnari, B., Mondesert, O., and Russell, P. (1999). Nuclear localization of Cdc25 is regulated by DNA damage and a 14-3-3 protein. *Nature* **397**(6715), 172–175.

Lu, Y. L., Spearman, P., and Ratner, L. (1993). Human immunodeficiency virus type 1 viral protein R localization in infected cells and virions. *J. Virol.* **67**(11), 6542–6550.

Lum, J. J., Cohen, O. J., Nie, Z., Weaver, J. G., Gomez, T. S., Yao, X. J., Lynch, D., Pilon, A. A., Hawley, N., Kim, J. E., Chen, Z., Montpetit, M., *et al.* (2003). Vpr R77Q is associated with long-term nonprogressive HIV infection and impaired induction of apoptosis. *J. Clin. Invest.* **111**(10), 1547–1554.

Madeo, F., Herker, E., Maldener, C., Wissing, S., Lachelt, S., Herlan, M., Fehr, M., Lauber, K., Sigrist, S. J., Wesselborg, S., and Frohlich, K. U. (2002). A caspase-related protease regulates apoptosis in yeast. *Mol. Cell* **9**(4), 911–917.

Mahalingam, S., Collman, R. G., Patel, M., Monken, C. E., and Srinivasan, A. (1995). Functional analysis of HIV-1 Vpr: Identification of determinants essential for subcellular localization. *Virology* **212**(2), 331–339.

Mansky, L. M., Preveral, S., Selig, L., Benarous, R., and Benichou, S. (2000). The interaction of vpr with uracil DNA glycosylase modulates the human immunodeficiency virus type 1 *in vivo* mutation rate. *J. Virol.* **74**(15), 7039–7047.

Marathi, U. K., Dahlen, M., Sunnerhagen, P., Romero, A. V., Ramagli, L. S., Siciliano, M. J., Li, L., and Legerski, R. J. (1998). RAD1, a human structural homolog of the *Schizosaccharomyces pombe* RAD1 cell cycle checkpoint gene. *Genomics* **54**(2), 344–347.

Masuda, M., Nagai, Y., Oshima, N., Tanaka, K., Murakami, H., Igarashi, H., and Okayama, H. (2000). Genetic studies with the fission yeast *Schizosaccharomyces pombe* suggest involvement of wee1, ppa2, and rad24 in induction of cell cycle arrest by human immunodeficiency virus type 1 Vpr. *J. Virol.* **74**(6), 2636–2646.

Matsuda, G., Nakajima, K., Kawaguchi, Y., Yamanashi, Y., and Hirai, K. (2003). Epstein-Barr virus (EBV) nuclear antigen leader protein (EBNA-LP) forms complexes with a cellular anti-apoptosis protein Bcl-2 or its EBV counterpart BHRF1 through HS1-associated protein X-1. *Microbiol. Immunol.* **47**(1), 91–99.

Matsuda, N., Tanaka, H., Yamazaki, S., Suzuki, J., Tanaka, K., Yamada, T., and Masuda, M. (2006). HIV-1 Vpr induces G2 cell cycle arrest in fission yeast associated with Rad24/14-3-3-dependent, Chk1/Cds1-independent Wee1 upregulation. *Microbes Infect.* **8**(12-13), 2736–2744.

Matsuoka, S., Huang, M., and Elledge, S. J. (1998). Linkage of ATM to cell cycle regulation by the Chk2 protein kinase. *Science* **282**(5395), 1893–1897.

McGowan, C. H., and Russell, P. (2004). The DNA damage response: Sensing and signaling. *Curr. Opin. Cell Biol.* **16**(6), 629–633.

Mils, V., Baldin, V., Goubin, F., Pinta, I., Papin, C., Waye, M., Eychene, A., and Ducommun, B. (2000). Specific interaction between 14-3-3 isoforms and the human CDC25B phosphatase. *Oncogene* **19**(10), 1257–1265.

Morellet, N., Bouaziz, S., Petitjean, P., and Roques, B. P. (2003). NMR structure of the HIV-1 regulatory protein VPR. *J. Mol. Biol.* **327**(1), 215–227.

Morgan, D. O. (1995). Principles of CDK regulation. *Nature* **374**(6518), 131–134.

Mothe, B. R., Horton, H., Carter, D. K., Allen, T. M., Liebl, M. E., Skinner, P., Vogel, T. U., Fuenger, S., Vielhuber, K., Rehrauer, W., Wilson, N., Franchini, G., *et al.* (2002). Dominance of CD8 responses specific for epitopes bound by a single major histocompatibility complex class I molecule during the acute phase of viral infection. *J. Virol.* **76**(2), 875–884.

Muller, B., Tessmer, U., Schubert, U., and Krausslich, H. G. (2000). Human immunodeficiency virus type 1 Vpr protein is incorporated into the virion in significantly smaller amounts than gag and is phosphorylated in infected cells. *J. Virol.* **74**(20), 9727–9731.

Munoz, M. J., Bejarano, E. R., Daga, R. R., and Jimenez, J. (1999). The identification of Wos2, a p23 homologue that interacts with Wee1 and Cdc2 in the mitotic control of fission yeasts. *Genetics* **153**(4), 1561–1572.

Muthumani, K., Hwang, D. S., Desai, B. M., Zhang, D., Dayes, N., Green, D. R., and Weiner, D. B. (2002a). HIV-1 Vpr induces apoptosis through caspase 9 in T cells and peripheral blood mononuclear cells. *J. Biol. Chem.* **277**(40), 37820–37831.

Muthumani, K., Zhang, D., Hwang, D. S., Kudchodkar, S., Dayes, N. S., Desai, B. M., Malik, A. S., Yang, J. S., Chattergoon, M. A., Maguire, H. C., Jr., and Weiner, D. B. (2002b). Adenovirus encoding HIV-1 Vpr activates caspase 9 and induces apoptotic cell death in both p53 positive and negative human tumor cell lines. *Oncogene* **21**(30), 4613–4625.

Muthumani, K., Desai, B. M., Hwang, D. S., Choo, A. Y., Laddy, D. J., Thieu, K. P., Rao, R. G., and Weiner, D. B. (2004). HIV-1 Vpr and anti-inflammatory activity. *DNA Cell Biol.* **23**(4), 239–247.

Muthumani, K., Choo, A. Y., Zong, W. X., Madesh, M., Hwang, D. S., Premkumar, A., Thieu, K. P., Emmanuel, J., Kumar, S., Thompson, C. B., and Weiner, D. B. (2006). The HIV-1 Vpr and glucocorticoid receptor complex is a gain-of-function interaction that prevents the nuclear localization of PARP-1. *Nat. Cell Biol.* **8**(2), 170–179.

Nagata, A., Igarashi, M., Jinno, S., Suto, K., and Okayama, H. (1991). An additional homolog of the fission yeast cdc25+ gene occurs in humans and is highly expressed in some cancer cells. *New Biol.* **3**(10), 959–968.

Nakielny, S., and Dreyfuss, G. (1999). Transport of proteins and RNAs in and out of the nucleus. *Cell* **99**(7), 677–690.

Nilsen, H., Otterlei, M., Haug, T., Solum, K., Nagelhus, T. A., Skorpen, F., and Krokan, H. E. (1997). Nuclear and mitochondrial uracil-DNA glycosylases are generated by alternative splicing and transcription from different positions in the UNG gene. *Nucleic Acids Res.* **25**(4), 750–755.

Norbury, C., Blow, J., and Nurse, P. (1991). Regulatory phosphorylation of the p34^{cdc2} protein kinase in vertebrates. *EMBO J.* **10**(11), 3321–3329.

Nurse, P. (1997). Checkpoint pathways come of age. *Cell* **91**, 865–867.

Olsen, L. C., Aasland, R., Krokan, H. E., and Helland, D. E. (1991). Human uracil-DNA glycosylase complements *E. coli ung* mutants. *Nucleic Acids Res.* **19**(16), 4473–4478.

O'Shea, C. C., Choi, S., McCormick, F., and Stokoe, D. (2005). Adenovirus overrides cellular checkpoints for protein translation. *Cell Cycle* **4**(7), 883–888.

Ozon, R. (1991). [From ovocyte to biochemistry of the cell cycle]. *Verh. K. Acad. Geneeskd. Belg.* **53**(4), 365–385.

Parikh, S. S., Walcher, G., Jones, G. D., Slupphaug, G., Krokan, H. E., Blackburn, G. M., and Tainer, J. A. (2000). Uracil-DNA glycosylase-DNA substrate and product structures: conformational strain promotes catalytic efficiency by coupled stereoelectronic effects. *Proc. Natl. Acad. Sci. USA* **97**(10), 5083–5088.

Park, H. U., Jeong, J. H., Chung, J. H., and Brady, J. N. (2004). Human T-cell leukemia virus type 1 Tax interacts with Chk1 and attenuates DNA-damage induced G2 arrest mediated by Chk1. *Oncogene* **23**(29), 4966–4974.

Parker, A. E., Van de Weyer, I., Laus, M. C., Verhasselt, P., and Luyten, W. H. (1998). Identification of a human homologue of the *Schizosaccharomyces pombe* rad17+

checkpoint gene. *J. Biol. Chem.* **273**(29), 18340–18346. [Erratum appears in *J. Biol. Chem.* (1999), **274**(34), 24438.]

Patel, C. A., Mukhtar, M., and Pomerantz, R. J. (2000). Human immunodeficiency virus type 1 Vpr induces apoptosis in human neuronal cells. *J. Virol.* **74**(20), 9717–9726.

Pemberton, L. F., and Paschal, B. M. (2005). Mechanisms of receptor-mediated nuclear import and nuclear export. *Traffic* **6**(3), 187–198.

Percival, K. J., Klein, M. B., and Burgers, P. M. (1989). Molecular cloning and primary structure of the uracil-DNA-glycosylase gene from *Saccharomyces cerevisiae*. *J. Biol. Chem.* **264**(5), 2593–2598.

Poon, B., Grovit-Ferbas, K., Stewart, S. A., and Chen, I. S. Y. (1998). Cell cycle arrest by Vpr in HIV-1 virions and insensitivity to antiretroviral agents. *Science* **281**(5374), 266–269.

Popov, S., Rexach, M., Ratner, L., Blobel, G., and Bukrinsky, M. (1998a). Viral protein R regulates docking of the HIV-1 preintegration complex to the nuclear pore complex. *J. Biol. Chem.* **273**(21), 13347–13352.

Popov, S., Rexach, M., Zybarth, G., Reiling, N., Lee, M. A., Ratner, L., Lane, C. M., Moore, M. S., Blobel, G., and Bukrinsky, M. (1998b). Viral protein R regulates nuclear import of the HIV-1 pre-integration complex. *EMBO J.* **17**(4), 909–917.

Priet, S., Gros, N., Navarro, J. M., Boretto, J., Canard, B., Querat, G., and Sire, J. (2005). HIV-1-associated uracil DNA glycosylase activity controls dUTP misincorporation in viral DNA and is essential to the HIV-1 life cycle. *Mol. Cell* **17**(4), 479–490.

Re, F., Braaten, D., Franke, E. K., and Luban, J. (1995). Human immunodeficiency virus type 1 Vpr arrests the cell cycle in G2 by inhibiting the activation of p34cdc2-cyclin B. *J. Virol.* **69**(11), 6859–6864.

Refaeli, Y., Levy, D. N., and Weiner, D. B. (1995). The glucocorticoid receptor type II complex is a target of the HIV-1 *vpr* gene product. *Proc. Natl. Acad. Sci. USA* **92**(8), 3621–3625.

Rhind, N., and Russell, P. (1998a). Mitotic DNA damage and replication checkpoints in yeast. *Curr. Opin. Cell Biol.* **10**(6), 749–758.

Rhind, N., and Russell, P. (1998b). Tyrosine phosphorylation of cdc2 is required for the replication checkpoint in Schizosaccharomyces pombe. *Mol. Cell. Biol.* **18**(7), 3782–3787.

Roopchand, D. E., Lee, J. M., Shahinian, S., Paquette, D., Bussey, H., and Branton, P. E. (2001). Toxicity of human adenovirus E4orf4 protein in *Saccharomyces cerevisiae* results from interactions with the Cdc55 regulatory B subunit of PP2A. *Oncogene* **20**(38), 5279–5290.

Roshal, M., Kim, B., Zhu, Y., Nghiem, P., and Planelles, V. (2003). Activation of the ATR-mediated DNA damage response by the HIV-1 viral protein R. *J. Biol. Chem.* **278**(28), 25879–25886.

Roumier, T., Vieira, H. L., Castedo, M., Ferri, K. F., Boya, P., Andreau, K., Druillennec, S., Joza, N., Penninger, J. M., Roques, B., and Kroemer, G. (2002). The C-terminal moiety of HIV-1 Vpr induces cell death via a caspase-independent mitochondrial pathway. *Cell Death Differ.* **9**(11), 1212–1219.

Sadhu, K., Reed, S. I., Richardson, H., and Russell, P. (1990). Human homolog of fission yeast cdc25 mitotic inducer is predominantly expressed in G2. *Proc. Natl. Acad. Sci. USA* **87**(13), 5139–5143.

Saka, Y., Esashi, F., Matsusaka, T., Mochida, S., and Yanagida, M. (1997). Damage and replication checkpoint control in fission yeast is ensured by interactions of Crb2, a protein with BRCT motif, with Cut5 and Chk1. *Genes Dev.* **11**(24), 3387–3400.

Sanchez, Y., Wong, C., Thoma, R. S., Richman, R., Wu, Z., Piwnica-Worms, H., and Elledge, S. J. (1997). Conservation of the Chk1 checkpoint pathway in mammals: Linkage of DNA damage to Cdk regulation through Cdc25. *Science* **277**(5331), 1497–1501.

Savitsky, K., Bar-Shira, A., Gilad, S., Rotman, G., Ziv, Y., Vanagaite, L., Tagle, D. A., Smith, S., Uziel, T., Sfez, S., *et al.* (1995). A single ataxia telangiectasia gene with a product similar to PI-3 kinase. *Science* **268**(5218), 1749–1753.

Schafer, E. A., Venkatachari, N. J., and Ayyavoo, V. (2006). Antiviral effects of mifepristone on human immunodeficiency virus type-1 (HIV-1): Targeting Vpr and its cellular partner, the glucocorticoid receptor (GR). *Antiviral Res.*

Schauber, C., Chen, L., Tongaonkar, P., Vega, I., Lamberston, D., Potts, W., and Madura, K. (1998). Rad 23 links DNA repair to the ubiquitin/proteasome pathway. *Nature* **391** (6668), 715–718.

Schrofelbauer, B., Yu, Q., Zeitlin, S. G., and Landau, N. R. (2005). Human immunodeficiency virus type 1 Vpr induces the degradation of the UNG and SMUG uracil-DNA glycosylases. *J. Virol.* **79**(17), 10978–10987.

Schuler, W., Wecker, K., de Rocquigny, H., Baudat, Y., Sire, J., and Roques, B. P. (1999). NMR structure of the (52–96) C-terminal domain of the HIV-1 regulatory protein Vpr: Molecular insights into its biological functions. *J. Mol. Biol.* **285**(5), 2105–2117.

Shiloh, Y. (2001). ATM and ATR: Networking cellular responses to DNA damage. *Curr. Opin. Genet. Dev.* **11**(1), 71–77.

Shtrichman, R., Sharf, R., Barr, H., Dobner, T., and Kleinberger, T. (1999). Induction of apoptosis by adenovirus E4orf4 protein is specific to transformed cells and requires an interaction with protein phosphatase 2A. *Proc. Natl. Acad. Sci. USA* **96**(18), 10080–10085.

Slupphaug, G., Markussen, F. H., Olsen, L. C., Aasland, R., Aarsaether, N., Bakke, O., Krokan, H. E., and Helland, D. E. (1993). Nuclear and mitochondrial forms of human uracil-DNA glycosylase are encoded by the same gene. *Nucleic Acids Res.* **21**(11), 2579–2584.

Stark, L. A., and Hay, R. T. (1998). Human immunodeficiency virus type 1 (HIV-1) viral protein R (Vpr) interacts with Lys-tRNA synthetase: Implications for priming of HIV-1 reverse transcription. *J. Virol.* **72**(4), 3037–3044.

Stewart, S. A., Poon, B., Jowett, J. B., and Chen, I. S. (1997). Human immunodeficiency virus type 1 Vpr induces apoptosis following cell cycle arrest. *J. Virol.* **71**(7), 5579–5592.

Subbramanian, R. A., Kessous-Elbaz, A., Lodge, R., Forget, J., Yao, X. J., Bergeron, D., and Cohen, E. A. (1998). Human immunodeficiency virus type 1 Vpr is a positive regulator of viral transcription and infectivity in primary human macrophages. *J. Exp. Med.* **187**(7), 1103–1111.

Tanaka, K., and Russell, P. (2001). Mrc1 channels the DNA replication arrest signal to checkpoint kinase Cds1. *Nat. Cell Biol.* **3**(11), 966–972.

Terada, Y., and Yasuda, Y. (2006). HIV-1 Vpr induces G2 checkpoint activation by interacting with the splicing factor SAP145. *Mol. Cell. Biol.*

Thotala, D., Schafer, E. A., Tungaturthi, P. K., Majumder, B., Janket, M. L., Wagner, M., Srinivasan, A., Watkins, S., and Ayyavoo, V. (2004). Structure-functional analysis of human immunodeficiency virus type 1 (HIV-1) Vpr: Role of leucine residues on Vpr-mediated transactivation and virus replication. *Virology* **328**(1), 89–100.

Tristem, M., Marshall, C., Karpas, A., and Hill, F. (1992). Evolution of the primate lentiviruses: Evidence from vpx and vpr. *EMBO J.* **11**(9), 3405–3412.

Tristem, M., Purvis, A., and Quicke, D. L. (1998). Complex evolutionary history of primate lentiviral vpr genes. *Virology* **240**(2), 232–237.

Turelli, P., Guiguen, F., Mornex, J. F., Vigne, R., and Querat, G. (1997). dUTPase-minus caprine arthritis-encephalitis virus is attenuated for pathogenesis and accumulates G-to-A substitutions. *J. Virol.* **71**(6), 4522–4530.

van Nocker, S., Walker, J. M., and Vierstra, R. D. (1996). The Arabidopsis thaliana UBC7/13/14 genes encode a family of multiubiquitin chain-forming E2 enzymes. *J. Biol. Chem.* **271** (21), 12150–12158.

Varadarajan, P., Mahalingam, S., Liu, P., Ng, S. B., Gandotra, S., Dorairajoo, D. S., and Balasundaram, D. (2005). The functionally conserved nucleoporins Nup124p from fission yeast and the human Nup153 mediate nuclear import and activity of the Tf1 retrotransposon and HIV-1 Vpr. *Mol. Biol. Cell* **16**(4), 1823–1838.

Varshney, U., Hutcheon, T., and van de Sande, J. H. (1988). Sequence analysis, expression, and conservation of *Escherichia coli* uracil DNA glycosylase and its gene (*ung*). *J. Biol. Chem.* **263**(16), 7776–7784.

Vodicka, M. A., Koepp, D. M., Silver, P. A., and Emerman, M. (1998). HIV-1 Vpr interacts with the nuclear transport pathway to promote macrophage infection. *Genes Dev.* **12**(2), 175–185.

Volkmer, E., and Karnitz, L. M. (1999). Human homologs of Schizosaccharomyces pombe rad1, hus1, and rad9 form a DNA damage-responsive protein complex. *J. Biol. Chem.* **274**(2), 567–570.

Wainberg, Z., Oliveira, M., Lerner, S., Tao, Y., and Brenner, B. G. (1997). Modulation of stress protein (hsp27 and hsp70) expression in CD4+ lymphocytic cells following acute infection with human immunodeficiency virus type-1. *Virology* **233**(2), 364–373.

Waldhuber, M. G., Bateson, M., Tan, J., Greenway, A. L., and McPhee, D. A. (2003). Studies with GFP-Vpr fusion proteins: Induction of apoptosis but ablation of cell-cycle arrest despite nuclear membrane or nuclear localization. *Virology* **313**(1), 91–104.

Walworth, N. C., and Bernards, R. (1996). rad-dependent response of the chk1-encoded protein kinase at the DNA damage checkpoint. *Science* **271**(5247), 353–356.

Wang, L., Mukherjee, S., Jia, F., Narayan, O., and Zhao, L. J. (1995). Interaction of virion protein Vpr of human immunodeficiency virus type 1 with cellular transcription factor Sp1 and trans-activation of viral long terminal repeat. *J. Biol. Chem.* **270**(43), 25564–25569.

Wang, Z., Wu, X., and Friedberg, E. C. (1997). Molecular mechanism of base excision repair of uracil-containing DNA in year cell-free extracts. *J. Biol. Chem.* **272**(38), 24064–24071.

Wilkinson, C. R., Seeger, M., Hartmann-Petersen, R., Stone, M., Wallace, M., Semple, C., and Gordon, C. (2001). Proteins containing the UBA domain are able to bind to multi-ubiquitin chains. *Nat. Cell. Biol.* **3**(10), 939–943.

Wecker, K., and Roques, B. P. (1999). NMR structure of the (1–51) N-terminal domain of the HIV-1 regulatory protein Vpr. *Eur. J. Biochem.* **266**(2), 359–369.

Wei, B. L., Arora, V. K., Foster, J. L., Sodora, D. L., and Garcia, J. V. (2003). *In vivo* analysis of Nef function. *Curr. HIV Res.* **1**(1), 41–50.

Wente, S. R. (2000). Gatekeepers of the nucleus. *Science* **288**(5470), 1374–1377.

Withers-Ward, E. S., Jowett, J. B., Stewart, S. A., Xie, Y. M., Garfinkel, A., Shibagaki, Y., Chow, S. A., Shah, N., Hanaoka, F., Sawitz, D. G., Armstrong, R. W., Souza, L. M., and Chen, I. S. (1997). Human immunodeficiency virus type 1 Vpr interacts with HHR23A, a cellular protein implicated in nucleotide excision DNA repair. *J. Virol.* **71**(12), 9732–9742.

Yao, X. J., Lemay, J., Rougeau, N., Clement, M., Kurtz, S., Belhumeur, P., and Cohen, E. A. (2002). Genetic selection of peptide inhibitors of human immunodeficiency virus type 1 Vpr. *J. Biol. Chem.* **277**(50), 48816–48826.

Yedavalli, V. S., Shih, H. M., Chiang, Y. P., Lu, C. Y., Chang, L. Y., Chen, M. Y., Chuang, C. Y., Dayton, A. I., Jeang, K. T., and Huang, L. M. (2005). Human immunodeficiency virus type 1 Vpr interacts with antiapoptotic mitochondrial protein HAX-1. *J. Virol.* **79**(21), 13735–13746.

Yuan, H., Kamata, M., Xie, Y. M., and Chen, I. S. (2004). Increased levels of Wee-1 kinase in G(2) are necessary for Vpr- and gamma irradiation-induced G(2) arrest. *J. Virol.* **78**(15), 8183–8190.

Zelivianski, S., Liang, D., Chen, M., Mirkin, B. L., and Zhao, R. Y. (2006). Suppressive effect of elongation factor 2 on apoptosis induced by HIV-1 viral protein R. *Apoptosis* **11**(3), 377–388.

Zeng, Y., Forbes, K. C., Wu, Z., Moreno, S., Piwnica-Worms, H., and Enoch, T. (1998). Replication checkpoint requires phosphorylation of the phosphatase Cdc25 by Cds1 or Chk1. *Nature* **395**(6701), 507–510.

Zhao, H., and Russell, P. (2004). DNA binding domain in the replication checkpoint protein Mrc1 of Schizosaccharomyces pombe. *J. Biol. Chem.* **279**(51), 53023–53027.

Zhao, L. J., Jian, H., and Zhu, H. (2004). HIV-1 auxiliary regulatory protein Vpr promotes ubiquitination and turnover of Vpr mutants containing the L64P mutation. *FEBS Lett.* **563**(1–3), 170–178.

Zhao, Y., Cao, J., O'Gorman, M. R. G., Yu, M., and Yogev, R. (1996). Effect of human immunodeficiency virus Type 1 protein R (*vpr*) gene expression on basic cellular functions of fission yeast Schizosaccharomyces pombe. *J. Virol.* **70**, 5821–5826.

Zhao, Y., Yu, M., Chen, M., Elder, R. T., Yamamoto, A., and Cao, J. (1998). Pleiotropic effects of HIV-1 protein R (Vpr) on morphogenesis and cell survival in fission yeast and antagonism by pentoxifylline. *Virology* **246**, 266–276.

Zhu, Y., Roshal, M., Li, F., Blackett, J., and Planelles, V. (2003). Upregulation of survivin by HIV-1 Vpr. *Apoptosis* **8**(1), 71–79.

Zimmerman, E. S., Chen, J., Andersen, J. L., Ardon, O., Dehart, J. L., Blackett, J., Choudhary, S. K., Camerini, D., Nghiem, P., and Planelles, V. (2004). Human immunodeficiency virus type 1 Vpr-mediated G2 arrest requires Rad17 and Hus1 and induces nuclear BRCA1 and gamma-H2AX focus formation. *Mol. Cell. Biol.* **24**(21), 9286–9294.

John M. Louis[*], Rieko Ishima[†],
Dennis A. Torchia[‡], and Irene T. Weber[§]

[*]Laboratory of Chemical Physics, National Institute of Diabetes
Digestive and Kidney Diseases, National Institutes of Health
Bethesda, Maryland 20892

[†]Department of Structural Biology, School of Medicine
University of Pittsburgh, Pittsburgh, Pennsylvania 15260

[‡]Molecular Structural Biology Unit
National Institute of Dental and Craniofacial Research
National Institutes of Health, Bethesda, Maryland 20892

[§]Department of Biology, Molecular Basis of Disease Program
Georgia State University, Atlanta, Georgia 30303

HIV-1 Protease: Structure, Dynamics, and Inhibition

I. Chapter Overview

The HIV-1 protease is synthesized as part of a large Gag-Pol precursor protein. It is responsible for its own release from the precursor and the processing of the Gag and Gag-Pol polyproteins into the mature structural and functional proteins required for virus maturation. Because of its indispensable role, the mature HIV-1 protease dimer has proven to be a successful target for the development of antiviral agents. In the last 5 years, a major emphasis in protease research has been to improve inhibitor design and treatment regimens, which include the highly active antiretroviral therapy (HAART), to overcome the problem of drug resistance and curb progress of

Advances in Pharmacology, Volume 55
1054-3589/07 $35.00
DOI: 10.1016/S1054-3589(07)55008-8

the disease. In this chapter, we focus on some new and evolving areas of protease research, namely (1) probing the structure and dynamics of the free and inhibited mature protease dimer by NMR to gain insights into specific regions of the dimer and their relationship to function, (2) determining crystal structures at atomic resolutions of wild-type and drug-resistant mutant proteases in complex with substrate analogues and comparison of structures using previous and new generations of active site inhibitors to understand the molecular mechanisms of drug resistance, and (3) mutational and structural studies aimed at characterizing the monomer of the mature protease and its precursor. The latter studies complement and form a basis for ongoing and future studies aimed at targeting protease dimerization, thus extending the target area of current inhibitors, all of which bind across the active site formed by both subunits in the active dimer.

II. Introduction

The HIV-1 protease is composed of 99 amino acids and is a member of the family of aspartic acid proteases (Oroszlan and Luftig, 1990; Pearl and Taylor, 1987). Unlike the cellular aspartic proteases that are active as monomers, catalytic activity of retroviral proteases including HIV protease requires dimer formation (Wlodawer and Erickson, 1993). The active site of the protease is formed along the dimer interface and each subunit contributes one of the two catalytic aspartic acid residues (D25; Fig. 1; Oroszlan and Luftig, 1990; Wlodawer and Erickson, 1993).

The mature wild-type protease (wt-PR) has served as one of the primary targets for the development of drugs against AIDS because of its indispensable role in processing the precursor proteins Gag and Gag-Pol into mature structural and functional proteins. Structure-based design of drugs targeted against the wt-PR has aided in the development of several potent inhibitors that bind specifically to the active site (Erickson and Burt, 1996). Hundreds of crystal structures of the protease dimer bound to various inhibitors have been solved (Erickson and Burt, 1996; Vondrasek *et al.*, 1997). Although several of these inhibitors are in clinical use and have curtailed the progression of the disease, the effectiveness of long-term treatment has been limited due to naturally selected protease variants exhibiting lower affinity to the drugs than the wt-PR, and this has been a challenge for the past decade (Fig. 2). Various drug-resistant mutants of the protease have been identified [Fig. 2; compiled from databases http://hiv.lanl.gov/content/hivdb/HTML/2005compendium.html (Leitner *et al.*, 2005) and http://hivdb.stanford.edu/cgi-bin/PIResiNote.cgi]. Different resistance mechanisms based on the observed structural and activity changes in drug-resistant mutants have been proposed. In general, the mutations modulate structure and interactions within and distant from the active site as well as inter- and intrasubunit flexibility (Erickson *et al.*, 1999; Mahalingam *et al.*, 1999; Rose *et al.*, 1998).

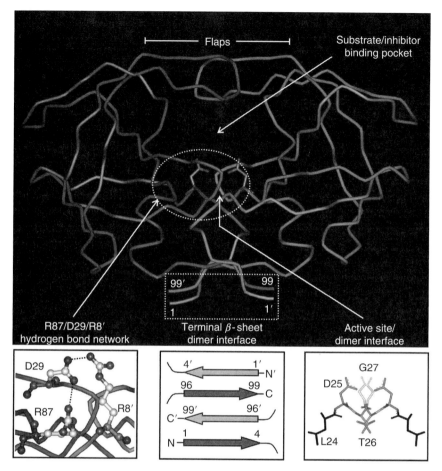

FIGURE 1   Ribbon drawing of the polypeptide backbone of the HIV-1 protease (PDB accession 1A30) with one protease monomer in green and the other in orange. The two major areas that constitute the dimer interface at the active site and the terminal regions, and the intra- and intersubunit contacts between R87-D29 and D29-R8′ residues, respectively, in the protease are indicated. Residues D25 are represented as stick models. The dotted black lines between R87, D29, and R8′ indicate hydrogen bonds (left bottom panel). A schematic drawing depicting the four-stranded terminal β-sheet of the mature protease dimer and the active site dimer interface hydrogen bond network formed by the triplet D25-T26-G27, also know as the "fireman's grip," are shown in the center and right bottom panels, respectively. The flaps essential for recruiting and binding the substrate or inhibitor are shown in a closed conformation. (See Color Insert.)

We had previously reviewed studies aimed at understanding the mechanism of maturation of the protease from the Gag-Pol precursor, enzyme specificity, and emerging issues of drug resistance (Louis *et al.*, 2000). Since then, a major emphasis in protease research has been to improve inhibitor

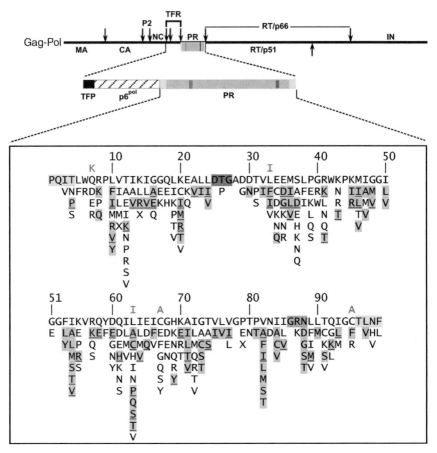

FIGURE 2 Organization of Gag-Pol polyprotein in HIV-1 (top). Straight arrows shown along the Gag-Pol polyprotein indicate specific sites of cleavage by the viral protease. The 99-amino acid protease is flanked at its N-terminus by the transframe region (TFR) consisting of the transframe peptide (TFP) FLREDLAF and 48 amino acids of p6^pol. TFP and p6^pol are separated by a protease cleavage site. Nomenclature of HIV-1 proteins is according to Leis *et al.* (1988). MA, matrix, CA, capsid; PR, protease; NC, nucleocapsid; RT, reverse transcriptase; RN, RNase; IN, integrase. Natural variation and selected drug-resistant mutations of mature HIV-1 protease (bottom). Natural variations in the protease sequence are listed alphabetically below the HXB2 sequence (wt-PR), selected drug-resistant mutations are indicated in cyan and residues common to both are underlined. The two highly conserved regions, the active site triad (DTG) common to all aspartic proteases and the C-terminal triad (GRN/D) unique to retroviral proteases are highlighted in red and gray, respectively. The N- and C-terminal residues involved in forming the dimer interface β-sheet (see Fig. 1) are highlighted in yellow. The optimized construct (pseudo-wild-type, termed PR) suitable for structural and kinetic studies bears five mutations, three mutations Q7K, L33I, L63I that restrict degradation (autoproteolysis) and two mutations C65A and C95A to avoid Cys-thiol oxidation are shown in red above the HXB2 sequence. TMPR bears only three mutations to restrict autoproteolysis used in some NMR studies. (See Color Insert.)

design and treatment regimens, which include the HAART, to overcome the problem of drug resistance and curb progress of the disease (Rodriguez-Barrios and Gago, 2004; Temesgen *et al.*, 2006). In this chapter, we focus on some new and evolving areas of advancement in protease research, namely, the structure and dynamics of the free and inhibited mature protease dimer, comparison of interactions of the protease dimer with previous and new generations of active site inhibitors and elucidation of molecular basis of drug resistance, and finally, mutational studies leading to dimer dissociation together with characterization and structure determination of the protease monomer and its precursor.

III. Mature Protease: Structure, Dynamics, and Relationship to Function

A. Optimization of the Mature Protease for Solution NMR Studies

Solution NMR studies of the wt-PR are difficult due to its rapid autoproteolysis at room temperature, which results in discrete cleavage products even at very low protein concentrations. This limitation has prevented NMR structural studies of the enzyme in the absence of inhibitors or in complex with active site inhibitors with low affinity. However, NMR studies of the protease in a complex with high-affinity inhibitors exhibiting K_i values in the low nanomolar range have been demonstrated (Yamazaki *et al.*, 1996). In this case, the inhibitor blocks autoproteolysis. The effect on protein integrity conferred by a tight binding inhibitor is readily appreciated from the Fig. 3 inset. Without inhibitor, autoproteolysis occurs within hours while inhibitor complexed protease is relatively stable.

The three major sites of autoproteloysis in the enzyme are L5/W6, L33/E34, and L63/I64 (Mildner *et al.*, 1994; Rose *et al.*, 1993). Extensive kinetic studies using peptides and proteins as substrates, together with the three-dimensional structure of the mature protease, have helped to establish and demonstrate that introduction of β-branched amino acids at P_1 or Lys at P_2' in the three autolysis sites greatly diminishes hydrolysis at corresponding P_1-P_1' positions (Dunn *et al.*, 1994; Tomaselli and Heinrikson, 1994). A mutant enzyme bearing the substitutions Q7K, L33I, and L63I (TMPR; Fig. 3) retains the specificity and kinetic properties of the wt-PR and is highly stabilized against autoproteolysis (Mildner *et al.*, 1994; Szeltner and Polgar, 1996). In addition to its resistance to autoproteolysis, TMPR exhibits a modest increase in its stability with regard to urea denaturation as compared to the wt-PR (Szeltner and Polgar, 1996). Figure 3 shows an ^{1}H-^{15}N HSQC spectrum of the TMPR at 0.5 mM. As is immediately apparent, the spectrum

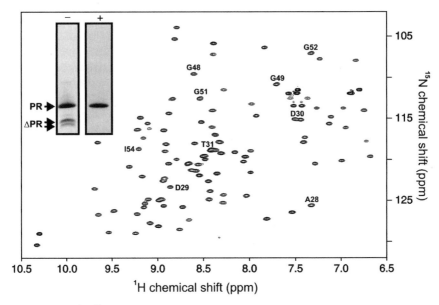

FIGURE 3 ^{1}H-^{15}N HSQC spectrum of TMPR (Fig. 2) in 10-mM phosphate buffer, pH 5.8, 2-mM DTT, 25°C. Selected cross peaks are identified by residue number in the mature protease sequence. Inset: analyses of uninhibited (−) and inhibited (+) C67A, C95A protease by SDS-PAGE. ΔPR denotes fragments of the protease resulting from autoproteolysis in the absence of the mutations Q7K, L33I, L63I.

is well dispersed and a large number of resonances exhibit very similar shifts to those reported for complexes with inhibitors (Yamazaki *et al.*, 1994). As expected, the largest chemical shift changes observed between the free-enzyme and drug complexes occur for residues at the active site and flap region surrounding the inhibitor.

Other factors to consider for long-term studies with respect to sample integrity are the presence of the Cys residues (C67 and C95) which have a tendency to form intermolecular disulfide bonds at concentrations commonly employed for NMR. It was shown that a Cys to Ala substitution at residue 95 of the mature protease greatly reduced the tendency of the protein to form intermolecular cross-links (Yamazaki *et al.*, 1996). Subsequent studies have demonstrated that both Cys residues, C67 and C95, of the protease can be exchanged to Ala without having significant effect on the kinetic parameters of the mutated enzyme as well as structure (Louis *et al.*, 1999a,b). The stability of the protease bearing these five mutations (pseudo-wild type, termed PR) is similar to that reported for TMPR (Szeltner and Polgar, 1996) with a midpoint transition of ~2-M urea (Louis *et al.*, 1999a).

B. Flap Dynamics

The crystal structure of the mature protease was first determined in 1989 (Miller *et al.*, 1989; Navia *et al.*, 1989). The protease forms nearly a symmetric dimer in which the subunits interface around the active site and the terminal regions (residues 1–4 and 96–99; Fig. 1). In the inhibitor-bound form of protease, the flaps (residues 47–56) cover the substrate or inhibitor and interact with each other (closed conformation). Initial studies monitoring fluorescence changes of the protease in the absence of inhibitor have shown that the flaps are flexible in solution (Furfine *et al.*, 1992; Rodriguez *et al.*, 1993). Based on the difference in the flap conformations between the free and inhibitor-bound forms as well as changes in the catalytic activity due to mutations of the flap residues (Tozser *et al.*, 1997), it has been long recognized that the flexibility of the protease flaps must play a role in inhibitor/substrate binding. Therefore, the flap dynamics have been investigated using NMR to pinpoint sites or regions involved in the motion and to estimate the timescales. Although both NMR and crystallography can determine atomic coordinates of protein structures, NMR is more suitable to study protein internal motion and equilibria involving multiple forms (e.g, monomer–dimer equilibrium), as there are no packing effects in solution NMR studies.

Using the optimized constructs described in the previous section, initial studies involved ^{1}H and ^{15}N relaxation experiments for the mature protease in its free form to understand flap dynamics experimentally at the atomic level. As shown in Fig. 4, in the free protease, residues G49, G51, G52, and I54 have significant values of ^{15}N R_{ex_diff}, while residues G48, G49, I50, G51, G52, F53, I54, and K55 have large values of ^{1}H R_{ex_diff} that is a difference in transverse relaxation rates measured at 92 Hz and 2 kHz effective field strength (Ishima *et al.*, 1999). Significant values of R_{ex_diff} indicate conformational exchange in millisecond timescale. Based on the ratio of the ^{15}N R_{ex_diff} and ^{1}H R_{ex_diff}, the sites that exhibit significant R_{ex_diff} values, except for G49 and F53, were suggested to undergo conformational exchange that involves changes in backbone angles rather than change in the relative orientation from the aromatic ring nearby. Assuming a two-site exchange, the correlation time for conformational exchange was estimated to be 0.1 ms for residues 48–55 in the flaps of the free protease at $20\,^\circ$C, pH 5.8.

In addition to this millisecond motion, the flap region of the free protease also undergoes sub-nanosecond motion, which was shown by applying the "model-free" analysis of ^{15}N relaxation (Freedberg *et al.*, 2002). Significant reduction of generalized order parameters, S^2, for the amide sites in the flap region (48–52) as well as an elbow region (38–42) was observed (Fig. 5A), indicating that these sites undergo motions faster than the overall tumbling of the molecule. The correlation time for internal motion of

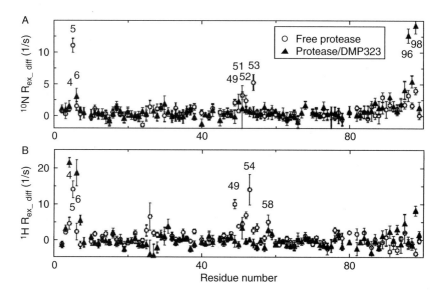

FIGURE 4   Comparison of (A) ^{15}N and (B) ^{1}H chemical exchange term, R_{ex_diff}, for the protease bound to DMP323 (closed triangle) with R_{ex_diff} observed for the free protease (circle). R_{ex_diff} indicates degree of ms-μs motion characterized by chemical exchange (Ishima *et al.*, 1999). The experiment was performed using ~0.4-mM PR dimer in 20-mM phosphate buffer, pH 5.8, 20°C.

the flap region was estimated to be ca. 1 ns by the model-free analysis (Fig. 5B). Based on these relaxation results, together with the observation of nuclear Overhauser effect (NOEs) that indicated a β-hairpin structure in the flap region of the free protease, a working model was proposed. In this model, the flap structures are mostly semi-open conformations, having a dynamic hydrogen-bonded hairpin structure that undergoes nanosecond timescale motion. In addition, the semi-open flaps also exhibit conformational exchange on the millisecond timescale.

The model-free analyses of the protease in the presence of two different types of active site inhibitors did not exhibit reduced S^2 values in the flap region (Nicholson *et al.*, 1995), which is consistent with the observation of a single closed flap conformation in the crystal structures of various protease-inhibitor complexes. However, even in the inhibitor-bound forms of PR, significant milli-microsecond motion was observed for residues 50 and 51 that are the tip of the flaps (Nicholson *et al.*, 1995). Similarly, the limited milli-micro second motion was also observed for residues I47 and G48 in one of the flaps in a protease–substrate complex (Katoh *et al.*, 2003). Comparison of the residues that were found to undergo milli-micro second motion in PR (or PR$_{D25N}$) bound to DMP323, P9941, KNI272 inhibitors, and substrate demonstrated that the flap conformational exchange on the

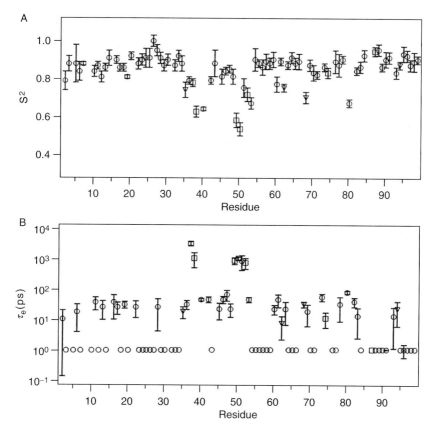

FIGURE 5 Generalized order parameter, S^2, which indicates degree of internal motion on sub-ns timescale (A), and a correlation time for internal motion (B) of the mature protease in the absence of inhibitors in 20-mM phosphate buffer, pH 5.8, 20°C (Freedberg *et al.*, 2002).

milli-microsecond timescale was not simply related to ligand-binding affinity and appears to be very sensitive to the chemical structure of the ligand (Katoh *et al.*, 2003).

Although NMR elucidated sites that undergo internal motion and the timescale of the motion, NMR did not provide information about the trajectories of the mobile atomic sites. Therefore, MD simulation is a useful complementary approach to obtain such information. Recent longtime simulations provide predictions of conformation changes on the nanosecond timescale. Published simulations have all predicted mobility in the flap regions, although there are differences in the predicted extent of the motion (Chen *et al.*, 2004; Hornak *et al.*, 2006; Perryman *et al.*, 2004; Scott and Schiffer, 2000). Accelerated MD or other longtime simulation approaches have predicted flap opening on slower than nanosecond timescale (Collins *et al.*, 1995; Hamelberg and McCammon, 2005; Rick *et al.*, 1998).

C. Dynamics at the Dimer Interface

The terminal residues 1–4 and 96–99 exhibit extensive subunit interaction forming the four-stranded β-sheet (Miller *et al.*, 1989; Weber, 1990). Earlier MD simulations have shown that the hydrogen bonds predicted in crystal structures for the terminal β-sheet are well maintained and that the terminal β-sheet is very stable in solution (Harte *et al.*, 1990; York *et al.*, 1993). Thermodynamic measurements have also suggested that the terminal β-sheet is the most stable region in the mature protease and that dimer formation is concomitant with protease folding (Todd *et al.*, 1998). Thus, all these experimental and theoretical studies demonstrated that the terminal β-sheet is very stable in the protease dimer. In contrast to these observations, NMR relaxation studies were the first to demonstrate conformational flexibility of the terminal β-sheet. As shown in Fig. 4, significant ^{15}N R_{ex_diff} values were observed for residues T4, W6, T96, and N98 in the PR particularly in its inhibitor-bound form (Ishima *et al.*, 1999). Since this region had been expected to be rigid, extensive systematic relaxation dispersion experiments (which are similar to R_{ex_diff} measurements but more quantitative) were performed to obtain more accurate dynamics information. Amide nitrogen, proton, and carbonyl carbon NMR results consistently indicated significant conformational exchange in the terminal β-sheet, with a minor population of 5–10% at 0.5 mM concentration at 20°C (Ishima and Torchia, 2003, 2005; Ishima *et al.*, 2004).

In the Gag-Pol polyprotein, the protease is flanked by the transframe region (TFR) and the reverse transcriptase domains at the N- and C-termini, respectively (Fig. 2; Louis *et al.*, 1998; Oroszlan and Luftig, 1990). Hence, the flexibility of the terminal residues seen on inhibitor binding may relate to accessibility for cleavage at the C-terminus of the protease during its maturation from Gag-Pol, which occurs via an intermolecular process (i.e., one dimer cleaves the PR–RT junction of another dimer) subsequent to the intramolecular cleavage at its N-terminus (TFR-PR junction; Louis *et al.*, 1994; Wondrak *et al.*, 1996). This interpretation is consistent with kinetic data showing that the second-order rate constant for the conversion of PR-ΔRT precursor (Δ denotes truncated) to the mature protease is ∼40-fold smaller, suggesting a restricted cleavage, than for the mature protease-catalyzed hydrolysis of a peptide substrate spanning the same C-terminal cleavage site (Wondrak *et al.*, 1996).

D. Side Chain Dynamics and Protease Packing

Although backbone dynamics studied by NMR elucidated flexible regions of the protease main chain, it is also important to characterize side chain dynamics in order to better understand protein-inhibitor interactions and to clarify the structural consequences of the drug-resistant mutations far from the active site region. Among the side chains, it is important to elucidate dynamics of methyl groups first because the protease contains an unusually high content (45%) of side chains containing methyl groups, and second because about 65% of the protease mutations associated with drug resistance involve such residues. Calculations using protease crystal structure coordinates reveal two methyl clusters in PR: the inner cluster that nearly surrounds the active site and the outer cluster that contains the hydrophobic core that stabilizes the inhibitor-free protease structure (Fig. 6; Ishima *et al.*, 2001b). Similar calculations for other retroviral proteases revealed that such two-methyl, inner and outer, cluster motifs appear to be a common structural feature unique to retroviral proteases.

NMR relaxation studies indicated that some protease methyl groups were flexible in solution. Sub-nanosecond motion of the methyl groups exposed to the solvent, such as residues L38, I50, and I54, was expected. Similarly, based on the backbone dynamics described in the previous paragraph, it was not surprising that buried methyl groups at the terminal β-sheet were also found to undergo conformational exchange on the milli-micro second timescale. An unexpected observation was the flexibility of methyl groups of V75 and L76 that are buried in the protease core and link the two methyl clusters (Fig. 6). Although L10 and L23 are partially exposed to the solvent, these

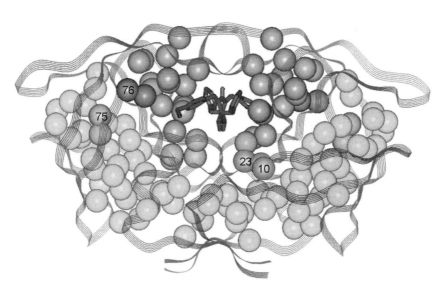

FIGURE 6   Methyl groups in inner (pink spheres) and outer (green spheres) clusters, and a ribbon diagram of the mature protease backbone. Yellow and orange spheres represent methyl groups undergoing motions on sub-ns and ms-μs timescales, respectively. The number on the sphere indicates residue position. The experiment was performed in 20-mM phosphate buffer, pH 5.8, 20 °C (Ishima *et al.*, 2001b). (See Color Insert.)

residues were also located at the cluster linker region and flexible on the sub-nanosecond timescale. Based on these observations, it is proposed that the flexibility at the cluster interface is a possible mechanism to minimize structural perturbations of mutations near and far from the active site.

IV. Active Site Inhibitors and Drug Resistance

A. Protease Interactions with Antiviral Inhibitors

Numerous crystal structures of mature protease with various inhibitors were used to guide designs during the development of clinical inhibitors (Wlodawer and Vondrasek, 1998). Antiviral protease inhibitors were first approved for clinical use in 1995. Nine protease inhibitors have been approved to date for treatment of HIV infection: saquinavir, indinavir, nelfinavir, ritonavir, atazanavir, lopinavir, amprenavir, tipranavir, and darunavir. These clinical inhibitors were designed to inhibit the wt-PR by binding to the active site. Crystal structures have demonstrated that the protease forms a substrate binding site consisting of subsites S3-S4′ spanning at least seven residues (P3-P4′) of a peptide substrate (Mahalingam *et al.*, 2001; Prabu-Jeyabalan *et al.*, 2002, 2003, 2004). Conserved hydrogen bond interactions are formed between the main chain amides and carbonyl oxygens of the peptide and the protease (Gustchina *et al.*, 1994; Louis *et al.*, 2000). In contrast, the clinical inhibitors are smaller than peptide substrates, and they bind mostly in the protease subsites S2-S2′ near the middle of the dimer (Chen *et al.*, 1994; Krohn *et al.*, 1991). They contain a central hydroxyl group that mimics the tetrahedral reaction intermediate and interacts with the side chain oxygens of the catalytic residues D25 and D25′ (Fig. 7). The large hydrophobic groups at P1 and P1′ on either side of the hydroxyl group increase the affinity for protease by binding in the hydrophobic S1 and S1 subsites. All the inhibitors contain polar groups that form several hydrogen bond interactions with the protease, similar to those observed for peptide analogues. Additionally, the hydrogen bond interactions mediated by the conserved water molecule (Gustchina *et al.*, 1994) are maintained in these clinical inhibitors. This highly conserved water has been proven to be important for catalysis (Grzesiek *et al.*, 1994; Wang *et al.*, 1996). Recent crystal structures have shown an altered flap conformation in complexes with peptide analogue and emphasize the important role of the flap region (Prabu-Jeyabalan *et al.*, 2006).

The first generation of clinical inhibitors, such as saquinavir and indinavir, provide high-affinity binding by maximizing the hydrophobic interactions with protease. However, they show fewer polar interactions than the peptide analogues. Indinavir, for example, has only two hydrogen bonds with main chain atoms of the protease and one with the side chain of D29

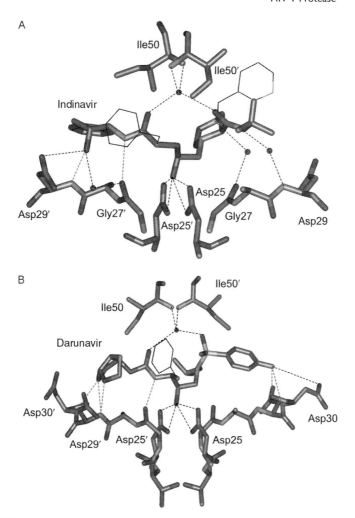

A

Ile50
Ile50'
Indinavir
Asp25
Asp29'   Gly27'   Gly27   Asp29
Asp25'

B

Ile50'
Ile50
Darunavir
Asp30'
Asp30
Asp29'   Asp25'   Asp25

FIGURE 7 Protease interactions with inhibitors indinavir (A) (Liu *et al.*, 2005; Mahalingam *et al.*, 2004) and darunavir (B) (Kovalevsky *et al.*, 2006a,b; Tie *et al.*, 2004). Water molecules are indicated by red spheres. Hydrogen bond interactions are shown as dashed lines. Red lines indicate hydrogen bonds with the main chain atoms of the protease and black lines indicate hydrogen bonds with side chain atoms of the protease or with water. (See Color Insert.)

(Fig. 7A) (Mahalingam *et al.*, 2004). Calorimetric studies have shown that the thermodynamics of binding of these first-generation inhibitors is entropically driven (Velazquez-Campoy *et al.*, 2000a,b). These crystallographic and thermodynamic data are valuable for the design of antiviral inhibitors to combat drug resistance (Ghosh *et al.*, 2006; Ohtaka and Freire, 2005; Ohtaka *et al.*, 2004). Ideally, the inhibitor should bind with high affinity to both the wt-PR and the drug-resistant variants. Thus, the general strategy is to optimize interactions between the inhibitor and conserved regions of the protease, and to introduce smaller or more flexible groups that will adapt to interact with variable regions of the protease. New, second-generation inhibitors, such as darunavir, have been designed to combat drug-resistant mutants by increasing the number of polar interactions with main chain atoms of the protease (Ghosh *et al.*, 2006). Darunavir binding to the protease is enthalpically driven, in contrast to the binding of the earlier drugs (King *et al.*, 2004). The crystal structure of protease in complex with darunavir showed six hydrogen bonds with main chain atoms and one with the side chain of D30 (Fig. 7B) Koh *et al.*, 2003; Tie *et al.*, 2004). These hydrogen bonds are similar to those of substrate analogues (Gustchina *et al.*, 1994; Tie *et al.*, 2005). Compared to other clinical inhibitors, darunavir has extra polar interactions with D29 and D30. These interactions resemble those of the P2′ Gln or Glu side chain of peptide analogues (Tie *et al.*, 2005; Weber *et al.*, 1997). These polar interactions of darunavir with D29 and D30 are predicted to be critical for its excellent resistance profile. The importance of preserving D29 and its interaction with the conserved R87 for the monomer–dimer equilibrium is discussed below. Interestingly, the 0.84- and 1.22-Å resolution structures of V32I and M46L mutant–darunavir complexes, respectively, showed a second binding site for darunavir on the protease surface in one flap region of the dimer (Kovalevsky *et al.*, 2006a). Remarkably, the shape of the flap site accommodates the diastereomer of darunavir with the *S*-enantiomeric nitrogen rather than the one with the *R*-enantiomeric nitrogen that is bound at the active site. The two diastereomers of darunavir are related by inversion of the sulfonamide nitrogen. The existence of this second site on the protease flap was proposed to assist in the effectiveness of darunavir on resistant HIV. The surface binding site in the flap provides another possible target for inhibitor design.

In summary, the initial antiviral protease inhibitors like indinavir were designed with large hydrophobic groups to maximize the hydrophobic interactions with the protease. Exposure to these drugs has resulted in development of high levels of resistance due to mutation of residues located in the protease active site, D30, G48, I50, V82, I84, and of nonactive site residues such as M46 and L90 (Mahalingam *et al.*, 2001) (Fig. 2). Combinations of several different mutations can be required to produce high levels of resistance. The newer antiviral inhibitors were designed to overcome resistance by reducing the size of the hydrophobic groups so that mutation of the active site residues will have less effect on inhibitor affinity and by adding favorable polar interactions with main chain atoms, which cannot be directly altered by mutation. Darunavir exemplifies both these design strategies, since the hydrophobic groups at P1 and P1′ are smaller than those of indinavir, and additional hydrogen bond interactions are formed with the main chain amides of D29 and D30. Moreover, darunavir was recently approved for clinical use, and so far no resistant mutants have been confirmed in clinical isolates.

B. Atomic Resolution Crystal Structures of Drug-Resistant Mutants

The structural effects of drug-resistant mutants of the protease have been illuminated by many crystal structures, especially several over the past few years that were solved at atomic (1.0–1.25 Å) (Kovalevsky *et al.*, 2006a,b; Liu *et al.*, 2005; Mahalingam *et al.*, 2004; Tie *et al.*, 2004, 2005) or subatomic (0.84 Å) resolution (Kovalevsky *et al.*, 2006a). The crystallographic analysis has benefited from the optimized protease construct with the five stabilizing mutations as described earlier. The diffraction data were obtained at very high resolution through the use of high-intensity synchrotron X-ray beamlines and optimization of different crystallization conditions. X-ray diffraction data were collected at the National Synchrotron Light Source, beamline X26C or the Advanced Photon Source, SER-CAT beamline. The screening for crystals was performed by the hanging drop vapor diffusion method using variations of the following two general conditions: 0.1-M sodium acetate buffer, pH 4.2–5.0, with precipitant of 0.4- to 1.2-M sodium chloride, or 0.1-M citrate phosphate buffer, pH 4.5–6.4, with 15–40% saturated ammonium sulfate as the precipitating agent. Possible additives to improve crystals are DMSO (which is usually needed to dissolve inhibitor), glycerol, methyl pentanediol, and dioxane. Varying these conditions has resulted in crystals for the majority of tested mutant/inhibitor combinations that diffract to high (better than 1.5 Å) or even subatomic resolution. These very accurate structures permit analysis of details of the protease-inhibitor interactions and changes introduced by the mutations.

The drug-resistant mutations observed in clinical isolates map to different regions of the three-dimensional protease structure. Many well-characterized mutations alter mostly hydrophobic residues, including D30N, V32I, G48V, I50V, V82A, and I84V that form the inhibitor-binding site or active site of the protease. Alternatively, mutations can alter residues that contribute to the interactions at the dimer interface such as R8Q, L24I, I50V, and F53L. A third category of mutations alters residues distal to the protease active site or dimer interface, including M46L, G71A, and G73S. High to atomic resolution structures have been analyzed for mutant complexes with indinavir (Liu *et al.*, 2005; Mahalingam *et al.*, 2004) or darunavir (Kovalevsky *et al.*, 2006a,b; Tie *et al.*, 2004), as well as with peptide analogues (Tie *et al.*, 2005). Crystallographic analysis has revealed distinct structural changes for each mutant relative to the wt-PR structure. The observed structural changes will be described separately for each category of resistant mutation.

I. Resistant Mutations of the Active Site Residues

Mutation of the active site residues showed varied effects in comparison with the wt-PR. The active site residues that are commonly observed to mutate in isolates with high-level resistance to one or more drugs are D30, V32, G48, I50, V82, and I84. Structural changes were observed at the site of mutation and depended on the type of mutation. The most obvious change was shown by mutation of the hydrophobic active site residue I84V, which resulted in the loss of van der Waals interactions due to the substitution of the smaller valine for isoleucine. Similar changes were observed in complexes with a peptide analogue (Tie *et al.*, 2005) and the clinical inhibitor darunavir (Tie *et al.*, 2004). I50V also showed reduced interactions with peptide analogue, indinavir, and darunavir (Kovalevsky *et al.*, 2006b; Liu *et al.*, 2005), and V32I also had reduced interactions with darunavir bound in the active site (Kovalevsky *et al.*, 2006a). In contrast, mutation V82A of another hydrophobic active site residue showed a shift in the protease main chain and compensation of van der Waals interactions with peptide analogues (Tie *et al.*, 2005), indinavir (Mahalingam *et al.*, 2004) and darunavir (Tie *et al.*, 2004), as illustrated in Fig. 8A. Mutation of the polar residue D30N in the protease active site showed an altered conformation of the side chain of D30/N30 in complexes with peptide analogues (Mahalingam *et al.*, 2001) and darunavir (Kovalevsky *et al.*, 2006b). The side chain of N30 formed a water-mediated interaction with inhibitor rather than a direct hydrogen bond. Therefore, resistant mutations of residues forming the active site show distinct effects including loss of favorable hydrophobic interactions and consequently lower affinity for inhibitor, adaptive shifts of the main chain atoms to provide compensating hydrophobic contacts, and altered side chain conformation and interaction with inhibitor. The structural flexibility of the protease active site can provide adaptation for the mutants to bind substrates and inhibitors. The drugs such as indinavir containing larger hydrophobic groups are likely to be most sensitive to mutation of the hydrophobic active site residues. Newer drugs like darunavir showed smaller changes in the interactions with mutant proteases and maintained higher affinity for the resistant protease.

2. Nonactive Site Mutations

The structures containing nonactive site mutations have revealed indirect effects on the protease active site. Mutation of residues outside of the active site has a significant role in drug resistance (Muzammil *et al.*, 2003). Unfortunately, there are fewer structural studies of the nonactive site mutations that are not located at the dimer interface. The nonactive site mutation L90M has consistently resulted in close repulsive contacts with the catalytic D25 in complexes with peptide analogues (Mahalingam, 2001; Shafer, 2002), indinavir (Mahalingam *et al.*, 2004) and darunavir (Kovalevsky *et al.*, 2006b). Moreover, the mutation L90M also resulted in additional

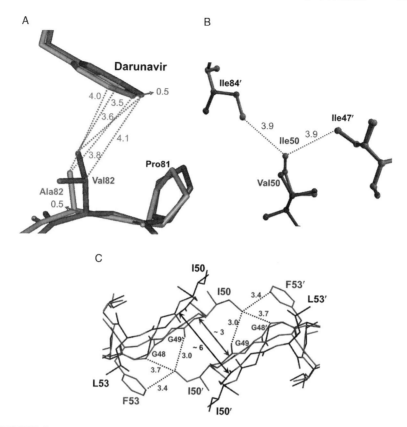

FIGURE 8   (A) Interactions of darunavir with V82 in wt-PR (magenta) and A82 in mutant (cyan). Hydrophobic contacts are indicated by dotted lines with the interatomic separation in angstroms. The structural shift of the C_α atom of residue 82 is shown as a red arrow with distance in angstroms. (B) Intersubunit interactions of I/V50 in crystal structures of I50V mutant (red) and wt-PR (green) with peptide analogue. Favorable van der Waals interactions are shown as dotted lines. Interatomic distances are shown in angstroms. (C) Comparison of intersubunit interactions of residue 53 in unliganded structures of wt (brown) and F53L mutant (black). (See Color Insert.)

interactions with indinavir (Mahalingam *et al.*, 2004) and darunavir (Kovalevsky *et al.*, 2006b) and showed increased inhibition of the mutant compared to the wt-PR. Residue M46 is commonly mutated in resistant isolates. This flap residue does not contribute directly to the inhibitor binding site, although the main chain atoms of M46 form hydrogen bond interactions with longer peptide analogues (Tie *et al.*, 2005). The structure of protease with the M46L mutation showed a loss of favorable interactions with darunavir at the active site (Kovalevsky *et al.*, 2006a). Mutation G73S, which is located far from the active site, introduced additional hydrogen bond interactions that were proposed to transmit changes to the substrate binding site and alter catalytic activity (Liu et al., 2005).

3. Mutations That Alter the Dimer Interface

Residues forming the dimer interface are conserved in protease sequences from HIV-infected patients. In vivo conservation of the protease in a large patient cohort in the absence and presence of pharmacological pressure has been reported (Ceccherini-Silberstein et al., 2004). Interestingly, conservation of the sequence decreases to about 45% in drug-treated patients as compared to 68% in untreated patients. While the terminal regions of the protease, P1-P9 and G94-F99, were conserved to about the same extent, in drug-treated individuals, regions within the protease are conserved to a smaller extent spanning residues D25-D29, G49-G52, G78-P81, and G86-R87 (Figs. 1 and 2). Exceptions to this conservation are mutations of I50, a residue that also interacts with inhibitor in the active site, as described in the previous section, and L24I adjacent to the catalytic Asp. Crystal structures have been analyzed for protease with mutations L24I, I50V, and F53L that alter residues at the dimer interface. Both L24I and I50V mutations had altered intersubunit contacts in complexes with a peptide analogue or indinavir (Liu et al., 2005). In agreement with these structural changes, mutants L24I and I50V showed higher dissociation of the dimer relative to wt-PR. Residue F53 does not form intersubunit contacts in the protease dimer in complex with inhibitor; however, the F53L mutation had an unexpected effect on the unliganded form of the protease (Liu et al., 2006). The F53L mutant had lost the intersubunit contact of the side chains of F53 with I50 that was observed in the wt-PR in the unliganded form (Fig. 8C). Increased dissociation of the F53L dimer was observed, which was consistent with the crystallographic data. Therefore, the dimer interface is particularly sensitive to mutation, which results in slightly increased dissociation of the dimer and altered intersubunit interactions both in the free (open) (Liu et al., 2006) and inhibitor-bound (closed) (Liu et al., 2005) protease dimer.

V. Dissociation of the Mature Protease Dimer and Characterization of the Monomeric Structure

It has long been recognized that disrupting the terminal β-sheet arrangement, which contributes to about 50% of the total dimer interface contacts, may provide an alternative avenue for inhibitor design thus extending the target area of current inhibitors, all of which bind across the active site formed by both subunits in the active dimer (Rodriguez-Barrios and Gago, 2004; Sluis-Cremer and Tachedjian, 2002; Weber, 1990). This presumably noncompetitive mode of inhibition might show a synergistic effect to the conventional active site–targeted compounds with the advantage of reducing the emergence of drug-resistant strains. Initial reports indicate that peptide analogues derived from the terminal regions of the protease inhibit enzymatic activity by blocking dimer formation (Babe *et al.*, 1992; Schramm *et al.*, 1991; Shultz and Chmielewski, 1999; Zhang *et al.*, 1991). Cross-linked interface peptides with semi-rigid or flexible spacers as well as analogues having lipophilic terminal groups have been developed as dimerization inhibitors (Bowman and Chmielewski, 2002; Merabet *et al.*, 2004; Rodriguez-Barrios and Gago, 2004; Schramm *et al.*, 1996, 1999; Sluis-Cremer and Tachedjian, 2002). Modular inhibitors, in which the active site–directed compound is tethered to a dimerization inhibitor, and non-peptide-based inhibitors of dimerization have also been described (Sluis-Cremer and Tachedjian, 2002; Uhlikova *et al.*, 1996). However, to date, such complexes have not been confirmed at atomic resolutions, by either X-ray crystallography or NMR. In addition, to our knowledge, none of these kinds of potential lead compounds have been developed further for possible clinical use.

The mature protease forms a stable dimer and exhibits a very low equilibrium dissociation constant ($K_d < 10 \times 10^{-9}$ M; Grant *et al.*, 1992; Louis *et al.*, 1999a; Todd *et al.*, 1998; Zhang *et al.*, 1991). Thus, studies targeting dimerization using peptides or non-peptide analogues will benefit from complementary structural and biophysical studies aimed at understanding the dissociation of the dimer and, in particular, the role of conserved regions in the protease required for a native fold and dimer formation. It is anticipated that insights derived from such studies will aid in the discovery and rational design of novel inhibitors aimed at binding to the monomer at the dimerization interface. Having established the conditions for solution NMR studies of the free protease as described above, several substitution and deletion mutations were introduced into the optimized construct, PR, for subsequent analysis by NMR, equilibrium sedimentation analysis, and kinetics. Results of the analysis of the various mutants of PR are summarized in Table I.

A. Identification and Characterization of the Monomer Fold

1. R87-D29-R8' Hydrogen Bond Network

While the active site triad D25-T26-G27 is common to all aspartic acid proteases, residues G86-R87-N/D88 in the α-helix are unique to retroviral proteases (Fig. 1) (Louis *et al.*, 1989; Pearl and Taylor, 1987). The very first identification of a folded monomer of the mature protease came from studies of the PR_{R87K} mutant. PR folds from a denatured state into an enzymatically active stable dimer similar to the wt-PR, when dialyzed from pH 2.8 to pH 4.2–5.8. In contrast, under the same folding conditions, the PR_{R87K} mutant folds as a monomer (Ishima *et al.*, 2001a). This was

TABLE I Summary of Folded Forms of Protease Constructs

Construct	Class	−I (Ratio by ESA)	+I (Ratio by ESA)
PR	Dimer (1.87/0.02)	Dimer-I complex (1.96/0.01)	
$PR_{D25N}^{a,b}$	A	Dimer	Dimer-I complex
$PR_{R8Q}^{c,d}$	A	Dimer	Dimer-I complex
PR_{D29N}^{d}	B	Monomer + Dimer	Dimer-I complex
PR_{T26A}^{d}	C	Monomer	Monomer+Dimer-I complex
PR_{R87K}^{e}	C	Monomer (0.98/0.05)	Monomer+ Dimer-I complex (1.57/0.09)
$PR_{1-95}^{b,e}$	D	Monomer (1.01/0.04)	Monomer (1.13/0.11)
PR_{5-99}^{e}	B	Monomer+ Dimer (1.04/0.01)	Dimer-I complex (1.87/0.06)
$TFP^{-P6}pol\text{-}PR_{D25N}^{b}$	C	Monomer	Monomer+ Dimer-I complex*
$TFP^{-P6}pol\text{-}PR_{1-95}^{b}$	D	Monomer	Monomer
$^{SFNF}PR_{D25N}^{b}$	C	Monomer	Dimer-I complex
$^{MI}PR^{b}$	B	Monomer > Dimer	Dimer-I complex
$^{MG}\text{-}PR^{b}$	B	Monomer < Dimer	Dimer-I complex

[a-e]Cited from references Katoh et al., 2003; Ishima et al., 2001a, 2003; Louis et al., 1999a, 2003, respectively.
*Under these conditions, <10% of $TFP^{-P6}pol\text{-}PR_{D25N}$ forms Dimer-I complex.
$1H$-^{15}N correlation spectra were acquired on ∼0.5-mM samples (in monomer) in 20-mM phosphate buffer, pH 5.8, 20°C either in the absence or approximately five-fold excess of the potent inhibitor DMP323 (denoted by I, K_i = ∼1 nM, Lam et al., 1996). Classes A to D define the effect of mutations on the K_d ranging from 0.5×10^{-6} M to 1×10^{-3} M, an increase of approximately two to five orders of magnitude as compared to the wild-type mature protease ($<10 \times 10^{-9}$ M). Ratio by ESA denotes molecular weight determined experimentally by equilibrium sedimentation analysis (ESA) divided by the calculated molecular weight.

initially suggested by the ^1H-^{15}N correlation spectrum recorded on a sample of PR_{R87K} which displays a set of well-dispersed signals indicating a folded conformation of the protein, but different from PR (Fig. 9A). Addition of the potent inhibitor DMP323 to PR_{R87K} results in two sets of signals (Fig. 9B) with the set having minor intensity belonging to free PR_{R87K}. The C_α chemical shifts of the major set for PR_{R87K} in the presence of DMP323 (Fig. 10B) are nearly identical to the C_α shifts in the PR–DMP323 complex suggesting that ternary complexes, PR dimer–DMP323 and PR_{R87K} dimer–DMP323, exhibit very similar structures.

Even in the absence of DMP323, the overall backbone C_α chemical shifts of PR_{R87K} residues are similar to those of PR (Fig. 10A). However, unlike the DMP323 bound forms of PR and PR_{R87K}, significant differences in chemical shifts of the free forms of PR and PR_{R87K} were noted for residues at the dimer interface, that is, near the active site (residues 24–29) and the N- and C-terminal regions (residues 1–10 and 90–99). In particular, the peaks for I3, Q92, I93, G94, and A95 that significantly shift in the dimer due to intermonomer and not DMP323 interaction are not observed

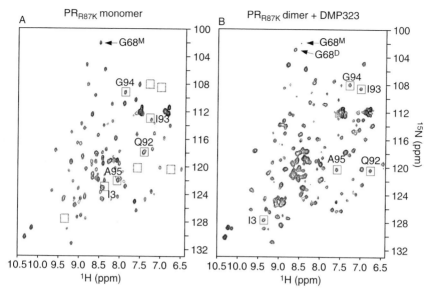

FIGURE 9   Amide ^{1}H-^{15}N HSQC spectra of (A) PR$_{R87K}$ and (B) PR$_{R87K}$ in the presence of inhibitor DMP323 measured in 20-mM phosphate buffer, pH 5.8, 20 °C (Ishima *et al.*, 2001a). Boxes in (A) and (B) delineate the location of peaks that exhibit significant changes due to dimer formation. Peaks of G68 for the dimer and monomer forms of PR$_{R87K}$ are labeled G68^D and G68^M, respectively.

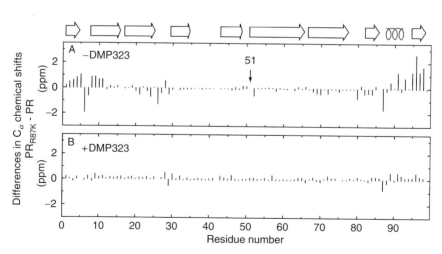

FIGURE 10   Differences in backbone C$_\alpha$ chemical shifts between PR and PR$_{R87K}$ in the (A) absence and (B) presence of DMP323 together with the secondary structure of PR (Ishima *et al.*, 2001a). The single α-helix and the β-strands are depicted as a coil and boxed arrows, respectively. Residue 51 whose C$_\alpha$ carbon was not assigned due to broadening of the signal in PR$_{R87K}$ is indicated.

in the corresponding positions in the free PR$_{R87K}$ spectrum (Figs. 9A and 10A). Additional approaches that include determining the relative translational diffusion by NMR, sedimentation equilibrium analysis (see Table I), and kinetics support the conclusion that PR$_{R87K}$ is a folded monomer at $\sim$0.5 mM in monomer concentration (Ishima *et al.*, 2001a). Thus, the most conservative change of the highly conserved R87 residue (R87K) leads to a drastic increase in the K_d by about five orders of magnitude.

Analysis of the ^{15}N relaxation experiments, as shown by the elevated T$_1$ and T$_2$ values and reduced NOE values, revealed significant motions on the sub-nanosecond timescale for both N- and C-terminal residues 2–10 and 93–99, respectively, the elbow residues 37–42 and the flap residues 48–53 in PR$_{R87K}$ (Ishima *et al.*, 2001a). Although the mobility of the flap and the elbow regions had been shown for free dimeric PR, increased sub-nanosecond motion of the termini had not been observed (Ishima *et al.*, 1999; Todd *et al.*, 1998). Inspection of a model of monomeric protease (Ishima *et al.*, 2001a) reveals that the mobile areas correspond to solvent-exposed regions, assuming the monomer structure remains essentially identical to that of a single subunit of the dimer.

The side chain of highly conserved R87 residue, residing on the sole α-helix (residues 87–91), forms a hydrogen bond with D29, a residue that is located near the active site and interacts with peptide analogues and inhibitors (Fig. 1; Wlodawer *et al.*, 1989). D29 is involved in two pivotal interactions: the first is a hydrogen bond between one of the carboxylate oxygens and the guanidinium group of R87 within the monomer, whereas the second is an intersubunit hydrogen bond across the dimer interface between the second D29 carboxylate oxygen and guanidine group of R8′ of the other monomer (Fig. 1; PDB accession 1A30; Louis *et al.*, 1998). Analysis of the complimentary mutants PR$_{D29N}$ and PR$_{R8Q}$ led to the conclusion that the intramonomer interaction between the side chains of D29 and R87 increases the K_d significantly more than the intermonomer interaction between D29 and R8′ (Table I; Louis *et al.*, 2003). In PR$_{R87K}$, chemical shift perturbations and sub-nanosecond timescale motions detected for the N-terminal residues of the α-helix increase further in the C-terminal β-strand. Taking into account the NMR results together with information from crystal structures that the C-terminal strands are in the interior of the four-stranded β-sheet, it is proposed that the disruption of the specific interactions involving the R87 side chain could induce enhanced mobility of the C-terminal strands at the dimer interface possibly leading to a destabilization of the terminal β-sheet.

2. Active Site and Terminal β-Sheet Dimer Interfaces

In the absence of an inhibitor, the active site and terminal residues that encompass the dimer interface are critical for maintaining the low K_d of the mature protease. Mutation of these residues increases the K_d from

~10^2-fold, as seen for PR_{D25N}, to >10^5-fold as in the case of PR_{1-95}, which carries a deletion of the four C-terminal residues (Table I). Based on the results of the analysis by NMR, sedimentation equilibrium analysis, and kinetics, the mutants can be grouped into four classes (Table I). Class A mutants (PR_{D25N}, PR_{R8Q}) are mostly dimeric at a concentration of ~0.5 μM and above. Class B mutants show significant monomer and dimer populations at ~0.5 mM whereas class C and D mutants are mostly monomeric at ~0.5 mM. Comparison of the ^1H-^{15}N HSQC spectra indicates that the active site interface mutant PR_{T26A} adopts a tertiary fold that is similar to that of the PR_{R87K} monomer. The nearly identical chemical shifts of the C-terminal residues T96 and F99 of PR_{T26A} monomer to those of PR_{R87K} suggest that the terminal strands of PR_{T26A} are also disordered and flexible similar to those of PR_{R87K}. Thus in the absence of a bound inhibitor, the highly conserved T26 residue of the active site DTG triad is as critical to dimer stability as are R87, D29, or the N-terminal residues 1–4.

Class B and C mutants, however, form mostly ternary complexes (dimer–inhibitor complex) with a tight binding inhibitor DMP323 similar to class A mutants and PR. ^{15}N and ^1H chemical shifts of the terminal residues of these mutant/DMP323 complexes are nearly identical to those of the PR-DMP323 complex implying very similar terminal β-sheet arrangements. Thus, interactions of the inhibitor with the active site/flap residues offset the effect of these mutations and restore the terminal β-sheet configuration. Class D mutants do not form significant concentrations of ternary complexes at monomer concentration of up to 1 mM even in the presence of excess inhibitor. Therefore, the loss of interaction between the two C-terminal strands has the major contribution to dimer stability.

The effect of single amino acid substitutions of the terminal β-sheet residues on dimerization and catalytic activity has been explored by coexpressing the mature protease in fusion with β-galactosidase bearing an internal protease cleavage site. The protease-catalyzed hydrolysis of β-galactosidase characterized, both by appearance of white colonies (fully cleaved product) and by product size, as determined by Western blotting, provides a semi-quantitative assessment of the effect of mutation on dimerization and catalytic activity of the protease (Choudhury et al., 2003). This study indicates that, while the N-terminal residues P1, Q2, and T4 tolerate Ala substitution mutations, C-terminal mutations T96A, L97A, and F99A, all lead to reduced activity (Choudhury et al., 2003). In accordance with this observation, the deletion mutant PR_{5-99} was shown to exhibit an increase in K_d by about 60-fold and a corresponding decrease in the k_{cat}/K_m value (~50-fold) as compared to PR (Louis et al., 1999a). Under the same conditions, the C-terminal deletion (PR_{1-95}), which exerts a much larger effect on the K_d, exhibits no catalytic activity (Ishima et al., 2001a).

B. Description of the Monomer Structure

The existence of PR_{1-95} as a monomer at a concentration of up to 1 mM with undetectable dimer allowed the three-dimensional structure determination of PR_{1-95} using heteronuclear multidimensional NMR spectroscopy. A backbone superposition of the average NMR structure with the monomer subunit of two different crystal structures of the free mature protease dimer (Freedberg *et al.*, 2002; Lapatto *et al.*, 1989) is shown in Fig. 11A. Residues 10–90 of the PR_{1-95} monomer exhibit a nearly identical fold to that of one subunit of the protease dimer. This similarity in structures is consistent with the backbone chemical shifts of the PR_{1-95} monomer compared to

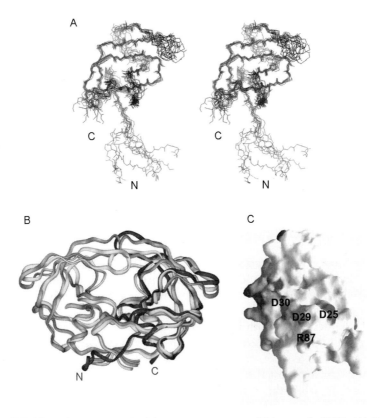

FIGURE 11   Solution structure of the protease monomer (Ishima *et al.*, 2003). (A) Overall stereo view of the PR_{1-95} structure showing the final ensemble of 10 NMR conformers. (B) Comparison of the average NMR structure of PR_{1-95} (blue) with one subunit of two free protease dimer crystal structures shown in green (Lapatto *et al.*, 1989) and yellow (Rick *et al.*, 1998). (C) Electrostatic surface potential of PR_{1-95} (excludes residues 1–10). Note: the crystal structure shown in green has a flap conformation that is more open than the crystal structure shown in yellow. (See Color Insert.)

those of the PR dimer (Ishima *et al.*, 2003). Characteristics that distinguish the PR_{1-95} structure from the monomer subunit of mature protease dimer are discussed below.

1. Terminal Residues

The absence of secondary structure of the N-terminal residues in the PR_{1-95} monomer is not surprising given that deletion of residues 96–99 precludes formation of the terminal interface β-sheet. Consistently, in the PR_{1-95} monomer, NOESY cross-peaks were not observed for the N-terminal residues 1–9 (Ishima *et al.*, 2003). Heteronuclear NOE experiments showed that these N-terminal residues are flexible on the sub-nanosecond timescale in the PR_{1-95} monomer. The chain flexibility and loss of the terminal β-sheet structure observed for PR_{1-95} (Fig. 11 and Ishima *et al.*, 2003) also occur in monomer constructs such as PR_{T26A} and PR_{R87K} that contain intact terminal sequences. Thus, in addition to interactions involving the termini, specific interactions distant from the terminal region also strongly influence the stability of the terminal β-sheet interface (Ishima *et al.*, 2001a; Louis *et al.*, 2003).

2. Flaps

The structure presented for PR_{1-95} monomer provides the first information about a flap conformation of free protease in solution. The flap in the PR_{1-95} monomer exhibits a β-hairpin structure, similar to the flap of the dimer, but with significant disorder in residues 48–53, and seems to adopt an open conformation (Fig. 11A). Evidence for flap flexibility on a sub-nanosecond timescale is provided by a decrease of the heteronuclear NOE values and increase in the transverse relaxation times of residues 49–53 (Ishima *et al.*, 2003). In addition, two sets of α-proton signals of G52 were observed in the monomer flap, suggesting a slow conformational change of this region presumably on a millisecond timescale. In contrast, a single set of α-proton signals for G52 was detected under equivalent conditions in the free protease dimer. The flap region in the free protease dimer was also found to undergo $\sim$100-μs conformational exchange at 20°C, pH 5.8 (Ishima *et al.*, 1999), suggesting a minor difference in flap dynamics between the monomer and the dimer. Although there may be differences in the timescale of the flap motion in monomer and dimer, both monomer and dimer flaps have dynamics undergoing slow conformational change in addition to fluctuations on the sub-nanosecond timescale (Freedberg *et al.*, 2002; Ishima *et al.*, 2003).

3. Active Site

The active site D25 residue in the dimer is involved in a β-1 turn termed the "fireman's grip" (Fig. 1; Pearl and Blundell, 1984; Strisovsky *et al.*, 2000). In the PR_{1-95} monomer structure, the region encompassing the β-1 turn region is somewhat disordered. Although NOE interactions typical of a β-1 turn are observed in the monomer, indicating that the β-1 turn exists, the decrease in transverse relaxation times suggests flexibility on the sub-nanosecond timescale in the active site region in the monomer (Ishima *et al.*, 2003). The accessible surface areas of side chains of residues L23, L24, T26, and D29 located in this β-turn region are 40% larger in the monomer than in the dimer. This increased flexibility of the β-turn region is most likely due to the loss of the intersubunit hydrogen bond network and a partial exposure of the turn to the solvent.

The active site β-turn region in the monomer contains a large number of exposed charged side chains. A negatively charged patch composed of D25, D29, and D30 side chains is adjacent to the positively charged R87 side chain (Fig. 11C). Because of the relatively low number of experimental structural constraints, orientations of the side chains of the residues were not determined; however, the side chains are expected to be mobile based on their solvent accessibility and chemical shifts.

VI. Insights into the Structure of the Protease Precursor and Its Maturation

A. Early Intermediates of the Gag-Pol Precursor During Protease Maturation

PR-mediated processing and particle maturation are complex events (for a review, see Vogt, 1996). In HIV-1, the structural and functional proteins are synthesized as two polyproteins, Gag and Gag-Pol, consisting of MA-CA-p2-NC-p1-p6 and MA-CA-p2-NC-TFR-PR-RT-IN, respectively (Leis *et al.*, 1988; Oroszlan and Luftig, 1990). In the precursors, the peptide bonds that connect each of the subdomains are specifically cleaved by the protease. The initial critical step in the maturation of the protease involves the folding and dimerization of the protease domain in the form of a Gag-Pol precursor in order to catalyze the hydrolysis of the peptide bonds at its termini and the other specific sites leading to the release of the mature structural and functional proteins. Kinetics of the maturation reaction clearly indicated that the cleavage at the N-terminus of the protease, which is concomitant with the appearance of mature-like enzymatic activity, precedes the cleavage at the C-terminus of the protease (Louis *et al.*, 1994; Wondrak *et al.*, 1996). The native TFR flanking the N-terminus of PR, comprises two domains, the conserved transframe octapeptide (TFP) followed by the 48 amino acid p6^{pol}, both separated by a protease cleavage site (Candotti *et al.*, 1994; Louis *et al.*, 1998). Reactions using the full-length TFP-P6^{pol}-PR precursor at pH 5.0, which is optimal for catalytic activity of the mature protease and the autocatalytic maturation reaction, showed that release of the protease occurs in two distinct steps (Louis *et al.*, 1999a,b). The first cleavage occurs at the TFP-P6^{pol} site to generate the intermediate precursor P6^{pol}-PR. In the second step, P6^{pol}-PR is converted to the mature protease concomitant with a large increase in catalytic activity. Thus, the two proteins, TFP-P6^{pol}-PR and P6^{pol}-PR, exhibit nearly the same very low catalytic activity and the rate-limiting intramolecular cleavage at the p6^{pol}-PR site is indeed concomitant with the appearance of mature-like enzymatic activity and stable tertiary structure formation characteristic of a stable protease dimer (Louis *et al.*, 1999a,b). These results are consistent with studies showing that HIV-1 particles of four different strains obtained from different cell lines contained only the 11-kDa mature protease and no p6^{pol}-PR precursor (Tessmer and Krausslich, 1998). Importantly, a mutation of the N-terminal protease cleavage site p6^{pol}/PR leading to the production of an N-terminally extended 17-kDa protease species caused a severe defect in Gag polyprotein processing and a complete loss of viral infectivity (Tessmer and Krausslich, 1998).

Monitoring the detailed kinetics of the maturation of the full-length Gag-Pol precursor is complex due to the presence of multiple cleavage sites. A recent study of the *in vitro* expression of the Gag-Pol protein (~160 kDa) had shown a primary cleavage at the P2/NC site followed by a slower cleavage at the TFP/p6^{pol} site leading to the accumulation of the processing intermediates MA-CA-P2 (42 kDa), NC-TFP (7.4 kDa), and p6^{pol}-PR-RT-IN (113 kDa; Pettit *et al.*, 2004). However, monitoring the *in vivo* processing in acutely infected, cultured T-lymphocytes in the presence of a potent inhibitor (1 μM) showed that Gag-Pol is cleaved in the vicinity of the N-terminus of TFR, presumably at the TFP-p6^{pol} site leading to the accumulation of a Pol intermediate, p6^{pol}-PR-RT-IN. This may point to TFP-p6^{pol} as the primary cleavage site in the processing of the Gag-Pol precursor that is insensitive to inhibition (Lindhofer *et al.*, 1995). In accordance with this result, preliminary studies of the inhibition of the maturation reaction of the precursor TFP-p6^{pol}-PR at pH 5.0 indicate that the two cleavages (TFP/p6^{pol} and p6^{pol}/PR) leading to the formation of the mature PR are inhibited differently by the substrate analogue inhibitor that is specific to the mature PR. IC$_{50}$ of cleavage at the TFP/p6^{pol} site (step 1) is less than two orders of magnitude larger than for the inhibition of the hydrolytic reaction catalyzed by the mature PR using the substrate analogue inhibitor (Louis *et al.*, 1999a). Thus, the maturation of the protease from the Gag-Pol polyprotein *in vivo* may resemble the *in vitro* two-step process described for the precursor TFP-p6^{pol}-PR$\leq$pH 6.0. Inhibition of the p6^{pol}/PR site is within the range of values reported for the inhibition of the wt-PR. Both sites, CA/P2 and TFP/p6^{pol}, that exhibit cleavage as the primary sites during the processing of the full-length Gag-Pol precursor *in vitro* also were relatively insensitive to inhibition with a potent inhibitor (Pettit *et al.*, 2004). Thus, from a combination of studies, it appears that the initial steps in the maturation of the protease appear to be a sequential multistep ordered process at pH 5 that involves at least two peptide bond cleavages upstream to PR domain prior to the generation of optimal enzymatic activity (Louis *et al.*, 1999b).

B. Tertiary Fold and Stability of the Protease Precursor

A systematic NMR structural study of the wild-type TFP-p6^{pol}-PR precursor bearing the native cleavage sites TFP/p6^{pol} and p6^{pol}/PR was not feasible due to its rapid autocatalytic maturation on folding to release the mature protease (Louis *et al.*, 1999a). Although maturation can be blocked with a large excess of inhibitor, it perturbs the monomer–dimer equilibrium of the free precursor and also contributes to undesirable effects such as the precipitation or aggregation of the protein at concentrations above 0.5 mM, thereby preventing detailed structural studies of the precursor. In earlier studies, it was shown that the mature protease bearing a mutation of the active site residue (Prabu-Jeyabalan *et al.*, 2000), PR$_{D25N}$, was highly suitable for long-term solution NMR studies of the mature protease dimer at a concentration of ∼0.5 mM (Katoh *et al.*, 2003; Louis *et al.*, 2003). In addition, the D25N mutation, unlike the T26A mutation (Louis *et al.*, 2003), has the least affect on the dimer stability of the mature protease. Thus in order to analyze the precursor protease by NMR in the absence of any inhibitor, an active site mutation D25N was introduced in the TFP-p6^{pol}-PR precursor to abolish its maturation. This construct was compared with the mature protease bearing the same D25N mutation, PR$_{D25N}$.

Figure 12 shows a comparison of ^{1}H-^{15}N HSQC spectra of PR$_{D25N}$ and TFP-P6^{pol}-PR$_{D25N}$ at identical conditions. Chemical shifts of most signals observed in a ^{1}H-^{15}N correlation spectrum of PR$_{D25N}$ are very similar to those of the active protease dimer (Freedberg *et al.*, 2002). In particular, signals of residues in the dimer interface of PR$_{D25N}$, such as I3, I84, Q92, and T96, exhibit shifts characteristic of the dimer (identified in stippled boxes in Fig. 12A). In the TFP-P6^{pol}-PR$_{D25N}$ spectrum, these peaks are absent and additional intense resonances are observed in the random coil region (8–8.5 ppm for protons; Fig. 12B). These intense signals likely arise from residues of the TFP-P6^{pol} domain, consistent with results indicating that the isolated TFR does not possess a stable secondary or tertiary structure (Beissinger *et al.*, 1996). In addition, less intense but well-dispersed signals (indicated in solid boxes in Fig. 12B) were observed in positions similar to those of signals in the spectra of the folded monomer PR$_{1-95}$ and other mutants that form monomers (Ishima *et al.*, 2001a, 2003; Louis *et al.*, 2003). Thus, the flanking transframe polypeptide influences the monomer–dimer equilibrium of the protease domain in accordance with the observation that TFP-P6^{pol}-PR$_{D25N}$ is predominantly a monomer whereas PR$_{D25N}$ is a dimer (Katoh *et al.*, 2003). Another precursor variant, TFP-P6^{pol}-PR$_{1-95}$,

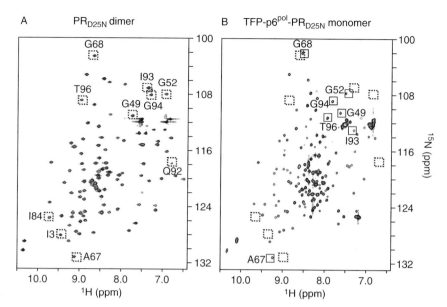

FIGURE 12 ^{1}H-^{15}N HSQC spectra of (A) PR$_{D25N}$ and (B) TFP-p6^{pol}-PR$_{D25N}$ acquired using ~0.5-mM protein (in monomer) in 20-mM phosphate buffer, pH 5.8, 20°C. Signals in boxes and stippled boxes are those that characterize the protease monomer and dimer folds, respectively (Ishima et al., 2003).

which lacks the same four C-terminal residues 96–99 as in PR$_{1-95}$, does not undergo maturation, which further emphasizes the fact that intersubunit interaction between the C-terminal β-strands is most critical to the dimerization of the protease precursor. The HSQC spectrum of TFP-P6^{pol}-PR$_{1-95}$ is similar to that of TFP-P6^{pol}-PR$_{D25N}$ exhibiting an unstructured TFP-p6^{Pol} domain and a monomeric fold of the protease domain.

It is apparent from the above results that the native TFR in fusion with the protease increases the K_d by several orders of magnitude. It is noteworthy that both the terminal regions of the TFR, the TFP and the C-terminal residues of p6^{pol}, are competitive inhibitors of the mature PR (Louis et al., 1998; Paulus et al., 1999). Comparison of the monomer spectra of the precursors TFP-p6^{pol}-PR$_{D25N}$ or TFP-p6^{pol}-PR$_{1-95}$ with that of PR$_{1-95}$ does not reveal significant differences indicative of an interaction between the TFP-p6^{pol} region and the protease monomer. We therefore believe that the dimeric precursor of the protease, in which the N-terminal cleavage site sequence is intramoleculary bound to the active site, is a transient form present in small amounts and thus undetectable in the HSQC spectrum (for a model see Fig. 5 in Louis et al., 1994).

It is likely that interactions between the two C-terminal strands are essential to produce transient dimeric folds of the protease precursor prior to maturation. This interpretation is supported by the result that deletion of the C-terminal residues 96–99 produced the most profound increase in the K_d of the mature protease. Studies showing that RT p66 homodimer is formed prior to the cleavage at the RT p66/p51 site by the protease to form the RT66/RT51 heterodimer (Sluis-Cremer *et al.*, 2004) suggest that RT66 dimerization may be a prerequisite for establishing the transient interaction between the C-terminal strands of the folded monomeric protease to partly stabilize the dimeric precursor leading to the intramolecular maturation of the protease at its N-terminus. We envision that it may be easier to design a drug that restricts dimer formation prior to the maturation of the protease from the Gag-Pol rather than the dimerization of the mature protease, which forms a far more stable dimer.

C. Influence of Local Interactions at the Termini of the Mature Protease on Dimer Stability

The protease is mainly monomeric when fused to relatively long sequences at its N-terminus (Ishima *et al.*, 2003; Louis *et al.*, 2000). To assess if dimerization is sensitive to local interactions involving a few residues of the flanking p6^{pol} sequence, the effect of just the SFNF extension (the C-terminal residues of p6^{pol}) on protease stability and enzymatic activity has been examined using the construct $^{SFNF}PR_{D25N}$. The HSQC spectrum of $^{SFNF}PR_{D25N}$ shows that it is mostly a folded monomer at ~0.6 mM (Ishima *et al.*, 2003) with signals in positions similar to those of PR_{1-95}. Comparison of the HSQC spectra of TFP-p6^{pol}-PR_{D25N} and ^{SFNF}-PR_{D25N} in the presence of approximately fivefold excess of DMP323 indicates that while nearly all the ^{SFNF}-PR_{D25N} is dimeric, a significant portion of TFP-p6^{pol}-PR_{D25N} precursor is monomeric. This observation suggests that a longer sequence, namely, the intact native TFP-p6^{pol}, hinders the dimerization of the protease to a larger extent than a 4-amino acid extension. This interpretation is also consistent with results showing that the active precursor TFP-p6^{pol}-PR is about 160-fold less active than the mature protease (Louis *et al.*, 1999b).

Subsequent studies have shown that even two residue extensions at the N-terminus of the protease also increase the K_d similar to $^{SFNF}PR_{D25N}$ (Ishima *et al.*, 2003). As noted from the crystal structure of the free protease dimer, P1 is relatively close to the A67-H69 loop as well to F99. We speculate that additional residues at the N-terminus of the protease may affect the local packing of side chains, thus lowering the dimer stability. The importance of the P1 residue is further emphasized in studies showing that the mutation of the P1 residue significantly alters the pattern of cleavage of the Gag-Pol precursor as compared to the wild type (Pettit *et al.*, 2005).

D. Pathway to the Maturation of the Protease in the Viral Replication Cycle

A plausible pathway for the regulation of the protease emerges taking into consideration several *in vivo* and *in vitro* studies of precursor processing. On its synthesis, the protease domain within the Gag-Pol precursor adopts a monomer fold at least spanning residues 10–90. It appears that the monomer–dimer equilibrium of the protease is modulated by the N-terminally flanking TFP-p6^{pol} domain such that prior to the cleavage at the p6^{pol}/PR junction the protease domain is mainly monomeric (K_d > 0.5 mM). The very low dimer stability of the protease precursor relative to the mature protease (K_d < 10 nM) may allow initial recruitment of the polyproteins and assembly of the particle to occur prior to the onset of limited proteolysis. The pH of the microenvironment and concentration effects leading to dimerization or oligomerization of the flanking domains, particularly that of the RT domain, may also modulate the autoprocessing reaction. Transient dimer formation of the precursor is facilitated by an interface requiring interactions of at least the active site and the C-terminal residues and possibly stabilized further by the interaction of the cleavage site sequence with the active site and flap residues. The concomitant increase in mature-like catalytic activity and stable dimer formation is consistent with a single rate-limiting step involving the intramolecular cleavage of the scissile bond at the p6^{pol}/PR junction. Intermediate precursor forms could be liberated either through an intramolecular process at a competing site (P2/NC or TFP/p6^{pol}) that becomes available for productive binding and hydrolysis below pH 5 or through an intermolecular process mediated by the accumulating released active protease, a reaction that becomes competitive with the intramolecular process. The formation of these intermediates under suboptimal conditions for the autoprocessing reaction is similar to that observed for the conversion of zymogen form of the gastric protease pepsinogen (Khan and James, 1998). In contrast to even 2–4 amino acids of the N-terminal flanking sequence that exert an effect on the K_d, the C-terminal reverse transcriptase sequence may not significantly affect either the kinetic parameters or the K_d (Cherry *et al.*, 1998; Sluis-Cremer *et al.*, 2004; Wondrak *et al.*, 1996). Subsequent cleavages in the Gag-Pol including the C-terminus of the protease occur via intermolecular processes (Wondrak *et al.*, 1996).

Finally, the existence of a monomer fold, both for the TFP-p6^{pol}-PR precursor and several mutants of the mature protease, indicates that folding and dimerization can occur independently. Future studies may enable targeting the folded precursor monomer or the folding process itself, prior to the maturation of the protease from the Gag-Pol precursor, for inhibitor design, in contrast to numerous ongoing and published studies aimed at inhibiting the dimerization of the mature protease. Furthermore, understanding structurally the molecular mechanism by which the TFP-p6^{pol} region increases the K_d of the protease may provide insights for rational drug design targeting dimerization.

Acknowledgments ─────────────────────────

Research sponsored by the NIH Intramural programs of NIDDK and NIDCR, NIH extramural awards GM62920 and AIDS-FIRCA TW01001, the Georgia State University Molecular Basis of Disease Program, the Georgia Research Alliance, and the Georgia Cancer Coalition. We thank A. Aniana for assistance in composing Fig. 2, and Y. Tie, F. Liu, and A. Kovalevsky for Figs. 7 and 8, and S. Oroszlan for many thoughtful and inspiring discussions during the course of our studies.

References ─────────────────────────

Babe, L. M., Rose, J., and Craik, C. S. (1992). Synthetic "interface" peptides alter dimeric assembly of the HIV 1 and 2 proteases. *Protein Sci.* 1, 1244–1253.

Beissinger, M., Paulus, C., Bayer, P., Wolf, H., Rosch, P., and Wagner, R. (1996). Sequence-specific resonance assignments of the 1H-NMR spectra and structural characterization in solution of the HIV-1 transframe protein p6. *Eur. J. Biochem.* 237, 383–392.

Bowman, M. J., and Chmielewski, J. (2002). Novel strategies for targeting the dimerization interface of HIV protease with cross-linked interfacial peptides. *Biopolymers* 66, 126–133.

Candotti, D., Chappey, C., Rosenheim, M., M'Pele, P., Huraux, J. M., and Agut, H. (1994). High variability of the gag/pol transframe region among HIV-1 isolates. *C. R. Acad. Sci. III* 317, 183–189.

Ceccherini-Silberstein, F., Erba, F., Gago, F., Bertoli, A., Forbici, F., Bellocchi, M. C., Gori, C., D'Arrigo, R., Marcon, L., Balotta, C., Antinori, A., Monforte, A. D., *et al.* (2004). Identification of the minimal conserved structure of HIV-1 protease in the presence and absence of drug pressure. *AIDS* 18, F11–F19.

Chen, X., Weber, I. T., and Harrison, R. W. (2004). Molecular dynamics simulations of 14 HIV protease mutants in complexes with indinavir. *J. Mol. Model.* 10, 373–381.

Chen, Z., Li, Y., Chen, E., Hall, D. L., Darke, P. L., Culberson, C., Shafer, J. A., and Kuo, L. C. (1994). Crystal structure at 1. 9-A resolution of human immunodeficiency virus (HIV) II protease complexed with L-735, 524, an orally bioavailable inhibitor of the HIV proteases. *J. Biol. Chem.* 269, 26344–26348.

Cherry, E., Liang, C., Rong, L., Quan, Y., Inouye, P., Li, X., Morin, N., Kotler, M., and Wainberg, M. A. (1998). Characterization of human immunodeficiency virus type-1 (HIV-1) particles that express protease-reverse transcriptase fusion proteins. *J. Mol. Biol.* 284, 43–56.

Choudhury, S., Everitt, L., Pettit, S. C., and Kaplan, A. H. (2003). Mutagenesis of the dimer interface residues of tethered and untethered HIV-1 protease result in differential activity and suggest multiple mechanisms of compensation. *Virology* 307, 204–212.

Collins, J. R., Burt, S. K., and Erickson, J. W. (1995). Flap opening in HIV-1 protease simulated by 'activated' molecular dynamics. *Nat. Struct. Biol.* 2, 334–338.

Dunn, B. M., Gustchina, A., Wlodawer, A., and Kay, J. (1994). Subsite preferences of retroviral proteinases. *Methods Enzymol.* 241, 254–278.

Erickson, J. W., and Burt, S. K. (1996). Structural mechanisms of HIV drug resistance. *Annu. Rev. Pharmacol. Toxicol.* 36, 545–571.

Erickson, J. W., Gulnik, S. V., and Markowitz, M. (1999). Protease inhibitors: Resistance, cross-resistance, fitness and the choice of initial and salvage therapies. *AIDS* 13(Suppl. A), S189–S204.

Freedberg, D. I., Ishima, R., Jacob, J., Wang, Y. X., Kustanovich, I., Louis, J. M., and Torchia, D. A. (2002). Rapid structural fluctuations of the free HIV protease flaps in solution: Relationship to crystal structures and comparison with predictions of dynamics calculations. *Protein Sci.* 11, 221–232.

Furfine, E. S., D'Souza, E., Ingold, K. J., Leban, J. J., Spector, T., and Porter, D. J. (1992). Two-step binding mechanism for HIV protease inhibitors. *Biochemistry* 31, 7886–7891.

Ghosh, A. K., Sridhar, P. R., Leshchenko, S., Hussain, A. K., Li, J., Kovalevsky, A. Y., Walters, D. E., Wedekind, J. E., Grum-Tokars, V., Das, D., Koh, Y., Maeda, K., *et al.* (2006). Structure-based design of novel HIV-1 protease inhibitors to combat drug resistance. *J. Med. Chem.* 49, 5252–5261.

Grant, S. K., Deckman, I. C., Culp, J. S., Minnich, M. D., Brooks, I. S., Hensley, P., Debouck, C., and Meek, T. D. (1992). Use of protein unfolding studies to determine the conformational and dimeric stabilities of HIV-1 and SIV proteases. *Biochemistry* 31, 9491–9501.

Grzesiek, S., Bax, A., Nicholson, L. K., Yamazaki, T., Wingfield, P., Stahl, S. J., Eyermann, C. J., Torchia, D. A., Hodge, C. N., Lam, P. Y. S., Jadhav, P. K., and Chang, C.-H. (1994). NMR evidence for the displacement of a conserved interior water molecule in HIV protease by a non-peptide cyclic urea-based inhibitor. *J. Am. Chem. Soc.* 116, 1581–1582.

Gustchina, A., Sansom, C., Prevost, M., Richelle, J., Wodak, S. Y., Wlodawer, A., and Weber, I. T. (1994). Energy calculations and analysis of HIV-1 protease-inhibitor crystal structures. *Protein Eng.* 7, 309–317.

Harte, W. E., Swaminathan, S., Mansuri, M. M., Martin, J. C., Rosenberg, I. E., and Beveridge, D. L. (1990). Domain communication in the dynamical structure of human immunodeficiency virus 1 Protease. *Proc. Natl. Acad. Sci.* 87, 8864–8868.

Hamelberg, D., and McCammon, J. A. (2005). Fast peptidyl cis-trans isomerization within the flexible Gly-rich flaps of HIV-1 protease. *J. Am. Chem. Soc.* 127, 13778–13779.

Hornak, V., Okur, A., Rizzo, R. C., and Simmerling, C. (2006). HIV-1 protease flaps spontaneously open and reclose in molecular dynamics simulations. *Proc. Natl. Acad. Sci. USA* 103, 915–920.

Ishima, R., and Torchia, D. A. (2003). Extending the range of amide proton relaxation dispersion experiments in proteins using a constant-time relaxation-compensated CPMG approach. *J. Biomol. NMR* 25, 243–248.

Ishima, R., and Torchia, D. A. (2005). Error estimation and global fitting in transverse-relaxation dispersion experiments to determine chemical-exchange parameters. *J. Biomol. NMR* 32, 41–54.

Ishima, R., Freedberg, D. I., Wang, Y. X., Louis, J. M., and Torchia, D. A. (1999). Flap opening and dimer-interface flexibility in the free and inhibitor-bound HIV protease, and their implications for function. *Structure* 7, 1047–1055.

Ishima, R., Ghirlando, R., Tozser, J., Gronenborn, A. M., Torchia, D. A., and Louis, J. M. (2001a). Folded monomer of HIV-1 protease. *J. Biol. Chem.* 276, 49110–49116.

Ishima, R., Louis, J. M., and Torchia, D. A. (2001b). Characterization of two hydrophobic methyl clusters in HIV-1 protease by NMR spin relaxation in solution. *J. Mol. Biol.* 305, 515–521.

Ishima, R., Torchia, D. A., Lynch, S. M., Gronenborn, A. M., and Louis, J. M. (2003). Solution structure of the mature HIV-1 protease monomer: Insight into the tertiary fold and stability of a precursor. *J. Biol. Chem.* 278, 43311–43319.

Ishima, R., Baber, J., Louis, J. M., and Torchia, D. A. (2004). Carbonyl carbon transverse relaxation dispersion measurements and ms-micros timescale motion in a protein hydrogen bond network. *J. Biomol. NMR* 29, 187–198.

Katoh, E., Louis, J. M., Yamazaki, T., Gronenborn, A. M., Torchia, D. A., and Ishima, R. (2003). A solution NMR study of the binding kinetics and the internal dynamics of an HIV-1 protease-substrate complex. *Protein Sci.* **12**, 1376–1385.

Khan, A. R., and James, M. N. (1998). Molecular mechanisms for the conversion of zymogens to active proteolytic enzymes. *Protein Sci.* **7**, 815–836.

King, N. M., Prabu-Jeyabalan, M., Nalivaika, E. A., Wigerinck, P., de Bethune, M. P., and Schiffer, C. A. (2004). Structural and thermodynamic basis for the binding of TMC114, a next-generation human immunodeficiency virus type 1 protease inhibitor. *J. Virol.* **78**, 12012–12021.

Koh, Y., Nakata, H., Maeda, K., Ogata, H., Bilcer, G., Devasamudram, T., Kincaid, J. F., Boross, P., Wang, Y. F., Tie, Y., Volarath, P., Gaddis, L., *et al.* (2003). Novel bis-tetrahydrofuranylurethane-containing nonpeptidic protease inhibitor (PI) UIC-94017 (TMC114) with potent activity against multi-PI-resistant human immunodeficiency virus *in vitro*. *Antimicrob. Agents Chemother.* **47**, 3123–3129.

Kovalevsky, A. Y., Liu, F., Leshchenko, S., Ghosh, A. K., Louis, J. M., Harrison, R. H., and Weber, I. T. (2006a). Ultra-high resolution crystal structure of HIV-1 protease reveals two binding sites for clinical inhibitor TMC114. *J. Mol. Biol.* **363**, 161–173.

Kovalevsky, A. Y., Tie, Y., Liu, F., Boross, P. I., Wang, Y. F., Leshchenko, S., Ghosh, A. K., Harrison, R. W., and Weber, I. T. (2006b). Effectiveness of nonpeptide clinical inhibitor TMC-114 on HIV-1 protease with highly drug resistant mutations D30N, I50V, and L90M. *J. Med. Chem.* **49**, 1379–1387.

Krohn, A., Redshaw, S., Ritchie, J. C., Graves, B. J., and Hatada, M. H. (1991). Novel binding mode of highly potent HIV-proteinase inhibitors incorporating the (R)-hydroxyethyla-mine isostere. *J. Med. Chem.* **34**, 3340–3342.

Lam, P. Y., Ru, Y., Jadhav, P. K., Aldrich, P. E., Delucca, G. V., Eyermann, C. J., Chang, C. H., Emmett, G., Holler, E. R., Daneker, W. F., Li, L., Confalone, P. N., *et al.* (1996). Cyclic HIV protease inhibitors: Synthesis, conformational analysis, P2/P2 structure-activity relationship, and molecular recognition of cyclic ureas. *J. Med. Chem.* **39**, 3514–3525.

Lapatto, R., Blundell, T., Hemmings, A., Overington, J., Wilderspin, A., Wood, S., Merson, J. R., Whittle, P. J., Danley, D. E., Geoghegan, K. F., Hawrylik, S. J., Lee, S., *et al.* (1989). X-ray analysis of HIV-1 proteinase at 2.7 Å resolution confirms structural homology among retroviral enzymes. *Nature* **342**, 299–302.

Leis, J., Baltimore, D., Bishop, J. M., Coffin, J., Fleissner, E., Goff, S. P., Oroszlan, S., Robinson, H., Skalka, A. M., and Temin, H. M. (1988). Standardized and simplified nomenclature for proteins common to all retroviruses. *J. Virol.* **62**, 1808–1809.

Leitner, T., Foley, B., Hahn, B., Marx, P., McCutchan, F., Mellors, J., Wolinsky, S., and Korber, B. (2005). HIV Sequence Compendium Published by the Theoretical Biology and Biophysics Group, Los Alamos National Laboratory, LA-UR number 06-0680.

Lindhofer, H., von der Helm, K., and Nitschko, H. (1995). *In vivo* processing of Pr160gag-pol from human immunodeficiency virus type 1 (HIV) in acutely infected, cultured human T-lymphocytes. *Virology* **214**, 624–627.

Liu, F., Boross, P. I., Wang, Y. F., Tozser, J., Louis, J. M., Harrison, R. W., and Weber, I. T. (2005). Kinetic, stability, and structural changes in high-resolution crystal structures of HIV-1 protease with drug-resistant mutations L24I, I50V, and G73S. *J. Mol. Biol.* **354**, 789–800.

Liu, F., Kovalevsky, A. Y., Louis, J. M., Boross, P. I., Wang, Y. F., Harrison, R. W., and Weber, I. T. (2006). Mechanism of drug resistance revealed by the crystal structure of the unliganded HIV-1 protease with F53L mutation. *J. Mol. Biol.* **358**, 1191–1199.

Louis, J. M., Smith, C. A., Wondrak, E. M., Mora, P. T., and Oroszlan, S. (1989). Substitution mutations of the highly conserved arginine 87 of HIV-1 protease result in loss of proteolytic activity. *Biochem. Biophys. Res. Commun.* **164**, 30–38.

Louis, J. M., Nashed, N. T., Parris, K. D., Kimmel, A. R., and Jerina, D. M. (1994). Kinetics and mechanism of autoprocessing of human immunodeficiency virus type 1 protease from an analog of the Gag-Pol polyprotein. *Proc. Natl. Acad. Sci. USA* **91**, 7970–7974.

Louis, J. M., Dyda, F., Nashed, N. T., Kimmel, A. R., and Davies, D. R. (1998). Hydrophilic peptides derived from the transframe region of Gag-Pol inhibit the HIV-1 protease. *Biochemistry* **37**, 2105–2110.

Louis, J. M., Clore, G. M., and Gronenborn, A. M. (1999a). Autoprocessing of HIV-1 protease is tightly coupled to protein folding. *Nat. Struct. Biol.* **6**, 868–875.

Louis, J. M., Wondrak, E. M., Kimmel, A. R., Wingfield, P. T., and Nashed, N. T. (1999b). Proteolytic processing of HIV-1 protease precursor, kinetics and mechanism. *J. Biol. Chem.* **274**, 23437–23442.

Louis, J. M., Weber, I. T., Tozser, J., Clore, G. M., and Gronenborn, A. M. (2000). HIV-1 protease: Maturation, enzyme specificity, and drug resistance. *Adv. Pharmacol.* **49**, 111–146.

Louis, J. M., Ishima, R., Nesheiwat, I., Pannell, L. K., Lynch, S. M., Torchia, D. A., and Gronenborn, A. M. (2003). Revisiting monomeric HIV-1 protease. Characterization and redesign for improved properties. *J. Biol. Chem.* **278**, 6085–6092.

Mahalingam, B., Louis, J. M., Reed, C. C., Adomat, J. M., Krouse, J., Wang, Y. F., Harrison, R. W., and Weber, I. T. (1999). Structural and kinetic analysis of drug resistant mutants of HIV-1 protease. *Eur. J. Biochem.* **263**, 238–245.

Mahalingam, B., Louis, J. M., Hung, J., Harrison, R. W., and Weber, I. T. (2001). Structural implications of drug-resistant mutants of HIV-1 protease: High-resolution crystal structures of the mutant protease/substrate analogue complexes. *Proteins* **43**, 455–464.

Mahalingam, B., Wang, Y. F., Boross, P. I., Tozser, J., Louis, J. M., Harrison, R. W., and Weber, I. T. (2004). Crystal structures of HIV protease V82A and L90M mutants reveal changes in the indinavir-binding site. *Eur. J. Biochem.* **271**, 1516–1524.

Merabet, N., Dumond, J., Collinet, B., Van Baelinghem, L., Boggetto, N., Ongeri, S., Ressad, F., Reboud-Ravaux, M., and Sicsic, S. (2004). New constrained "molecular tongs" designed to dissociate HIV-1 protease dimer. *J. Med. Chem.* **47**, 6392–6400.

Mildner, A. M., Rothrock, D. J., Leone, J. W., Bannow, C. A., Lull, J. M., Reardon, I. M., Sarcich, J. L., Howe, W. J., Tomich, C. S., and Smith, C. W. (1994). The HIV-1 protease as enzyme and substrate: Mutagenesis of autolysis sites and generation of a stable mutant with retained kinetic properties. *Biochemistry* **33**, 9405–9413.

Miller, M., Schneider, J., Sathyanarayana, B. K., Toth, M. V., Marshall, G. R., Clawson, L., Selk, L., Kent, S. B., and Wlodawer, A. (1989). Structure of complex of synthetic HIV-1 protease with a substrate-based inhibitor at 2.3 Å resolution. *Science* **246**, 1149–1152.

Muzammil, S., Ross, P., and Freire, E. (2003). A major role for a set of non-active site mutations in the development of HIV-1 protease drug resistance. *Biochemistry* **42**, 631–638.

Navia, M. A., Fitzgerald, P. M., McKeever, B. M., Leu, C. T., Heimbach, J. C., Herber, W. K., Sigal, I. S., Darke, P. L., and Springer, J. P. (1989). Three-dimensional structure of aspartyl protease from human immunodeficiency virus HIV-1. *Nature* **337**, 615–620.

Nicholson, L. K., Yamazaki, T., Torchia, D. A., Grzesiek, S., Bax, A., Stahl, S. J., Kaufman, J. D., Wingfield, P. T., Lam, P. Y., and Jadhav, P. K. (1995). Flexibility and function in HIV-1 protease [see comments]. *Nat. Struct. Biol.* **2**, 274–280.

Ohtaka, H., and Freire, E. (2005). Adaptive inhibitors of the HIV-1 protease. *Prog. Biophys. Mol. Biol.* **88**, 193–208.

Ohtaka, H., Muzammil, S., Schon, A., Velazquez-Campoy, A., Vega, S., and Freire, E. (2004). Thermodynamic rules for the design of high affinity HIV-1 protease inhibitors with adaptability to mutations and high selectivity towards unwanted targets. *Int. J. Biochem. Cell Biol.* **36**, 1787–1799.

Oroszlan, S., and Luftig, R. B. (1990). Retroviral proteinases. *Curr. Top. Microbiol. Immunol.* **157**, 153–185.

Paulus, C., Hellebrand, S., Tessmer, U., Wolf, H., Krausslich, H. G., and Wagner, R. (1999). Competitive inhibition of human immunodeficiency virus type-1 protease by the Gag-Pol transframe protein. *J. Biol. Chem.* **274**, 21539–21543.

Pearl, L., and Blundell, T. (1984). The active site of aspartic proteinases. *FEBS Lett.* **174**, 96–101.

Pearl, L. H., and Taylor, W. R. (1987). A structural model for the retroviral proteases. *Nature* **329**, 351–354.

Perryman, A. L., Lin, J. H., and McCammon, J. A. (2004). HIV-1 protease molecular dynamics of a wild-type and of the V82F/I84V mutant: Possible contributions to drug resistance and a potential new target site for drugs. *Protein Sci.* **13**, 1108–1123.

Pettit, S. C., Everitt, L. E., Choudhury, S., Dunn, B. M., and Kaplan, A. H. (2004). Initial cleavage of the human immunodeficiency virus type 1 GagPol precursor by its activated protease occurs by an intramolecular mechanism. *J. Virol.* **78**, 8477–8485.

Pettit, S. C., Clemente, J. C., Jeung, J. A., Dunn, B. M., and Kaplan, A. H. (2005). Ordered processing of the human immunodeficiency virus type 1 GagPol precursor is influenced by the context of the embedded viral protease. *J. Virol.* **79**, 10601–10607.

Prabu-Jeyabalan, M., Nalivaika, E., and Schiffer, C. A. (2000). How does a symmetric dimer recognize an asymmetric substrate? A substrate complex of HIV-1 protease. *J. Mol. Biol.* **301**, 1207–1220.

Prabu-Jeyabalan, M., Nalivaika, E., and Schiffer, C. A. (2002). Substrate shape determines specificity of recognition for HIV-1 protease: Analysis of crystal structures of six substrate complexes. *Structure* **10**, 369–381.

Prabu-Jeyabalan, M., Nalivaika, E. A., King, N. M., and Schiffer, C. A. (2003). Viability of a drug-resistant human immunodeficiency virus type 1 protease variant: Structural insights for better antiviral therapy. *J. Virol.* **77**, 1306–1315.

Prabu-Jeyabalan, M., Nalivaika, E. A., King, N. M., and Schiffer, C. A. (2004). Structural basis for coevolution of a human immunodeficiency virus type 1 nucleocapsid-p1 cleavage site with a V82A drug-resistant mutation in viral protease. *J. Virol.* **78**, 12446–12454.

Prabu-Jeyabalan, M., Nalivaika, E. A., Romano, K., and Schiffer, C. A. (2006). Mechanism of substrate recognition by drug-resistant human immunodeficiency virus type 1 protease variants revealed by a novel structural intermediate. *J. Virol.* **80**, 3607–3616.

Rick, S. W., Erickson, J. W., and Burt, S. K. (1998). Reaction path and free energy calculations of the transition between alternate conformations of HIV-1 protease. *Proteins* **32**, 7–16.

Rodriguez, E. J., Debouck, C., Deckman, I. C., Abu-Soud, H., Raushel, F. M., and Meek, T. D. (1993). Inhibitor binding to the Phe53Trp mutant of HIV-1 protease promotes conformational changes detectable by spectrofluorometry. *Biochemistry* **32**, 3557–3563.

Rodriguez-Barrios, F., and Gago, F. (2004). HIV protease inhibition: Limited recent progress and advances in understanding current pitfalls. *Curr. Top. Med. Chem.* **4**, 991–1007.

Rose, J. R., Salto, R., and Craik, C. S. (1993). Regulation of autoproteolysis of the HIV-1 and HIV-2 proteases with engineered amino acid substitutions. *J. Biol. Chem.* **268**, 11939–11945.

Rose, R. B., Craik, C. S., and Stroud, R. M. (1998). Domain flexibility in retroviral proteases: Structural implications for drug resistant mutations. *Biochemistry* **37**, 2607–2621.

Schramm, H. J., Nakashima, H., Schramm, W., Wakayama, H., and Yamamoto, N. (1991). HIV-1 reproduction is inhibited by peptides derived from the N- and C-termini of HIV-1 protease. *Biochem. Biophys. Res. Commun.* **179**, 847–851.

Schramm, H. J., Boetzel, J., Buttner, J., Fritsche, E., Gohring, W., Jaeger, E., Konig, S., Thumfart, O., Wenger, T., Nagel, N. E., and Schramm, W. (1996). The inhibition of human immunodeficiency virus proteases by 'interface peptides.' *Antiviral Res.* **30**, 155–170.

Schramm, H. J., de Rosny, E., Reboud-Ravaux, M., Buttner, J., Dick, A., and Schramm, W. (1999). Lipopeptides as dimerization inhibitors of HIV-1 protease. *Biol. Chem.* **380**, 593–596.

Scott, W. R., and Schiffer, C. A. (2000). Curling of flap tips in HIV-1 protease as a mechanism for substrate entry and tolerance of drug resistance. *Structure* **8**, 1259–1265.

Shafer, R. W. (2002). Genotypic testing of human immunodeficiency virus type 1 drug resistance. *Clin. Microbiol. Rev.* **15**, 247–277.

Shultz, M. D., and Chmielewski, J. (1999). Probing the role of interfacial residues in a dimerization inhibitor of HIV-1 protease. *Bioorg. Med. Chem. Lett.* **9**, 2431–2436.

Sluis-Cremer, N., and Tachedjian, G. (2002). Modulation of the oligomeric structures of HIV-1 retroviral enzymes by synthetic peptides and small molecules. *Eur. J. Biochem.* **269**, 5103–5111.

Sluis-Cremer, N., Arion, D., Abram, M. E., and Parniak, M. A. (2004). Proteolytic processing of an HIV-1 pol polyprotein precursor: Insights into the mechanism of reverse transcriptase p66/p51 heterodimer formation. *Int. J. Biochem. Cell Biol.* **36**, 1836–1847.

Strisovsky, K., Tessmer, U., Langner, J., Konvalinka, J., and Krausslich, H. G. (2000). Systematic mutational analysis of the active-site threonine of HIV-1 proteinase: Rethinking the "fireman's grip" hypothesis. *Protein Sci.* **9**, 1631–1641.

Szeltner, Z., and Polgar, L. (1996). Conformational stability and catalytic activity of HIV-1 protease are both enhanced at high salt concentration. *J. Biol. Chem.* **271**, 5458–5463.

Temesgen, Z., Warnke, D., and Kasten, M. J. (2006). Current status of antiretroviral therapy. *Expert Opin. Pharmacother.* **7**, 1541–1554.

Tessmer, U., and Krausslich, H. G. (1998). Cleavage of human immunodeficiency virus type 1 proteinase from the N-terminally adjacent p6* protein is essential for efficient Gag polyprotein processing and viral infectivity. *J. Virol.* **72**, 3459–3463.

Tie, Y., Boross, P. I., Wang, Y. F., Gaddis, L., Hussain, A. K., Leshchenko, S., Ghosh, A. K., Louis, J. M., Harrison, R. W., and Weber, I. T. (2004). High resolution crystal structures of HIV-1 protease with a potent non-peptide inhibitor (UIC-94017) active against multi-drug-resistant clinical strains. *J. Mol. Biol.* **338**, 341–352.

Tie, Y., Boross, P. I., Wang, Y. F., Gaddis, L., Liu, F., Chen, X., Tozser, J., Harrison, R. W., and Weber, I. T. (2005). Molecular basis for substrate recognition and drug resistance from 1.1 to 1.6 angstroms resolution crystal structures of HIV-1 protease mutants with substrate analogs. *FEBS J.* **272**, 5265–5277.

Todd, M. J., Semo, N., and Freire, E. (1998). The structural stability of the HIV-1 protease. *J. Mol. Biol.* **283**, 475–488.

Tomaselli, A. G., and Heinrikson, R. L. (1994). Specificity of retroviral proteases: An analysis of viral and nonviral protein substrates. *Methods Enzymol.* **241**, 279–301.

Tozser, J., Yin, F. H., Cheng, Y. S., Bagossi, P., Weber, I. T., Harrison, R. W., and Oroszlan, S. (1997). Activity of tethered human immunodeficiency virus 1 protease containing mutations in the flap region of one subunit. *Eur. J. Biochem.* **244**, 235–241.

Uhlikova, T., Konvalinka, J., Pichova, I., Soucek, M., Krausslich, H. G., and Vondrasek, J. (1996). A modular approach to HIV-1 proteinase inhibitor design. *Biochem. Biophys. Res. Commun.* **222**, 38–43.

Velazquez-Campoy, A., Luque, I., Todd, M. J., Milutinovich, M., Kiso, Y., and Freire, E. (2000a). Thermodynamic dissection of the binding energetics of KNI-272, a potent HIV-1 protease inhibitor. *Protein Sci.* **9**, 1801–1809.

Velazquez-Campoy, A., Todd, M. J., and Freire, E. (2000b). HIV-1 protease inhibitors: Enthalpic versus entropic optimization of the binding affinity. *Biochemistry* **39**, 2201–2207.

Vogt, V. M. (1996). Proteolytic processing and particle maturation. *Curr. Top. Microbiol. Immunol.* **214**, 95–131.

Vondrasek, J., van Buskirk, C. P., and Wlodawer, A. (1997). Database of three-dimensional structures of HIV proteinases. *Nat. Struct. Biol.* **4**, 8.

Wang, Y. X., Freedberg, D. I., Grzesiek, S., Torchia, D. A., Wingfield, P. T., Kaufman, J. D., Stahl, S. J., Chang, C. H., and Hodge, C. N. (1996). Mapping hydration water molecules in the HIV-1 protease/DMP323 complex in solution by NMR spectroscopy. *Biochemistry* 35, 12694–12704.

Weber, I. T. (1990). Comparison of the crystal structures and intersubunit interactions of human immunodeficiency and Rous sarcoma virus proteases. *J. Biol. Chem.* 265, 10492–10496.

Weber, I. T., Wu, J., Adomat, J., Harrison, R. W., Kimmel, A. R., Wondrak, E. M., and Louis, J. M. (1997). Crystallographic analysis of human immunodeficiency virus 1 protease with an analog of the conserved CA-p2 substrate-interactions with frequently occurring glutamic acid residue at P2' position of substrates. *Eur J. Biochem.* 249, 523–530.

Wlodawer, A., and Erickson, J. (1993). Structure-based inhibitors of HIV-1 protease. *Annu. Rev. Biochem.* 62, 543–585.

Wlodawer, A., and Vondrasek, J. (1998). Inhibitors of HIV-1 protease: A major success of structure-assisted drug design. *Annu. Rev. Biophys. Biomol. Struct.* 27, 249–284.

Wlodawer, A., Miller, M., Jaskolski, M., Sathyanarayana, B. K., Baldwin, E., Weber, I. T., Selk, L. M., Clawson, L., Schneider, J., and Kent, S. B. (1989). Conserved folding in retroviral proteases: Crystal structure of a synthetic HIV-1 protease. *Science* 245, 616–621.

Wondrak, E. M., Nashed, N. T., Haber, M. T., Jerina, D. M., and Louis, J. M. (1996). A transient precursor of the HIV-1 protease. Isolation, characterization, and kinetics of maturation. *J. Biol. Chem.* 271, 4477–4481.

Yamazaki, T., Nicholson, L. K., Torchia, D. A., Stahl, S. J., Kaufman, J. D., Wingfield, P. T., Domaille, P. J., and Campbell-Burk, S. (1994). Secondary structure and signal assignments of human-immunodeficiency-virus-1 protease complexed to a novel, structure-based inhibitor. *Eur. J. Biochem.* 219, 707–712.

Yamazaki, T., Hinck, A. P., Wang, Y. X., Nicholson, L. K., Torchia, D. A., Wingfield, P., Stahl, S. J., Kaufman, J. D., Chang, C. H., Domaille, P. J., and Lam, P. Y. (1996). Three-dimensional solution structure of the HIV-1 protease complexed with DMP323, a novel cyclic urea-type inhibitor, determined by nuclear magnetic resonance spectroscopy. *Protein Sci.* 5, 495–506.

York, D. M., Darden, T. A., Pedersen, L. G., and Anderson, M. W. (1993). Molecular dynamics simulation of HIV-1 protease in a crystalline environment and in solution. *Biochemistry* 32, 1443–1453.

Zhang, Z. Y., Poorman, R. A., Maggiora, L. L., Heinrikson, R. L., and Kezdy, F. J. (1991). Dissociative inhibition of dimeric enzymes. Kinetic characterization of the inhibition of HIV-1 protease by its COOH-terminal tetrapeptide. *J. Biol. Chem.* 266, 15591–15594.

Jean-Luc Darlix*, José Luis Garrido*, Nelly Morellet[‡], Yves Mély[†], and Hugues de Rocquigny[†]

*LaboRetro, Unité INSERM de Virologie Humaine, IFR128, ENS Sciences de Lyon
46 allée d'Italie, 69364 Lyon, France

[†]Institut Gilbert Laustriat, Pharmacologie et Physico-Chimie des Interactions
Cellulaires et Moléculaires, UMR 7034 CNRS, Faculté de Pharmacie
Université Louis Pasteur, Strasbourg 1, 74, Route du Rhin
67401 ILLKIRCH Cedex, France

[‡]Unité de Pharmacologie Chimique et Génétique, INSERM U640-CNRS UMR 8151
UFR des Sciences Pharmaceutiques et Biologiques
4, avenue de l'Observatoire, 75270 Paris Cedex 06, France

Properties, Functions, and Drug Targeting of the Multifunctional Nucleocapsid Protein of the *Human Immunodeficiency Virus*

I. Chapter Overview

Retroviral nucleocapsid (NC) proteins are small proteins generated by the cleavage of the Gag structural polyprotein by the viral protease, and are characterized by one or two copies of a highly conserved CCHC zinc finger (ZF), flanked by basic residues. Retroviral NC proteins are nucleic acid–binding proteins with potent RNA-chaperoning properties, enabling

Advances in Pharmacology, Volume 55
1054-3589/07 $35.00
DOI: 10.1016/S1054-3589(07)55009-X

important structural rearrangements that are required for genomic RNA replication and its packaging during virion assembly.

This chapter reviews the structure and functions of the HIV-1 NC protein, and the rational for a simple, rapid screening of anti-NC drugs aimed at inhibiting virion production. The three-dimensional (3D) conformation of HIV-1 NC shows that the central domain folds into a hydrophobic plateau flanked by disordered basic sequences. The hydrophobic plateau appears to orchestrate the NC functions network such as chaperoning the conversion of the genomic RNA into viral DNA by reverse transcriptase (RT) and balancing misincorporations of nucleotides into cDNA, thus exerting a control over HIV-1 variability during the early phase of virus replication. In the late phase, the NC hydrophobic plateau pilots the selection, dimerization, and packaging of the genomic RNA during the virion assembly process, which ensures formation of a mature functional inner capsid structure. A new one-step screening assay is described, which allows for the rapid *in vitro* identification of anti-NC compounds aimed at binding to the hydrophobic plateau, thus inhibiting NC during the early and late steps of HIV-1 replication.

II. The NC Protein: The Story So Far

During the twentieth century, studies on retroviruses led the way to remarkable discoveries seminal to our understanding of living organisms. Research on retroviruses has triggered fundamental discoveries such as that of oncogenes and their implication in cancer (Bishop, 1983; Brugge and Erikson, 1977; Hanafusa, 1969; Hu and Temin, 1990; Huebner and Todaro, 1969) and the role of retroelements in the plasticity and possibly the evolution of eukaryotic genomes (Baltimore, 1970; Garfinkel *et al.*, 1985; Hansen *et al.*, 1988; Huebner and Todaro, 1969). In this context, our understanding of the role of retroviral nucleocapsid protein, commonly referred to as NC, has come a long way since the first descriptions of oncoretroviruses and the oncoviral nucleoprotein (Ellermann and Bang, 1908; Rous, 1910). Elucidation of HIV-1 NC functions has largely benefited from the study of the NC protein of alpharetroviruses and gammaretroviruses, namely avian sarcoma leukosis viruses (ASLV) and the murine leukemia viruses (MuLV), respectively.

The NC story began with the isolation of ribonucleoprotein (RNP) complexes (Davis and Rueckert, 1972) from virions of ASLV and MuLV, which were able to support viral DNA synthesis. These RNP complexes, consisting of the 70S genomic RNA dimer coated by about 2000–2500 NC molecules, represent the most stable component of the viral particle, providing a chromatin-like structure with a circular conformation (Chen *et al.*, 1980; Pager *et al.*, 1994). These viral RNPs or nucleocores also contain molecules of the viral RT and integrase (IN) enzymes as well as molecules of cellular tRNAs and ribosomal RNA (Chen *et al.*, 1980; Darlix *et al.*, 1995; Dickson *et al.*, 1985). NC was first isolated from purified virions and shown to be a nucleic acid–binding protein (NABP) with preference for single-stranded sequences within structured RNA domains (Davis *et al.*, 1976). In the virus context, NC was shown to tightly bind a small number of genomic RNA sites rich in U and G residues, located in the 5′ untranslated leader region (5′ UTR) (Dannull *et al.*, 1994; Darlix and Spahr, 1982; Meric *et al.*, 1984; Tanchou *et al.*, 1995).

In the 1980s, two series of findings effectively started the NC story. First, NC was shown to be the driving force in genomic RNA selection, dimerization, and packaging during ASLV and MuLV assembly (Gorelick *et al.*, 1999; Meric *et al.*, 1988). Second, NC was found to direct viral RNA dimerization *in vitro* and annealing of the replication primer tRNA to the genomic primer-binding site (PBS) both *in vitro* and in ASLV and MuLV virions (Darlix *et al.*, 1990; Prats *et al.*, 1988, 1991). This second series of observations led to the discovery that NC was a viral protein with potent nucleic acid–chaperoning properties that were later found to be necessary for *bona fide* proviral DNA synthesis (reviewed in Darlix *et al.*, 1995; Rein *et al.*, 1998). These findings have since been borne out (Allain *et al.*, 1994; Auxilien *et al.*, 1999; Barat *et al.*, 1989; Buckman *et al.*, 2003; Darlix *et al.*, 1993; Gao *et al.*, 1997, 2003; Gorelick *et al.*, 1990; Shubsda *et al.*, 2002; You and McHenry, 1994; Yu and Darlix, 1996) paving the way for attempts to identify anti-HIV drugs specifically targeting NC (Druillennec *et al.*, 1999a,b; Rice *et al.*, 1995; Druillennec and Roques, 2000).

In the following sections we will briefly review HIV-1 NC, including its structure either in its free state or when bound to a small viral nucleic acid molecule, its DNA/RNA-chaperoning properties, its roles in the early and late phases of virus replication, and viral fitness. Emphasis will be given to the role of NC in nucleotide misincorporation during proviral DNA synthesis by RT and to the screening strategies aimed at identifying anti-HIV drugs targeting NC.

III. The Structure of HIV-1 NC

Retroviral NC proteins are small proteins generated by the viral protease–mediated cleavage of the Gag structural polyprotein precursor and are characterized by one or two copies of a highly conserved ZF motif of the CCHC type, flanked by basic regions. Spumaretroviruses and the Gypsy retrovirus of the fruit fly *Drosophila melanogaster* are rare exceptions to this rule since the corresponding Gag precursor in these cases is not processed by the viral protease and only contain an NC-like domain characterized by a large number of basic residues but no ZF motif (Fig. 1).

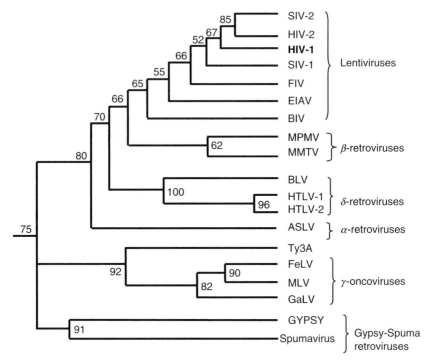

FIGURE I   Retroviral phylogeny based on NC proteins. The tree was constructed on NC proteins alignment of retrovirus families as indicated, using the protein sequence aligned by the clustalX and phylip program and displayed using the Tree View application, rooted to the CaMV NC-like protein. The figure on each branch represents percentage of bootstrap support, and the unsolved branches have been collapsed.

Retroviral NCs bind with high affinity to a large variety of nucleic acids, yet exhibit a high preference for single-stranded sequences rich in U and G residues (discussed in Section IV).

A. The ZF Structure

Each retroviral ZF coordinates one zinc ion with high affinity via CCHC–Zn^{2+} interactions (Berg, 1986; Mely *et al.*, 1991, 1996), which act as the main driving force behind the folded structure of this small peptidic domain. A large number of ZF and complete NC structures have been solved by nuclear magnetic resonance (NMR) spectroscopy and not surprisingly, ZFs from different retroviruses show similar structures. Specifically, the N-terminal part of each ZF adopts a rubredoxin-type turn, while the central amino acids fold into a loop and NH...S hydrogen bonds are formed between amide protons of the backbone and the zinc-chelating Cys residues

(Omichinski *et al.*, 1991; South *et al.*, 1991; Summers *et al.*, 1990; Turner and Summers, 1999). In the case of HIV-1 NCp7, the conformation of [29]RAPRKKG located downstream of the first CCHC box is responsible for the close proximity of the two zinc fingers (Morellet *et al.*, 1992; Summers *et al.*, 1992). However, the subtle differences between the two HIV-1 NC ZFs are clearly more than cosmetic as highlighted by a loss of NC functions on substitution of either of the ZFs by an identical counterpart (Gorelick *et al.*, 1993). Both proximal and distal HIV-1 NC ZFs are required and probably act in concert during virus replication (Figs. 3 and 4) (Section IV).

Structural differences also exist between the tandemly linked ZFs in SIV-1hoest NCp8, MMTV, and MPMV NCp9 (Gao *et al.*, 1998; Klein *et al.*, 2000). While the proximal NC ZF of the beta-retroviruses MMTV and MPMV can be superimposed on that of HIV-1 NC, SIV-1hoest NCp8, and NCp10 from the gammaretrovirus MuLV, their distal NC ZF contains an additional β-hairpin structure. This peculiarity within the distal ZFs of MMTV and MPMV may be responsible for a circular conformation, exposing residues necessary for RNA recognition and may thus be important for genomic RNA selection and packaging. However, this remains to be experimentally confirmed.

On a more general note, the ZF motifs of HIV and SIV-1hoest NC, of the betaretroviruses MMTV and MPMV NCp9, and the single NC ZF of the gammaretrovirus MuLV (Demene *et al.*, 1994b) all show high structural homology in spite of significant sequence differences (Figs. 2 and 3). This observation points to a common ancestor for the retroviral NC ZF motifs with the NC ZF of the yeast retroelement TY3 as a possible candidate (Fig. 2).

B. The 3D Structure of NC

In HIV-1 NCp7 as well as in other retroviral NCs with two ZFs, a short basic and flexible linker of 5–13 residues bridges the two ZFs (Fig. 2). In the case of HIV-1 NCp7, the conformation of [29]RAPRKKG located downstream of the first CCHC box is responsible for the proximity of the two ZFs (Morellet *et al.*, 1992; Summers *et al.*, 1992). Most linkers contain a Pro residue as is the case in HIV-1, HIV-2, SIV, MPMV, MMTV, and ASLV, while others do not such as in FIV and EIAV.

The flexible linker appears to be responsible for the transient globular structure of NC since weak and strong interfinger nuclear overhauser effect (NOE) in HIV-1 NCp7 and SIV-1hoest NCp8, respectively, indicate that the two independently folded ZFs can be in proximity in the free protein (Lee *et al.*, 1998; Morellet *et al.*, 1992, 1994, 2006). This proximity was confirmed by FRET and NMR using ^{15}N, ^{13}C-enriched NC samples (Lee *et al.*, 1998; Mely *et al.*, 1994; Ramboarina *et al.*, 2002). In contrast, the central domain of MMTV and MPMV NCs presents a higher degree of flexibility

```
HIV-1    --IQKGNFRNQRKT-VKCFNCGKEGHIAK-NCRAPRKKGCWKCGKEGHQMKDCTERQANFLGKIWPSHKGRPGNFL---  72
HIV-2    --PIPFAAAQQRRA-IRCWNCGKEGHSAK-QCRAPRRQGCWKCGKSHIMANCPERQAGFLG-MGPRGK-QPRNFP---  72
SIV-2    --PPRGPPRQPPRN-IRCFNCGKFGHLGLR-DSPRKKGCFKCGDLGHIMRNCP-KMVNFLG-NTPWGSGKPRNFPAM-  72
SIV-1    --QVGPQKKGPRGPLKEN-FEMQR-EKAPLQIKCFKCGKIHMAKDCKNGQANFLG-YGHWGGAKPRNFVQ---  72
FIV      --TKVQVVQSKGSGPVCFNKPGHLAR-QCREV--KKCNKCGKPGHVAAKWQGNRKNSGNWKAGRAAAPVNQMQQ---  72
BIV      ------PEDGRRGCGHTHLKR-NKQ---QKCYHCGKPGHQARNCRS--KN---  42
EIAV     ------PLKAAQTGNCGHPHLSS-QCAP--KVFFKCGKPGHFSKQCR------SVPKNGKQ---  49

Consensus ----------------*-**-*-***---*!*-------!**!*--!:---  80

Yeast Ty3 NC ---TVRTRRSYNKPMSNHRNRNNNPSREEIKN--RICFYCKKECHRLNECR-------ARKASSNRS----  57
```

FIGURE 2 Sequence alignment between lentiviral NC proteins and yeast retrotransposon Ty3 NC. Alignment of amino acid sequences of lentiviral NC proteins as indicated on the left: HIV-1, *Human immunodeficiency virus type 1*; HIV-2, *Human immunodeficiency virus type 2*; SIV-2, *Simian immunodeficiency virus type 2*; SIV-1, *Simian immunodeficiency virus type 1*; EIAV, *Equine infectious anemia virus*; FIV, *Feline immunodeficiency virus*; BIV, *Bovine immunodeficiency virus*; Ty3, yeast TY3 retrotransposon. For conserved residues the baseline has been set at 42% similarity. For residues under the 42% baseline, symbols are indicated for similar residues and for conserved residues (* for consensus), and for identical residues (! for consensus). Note that all sequences are rich in basic residues and contain at least one CCHC zinc finger motif which is entirely conserved (in dark shaded blocks) for coordinating a Zn^{2+}.

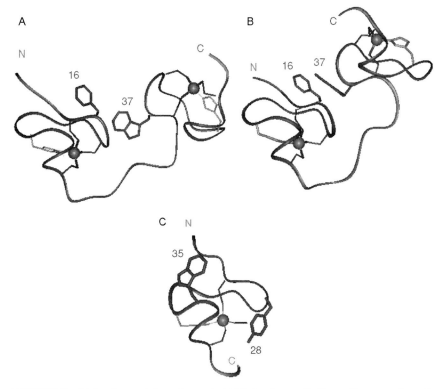

FIGURE 3 Molecular modeling of retroviral NC zinc fingers (I). Figure illustrates the well-conserved ZF backbone (in blue) based on the first ZF of HIV-1 NCp7 (A), in comparison with SIV NCp8 (B) and MuLV NCp10 (C). Aromatic residues essential for NC functions *in vivo* are in red (see numbers) and the N- and C-terminal ends are indicated by orange N and C letters. Zn^{2+} are represented by orange marbles. (See Color Insert.)

since no ZF interaction was found (Gao *et al.*, 1998; Klein *et al.*, 2000). Such structural differences in NCs from different retroviruses could result from the size of the linker, which is 7 amino acids for HIV and SIV NCs, and 13–15 residues for MMTV and MPMV NCs. Moreover in the HIV-1 and SIV NC structures, the proximity between the two zinc fingers is probably induced by the presence of a proline located in the linker, which favours the formation of a bend between the two ZFs. This relative orientation is stabilized by hydrophobic and aromatic interactions between the two ZFs, namely, Phe16, Ala25, Trp37 and Met46 in HIV-1 NCp7, and Thr14, Phe16, Thr24, Ala25, Trp37, Phe46 and Ala47 in SIV NCp8. In a manner different from NCp7, the two ZFs are strongly locked to each other in NCp8. This is directly related to the number of hydrophobic and aromatic residues at the interface between the two ZFs. The major consequence of such ZF interactions is that the basic residues spread in the sequence are

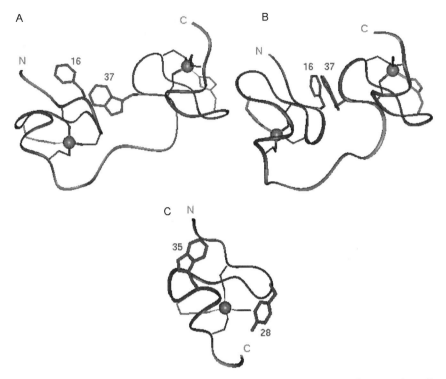

FIGURE 4 Molecular modeling of retroviral NC zinc fingers (II). Figure illustrates the well-conserved ZF backbone (in blue) based on the second ZF of HIV-1 NCp7 (A), in comparison with SIV NCp8 (B) and MoMuLV NCp10 (C). Aromatic residues essential for NC functions *in vivo* are in red (see numbers) and the N- and C-terminal ends are indicated by orange N and C letters. Zn^{2+} are represented by orange marbles. (See Color Insert.)

found in close proximity. In HIV-1 NCp7, Lys14, 20 and 38 on one hand, and Lys26, Arg29 and Arg32, on the other hand, are clustered and in the vicinity of the Phe16 and Trp37 aromatic residues. Similar observations can be done on the unique ZF of MuLV NCp10 where the basic residues Arg23 and Lys30, 32, 37, 41 and 42 are close to the aromatic residues at the surface of the ZF structure (Deméné *et al.*, 1994b). (Figs. 3 and 4)

In the case of the betaretrovirus MPMV, the structure of ^{50}P-^{52}L in NCp9 is stabilized by hydrophobic interactions involving the W62 side chain that is largely exposed to the solvent in the ZF structure (Gao *et al.*, 1998). Furthermore, the conserved hydrophobic residue I77 located downstream of the distal ZF is found in proximity with the C56 residue of the ZF. Nevertheless, as described for MMTV (Klein *et al.*, 2000), the total absence of NOEs between the two ZFs in this case is probably due to the lengthy sequence (11–15 residues) between them, preventing the immediate observation of an hydrophobic plateau. NMR studies of the two proteins in interaction with their cognate RNA will probably bring to light a pinch shaped by aromatic rings present in the NCp9 ZFs, surrounded by numerous basic residues.

We can provisionally conclude that the central ZF domain of the HIV-1 NCp7 folds into a tight structure while the flanking N- and C-terminal regions are rather disordered and independent from the central ZF (Figs. 3 and 4). This has led to the classification of HIV-1 NCp7 and retroviral NCs in general within the large family of proteins possessing extended intrinsically disordered/flexible regions (reviewed in Ivanyi-Nagy et al., 2005). It may be no coincidence that NC encoded by the ancient yeast TY3 retrotransposon—a possible ancestor of HIV NC based on observations of similar property and function (Gabus et al., 1998)—was found to be largely unstructured (unpublished data). This intrinsic disorder extends well beyond the retroviral NCs since it appears to be a hallmark of most if not all RNA chaperones (Cristofari and Darlix, 2002). The disordered NC regions may allow for the observed interactions of NC with a large panel of targeted viral nucleic acid sequences, such as the HIV-1 psi-packaging stem loops (SL), the PBS, and the TAR (see below), while the main aim of the folded ZFs is to properly present several amino acids critical for nucleic acid recognition and genomic RNA packaging into virion.

C. The Structure of NC in Small Nucleic Acid Molecular Complexes

The structure of HIV-1 NCp7 and MuLV NCp10 was explored by NMR in a 1:1 complex with either DNA (dACGCC) (Morellet et al., 1998; Roques et al., 1997; Schuler et al., 1999) or RNA (HIV-1 SL2 and SL3) (Amarasinghe et al., 2000a,b; De Guzman et al., 1998). According to the structural data obtained, the mode of interaction of NCp7 with single-stranded DNA or RNA is roughly the same with respect to the amino acids involved and the globular structure of the ZF domain. Once more the functional importance of the ZFs is revealed since they direct the recognition of DNA/RNA while the N- and C-terminal regions stabilize the nucleoprotein complex. Binding of NCp7 to an oligonucleotide modifies the backbone architecture of NC notably at the level of the linker and the N-terminal region. The linker becomes orthogonal to the ribose phosphate backbone and locates the ZFs in preparedness to pinch the oligonucleotide. The interaction is mainly due to the ZF tips so that a part of the ZF structure remains accessible for additional interactions that are critical for viral replication (i.e., RT, see Section IV). In addition, the spatial proximity of the two ZFs is reinforced on oligonucleotide binding. The NMR structures also show that the hydrophobic plateau at the surface of the ZFs represents the oligonucleotide-binding motif. Interestingly, a similar hydrophobic cluster composed of L21, A27, W35, and A36 participates in the nucleic acid recognition by MuLV NCp10 (Schuler et al., 1999). A similar ZF plateau is thought to present W37 of HIV NC and W35 of MLV NC to the nucleic acid molecule and to promote G stacking, a suggestion confirmed by fluorescence and phosphorescence studies (Bombarda *et al.*, 1999; Casas-Finet *et al.*, 1988; Khan and Giedroc, 1994; Mely *et al.*, 1995; Vuilleumier *et al.*, 1999; Wu *et al.*, 1997). Additional structural similarities between these HIV NC complexes have been noted. For instance, the Nε-H proton of R32 in the linker is hydrogen bonded to A8 of SL3 (De Guzman *et al.*, 1998) and to C4 of G3 in ACGCC (Morellet *et al.*, 1998). At the same time there are also clear differences between the structures. In the SL2/NCp7 and SL3/NCp7 complexes, the oligonucleotides bind in opposite direction to NCp7 as compared with the complex with d(ACGCC).

With respect to the basic N-terminal domain, binding of NCp7 to the oligonucleotide causes the formation of a 3_{10} helix resulting in its packing near the proximal ZF, while N8 and Q9 form H bonds with the carbonyl groups of T12 and G22, respectively. Such structural modifications are also observed with MuLV NCp10 where binding to a DNA/RNA molecule results in the folding of the N-terminal (A18-D24) sequence located upstream of its unique ZF (D'Souza and Summers, 2004; Schuler *et al.*, 1999).

The structure of the oligonucleotide backbone on NCp7 binding has also been explored by NMR. Structural changes in the loop of SL2 and SL3 that are part of the HIV-1 Psi packaging signal were observed, but NC does not affect significantly the structure of the stem. Slight structural changes can be seen with a small DNA molecule since stacking of W37 with the G3 residue of dACGCC increases the distance between C2 and G3 and results in a limited extension of the phosphate backbone. This limited RNA modification was also observed when NCp7 binds the HIV replication primer tRNA^{Lys3} (Gregoire *et al.*, 1997; Tisne *et al.*, 2003). Similar observations were made with MuLV NCp10 where its binding to the DIS-2, SL-C, and SL-D sequences of the MLV psi signal did not significantly affect folding (D'Souza and Summers, 2004).

In conclusion, the mutual recognition between NCp7 and a nucleic acid molecule necessitates the W37 residue, which represents a key signal on the hydrophobic ZF plateau and the surrounding basic residues that are present in the disordered N-terminal region and in the linker. The stacking of W37 with a G residue in a single-stranded sequence appears to be the key determinant for nucleic acid recognition while the basic residues would reinforce and modulate the binding. Thus, W37 in the ZF plateau may specifically select an RNA or DNA-binding site, while the basic flexible regions allow for variability in the surrounding sequence and structure contexts. This has important consequences in HIV-1 assembly and genomic RNA packaging (Section IV). However, structures obtained to date are limited to a single HIV-1 NC molecule interacting with short oligonucleotides. More sophisticated complexes involving several NC molecules interacting with a large RNA should undoubtedly provide new insights into NC–NC interactions and structural rearrangements of nucleic acid molecules (see future prospects).

IV. The Network of NC Functions

A. RNA Chaperone Proteins and Rearrangement of Nucleic Acid Structures

Retroviral NC proteins belong to a large class of NABPs named RNA chaperones that are ubiquitous in all living organisms and viruses where they perform seminal functions ranging from gene transcription and regulation to RNA translation and maintenance (Cristofari and Darlix, 2002; Herschlag, 1995; Schroeder *et al.*, 2004; Tompa and Csermely, 2004). These proteins contain flexible/disordered domains (Dunker *et al.*, 2001; Uversky, 2002; Wright and Dyson, 1999) rich in basic residues and bind nucleic acids with broad sequence specificity (Cristofari and Darlix, 2002; Schroeder *et al.*, 2004).

But why are RNA chaperones indispensable partners of nucleic acids? In fact RNA molecules can easily be trapped in a large variety of stable but nonfunctional conformations and it is the RNA chaperone proteins that assist RNA folding by preventing misfolding or by resolving misfolded RNA species (Cristofari and Darlix, 2002; Herschlag, 1995; Schroeder *et al.*, 2004). RNA-folding assistance is essential to ensure that RNA species reach their proper functional conformation in a rapid manner in physiological conditions (Cristofari and Darlix, 2002; Schroeder *et al.*, 2004). Examples of well-known RNA chaperones include the tumor suppressor P53, hnRNP A1, the major mRNA-binding protein YB1/P50, the fragile X mental retardation protein FMRP, and the prion protein (PrP), to name a few (Cristofari and Darlix, 2002; Evdokimova *et al.*, 2006; Gabus *et al.*, 2001; Ivanyi-Nagy *et al.*, 2005). Retroviral NCs represent canonical examples of multifunctional RNA chaperones that drive the necessary structural rearrangements of the genomic RNA during the early and late phases of virus replication (see below; reviewed in Darlix *et al.*, 1995, 2000). Other viral nucleoproteins with chaperone activities have been discovered in the *Human hepatitis C virus* (HCV) (Cristofari *et al.*, 2004; Ivanyi-Nagy *et al.*, 2006) and *Hantavirus* (Mir and Panganiban, 2005), yet their function in virus replication remains to be experimentally determined.

Both simple and advanced assays have been developed to examine some of the properties of RNA chaperones that involve rearrangement of nucleic acid structures in physiological conditions (Cristofari and Darlix, 2002; Schroeder *et al.*, 2004). Assays include annealing of two complementary sequences, DNA strand exchange, hammerhead ribozyme-directed cleavage of an RNA substrate, and *trans* RNA splicing. HIV-1 NC was shown to be very active in all nucleic acid–chaperoning assays and optimal activity required both the ZFs and the basic domains. However, data on HIV-1 and more generally on RNA chaperones may vary greatly as a function of the experimental conditions used. For instance, results can be at variance depending on the NC to RNA/DNA molar ratio in the assay, which determines the level of RNA occupancy (Ivanyi-Nagy *et al.*, 2005).

How then does HIV-1 NC function? The current view is that firstly NC recognizes RNA through multiple interactions (see above). This leads NC to make contact with six to seven nucleotides that represent the NC-binding site (Dib-Hajj *et al.*, 1993; Khan and Giedroc, 1994; Mely *et al.*, 1995). Secondly, the molar ratio of NC to RNA determines at least three levels of RNA occupancy and thus three discrete modes of activity and function (Ivanyi-Nagy *et al.*, 2005): (1) At limiting NC concentrations, a simple nucleoprotein complex is formed corresponding to the "binding mode." (2) If more NC is available, the RNA molecule becomes coated with NC. This high degree of RNA occupancy corresponds to the "chaperoning mode" whereby RNA molecules can undergo structural rearrangements, and possibly recruit other protein and nucleic factors (see section on functions). (3) If saturating levels of NC are present, the RNA molecules are entirely coated by NC, resulting in the unwinding of most if not all RNA structures by NC molecules. At this "saturating mode," the completeness of RNA occupancy by NC is a state that is believed to preclude any further interactions.

B. *In Vitro* Assays to Explore the Early Functions of NC

To simulate the functions of HIV-1 NC during the course of genome replication, specific *in vitro* assays have been designed using 5' and 3' RNA accurately representing the terminal regions of the genomic RNA. In fact they contain sequences and SL structures indispensable to virus replication, namely the PBS and PPT for the initiation of (−) and (+)strand DNA synthesis, respectively, TAR for cDNA strand transfer, and the stem loops SL1 to SL4 required for the selection, dimerization, and packaging of the genomic RNA and that are also required for the initiation of the full-length viral RNA translation (Brasey *et al.*, 2003; Buck *et al.*, 2001; Ohlmann *et al.*, 2000).

I. Viral DNA Synthesis

The early phase of virus replication spans virus-cell recognition and entry to viral DNA synthesis and integration into the host genome. The double-stranded viral DNA is synthesized by the viral RT during a succession of specific events that take place in an RT complex most probably corresponding to the viral NC (reviewed in Darlix *et al.*, 1995; Rein *et al.*, 1998). Needless to say the conversion of the genomic RNA into the viral

DNA with long terminal repeats (LTRs) has been extensively studied and reviewed (see, e.g., above cited reviews; Levin *et al.*, 2005). The overall process of reverse transcription necessitates profound structural rearrangements of the genomic RNA, the cellular primer tRNA, and the newly made viral DNA, and which are all orchestrated by NC. For example, NC chaperones the annealing of primer tRNA to the PBS for initiation (Cen *et al.*, 2000; Darlix *et al.*, 1990; De Rocquigny *et al.*, 1992, 1993; Hargittai *et al.*, 2001, 2004; Huang *et al.*, 1997; Li *et al.*, 1996; Liang *et al.*, 1997; Prats *et al.*, 1988), of TAR(–) DNA to TAR(+) RNA annealing for the obligatory (–) strand DNA transfer (Beltz *et al.*, 2003, 2004, 2005; Bernacchi *et al.*, 2002; Godet *et al.*, 2006; Guo *et al.*, 1997), and of PBS(+) DNA to PBS(–) DNA annealing for the obligatory (+)strand transfer (Egele *et al.*, 2004, 2005). At the same time binding of NC to the viral RNA and cDNA prevents false initiation and elongation reactions caused by 3′ terminal SLs (Beltz *et al.*, 2005; Lapadat-Tapolsky *et al.*, 1997). Thus, NC appears to chaperone the RT-mediated synthesis of a complete *bona fide* proviral DNA by means of specific intermolecular nucleic acid interactions dictated by their sequence (Lapadat-Tapolsky *et al.*, 1997; Levin *et al.*, 2005 and reviews cited above).

From a mechanistic perspective, the NC-chaperoning properties can be separated in two distinct but related components: (1) the intramolecular destabilization of the folded complementary sequences and (2) the activation of their intermolecular annealing. Importantly, optimal NC activity is reached at a protein to nucleic acid molar ratio of between 1:8 and 1:6 nt, which corresponds to the "chaperoning mode" (described above) whereby the template is coated with NC molecules in a proportion similar to that existing in the virion NC (i.e., about 1500 NC molecules per dimeric genome).

a. Initiation At the initiation step, NC destabilizes the G6-U67 and T54-A58 pairs of tRNA^{Lys3} primer structure (Chan *et al.*, 1999; Hargittai *et al.*, 2001; Tisne *et al.*, 2001). The NC-promoted destabilization of the first of these base pairs likely brings about access by the PBS sequence to the weak bases at the four-way junction within the tRNA^{Lys3} cloverleaf (Tisne *et al.*, 2004). NC then facilitates strand exchange at the level of the tRNA acceptor stem, presumably via its basic N- and C-terminal extensions. Next, NC unlocks via probably its ZFs the highly stable interactions at the TΨC loop to promote the opening of the tRNA tertiary structure, enabling the complete annealing to the genomic RNA. The hybridization follows a second-order kinetics, consistent with the nucleation of the intermolecular duplex being the rate-limiting step (Hargittai *et al.*, 2004), which is subsequently followed by a much accelerated zipping of the remaining 18 bp duplex.

b. Minus cDNA Transfer The first strand transfer during cDNA synthesis requires both cTAR DNA and TAR RNA, which are imperfect SLs with numerous conserved bulges, mismatches, and internal loops delineating contiguous double-stranded segments. In the absence of NC, the fully closed cTAR species is in equilibrium with short lived, partially melted species where either the terminal double-stranded segment, the lower half of the stem or the full stem are melted (Beltz *et al.*, 2003; Bernacchi *et al.*, 2002). NC activates the transient opening of cTAR terminal base pairs that propagates up to the middle of the stem (Beltz *et al.*, 2003; Bernacchi *et al.*, 2002; Cosa *et al.*, 2004, 2006). NC also promotes the destabilization of cTAR, which is strongly dependent on the destabilizing motifs that are scattered along the structure of cTAR (Beltz *et al.*, 2003, 2004). Since these motifs are highly conserved, a coevolutionary relationship between TAR and NC activity is likely required to activate strand transfer. NC also melts TAR but less efficiently than cTAR due to the higher stability of TAR as compared with cTAR (Bernacchi *et al.*, 2002). The ability of NC to destabilize nucleic acid structures is supported by its two fingers in their proper context, and the basic linker (Beltz *et al.*, 2005). This strict requirement seems to result from the interaction of cTAR with the hydrophobic plateau present at the surface of the NC structure (Figs. 3–5), only if the ZFs are properly folded and oriented (Morellet *et al.*, 1992, 1994; Stote *et al.*, 2004). This plateau is crucial for the progressive melting of the cTAR from the ends up to the middle of the stem, in order to generate the single-stranded complementary regions for nucleating the duplexes. The kinetics and mechanism of the formation of cTAR/TAR extended duplex (ED) are still debated. Initial studies (You and McHenry, 1994) showed that ED formation follows first-order kinetics, consistent with an unusually slow unfolding of the secondary structure as the rate-limiting step followed by a more rapid nucleation step. In contrast, more recent studies (Godet *et al.*, 2006; Liu *et al.*, 2005) suggest that ED forms through a second-order "zipper" pathway that is kinetically limited by the nucleation of residues located mainly within the central double-stranded segment of both cTAR and TAR stems. An alternative mechanism involving a "kissing-loop" interaction between TAR and cTAR top loops is also observed but its relative importance with respect to the "zipper" pathway seems to vary according to the experimental conditions (Godet *et al.*, 2006; Kanevsky *et al.*, 2005; Liu *et al.*, 2005).

c. Plus DNA Strand Transfer   Soon after the initiation of (+)strand DNA by RT, NC directs the annealing of the (−)PBS and (+)PBS DNA sequences, which are required for the second strand transfer. It induces only a limited destabilization of the stem of both sequences, activating the transient melting of the final G-C pair (Egele *et al.*, 2004, 2005). By binding the 5-CTG-7 sequence of (−)PBS, NC induces a stretching of the loop, and a perturbation of the C5-G11 base pair next to the loop that could favor annealing with the complementary (+)PBS sequence through a "kissing complex" (Morellet *et al.*, unpublished data, Ramalanjaona *et al.*, unpublished data).

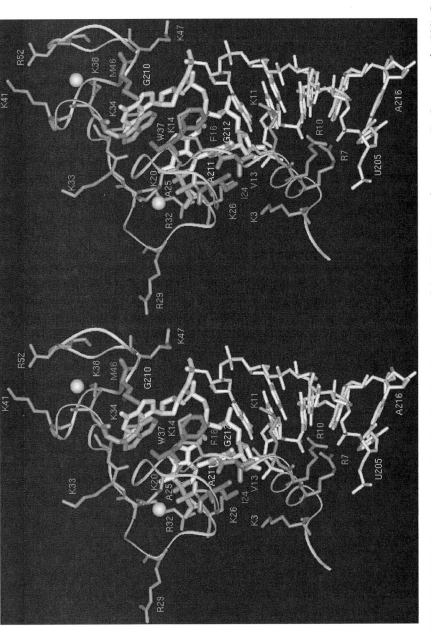

FIGURE 5 HIV-1 NCp7 bound to a small nucleic acid molecule. Stereoview of the NCp7/SL3 complex structure (De Guzman *et al.*, 1998). Only the lysine, arginine, and hydrophobic residues V13, F16, I24, A25, W37, M46, and the 205–216 domain of the HIV-1 SL3 sequence are represented. The zinc ions are in yellow. NCp7 is illustrated as a green ribbon. The nucleotides in interaction with the ZF domain of NCp7 are in light yellow. (See Color Insert.)

This NC-promoted hybridization of PBS(−):(+)PBS appears kinetically limited by the conversion of the "kissing" complex to the ED. Along this line, NC directs formation of a "kissing" TAR homodimer complex (Andersen *et al.*, 2004; Egele *et al.*, 2004, 2005). This propensity of NC to facilitate the dimerization of partly complementary sequences may favor secondary contacts between viral sequences, and thus recombination during viral DNA synthesis, which fuels viral diversity (Section VI).

d. NC–RT Interactions   Direct NC–RT interactions are believed to facilitate this complex series of reactions leading to the synthesis of a complete proviral DNA by RT (Druillennec *et al.*, 1999a; Lener *et al.*, 1998). Illustration of a globular replicating complex proposes that the template and the newly made cDNA are at the interface between two hemispheres corresponding to bound NC molecules on the one hand and a heterodimeric RTp66/p51 on the other (Fig. 6). Accordingly, RT would easily access the genomic template and convert it into cDNA in a reaction that NC facilitates by increasing the time of residency of RT on the template and by preventing false initiation and elongation events (Bampi *et al.*, 2006; Lapadat-Tapolsky *et al.*, 1997; Lener *et al.*, 1998) (Fig. 6).

2. Viral DNA Integration

At the end of the reverse transcription process, NC molecules coat the newly made viral DNA in a nucleoprotein complex found to be partially resistant to nuclease degradation (Lapadat-Tapolsky *et al.*, 1993). In addition, the inverted repeat sequences "ir" at the very end of the LTR were shown to become protected due to the binding of NC and IN (Bampi *et al.*, 2004), favoring the view that NC and IN cooperate to ensure the maintenance of the proviral DNA. The existence of functional interactions between NC and IN is further supported by the fact that NC can strongly stimulate LTR DNA integration by IN under physiological conditions *in vitro* (Buckman *et al.*, 2003; Carteau *et al.*, 1997; Poljak *et al.*, 2003; Thomas *et al.*, 2006).

C. The Functions of NC During the Early Phase of Virus Replication

The role of NC in HIV-1 replication has been extensively studied, mostly using molecular biology and human cell lines since these are easy to culture and transfect with DNA (review in Darlix *et al.*, 1995; Levin *et al.*, 2005). The emerging view is that NC coordinates multiple processes both during the early steps as the mature NC protein and during the late steps as the C-terminal domain of the structural Gag precursor. Since the role of NC in

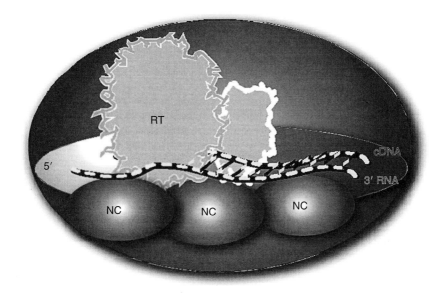

FIGURE 6 Schematic representation of the reverse transcription complex. NC protein molecules (in white-blue) coat the genomic RNA (in yellow with black bars) in the form of NC oligomers, ensuring faithful cDNA synthesis (in yellow) at the initiation and strand transfers steps, and providing protection of the complex against degradation by proteases and nucleases. Heterodimeric RTp66-p51 (in orange) copies the genome to generate a double-stranded DNA flanked by two LTRs.

viral DNA synthesis has been amply described, we will focus on the biological relevance of NC structure in viral DNA synthesis.

The ZF hydrophobic plateau is most probably required for the synthesis of the complete viral DNA with LTRs and for its maintenance, and possibly its integration into the host genome (Buckman *et al.*, 2003; Tanchou *et al.*, 1997). Indeed, subtle structural changes in the first or second ZF caused by the H23C or H44C mutation have drastic consequences since the mutant virus is replication defective. Further investigation revealed that viral DNA synthesis is impaired and results in the production of an incomplete and/or unstable viral DNA (Demene *et al.*, 1994a; Gorelick *et al.*, 1996, 1999). Recent results by Gorelick *et al.* also indicate that the integration reaction is partially impaired (Buckman *et al.*, 2003; Thomas *et al.*, 2006), supporting the view that functional interactions exist between NC and IN. From a structural point of view, analyses of the H23C mutant show that residues V13, F16, T24, and A25 have a spatial orientation different from the wild type resulting in loose interactions between the ZF plateau and the RNA (Remy *et al.*, 1998). In addition, mutations in the ZF strongly diminish

NC–RT interactions (Lener *et al.*, 1998). On the other hand, mutating the disordered regions flanking the ZF appears to be much less detrimental to virus replication since several basic residues need to be changed to neutral ones in order to cause a drastic reduction in viral DNA synthesis (Berthoux *et al.*, 1997; Cimarelli and Darlix, 2002).

Taken together, these findings suggest that the ZF hydrophobic plateau coordinates the early functions of NC in viral DNA synthesis, maintenance, and integration, while the basic regions are probably redundant and act in support of the ZFs (see also below the late functions of NC).

V. The Role of NC in HIV-1 Assembly _____

A. Overview of the Assembly Process

Two distinct mechanisms of retrovirus assembly have long been described. Retroviral particles are preformed in the cytoplasm of infected cells and transported to the plasma membrane such as in the case of betaretroviruses (MMTV, MPMV), or they directly assemble underneath the plasma membrane as for alpha- and gammaretroviruses (ASLV and MLV, respectively). Until recently, HIV-1 assembly was thought to follow the second mode (Ono *et al.*, 2004), but recent findings indicate that this may not be the case. Several reports indicate that HIV assembly can also take place in intracellular vesicles in human macrophages and in T cells (Grigorov *et al.*, 2006; Ono and Freed, 2004; Pelchen-Matthews *et al.*, 2003; Rudner *et al.*, 2005). Since the mature Gag proteins are the major components of the virus and because Gag on its own is capable of assembling into virus-like particles (VLP) (Freed, 2002, 2004; Gheysen *et al.*, 1989; Göttlinger, 2001; Ono and Freed, 2004; Ono *et al.*, 2004; Pornillos *et al.*, 2002; Resh, 2005), the remaining discussion will focus on Gag.

B. Gag Synthesis

The Gag polyprotein precursor contains all the signals and domains required for particle assembly, and consequently is viewed as the major player in the entire assembly process that goes from synthesis to assembly and release of virions (Darlix *et al.*, 1995; Göttlinger, 2001). In infected cells, the unspliced viral RNA acts both as the messenger coding for Gag and Gag-Pol and as the genome to be selected, dimerized, and packaged into assembling particles (Levin *et al.*, 2005; Muriaux *et al.*, 1996). Since the genomic RNA cannot fulfill these two key functions at the same time, this raises the question on how genomic RNA translation and packaging are regulated

(Brasey *et al.*, 2003; Lopez-Lastra *et al.*, 2005). As previously shown for alpha- and gammaretroviruses and more recently for lentiviruses (Attal *et al.*, 1996; Berlioz and Darlix, 1995; Berlioz *et al.*, 1995; Brasey *et al.*, 2003; Buck *et al.*, 2001; Deffaud and Darlix, 2000; Herbreteau *et al.*, 2005; Lopez-Lastra *et al.*, 1997; Ohlmann *et al.*, 2000; Vagner *et al.*, 1995), Gag is synthesized by an original mechanism whereby the cellular translation machinery has a direct access to sequences within the viral RNA, upstream of the initiator AUG of Gag, a region called the internal ribosome entry signal or IRES. For HIV, two IRESs have been described one spanning the packaging signal, SL1 to SL4, up to the Gag initiation codon and the second entirely located within the Gag-coding region (Brasey *et al.*, 2003; Buck *et al.*, 2001; Herbreteau *et al.*, 2005; reviewed by Prevot *et al.*, 2003). Importantly, these two HIV IRESs can function during the G2-M phase of the cell cycle during which most 5′ Cap-dependent translation is halted (Brasey *et al.*, 2003; Pyronnet and Sonenberg, 2001). This has important consequences for the level of HIV translation because the viral protein R(VPR) protein tends to block infected cells into the G2-M phase (Goh *et al.*, 1998; He *et al.*, 1995; Jowett *et al.*, 1995; Levy *et al.*, 1993; McCarthy, 1995). As newly made Gag molecules accumulate at the site of synthesis, it is conceivable that they will bind the full-length viral RNA via specific inter-actions between NC and the high-affinity binding sites present on the IRES/packaging region (Aldovini and Young, 1990; Baudin *et al.*, 1993; Berkhout, 1996; Clever *et al.*, 1995, 2002; Hayashi *et al.*, 1992; Lever *et al.*, 1989; McBride and Panganiban, 1996; Sakaguchi *et al.*, 1993). In fact, NC binds with a high affinity, in the order of 10^7 M^{-1}, to each SL *in vitro* where it recognizes a consensus GXG motif (Fisher *et al.*, 1998; Vuilleumier *et al.*, 1999). Moreover, it is important to note that recombinant Gag-NC has a tenfold higher affinity than NC for such sequences *in vitro* (Cruceanu *et al.*, 2006). Taken together, these findings favor a mechanism where binding of several neosynthesized Gag-NC molecules to the SL1–SL4 region of the full-length viral RNA would render it inaccessible to active ribosomes due to structural rearrangements and the presence of bound Gag molecules (Huthoff and Berkhout, 2001a,b, 2002), and reorient the genomic RNA toward dimerization and packaging, effectively starting the assembly process (reviewed in Butsch and Boris-Lawrie, 2000, 2002; Darlix *et al.*, 1995, 2000). In agreement with this proposed mechanism, recent data suggest that RNA structural modifications are not sufficient on their own to inhibit Gag protein synthesis (Abbink *et al.*, 2005), but they most probably act in concert with NC to reorient the genomic RNA from messenger toward dimerization (Dardel *et al.*, 1998; Ennifar *et al.*, 2001) and ultimately to packaging (Abbink *et al.*, 2005). In consequence, it is conceivable that NC has a major contribution in determining the fate of HIV genomic RNA and that this contribution will not exclusively depend on NC-induced RNA structural rearrangements as previously assumed (Abbink and Berkhout, 2003; Brasey *et al.*, 2003, Darlix *et al.*, 1995).

C. HIV Gag Assembly

How and Where is Gag assembly taking place?

I. How?

The binding of several Gag-NC molecules to the SL1–SL4 RNA-packaging region may effectively kick-start HIV assembly by concentrating Gag on a single dimeric RNA, a process known as nucleation (see above refs., reviewed in Darlix *et al.*, 2003). This nucleation event can then favor protein–protein interactions via the different Gag domains to orchestrate virus assembly. In this model of virus assembly, the genomic RNA acts as platform for the recruitment of Gag molecules via specific interactions between NC and the SL1–SL4-packaging/dimerization signal (Echols, 1990; Kaye and Lever, 1999; Muriaux *et al.*, 2001; Tanchou *et al.*, 1995) and concomitantly Gag-Pol precursor molecules, which will result in protease activation and precursor processing due to the high local protease concentration (Gelderblom *et al.*, 1987). This will ultimately lead to the coating of the dimeric RNA genome with NC molecules, and hybridization of the primer tRNA to the PBS to initiate cDNA synthesis (Barat *et al.*, 1989; Cen *et al.*, 2000; De Rocquigny *et al.*, 1992; Hargittai *et al.*, 2001; Lori *et al.*, 1992; Trono, 1992; Zhang *et al.*, 1994).

Under these conditions, what is the biological relevance of the 3D structure of NC? As described above, NC is characterized by a ZF hydrophobic plateau flanked by disordered basic regions. Subtle structural changes of the plateau caused by mutating the Cys or Histine residues of either ZF, or replacing the critical W37 by an Ala have drastic consequences, rendering the virus noninfectious and impairing, but not completely eliminating, genomic RNA packaging (Deméné *et al.*, 1994a; Dorfman *et al.*, 1993). The basic NC regions have a similar, but not identical role because at least two to three basic residues need to be substituted by neutral ones in order to cause a drastic—though not preclusion—of virus infectivity (Deméné *et al.*, 1994; Tanchou *et al.*, 1997). In addition, changing the ZF or the basic regions can cause drastic alterations in Gag trafficking, the level of virus production, and in the overall structure of the virion core (Berthoux *et al.*, 1999; Ottmann *et al.*, 1995).

This body of evidence favors the idea that the NC ZF plateau is present in the Gag polyprotein and orchestrates the nucleation event corresponding to the start of assembly. It is also tempting to conclude that the specific interactions between Gag-NC molecules and the packaging/dimerization element chaperone correct Gag–Gag interactions and the capture of more Gag molecules into the growing viral globule.

2. Where?

The currently accepted model of HIV assembly posits that in addition to the genomic RNA platform, a second platform is needed. While the genomic RNA acts as an inner scaffold (see above), a membrane is the outer platform in which Gag molecules are anchored through interactions between the phospholipids and the N-terminal part of the matrix domain (reviewed in Cimarelli and Darlix, 2002; Freed, 2002; Zhou *et al.*, 1994). The plasma membrane was until recently considered to be the major, if not the sole membrane where assembly took place (Cimarelli and Darlix, 2002; Ono and Freed, 2004; Ono *et al.*, 2004). However, this canonical view has been called into question by the observation that HIV assembly mostly occurs on endosomal membranes in the interior of infected human macrophages and T lymphocytes (Basyuck *et al.*, 2003; Fevrier and Raposo, 2004; Grigorov *et al.*, 2006; Kramer *et al.*, 2005; Pelchen-Matthews *et al.*, 2003; Raposo *et al.*, 2002). In fact, large amounts of Gag, the genomic RNA, and Env are found in endosomal compartments where infectious virions accumulate (Fig. 7). These recent findings favor the view that newly synthesized Gag molecules specifically bind the genomic RNA in the cytosol, possibly in proximity to translating ribosomes, then viral core complexes are targeted to late endosomes together with the Env proteins where infectious HIV-1 particles are completed and subsequently released from the infected cell by active exocytosis with the help of the cellular factors including TSG101 (Strack *et al.*, 2003; Stuchell *et al.*, 2004; Von Schwedler *et al.*, 2003; reviewed in Marsh and Thali, 2003) (Fig. 7). In support of this original

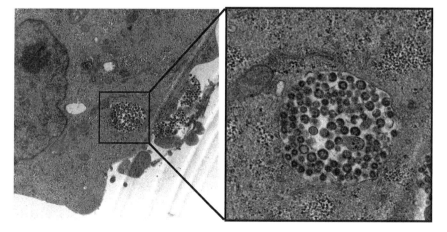

FIGURE 7   HIV-1 in endosomes of infected T CD4+ cells. Electron microscopy pictures showing the accumulation of HIV-1 particles (see insert on the left) within endosomes of chronically infected human TCD4+ cells (see right panel where about 50 virions with a diameter of 110–130 nm can be seen) (Grigorov *et al.*, 2006).

mechanism, NC ZF mutations cause an accumulation of Gag either at the plasma membrane or within the cytoplasm but not at the level of endosomes (Muriaux *et al.*, unpublished data).

Specific interactions between the Gag ZFs and the genomic RNA thus comprise the essential initial nucleation reaction that subsequently determines the correct assembly of HIV Gag. And at the opposite end of Gag, tight interactions between MA-Gag and a cellular membrane are further required for efficient Gag assembly and trafficking, as well as virus release by budding and exocytosis.

VI. The Role of NC in HIV-1 Variability and Fitness

The virulence and the fitness of any given pathogen influence its capacity to replicate *in vivo* and consequently the progression to disease of the infected host. In retroviruses, notably in HIV, both historic and more recent studies have amply shown that numerous viral and cellular factors contribute to virus replication capacity and fitness *in vivo* and in cell culture (reviewed in Coffin, 1995; Darlix *et al.*, 1995; Hu and Temin, 1990; Temin, 1991; Zhang and Temin, 1993). Additional work reveals that variability in these viral and cellular factors appears to influence virus replication and dissemination and thus disease progression. In HIV, the emergence of virus quasispecies in single individuals poses major issues for AIDS treatment (highly active antiretroviral therapy named HAART) and vaccine development (Barbaro *et al.*, 2005; Berkhout, 1999; Girard *et al.*, 2006; Kulkosky and Bray, 2006; McMichael, 2006; Shehu-Xhilaga *et al.*, 2005). However, variability in the viral factors could potentially be altered by antiretroviral therapies (HAART), both of which can influence the viral fitness (Barbour and Grant, 2005; reviewed in Lucas, 2005).

In this section, we will review how the multiple functions of NC might influence HIV variability and fitness and the possible molecular mechanisms underlying such effects.

A. The Dual Role of NC in Viral DNA Synthesis

The process of viral DNA synthesis is the major source of HIV variability. The viral DNA polymerase, commonly named RT, is considered to be highly error prone because it is capable of commencing cDNA synthesis at false sites and to misincorporate nucleotides during cDNA extension, as well as to extend mispaired nucleotides *in vitro*. However, the extensive accumulation of mutations, insertions, and deletions should rapidly lead to a replication defective provirus (Darlix, 1986; Katz and Skalka, 1990) unless the genetic variability brought about by RT is at least partially suppressed. NC may play precisely this role since it suppresses false initiations by RT and chaperones the two obligatory strand transfers at the TAR and PBS sequences (see reviews cited above). Recently, it was reported that NC triggers an RT excision-repair activity whereby misincorporated nucleotides are removed from the growing cDNA chain *in vitro* (Bampi *et al.*, 2006). On the other hand, NC chaperones random interstrand transfers during the conversion of the dimeric genome to proviral DNA by RT, which generate new recombinant viruses (Galetto and Negroni, 2005; Galetto *et al.*, 2006; Katz and Skalka, 1990; Negroni and Buc, 2001). Such strand-switching events can occur at pauses during cDNA synthesis due to stable RNA secondary structures or nicks in the genome and, in 30% of cases, are coupled with mutations at the transfer site (Darlix *et al.*, 2000; review of Darlix *et al.*, 1995, 2000; Galetto and Negroni, 2005). These mutations probably correspond to nontemplate addition of nucleotides by RT in the presence of NC (Bampi *et al.*, 2006).

Thus, the dual role of NC during viral DNA synthesis by RT ensures faithful and efficient virus replication, yet permits sufficient genetic diversity for the virus to escape HAART treatments and an immune response. Recent data show that AZT- and ddI-resistant RTs retain their nontemplate addition and nucleotide excision-repair activities in the presence of NC *in vitro*, suggesting that variability of AZT- and ddI-resistant viruses should be achieved using the same mechanism (Bampi *et al.*, 2006).

B. NC, APOBEC3G, and VIF

The human APOBEC3G deaminase belongs to the family of cellular Cytidine deaminase-editing enzymes with potent anti-HIV activity because it can deaminate Cytidine residues newly incorporated into nascent cDNAs in the absence of virus infectivity factor (VIF) (Chiu *et al.*, 2005; Mangeat *et al.*, 2003, 2004; Perez and Hope, 2006; Soros and Greene, 2006). The antiretroviral activity of APOBEC3G requires its incorporation into nascent virions and its presence in close association with the reverse transcription complex within the virion nucleocapsid. It has been reported that APOBEC3G is indeed packaged into assembling virions via specific interactions with Gag, which occur on membranes of late endosomes and multivesicular bodies (see section on virus assembly) (Cen *et al.*, 2004; Liu *et al.*, 2004; Popik and Alce, 2004). This Gag–APOBEC3G interaction may be directed by NC, ensuring a close contact with RT and thus activates Cytidine deamination (Luo *et al.*, 2004).

The HIV-1 infectivity factor VIF has a crucial role in regulating virus infectivity, at various levels (Goncalves and Santa-Marta, 2004; Kremer and Schnierle, 2005; Navarro and Landau, 2004). However, the molecular mechanisms by which VIF exerts its role are still somewhat controversial. First, VIF is thought to prevent APOBEC3G encapsidation into virions through direct interactions, which then promote rapid proteasome-mediated degradation of both APOBEC3G and VIF (Kobayashi *et al.*, 2005; Shirakawa *et al.*, 2006). Or else, if VIF were copackaged with APOBEC3G into newly formed virions it would inhibit its deaminase activity (Mangeat *et al.*, 2003). In either case, VIF contributes to the faithful synthesis of the proviral DNA. Second, virion packaging of VIF can occur under certain circumstances via interactions with NC and the genomic RNA (Bardy et al., 2001, p. 2719; Henriet et al., 2005; Khan et al., 2001), which results in the modulation of Gag processing by the protease at the NC-flanking sites, and virus infectivity (Dettenhofer et al., 2000).

C. NC and VPR

The viral factor VPR is a 96-amino acid basic protein folded into three well-defined α-helices and surrounded by flexible N- and C-terminal domains (Morellet et al., 2006; Wecker et al., 2002). In vitro assays revealed that different parts of the protein spanning the N- or the C-terminus were involved in the formation of protein–protein contacts by a leucine zipper mode (Bourbigot et al., 2005; Wang et al., 1996; Zhao et al., 1994). This leucine zipper-like structure could account for the formation of ion channels in the outer membrane (Piller et al., 1996) and for the interaction with cellular proteins (Le Rouzic et al., 2002; Popov et al., 1998; Sabbah et al., 2006; Vieira et al., 2000; Zander et al., 2003). VPR exerts several functions affecting both the host and the virus; indeed, VPR was described as a transactivator of HIV and cellular genes (Agostini et al., 1996; Varin et al., 2005; Wang et al., 1995). Moreover, VPR induces apoptotic death of infected cells (Poon et al., 1998) and bystander cells, and arrests the cells in the G2-M phase of the cell cycle (Andersen and Planelles, 2005; Goh et al., 1998; Hrimech et al., 2000; Jowett et al., 1995; Levy et al., 1993; McCarthy, 1995; Vodicka et al., 1998) to the benefit of genomic RNA expression and viral protein synthesis (see also Section V.B). Additionally, VPR participates in the nuclear import of the newly made viral DNA through interactions with the RT complex (Fouchier and Malim, 1999; Le Rouzic et al., 2002; Popov et al., 1998; Vodicka et al., 1998). To this end, VPR is incorporated into virions via interactions with Gag p6 (Cohen et al., 1990; Kondo and Gottlinger, 1996; Kondo et al., 1995; Lu et al., 1995) and NC (Accola et al., 2000; de Rocquigny et al., 1997; Selig et al., 1999), ensuring a close contact between VPR and the RT complex. VPR has also been reported to partially limit the mutation rate of HIV-1 by interacting with Uracyl DNA glycosylase (UNG), a DNA repair enzyme (Bouhamdan et al., 1996), an observation which is in agreement with its presence in the virion nucleocapsid (Mansky et al., 2000).

D. NC and the PrP

Although the cellular prion protein, PrPc, is ubiquitous in all vertebrates, its function remains a matter of speculation and controversy (Aguzzi et al., 2004; Chiti and Dobson, 2006; Harris and True, 2006; Priola and Vorberg, 2006). In its pathologic form called scrapie prion or PrPSc, it is considered to be a major component of the causative agent of prion diseases that are fatal transmissible spongiform encephalopathies associated with the accumulation of a protease-resistant form of the PrP (Aguzzi and Miele, 2004; Aguzzi *et al.*, 2004). A serendipitous discovery found that recombinant PrP binds the HIV genomic RNA and exhibits RNA-chaperoning properties similar to that of HIV-1 NC in viral replicating complexes formed *in vitro* (Gabus *et al.*, 2001). Moreover, in HIV-1 producing cells PrPc can strongly interfere with Gag assembly and trafficking, and virus infectivity (Leblanc *et al.*, 2004), suggesting that this ubiquitous cellular factor could be a line of defense acting at the level of virus formation. Interestingly enough, PrPc and PrPSc can be incorporated into retroviral particles, notably HIV and MLV, which assemble on late endosomal membranes (see section on assembly) and would thus function as prion-spreading vehicles (Leblanc *et al.*, 2006). The molecular mechanism governing PrP incorporation into retroviral particles seems to be dependent on direct interactions between Gag and PrP, more precisely the NC domain (Leblanc *et al.*, 2006).

In conclusion, the emergence of viral populations consisting of well-suited replicating HIV quasispecies is dependent on a large number of factors, and is a dynamic, multistep process (Berkhout, 1999; Daar *et al.*, 2005; Darlix *et al.*, 2000). The founding event is virus variability whereby a large panel of viable viral clones are generated via point mutations, insertions, substitutions and deletions, and recombinations due to multiple HIV infections of single cells (Bocharov *et al.*, 2005; Chin *et al.*, 2005; Jung *et al.*, 2002; Hu *et al.*, 2003; Rhodes *et al.*, 2005; Wain-Hobson *et al.*, 2003). However, there is a fine balance to be struck for the virus between self-destructive levels of genetic variability leading to defective viral clones and a rate of variability capable of conferring an ability to evade the onslaught of an immune response and/or of antiviral drugs. And it is in this context that the network of NC functions seems to be seminal in generating and controlling virus variability (Fig. 8). In fact, NC achieves a tight control over the fidelity of viral DNA synthesis at several levels, namely at initiation, (−) and (+)DNA strand transfers, excision-repair of misincorporated nucleotides by RT, and via the recruitment of VIF and VPR. On the other hand, NC fuels variability by several mechanisms starting with the dimerization of the viral genome generating both homozygous and heterozygous viruses (Galetto and Negroni, 2005; Hu and Temin, 1990; Jung *et al.*, 2002; Negroni and Buc, 2001), nontemplate addition of nucleotides coupled with forced cDNA elongation by RT (Bampi *et al.*, 2006), recombinations by random strand transfers and rapid creation of recombinant quasispecies, and the recruitment of APOBEC3G. The fitness and diversity of a given viral population in individuals will result from the selection pressures imposed by the *in vivo* milieu at the start of infection including the initial infectious dose, the character of the immune response, the prevalence of co- and superinfections, and the nature of HAART treatments (Fig. 8) (Brenner *et al.*, 2002; Doualla-Bell *et al.*, 2004; Gallant *et al.*, 2003; Miller *et al.*, 2002, 2005).

VIRUS: heterozygous, two different RNA - homozygous, two identical RNA

**1. VIRUS Formation
in HIV infected cells:**

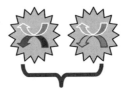

Virus replication and variability
(i) Genomic RNA copied into DNA by error-prone RT; control by NC.
(ii) Recombinations and the role of the dimeric genome and NC;
(iii) Trans-complementations between quasi-species;
(iv) Pseudo-typing and coinfections (HCV);
(v) HAART and emergence of resistances (RT and NC).

**2. Virus infection by
adapted quasi-species**

**3. Circulating
viral populations**

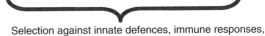

Selection against innate defences, immune responses,
and HAART (NRTI, NNRTI–,and PRI);
 viral co-infections (i.e. HCV, HBV) and reservoirs
--> Highly dynamic viral populations

FIGURE 8   HIV variability and fitness. Viruses produced by HIV-1-infected cells can be homozygous with two identical RNAs or heterozygous with different RNAs(1). A high level of virus variablity results from several processes as outlined in(2; i–v). Circulating viral populations result from selection processes, natural ones, and because of co-infections and HAART(3).

VII. Anti-NC Drug Screening

A. Anti-NC Drug Design

Emerging resistance to antiviral strategies targeting RT and PR has led to an overwhelming urgency for an extended panel of new anti-HIV drugs directed at new viral targets. Among the potential targets, NCp7 stands out since it, and especially the ZFs plateau, is highly conserved among HIV isolates and plays seminal roles in the early stages of viral DNA synthesis by chaperoning RT, in the course of intracellular preintegration complex (PIC) migration and integration processes and in assembly within the Gag precursor, as extensively outlined in this chapter. Viruses containing mutations of residues involved in NCp7–RNA recognition fail to replicate due notably to defects in genomic RNA encapsidation. Moreover, the interaction of ZFs with structural elements within the RNA leader sequence should be specific. Promising anti-NCp7 molecules would thus be those that interfere with RNA recognition and/or its chaperone activities. On the basis of these appealing possibilities, three strategies aimed at targeting HIV NCp7 are currently being pursued.

B. Zinc Ejectors

The first approach is based on zinc ejection to induce NCp7 unfolding. Zinc ejection was first obtained with 3-nitrobenzamide (NOBA) (Rice *et al.*, 1993) and the 2,2′-dithiobis(benzamide) disulfide (DIBA) family

(Rice *et al.*, 1995). In the later family, the two benzamide moieties are held together through a disulfide bridge. To avoid a loss of activity following the reduction of the S–S bond, substitution for a thioester link led to the generation of the PATEs family (Turpin *et al.*, 1999) that exhibits an increased antiviral potency and water solubility without increase of cell toxicity (Song *et al.*, 2002). An alternative strategy to prevent disulfide reduction involved dithiane compounds (Rice *et al.*, 1997a,b). The S–S bond in this approach is tethered to a ring structure and these compounds maintain antiviral activity in the presence of glutathion reductase, even at high concentrations. Moreover, an azodicarbonamide derivative was described as possessing anti-HIV activity and this compound was assessed in clinical I and II trials, in Europe in spite of an unknown mechanism of action (Vandevelde *et al.*, 1996). The target of azodicarbonamide was found to be NCp7 (Rice *et al.*, 1997b). Interestingly, there is no disulfide bond in this structure which circumvents any loss of activity by reduction.

All these zinc ejectors inhibit a large range of HIV-1 isolates whether expressed from acutely, latently, or chronically infected cells (Berthoux *et al.*, 1999). These compounds also inhibit MLV replication but have no effect on spumaretroviruses lacking ZFs in their NCs (Rein *et al.*, 1996), supporting the notion that ZFs are the targets for MuLV and HIV-1 inactivation. Moreover, these compounds exhibit a synergistic effect when combined with AZT or other retroviral agents (Chuang *et al.*, 1993). Mechanistic studies using density-functional theory (Maynard *et al.*, 1998) or DTNB as competitor (Tummino *et al.*, 1997) show that zinc ejection resulted from an electrophilic attack of Cys 49 residue, in line with the higher reactivity of this residue (Bombarda *et al.*, 2002) and the lower stability of the distal ZF as compared with the proximal one (Mely *et al.*, 1996; Morellet *et al.*, 1994). The loss of one zinc coordinating residue decreases the affinity for zinc and allows intra- and intermolecular cross linking in either mature NCp7 or the Gag-NC precursor. Even though these compounds show a degree of selectivity for NCp7 over cellular enzymes containing zinc ions such as poly(ADP-ribose) polymerase and various transcription factors (Huang *et al.*, 1998), their failure in clinical trials is probably due to cell toxicity or to the short intracellular half-life of these drugs (Druillennec and Roques, 2000).

C. Drugs Targeting NC Structure

The second approach involves targeting NCp7 via its binding to a nucleic acid target. This approach is illustrated by NCp7 peptidomimetics, rationally designed based on a cyclic scaffold deduced from the NCp7 3D structure (Druillennec *et al.*, 1999b). In these, the W37 and F16 residues adopt the spatial orientation found in the native protein, and basic residues were introduced to enhance peptide-nucleic acid affinity. The most efficient peptide is able to disrupt the functional complex involving NC, DNA, and RT without zinc removal. Recently, a Trp-rich peptide was found to bind with affinities similar to NC to its nucleic acid targets, and to compete out the NC chaperone activity (Pustowka *et al.*, 2003; Raja *et al.*, 2006). These peptides need to be made more specific but the approach holds promise for the development of a broad spectrum of antiviral compounds. Nevertheless, the ideal strategy would be to find small molecules that specifically recognize NCp7 itself rather than its RNA or DNA target. Since in all described structures, Trp 37 is intercalated between two successive bases, one of them being always a G moiety, pseudonucleotides linked by an amide bond instead of a phosphate bond were synthesized (Druillennec *et al.*, 1999b). These derivatives interact with the ZFs mainly through hydrophobic contacts and are able to disrupt NCp7-SL3 recognition. However, only a weak antiviral activity is observed probably due to their low bioavailability. The identification of antagonists of the interaction between NCp7 and oligonucleotides was also used for the screening of NCI's pharmacophore repository, which identified fluorescein or gallein-like compounds as potential anti-NC agents (Stephen *et al.*, 2002). In contrast to nucleomimetics, the interaction with these compounds is mainly stabilized by electrostatic contacts despite the fact that these compounds contain several aromatic rings. Since NCp7 is highly basic, this could explain the observed 2:1 stoichiometry. Nevertheless, this first generation of nonchelating molecules does indeed show antiviral activity in cell-based assays and may lead to a new class of antiviral compounds. In further pursuit of this strategy, a more specific assay was developed taking advantage of the chaperone activity of NCp7.

D. Antichaperone

The assay for chaperone activity is based on the transient melting of the secondary structure of cTAR by NCp7 (Beltz *et al.*, 2005; Bernacchi *et al.*, 2002). The specificity of this assay relies on the exquisite dependence of NC melting activity on the native structure of its ZF domain since either the SSHS mutant or EDTA-treated NC derivatives remain capable of interaction but fail to melt cTAR. Using this assay, an "in-house" chemical library containing 5000 molecules was screened (Ramstrom *et al.*, 2004). Several lead compounds have been selected and are currently under intensive study (Fig. 9).

VIII. Conclusions and Future Prospects

It is clear from the above account that the NC protein of HIV represents a small viral peptide with a multitude of functions. NC may indeed be considered as the high-fidelity chaperoning partner for viral genomic RNA, acting on all stages of virus replication and dissemination.

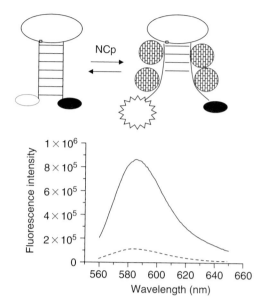

FIGURE 9 Basic principle of anti-NC screening. Destabilization of cTAR by NCp7 as monitored by fluorescence: the cTAR 5′ and 3′ ends are labeled by a fluorophore and a quencher, respectively. In the closed form of cTAR, fluorophore emission is quenched (bottom spectrum). Addition of NCp7 transiently destabilizes the stem, increasing the distance between the two dyes, thus causing fluorophore emission (top spectrum). Positive screening hits are detected through the decrease of the fluorophore emission (bottom spectrum).

Firstly, NC variously exerts its functions in the form of the Gag-NC precursor and, as recently discovered, in the form of Gag-NC isoforms (Buck *et al.*, 2001; Herbreteau *et al.*, 2005), during the course of Gag trafficking and virus assembly bringing about formation of stable virions containing a replication-recombination competent dimeric RNA genome. Secondly, in the "just made" infectious virus population NC exists in several mature isoforms of NCp15, NC(1–71), and NC(1–55). These NC chaperone essential structural rearrangements of the genomic RNA and of the newly made cDNA to generate a complete proviral DNA with two LTRs while fueling genetic variability.

Importantly HIV NC should be pictured as operating within small Gag-NC oligomeric complexes for genomic RNA selection and dimerization (Feng *et al.*, 1996; Fu *et al.*, 1994), then in ever growing complexes during assembly of the viral globule, in highly packed NC oligomeric complexes during maturation and core condensation, and ultimately in the process of genomic RNA conversion to DNA to generate a *bona fide* provirus (Darlix *et al.*, 1995, 2000; Tanchou *et al.*, 1995). Several specific stages of this mode of action deserve closer attention as outlined below.

We hope that the years ahead will bring significant advances in our understanding of the molecular mechanisms underlying HIV assembly and further detailed refinement on the precise roles of NC from viral translation to virus production and dissemination.

A. Translational Regulation

Little is presently known about the extent of translational regulations in HIV, which, in addition to the full-length viral RNA, codes for 20 or so different, singly and doubly spliced viral mRNAs. What are the viral sequences, and cellular and viral factors governing the translational balance between all these viral mRNAs to ensure optimal virus production, especially in the G2-M phase of the cell cycle? What could be the functions of the Gag-NC isoforms that are conserved in all HIV strains (Buck *et al.*, 2001; Herbreteau *et al.*, 2005; reviewed in Lopez-Lastra *et al.*, 2005). How do the newly made Gag-NC molecules regulate the early metabolism of the genomic RNA from translation to dimerization and packaging (Feng *et al.*, 1996)? Does this switch occur at the level of active polysomes, which would act as the initial assembly site? In that context what is the exact role of the viral protease, which cleaves the translation initiation factor eIF4G in cells expressing a high level of HIV-1, thus causing cell apoptosis (Prevot *et al.*, 2003)?

B. The 5′ UTR and the Switch from Translation to Packaging

The HIV-1 5′ untranslated region, also called Leader, contains multiple genetic determinants, often represented as SLs, such as TAR, polyA SL, PBS, SL1 to SL4, which are essential at all stages of the virus replication cycle. However, the possibility of long range interactions between the 5′ and 3′ UTRs deserves much closer attention since they may equally regulate genomic RNA translation, packaging, and replication, as indicated by data on ASLV and yeast TY retrotransposons (Abbink *et al.*, 2005; Cristofari and Darlix, 2002; Darlix *et al.*, 1995; Gabus *et al.*, 1998). What might be the extent of the chaperoning role for NC (and implicating which NC isoforms?), in linking the 5′ and 3′ ends of the genomic RNA possibly via the TAR sequences (Kanevsky *et al.*, 2005).

C. Structure of the 5′ UTR

Comprehensive and compelling pictures of NC bound to small viral sequences have been published, together with proposed conformations for the dimer initiation sequence (DIS) and the 5′ UTR. However, a clear mechanism of genomic RNA selection and dimerization by Gag-NC necessitates a clear view of the 3D structure of the HIV-1 psi-packaging signal and 5′UTR in the monomeric and dimeric forms, either alone or with bound NC molecules.

D. HIV Assembly in Endosomes

Advances have recently been achieved in delineating virus dynamics, from Gag assembly to virus formation and budding. In fact, large amounts of HIV virions can accumulate in late endosomes/MVB of infected human macrophages and T cells, and subvert the cellular vesicular trafficking pathway to leave the infected cell by exocytosis (Grigorov *et al.*, 2006; Pelchen-Matthews *et al.*, 2003; Raposo *et al.*, 2002). At first sight this novel mechanism of virion formation might be considered as disputing the canonical mechanism where assembly and budding occur at the plasma membrane. However, it may provide a route for the newly formed virus to escape the attention of the immune responses, thus facilitating virus spread probably via the viral synapse (Blanco *et al.*, 2004; Piguet and Sattentau, 2004). Therefore, pursuing this key area of research on HIV-1 seems to be a priority.

E. New Anti-HIV Drugs Targeting NC

In a provocative review on the development of an anti-HIV vaccine, N. Sheppard and Q. Sattentau asked *"is-it more than a field of long-term nonprogression?"* (Sheppard and Sattentau, 2005). Fortunately enough, regimens of HAART are indisputably efficient for people living with HIV, but at the same time resistance and treatment escapes are becoming more and more frequent. Thus it is of the utmost importance to widen the portfolio of potent antiviral targets merely to maintain our present ability to control HIV replication in AIDS patients (Mély *et al.*, submitted for publication; Stephen *et al.*, 2002). A simple and efficient strategy using NC and the TAR sequence has recently been developed to screen for lead compounds capable of irreversibly interfering with the ZFs of HIV-1 NC (Mély *et al.*). Due to high sequence conservation in the ZFs, such compounds should also inhibit NC activity in other pathogenic lentiviruses and in the closely related human retrovirus XMRV associated with prostate tumors (Urisman *et al.*, 2006). It is hoped that in the years ahead simple molecules targeting the NC ZFs will find their way into clinic.

Acknowledgments _____

We wish to thank M. Summers for figure 5 and M. Lopez-Lastra for comments and discussions. ANRS, CNRS, INSERM, the European community (TRIOH of the 6th PCRDT), and Sidaction are acknowledged for their strong continuous support. Thanks are due to B. Grigorov, D. Muriaux (Lyon) and P. Roingeard (Tours) for providing us with EM pictures of HIV-1 in endosomes. J.L.G. is supported by a TRIOH Ph.D. fellowship.

References

Abbink, T. E., and Berkhout, B. (2003). A novel long distance base-pairing interaction in human immunodeficiency virus type 1 RNA occludes the Gag start codon. *J. Biol. Chem.* **278**, 11601–11611.

Abbink, T. E., Ooms, M., Haasnoot, P. C., and Berkhout, B. (2005). The HIV-1 leader RNA conformational switch regulates RNA dimerization but does not regulate mRNA translation. *Biochemistry* **44**, 9058–9066.

Accola, M. A., Ohagen, A., and Gottlinger, H. G. (2000). Isolation of human immunodeficiency virus type 1 cores: Retention of Vpr in the absence of p6(gag). *J. Virol.* **74**, 6198–6202.

Agostini, I., Navarro, J. M., Rey, F., Bouhamdan, M., Spire, B., Vigne, R., and Sire, J. (1996). The human immunodeficiency virus type 1 Vpr transactivator: Cooperation with promoter-bound activator domains and binding to TFIIB. *J. Mol. Biol.* **261**, 599–606.

Aguzzi, A., and Miele, G. (2004). Recent advances in prion biology. *Curr. Opin. Neurol.* **17**, 337–342.

Aguzzi, A., Heikenwalder, M., and Miele, G. (2004). Progress and problems in the biology, diagnostics, and therapeutics of prion diseases. *J. Clin. Invest.* **114**, 153–160.

Aldovini, A., and Young, R. A. (1990). Mutations of RNA and protein sequences involved in human immunodeficiency virus type 1 packaging result in production of noninfectious virus. *J. Virol.* **64**, 1920–1926.

Allain, B., Lapadat-Tapolsky, M., Berlioz, C., and Darlix, J. L. (1994). Transactivation of the minus-strand DNA transfer by nucleocapsid protein during reverse transcription of the retroviral genome. *EMBO J.* **13**, 973–981.

Amarasinghe, G. K., De Guzman, R. N., Turner, R. B., Chancellor, K. J., Wu, Z. R., and Summers, M. F. (2000a). NMR structure of the HIV-1 nucleocapsid protein bound to stem-loop SL2 of the psi-RNA packaging signal. Implications for genome recognition. *J. Mol. Biol.* **301**, 491–511.

Amarasinghe, G. K., De Guzman, R. N., Turner, R. B., and Summers, M. F. (2000b). NMR structure of stem-loop SL2 of the HIV-1 psi RNA packaging signal reveals a novel A-U-A base-triple platform. *J. Mol. Biol.* **299**, 145–156.

Andersen, E. S., Contera, S. A., Knudsen, B., Damgaard, C. K., Besenbacher, F., and Kjems, J. (2004). Role of the trans-activation response element in dimerization of HIV-1 RNA. *J. Biol. Chem.* **279**, 22243–22249.

Andersen, J. L., and Planelles, V. (2005). The role of Vpr in HIV-1 pathogenesis. *Curr. HIV Res.* **3**, 43–51.

Attal, J., Theron, M. C., Taboit, F., Cajero-Juarez, M., Kann, G., Bolifraud, P., and Houdebine, L. M. (1996). The RU5 ('R') region from human leukaemia viruses (HTLV-1) contains an internal ribosome entry site (IRES)-like sequence. *FEBS Lett.* **392**, 220–224.

Auxilien, S., Keith, G., Le Grice, S. F., and Darlix, J. L. (1999). Role of post-transcriptional modifications of primer tRNALys, 3 in the fidelity and efficacy of plus strand DNA transfer during HIV-1 reverse transcription. *J. Biol. Chem.* **274**, 4412–4420.

Baltimore, D. (1970). RNA-dependent DNA polymerase in virions of RNA tumour viruses. *Nature* **226**, 1209–1211.

Bampi, C., Jacquenet, S., Lener, D., Decimo, D., and Darlix, J. L. (2004). The chaperoning and assistance roles of the HIV-1 nucleocapsid protein in proviral DNA synthesis and maintenance. *Int. J. Biochem. Cell Biol.* **36**, 1668–1686.

Bampi, C., Bibillo, A., Wendeler, M., Divita, G., Gorelick, R. J., Le Grice, S. F., and Darlix, J. L. (2006). Nucleotide excision repair and template-independent addition by HIV-1 reverse transcriptase in the presence of nucleocapsid protein. *J. Biol. Chem.* **281**, 11736–11743.

Barat, C., Lullien, V., Schatz, O., Keith, G., Nugeyre, M. T., Gruninger-Leitch, F., Barre-Sinoussi, F., LeGrice, S. F., and Darlix, J. L. (1989). HIV-1 reverse transcriptase specifically interacts with the anticodon domain of its cognate primer tRNA. *EMBO J.* **8**, 3279–3285.

Barbaro, G., Scozzafava, A., Mastrolorenzo, A., and Supuran, C. T. (2005). Highly active antiretroviral therapy: Current state of the art, new agents and their pharmacological interactions useful for improving therapeutic outcome. *Curr. Pharm. Des.* **11**, 1805–1843.

Barbour, J. D., and Grant, R. M. (2005). The role of viral fitness in HIV pathogenesis. *Curr. HIV/AIDS Rep.* **2**, 29–34.

Bardy, M., Gay, B., Pebernard, S., Chazal, N., Courcoul, M., Vigne, R., Decroly, E., and Boulanger, P. (2001). Interaction of human immunodeficiency virus type 1 Vif with Gag and Gag-Pol precursors: Co-encapsidation and interference with viral protease-mediated Gag processing. *J. Gen. Virol.* **82**, 2719–2733.

Basyuk, E., Galli, T., Mougel, M., Blanchard, J. M., Sitbon, M., and Bertrand, E. (2003). Retroviral genomic RNAs are transported to the plasma membrane by endosomal vesicles. *Dev. Cell* 161–174.

Baudin, F., Marquet, R., Isel, C., Darlix, J. L., Ehresmann, B., and Ehresmann, C. (1993). Functional sites in the 5' region of human immunodeficiency virus type 1 RNA form defined structural domains. *J. Mol. Biol.* **229**, 382–397.

Beltz, H., Azoulay, J., Bernacchi, S., Clamme, J. P., Ficheux, D., Roques, B., Darlix, J. L., and Mely, Y. (2003). Impact of the terminal bulges of HIV-1 cTAR DNA on its stability and the destabilizing activity of the nucleocapsid protein NCp7. *J. Mol. Biol.* **328**, 95–108.

Beltz, H., Piemont, E., Schaub, E., Ficheux, D., Roques, B., Darlix, J. L., and Mely, Y. (2004). Role of the structure of the top half of HIV-1 cTAR DNA on the nucleic acid destabilizing activity of the nucleocapsid protein NCp7. *J. Mol. Biol.* **338**, 711–723.

Beltz, H., Clauss, C., Piemont, E., Ficheux, D., Gorelick, R. J., Roques, B., Gabus, C., Darlix, J. L., de Rocquigny, H., and Mely, Y. (2005). Structural determinants of HIV-1 nucleocapsid protein for cTAR DNA binding and destabilization, and correlation with inhibition of self-primed DNA synthesis. *J. Mol. Biol.* **348**, 1113–1126.

Berg, J. M. (1986). Potential metal-binding domains in nucleic acid binding proteins. *Science* **232**, 485–487.

Berkhout, B. (1996). Structure and function of the human immunodeficiency virus leader RNA. *Prog. Nucleic Acid Res. Mol. Biol.* **54**, 1–34.

Berkhout, B. (1999). HIV-1 evolution under pressure of protease inhibitors: Climbing the stairs of viral fitness. *J. Biomed. Sci.* **6**, 298–305.

Berlioz, C., and Darlix, J. L. (1995). An internal ribosomal entry mechanism promotes translation of murine leukemia virus gag polyprotein precursors. *J. Virol.* **69**, 2214–2222.

Berlioz, C., Torrent, C., and Darlix, J. L. (1995). An internal ribosomal entry signal in the rat VL30 region of the Harvey murine sarcoma virus leader and its use in dicistronic retroviral vectors. *J. Virol.* **69**, 6400–6407.

Bernacchi, S., Stoylov, S., Piemont, E., Ficheux, D., Roques, B. P., Darlix, J. L., and Mely, Y. (2002). HIV-1 nucleocapsid protein activates transient melting of least stable parts of the secondary structure of TAR and its complementary sequence. *J. Mol. Biol.* **317**, 385–399.

Berthoux, L., Pechoux, C., Ottmann, M., Morel, G., and Darlix, J. L. (1997). Mutations in the N-terminal domain of human immunodeficiency virus type 1 nucleocapsid protein affect virion core structure and proviral DNA synthesis. *J. Virol.* **71**, 6973–6981.

Berthoux, L., Pechoux, C., and Darlix, J. L. (1999). Multiple effects of an anti-human immunodeficiency virus nucleocapsid inhibitor on virus morphology and replication. *J. Virol.* **73**, 10000–10009.

Bishop, J. M. (1983). Oncogenes and proto-oncogenes. *Hosp. Pract. (Off Ed)* **18**, 67–74.

Blanco, J., Bosch, B., Fernandez-Figueras, M. T., Barretina, J., Clotet, B., and Este, J. A. (2004). High level of coreceptor-independent HIV transfer induced by contacts between primary CD4 T cells. *J. Biol. Chem.* **279**, 51305–51314.

Bocharov, G., Ford, N. J., Edwards, J., Breinig, T., Wain-Hobson, S., and Meyerhans, A. (2005). A genetic-algorithm approach to simulating human immunodeficiency virus evolution reveals the strong impact of multiply infected cells and recombination. *J. Gen. Virol.* **86**, 3109–3118.

Bombarda, E., Ababou, A., Vuilleumier, C., Gerard, D., Roques, B. P., Piemont, E., and Mely, Y. (1999). Time-resolved fluorescence investigation of the human immunodeficiency virus type 1 nucleocapsid protein: Influence of the binding of nucleic acids. *Biophys. J.* **76**, 1561–1570.

Bombarda, E., Cherradi, H., Morellet, N., Roques, B. P., and Mely, Y. (2002). Zn(2+) binding properties of single-point mutants of the C-terminal zinc finger of the HIV-1 nucleocapsid protein: Evidence of a critical role of cysteine 49 in Zn(2+) dissociation. *Biochemistry* **41**, 4312–4320.

Bouhamdan, M., Benichou, S., Rey, F., Navarro, J. M., Agostini, I., Spire, B., Camonis, J., Slupphaug, G., Vigne, R., Benarous, R., and Sire, J. (1996). Human immunodeficiency virus type 1 Vpr protein binds to the uracil DNA glycosylase DNA repair enzyme. *J. Virol.* **70**, 697–704.

Bourbigot, S., Beltz, H., Denis, J., Morellet, N., Roques, B. P., Mely, Y., and Bouaziz, S. (2005). The C-terminal domain of the HIV-1 regulatory protein Vpr adopts an antiparallel dimeric structure in solution via its leucine-zipper-like domain. *Biochem. J.* **387**, 333–341.

Brasey, A., Lopez-Lastra, M., Ohlmann, T., Beerens, N., Berkhout, B., Darlix, J. L., and Sonenberg, N. (2003). The leader of human immunodeficiency virus type 1 genomic RNA harbors an internal ribosome entry segment that is active during the G2/M phase of the cell cycle. *J. Virol.* **77**, 3939–3949.

Brenner, B. G., Turner, D., and Wainberg, M. A. (2002). HIV-1 drug resistance: Can we overcome? *Expert Opin. Biol. Ther.* **2**, 751–761.

Brugge, J. S., and Erikson, R. L. (1977). Identification of a transformation-specific antigen induced by an avian sarcoma virus. *Nature* **269**, 346–348.

Buck, C. B., Shen, X., Egan, M. A., Pierson, T. C., Walker, C. M., and Siliciano, R. F. (2001). The human immunodeficiency virus type 1 gag gene encodes an internal ribosome entry site. *J. Virol.* **75**, 181–191.

Buckman, J. S., Bosche, W. J., and Gorelick, R. J. (2003). Human immunodeficiency virus type 1 nucleocapsid Zn(2+) fingers are required for efficient reverse transcription, initial integration processes, and protection of newly synthesized viral DNA. *J. Virol.* **77**, 1469–1480.

Butsch, M., and Boris-Lawrie, K. (2000). Translation is not required to generate virion precursor RNA in human immunodeficiency virus type 1-infected T cells. *J. Virol.* **74**, 11531–11537.

Butsch, M., and Boris-Lawrie, K. (2002). Destiny of unspliced retroviral RNA: Ribosome and/or virion? *J. Virol.* **76**, 3089–3094.

Carteau, S., Batson, S. C., Poljak, L., Mouscadet, J. F., de Rocquigny, H., Darlix, J. L., Roques, B. P., Kas, E., and Auclair, C. (1997). Human immunodeficiency virus type 1 nucleocapsid protein specifically stimulates Mg2+-dependent DNA integration *in vitro*. *J. Virol.* **71**, 6225–6229.

Casas-Finet, J. R., Jhon, N. I., and Maki, A. H. (1988). p10, a low molecular weight single-stranded nucleic acid binding protein of murine leukemia retroviruses, shows stacking interactions of its single tryptophan residue with nucleotide bases. *Biochemistry* **27**, 1172–1178.

Cen, S., Khorchid, A., Gabor, J., Rong, L., Wainberg, M. A., and Kleiman, L. (2000). Roles of Pr55(gag) and NCp7 in tRNA(3)(Lys) genomic placement and the initiation step of reverse transcription in human immunodeficiency virus type 1. *J. Virol.* **74**, 10796–10800.

Cen, S., Guo, F., Niu, M., Saadatmand, J., Deflassieux, J., and Kleiman, L. (2004). The interaction between HIV-1 Gag and APOBEC3G. *J. Biol. Chem.* **279**, 33177–33184.

Chan, B., Weidemaier, K., Yip, W. T., Barbara, P. F., and Musier-Forsyth, K. (1999). Intra-tRNA distance measurements for nucleocapsid protein dependent tRNA unwinding during priming of HIV reverse transcription. *Proc. Natl. Acad. Sci. USA* 96, 459–464.

Chen, M., Garon, C. F., and Papas, T. S. (1980). Native ribonucleoprotein is an efficient transcriptional complex of avian myeloblastosis virus. *Proc. Natl. Acad. Sci. USA* 77, 1296–1300.

Chin, M. P., Rhodes, T. D., Chen, J., Fu, W., and Hu, W. S. (2005). Identification of a major restriction in HIV-1 intersubtype recombination. *Proc. Natl. Acad. Sci. USA* 102, 9002–9007.

Chiti, F., and Dobson, C. M. (2006). Protein misfolding, functional amyloid, and human disease. *Annu. Rev. Biochem.* 75, 333–366.

Chiu, Y. L., Soros, V. B., Kreisberg, J. F., Stopak, K., Yonemoto, W., and Greene, W. C. (2005). Cellular APOBEC3G restricts HIV-1 infection in resting CD4+ T cells. *Nature* 435, 108–114.

Chuang, A. J., Killam, K. F., Jr., Chuang, R. Y., Rice, W. G., Schaeffer, C. A., Mendeleyev, J., and Kun, E. (1993). Inhibition of the replication of native and 3′-azido-2′,3′-dideoxythymidine (AZT)-resistant simian immunodeficiency virus (SIV) by 3-nitroso-benzamide. *FEBS Lett.* 326, 140–144.

Cimarelli, A., and Darlix, J. L. (2002). Assembling the human immunodeficiency virus type 1. *Cell. Mol. Life Sci.* 59, 1166–1184.

Clever, J., Sassetti, C., and Parslow, T. G. (1995). RNA secondary structure and binding sites for gag gene products in the 5′ packaging signal of human immunodeficiency virus type 1. *J. Virol.* 69, 2101–2109.

Clever, J. L., Mirandar, D., Jr., and Parslow, T. G. (2002). RNA structure and packaging signals in the 5′ leader region of the human immunodeficiency virus type 1 genome. *J. Virol.* 76, 12381–12387.

Coffin, J. M. (1995). HIV Population dynamics *in vivo*: Implications for genetic variation, pathogenesis, and therapy. *Science* 267, 483–489.

Cohen, E. A., Terwilliger, E. F., Jalinoos, Y., Proulx, J., Sodroski, J. G., and Haseltine, W. A. (1990). Identification of HIV-1 vpr product and function. *J. Acquir. Immune Defic. Syndr.* 3, 11–18.

Cosa, G., Harbron, E. J., Zeng, Y., Liu, H. W., O'Connor, D. B., Eta-Hosokawa, C., Musier-Forsyth, K., and Barbara, P. F. (2004). Secondary structure and secondary structure dynamics of DNA hairpins complexed with HIV-1 NC protein. *Biophys. J.* 87, 2759–2767.

Cosa, G., Zeng, Y., Liu, H. W., Landes, C. F., Makarov, D. E., Musier-Forsyth, K., and Barbara, P. F. (2006). Evidence for non-two-state kinetics in the nucleocapsid protein chaperoned opening of DNA hairpins. *J. Phys. Chem. B Condens. Matter Mater. Surf. Interfaces Biophys.* 110, 2419–2426.

Cristofari, G., and Darlix, J. L. (2002). The ubiquitous nature of RNA chaperone proteins. *Prog. Nucleic Acid Res. Mol. Biol.* 72, 223–268.

Cristofari, G., Ivanyi-Nagy, R., Gabus, C., Boulant, S., Lavergne, J. P., Penin, F., and Darlix, J. L. (2004). The hepatitis C virus Core protein is a potent nucleic acid chaperone that directs dimerization of the viral (+) strand RNA *in vitro*. *Nucleic Acids Res.* 32, 2623–2631.

Cruceanu, M., Urbaneja, M. A., Hixson, C. V., Johnson, D. G., Datta, S. A., Fivash, M. J., Stephen, A. G., Fisher, R. J., Gorelick, R. J., Casas-Finet, J. R., Rein, A., Rouzina, I., *et al.* (2006). Nucleic acid binding and chaperone properties of HIV-1 Gag and nucleocapsid proteins. *Nucleic Acids Res.* 34, 593–605.

Daar, E. S., Lynn, H. S., Donfield, S. M., Lail, A., O'Brien, S. J., Huang, W., and Winkler, C. A. (2005). Stromal cell-derived factor-1 genotype, coreceptor tropism, and HIV type 1 disease progression. *J. Infect. Dis.* 192, 1597–1605.

Dannull, J., Surovoy, A., Jung, G., and Moelling, K. (1994). Specific binding of HIV-1 nucleocapsid protein to PSI RNA *in vitro* requires N-terminal zinc finger and flanking basic amino acid residues. *EMBO J.* **13**, 1525–1533.

Dardel, F., Marquet, R., Ehresmann, C., Ehresmann, B., and Blanquet, S. (1998). Solution studies of the dimerization initiation site of HIV-1 genomic RNA. *Nucleic Acids Res.* **26**, 3567–3571.

Darlix, J. L. (1986). Control of Rous sarcoma virus RNA translation and packaging by the 5′ and 3′ untranslated sequences. *J. Mol. Biol.* **189**, 421–434.

Darlix, J. L., and Spahr, P. F. (1982). Binding sites of viral protein P19 onto Rous sarcoma virus RNA and possible controls of viral functions. *J. Mol. Biol.* **160**, 147–161.

Darlix, J. L., Gabus, C., Nugeyre, M. T., Clavel, F., and Barre-Sinoussi, F. (1990). Cis elements and trans-acting factors involved in the RNA dimerization of the human immunodeficiency virus HIV-1. *J. Mol. Biol.* **216**, 689–699.

Darlix, J. L., Vincent, A., Gabus, C., de Rocquigny, H., and Roques, B. (1993). Transactivation of the 5′ to 3′ viral DNA strand transfer by nucleocapsid protein during reverse transcription of HIV1 RNA. *C. R. Acad. Sci. III* **316**, 763–771.

Darlix, J. L., Lapadat-Tapolsky, M., de Rocquigny, H., and Roques, B. P. (1995). First glimpses at structure-function relationships of the nucleocapsid protein of retroviruses. *J. Mol. Biol.* **254**, 523–537.

Darlix, J. L., Cristofari, G., Rau, M., Pechoux, C., Berthoux, L., and Roques, B. (2000). Nucleocapsid protein of human immunodeficiency virus as a model protein with chaperoning functions and as a target for antiviral drugs. *Adv. Pharmacol.* **48**, 345–372.

Davis, J., Scherer, M., Tsai, W. P., and Long, C. (1976). Low-molecular- weight Rauscher leukemia virus protein with preferential binding for single-stranded RNA and DNA. *J. Virol.* **18**, 709–718.

Davis, N. L., and Rueckert, R. R. (1972). Properties of a ribonucleoprotein particle isolated from Nonidet P-40-treated Rous sarcoma virus. *J. Virol.* **10**, 1010–1020.

De Guzman, R. N., Wu, Z. R., Stalling, C. C., Pappalardo, L., Borer, P. N., and Summers, M. F. (1998). Structure of the HIV-1 nucleocapsid protein bound to the SL3 psi-RNA recognition element. *Science* **279**, 384–388.

De Rocquigny, H., Gabus, C., Vincent, A., Fournie-Zaluski, M. C., Roques, B., and Darlix, J. L. (1992). Viral RNA annealing activities of human immunodeficiency virus type 1 nucleocapsid protein require only peptide domains outside the zinc fingers. *Proc. Natl. Acad. Sci. USA* **89**, 6472–6476.

De Rocquigny, H., Ficheux, D., Gabus, C., Allain, B., Fournie-Zaluski, M. C., Darlix, J. L., and Roques, B. P. (1993). Two short basic sequences surrounding the zinc finger of nucleocapsid protein NCp10 of Moloney murine leukemia virus are critical for RNA annealing activity. *Nucleic Acids Res.* **21**, 823–829.

de Rocquigny, H., Petitjean, P., Tanchou, V., Decimo, D., Drouot, L., Delaunay, T., Darlix, J. L., and Roques, B. P. (1997). The zinc fingers of HIV nucleocapsid protein NCp7 direct interactions with the viral regulatory protein Vpr. *J. Biol. Chem.* **272**, 30753–30759.

Deffaud, C., and Darlix, J. L. (2000). Characterization of an internal ribosomal entry segment in the 5′ leader of murine leukemia virus env RNA. *J. Virol.* **74**, 846–850.

Demene, H., Dong, C. Z., Ottmann, M., Rouyez, M. C., Jullian, N., Morellet, N., Mely, Y., Darlix, J. L., Fournie-Zaluski, M. C., and Saragosti, S. (1994a). 1H NMR structure and biological studies of the His23 –> Cys mutant nucleocapsid protein of HIV-1 indicate that the conformation of the first zinc finger is critical for virus infectivity. *Biochemistry* **33**, 11707–11716.

Demene, H., Jullian, N., Morellet, N., de Rocquigny, H., Cornille, F., Maigret, B., and Roques, B. P. (1994b). Three-dimensional 1H NMR structure of the nucleocapsid protein NCp10 of Moloney murine leukemia virus. *J. Biomol. NMR* **4**, 153–170.

Dettenhofer, M., Cen, S., Carlson, B. A., Kleiman, L., and Yu, X. F. (2000). Association of human immunodeficiency virus type 1 Vif with RNA and its role in reverse transcription. *J. Virol.* **74**, 8938–8945.

Dib-Hajj, F., Khan, R., and Giedroc, D. P. (1993). Retroviral nucleocapsid proteins possess potent nucleic acid strand renaturation activity. *Protein Sci.* **2**, 231–243.

Dickson, C., Eisenman, R., Fan, H., Hunter, E., and Reich, N. (1985). Protein biosynthesis and assembly. *In* "RNA tumor viruses" (R. Weiss, N. Teich, H. Varmus, and J. Coffin, Eds.), Part 2, 2nd edn., pp. 513–648. Cold Spring Harbor Laboratory, Cold Spring Harbor, New York.

Dorfman, T., Luban, J., Goff, S. P., Haseltine, W. A., and Gottlinger, H. G. (1993). Mapping of functionally important residues of a cysteine-histidine box in the human immunodeficiency virus type 1 nucleocapsid protein. *J. Virol.* **67**, 6159–6169.

Doualla-Bell, F., Turner, D., Loemba, H., Petrella, M., Brenner, B., and Wainberg, M. A. (2004). HIV drug resistance and optimization of antiviral treatment in resource-poor countries. *Med. Sci. (Paris)* **20**, 882–886.

Druillennec, S., and Roques, B. P. (2000). HIV-1 NCp7 as a target for the design of novel antiviral agents. *Drug News Perspect.* **13**, 337–349.

Druillennec, S., Caneparo, A., de Rocquigny, H., and Roques, B. P. (1999a). Evidence of interactions between the nucleocapsid protein NCp7 and the reverse transcriptase of HIV-1. *J. Biol. Chem.* **274**, 11283–11288.

Druillennec, S., Meudal, H., Roques, B. P., and Fournie-Zaluski, M. C. (1999b). Nucleomimetic strategy for the inhibition of HIV-1 nucleocapsid protein NCp7 activities. *Bioorg. Med. Chem. Lett.* **9**, 627–632.

D'Souza, V., and Summers, M. F. (2004). Structural basis for packaging the dimeric genome of Moloney murine leukaemia virus. *Nature* **431**, 586–590.

Dunker, A. K., Lawson, J. D., Brown, C. J., Williams, R. M., Romero, P., Oh, J. S., Oldfield, C. J., Campen, A. M., Ratliff, C. M., Hipps, K. W., Ausio, J., Nissen, M. S., *et al.* (2001). Intrinsically disordered protein. *J. Mol. Graph. Model.* **19**, 26–59.

Echols, H. (1990). Nucleoprotein structures initiating DNA replication, transcription, and site-specific recombination. *J. Biol. Chem.* **265**, 14697–14700.

Egele, C., Schaub, E., Ramalanjaona, N., Piemont, E., Ficheux, D., Roques, B., Darlix, J. L., and Mely, Y. (2004). HIV-1 nucleocapsid protein binds to the viral DNA initiation sequences and chaperones their kissing interactions. *J. Mol. Biol.* **342**, 453–466.

Egele, C., Schaub, E., Piemont, E., de Rocquigny, H., and Mely, Y. (2005). Investigation by fluorescence correlation spectroscopy of the chaperoning interactions of HIV-1 nucleocapsid protein with the viral DNA initiation sequences. *C. R. Biol.* **328**, 1041–1051.

Ellermann, V., and Bang, O. (1908). Experimentelle Leukämie bei hühnern. *Zentralbl. Backteriol.* **46**, 595–609.

Ennifar, E., Walter, P., Ehresmann, B., Ehresmann, C., and Dumas, P. (2001). Crystal structures of coaxially stacked kissing complexes of the HIV-1 RNA dimerization initiation site. *Nat. Struct. Biol.* **8**, 1064–1068.

Evdokimova, V., Ovchinnikov, L. P., and Sorensen, P. H. (2006). Y-box binding protein 1: Providing a new angle on translational regulation. *Cell cycle* **5**, 1143–1147.

Feng, Y. X., Copeland, T. D., Henderson, L. E., Gorelick, R. J., Bosche, W. J., Levin, J. G., and Rein, A. (1996). HIV-1 nucleocapsid protein induces "maturation" of dimeric retroviral RNA *in vitro*. *Proc. Natl. Acad. Sci. USA* **93**, 7577–7581.

Fevrier, B., and Raposo, G. (2004). Exosomes: Endosomal-derived vesicles shipping extracellular messages. *Curr. Opin. Cell Biol.* **16**, 415–421.

Fisher, R. J., Rein, A., Fivash, M., Urbaneja, M. A., Casas-Finet, J. R., Medaglia, M., and Henderson, L. E. (1998). Sequence-specific binding of human immunodeficiency virus type 1 nucleocapsid protein to short oligonucleotides. *J. Virol.* **72**, 1902–1909.

Fouchier, R. A., and Malim, M. H. (1999). Nuclear import of human immunodeficiency virus type-1 preintegration complexes. *Adv. Virus Res.* **52**, 275–299.

Freed, E. O. (2002). Viral late domains. *J. Virol.* **76**, 4679–4687.

Freed, E. O. (2004). HIV-1 and the host cell: An intimate association. *Trends Microbiol.* **12**, 170–177.

Fu, W., Gorelick, R. J., and Rein, A. (1994). Characterization of human immunodeficiency virus type 1 dimeric RNA from wild-type and protease-defective virions. *J. Virol.* **68**, 5013–5018.

Gabus, C., Ficheux, D., Rau, M., Keith, G., Sandmeyer, S., and Darlix, J. L. (1998). The yeast Ty3 retrotransposon contains a 5′-3′ bipartite primer-binding site and encodes nucleocapsid protein NCp9 functionally homologous to HIV-1 NCp7. *EMBO J.* **17**, 4873–4880.

Gabus, C., Auxilien, S., Pechoux, C., Dormont, D., Swietnicki, W., Morillas, M., Surewicz, W., Nandi, P., and Darlix, J. L. (2001). The prion protein has DNA strand transfer properties similar to retroviral nucleocapsid protein. *J. Mol. Biol.* **307**, 1011–1021.

Galetto, R., Giacomoni, V., Veron, M., and Negroni, M. (2006). Dissection of a circumscribed recombination hot spot in HIV-1 after a single infectious cycle. *J. Biol. Chem.* **281**, 2711–2720.

Galetto, R., and Negroni, M. (2005). Mechanistic features of recombination in HIV. *AIDS Rev.* **7**, 92–102.

Gallant, J. E., Gerondelis, P. Z., Wainberg, M. A., Shulman, N. S., Haubrich, R. H., St. Clair, M., Lanier, E. R., Hellmann, N. S., and Richman, D. D. (2003). Nucleoside and nucleotide analogue reverse transcriptase inhibitors: A clinical review of antiretroviral resistance. *Antivir. Ther.* **8**, 489–506.

Gao, K., Gorelick, R. J., Johnson, D. G., and Bushman, F. (2003). Cofactors for human immunodeficiency virus type 1 cDNA integration *in vitro*. *J. Virol.* **77**, 1598–1603.

Gao, Y., Kaluarachchi, K., and Giedroc, D. P. (1998). Solution structure and backbone dynamics of Mason-Pfizer monkey virus (MPMV) nucleocapsid protein. *Protein Sci.* **7**, 2265–2280.

Garfinkel, D. J., Boeke, J. D., and Fink, G. R. (1985). Ty element transposition: Reverse transcriptase and virus-like particles. *Cell* **42**, 507–517.

Gelderblom, H. R., Hausmann, E. H., Ozel, M., Pauli, G., and Koch, M. A. (1987). Fine structure of human immunodeficiency virus (HIV) and immunolocalization of structural proteins. *Virology* **156**, 171–176.

Gheysen, D., Jacobs, E., de Foresta, F., Thiriart, C., Francotte, M., Thines, D., and De Wilde, M. (1989). Assembly and release of HIV-1 precursor Pr55gag virus-like particles from recombinant baculovirus-infected insect cells. *Cell* **59**, 103–112.

Girard, M. P., Osmanov, S. K., and Kieny, M. P. (2006). A review of vaccine research and development: The human immuno-deficiency virus (HIV). *Vaccine* **24**, 4062–4081.

Godet, J., de Rocquigny, H., Raja, C., Glasser, N., Ficheux, D., Darlix, J. L., and Mely, Y. (2006). During the early phase of HIV-1 DNA synthesis, nucleocapsid protein directs hybridization of the TAR complementary sequences via the ends of their double-stranded stem. *J. Mol. Biol.* **356**, 1180–1192.

Goh, W. C., Rogel, M. E., Kinsey, C. M., Michael, S. F., Fultz, P. N., Nowak, M. A., Hahn, B. H., and Emerman, M. (1998). HIV-1 Vpr increases viral expression by manipulation of the cell cycle: A mechanism for selection of Vpr *in vivo*. *Nat. Med.* **4**, 65–71.

Goncalves, J., and Santa-Marta, M. (2004). HIV-1 Vif and APOBEC3G: Multiple roads to one goal. *Retrovirology* **1**, 28.

Gorelick, R. J., Nigida, S. M., Jr., Bess, J. W., Jr., Arthur, L. O., Henderson, L. E., and Rein, A. (1990). Noninfectious human immunodeficiency virus type 1 mutants deficient in genomic RNA. *J. Virol.* **64**, 3207–3211.

Gorelick, R. J., Chabot, D. J., Rein, A., Henderson, L. E., and Arthur, L. O. (1993). The two zinc fingers in the human immunodeficiency virus type 1 nucleocapsid protein are not functionally equivalent. *J. Virol.* **67**, 4027–4036.

Gorelick, R. J., Chabot, D. J., Ott, D. E., Gagliardi, T. D., Rein, A., Henderson, L. E., and Arthur, L. O. (1996). Genetic analysis of the zinc finger in the Moloney murine leukemia virus nucleocapsid domain: Replacement of zinc-coordinating residues with other zinc-coordinating residues yields noninfectious particles containing genomic RNA. *J. Virol.* **70**, 2593–2597.

Gorelick, R. J., Fu, W., Gagliardi, T. D., Bosche, W. J., Rein, A., Henderson, L. E., and Arthur, L. O. (1999). Characterization of the block in replication of nucleocapsid protein zinc finger mutants from moloney murine leukemia virus. *J. Virol.* **73**, 8185–8195.

Gottlinger, H. G. (2001). The HIV-1 assembly machine. *Aids* **15**(Suppl. 5), S13–S20.

Gregoire, C. J., Gautheret, D., and Loret, E. P. (1997). No tRNA3Lys unwinding in a complex with HIV NCp7. *J. Biol. Chem.* **272**, 25143–25148.

Grigorov, B., Arcanger, F., Roingeard, P., Darlix, J. L., and Muriaux, D. (2006). Assembly of infectious HIV-1 in human epithelial and T-lymphoblastic cell lines. *J. Mol. Biol.* **359**, 848–862.

Guo, J., Henderson, L. E., Bess, J., Kane, B., and Levin, J. G. (1997). Human immunodeficiency virus type 1 nucleocapsid protein promotes efficient strand transfer and specific viral DNA synthesis by inhibiting TAR-dependent self-priming from minus-strand strong-stop DNA. *J. Virol.* **71**, 5178–5188.

Hanafusa, H. (1969). Rapid transformation of cells by Rous sarcoma virus. *Proc. Natl. Acad. Sci. USA* **63**, 318–325.

Hansen, L. J., Chalker, D. L., and Sandmeyer, S. B. (1988). Ty3, a yeast retrotransposon associated with tRNA genes, has homology to animal retroviruses. *Mol. Cell. Biol.* **8**, 5245–5256.

Hargittai, M. R., Mangla, A. T., Gorelick, R. J., and Musier-Forsyth, K. (2001). HIV-1 nucleocapsid protein zinc finger structures induce tRNA(Lys,3) structural changes but are not critical for primer/template annealing. *J. Mol. Biol.* **312**, 985–997.

Hargittai, M. R., Gorelick, R. J., Rouzina, I., and Musier-Forsyth, K. (2004). Mechanistic insights into the kinetics of HIV-1 nucleocapsid protein-facilitated tRNA annealing to the primer binding site. *J. Mol. Biol.* **337**, 951–968.

Harris, D. A., and True, H. L. (2006). New insights into prion structure and toxicity. *Neuron* **50**, 353–357.

Hayashi, T., Shioda, T., Iwakura, Y., and Shibuta, H. (1992). RNA packaging signal of human immunodeficiency virus type 1. *Virology* **188**, 590–599.

He, J., Choe, S., Walker, R., Di Marzio, P., Morgan, D. O., and Landau, N. R. (1995). Human immunodeficiency virus type 1 viral protein R (Vpr) arrests cells in the G2 phase of the cell cycle by inhibiting p34cdc2 activity. *J. Virol.* **69**, 6705–6711.

Henriet, S., Richer, D., Bernacchi, S., Decroly, E., Vigne, R., Ehresmann, B., Ehresmann, C., Paillart, J. C., and Marquet, R. (2005). Cooperative and specific binding of Vif to the 5′ region of HIV-1 genomic RNA. *J. Mol. Biol.* **354**, 55–72.

Herbreteau, C. H., Weill, L., Decimo, D., Prevot, D., Darlix, J. L., Sargueil, B., and Ohlmann, T. (2005). HIV-2 genomic RNA contains a novel type of IRES located downstream of its initiation codon. *Nat. Struct. Mol. Biol.* **12**, 1001–1007.

Herschlag, D. (1995). RNA chaperones and the RNA folding problem. *J. Biol. Chem.* **270**, 20871–20874.

Hrimech, M., Yao, X. J., Branton, P. E., and Cohen, E. A. (2000). Human immunodeficiency virus type 1 Vpr-mediated G(2) cell cycle arrest: Vpr interferes with cell cycle signaling cascades by interacting with the B subunit of serine/threonine protein phosphatase 2A. *EMBO J.* **19**, 3956–3967.

Hu, W. S., Rhodes, T., Dang, Q., and Pathak, V. (2003). Retroviral recombination: Review of genetic analyses. *Front. Biosci.* **8**, d143–d155.

Hu, W. S., and Temin, H. M. (1990). Retroviral recombination and reverse transcription. *Science* **250**, 1227–1233.

Huang, M., Maynard, A., Turpin, J. A., Graham, L., Janini, G. M., Covell, D. G., and Rice, W. G. (1998). Anti-HIV agents that selectively target retroviral nucleocapsid protein zinc fingers without affecting cellular zinc finger proteins. *J. Med. Chem.* **41**, 1371–1381.

Huang, Y., Khorchid, A., Wang, J., Parniak, M. A., Darlix, J. L., Wainberg, M. A., and Kleiman, L. (1997). Effect of mutations in the nucleocapsid protein (NCp7) upon Pr160 (gag-pol) and tRNA(Lys) incorporation into human immunodeficiency virus type 1. *J. Virol.* **71**, 4378–4384.

Huebner, R. J., and Todaro, G. J. (1969). Oncogenes of RNA tumor viruses as determinants of cancer. *Proc. Natl. Acad. Sci. USA* **64**, 1087–1094.

Huthoff, H., and Berkhout, B. (2001a). Mutations in the TAR hairpin affect the equilibrium between alternative conformations of the HIV-1 leader RNA. *Nucleic Acids Res.* **29**, 2594–2600.

Huthoff, H., and Berkhout, B. (2001b). Two alternating structures of the HIV-1 leader RNA. *RNA* **7**, 143–157.

Huthoff, H., and Berkhout, B. (2002). Multiple secondary structure rearrangements during HIV-1 RNA dimerization. *Biochemistry* **41**, 10439–10445.

Ivanyi-Nagy, R., Davidovic, L., Khandjian, E. W., and Darlix, J. L. (2005). Disordered RNA chaperone proteins: From functions to disease. *Cell. Mol. Life Sci.* **62**, 1409–1417.

Ivanyi-Nagy, R., Kanevsky, I., Gabus, C., Lavergne, J. P., Ficheux, D., Penin, F., Fosse, P., and Darlix, J. L. (2006). Analysis of hepatitis C virus RNA dimerization and core-RNA interactions. *Nucleic Acids Res.* **34**, 2618–2633.

Jowett, J. B., Planelles, V., Poon, B., Shah, N. P., Chen, M. L., and Chen, I. S. (1995). The human immunodeficiency virus type 1 vpr gene arrests infected T cells in the G2 + M phase of the cell cycle. *J. Virol.* **69**, 6304–6313.

Jung, A., Maier, R., Vartanian, J. P., Bocharov, G., Jung, V., Fischer, U., Meese, E., Wain-Hobson, S., and Meyerhans, A. (2002). Multiply infected spleen cells in HIV patients. *Nature* **418**, 144.

Kanevsky, I., Chaminade, F., Ficheux, D., Moumen, A., Gorelick, R., Negroni, M., Darlix, J. L., and Fosse, P. (2005). Specific interactions between HIV-1 nucleocapsid protein and the TAR element. *J. Mol. Biol.* **348**, 1059–1077.

Katz, R. A., and Skalka, A. M. (1990). Generation of diversity in retroviruses. *Annu. Rev. Genet.* **24**, 409–445.

Kaye, J. F., and Lever, A. M. (1999). Human immunodeficiency virus types 1 and 2 differ in the predominant mechanism used for selection of genomic RNA for encapsidation. *J. Virol.* **73**(4), 3023–3031.

Khan, M. A., Aberham, C., Kao, S., Akari, H., Gorelick, R., Bour, S., and Strebel, K. (2001). Human immunodeficiency virus type 1 Vif protein is packaged into the nucleoprotein complex through an interaction with viral genomic RNA. *J. Virol.* **75**, 7252–7265.

Khan, R., and Giedroc, D. P. (1994). Nucleic acid binding properties of recombinant Zn2 HIV-1 nucleocapsid protein are modulated by COOH-terminal processing. *J. Biol. Chem.* **269**, 22538–22546.

Klein, D. J., Johnson, P. E., Zollars, E. S., De Guzman, R. N., and Summers, M. F. (2000). The NMR structure of the nucleocapsid protein from the mouse mammary tumor virus reveals unusual folding of the C-terminal zinc knuckle. *Biochemistry* **39**, 1604–1612.

Kobayashi, M., Takaori-Kondo, A., Miyauchi, Y., Iwai, K., and Uchiyama, T. (2005). Ubiquitination of APOBEC3G by an HIV-1 Vif-Cullin5-Elongin B-Elongin C complex is essential for Vif function. *J. Biol. Chem.* **280**, 18573–18578.

Kondo, E., and Gottlinger, H. G. (1996). A conserved LXXLF sequence is the major determinant in p6gag required for the incorporation of human immunodeficiency virus type 1 Vpr. *J. Virol.* **70**, 159–164.

Kondo, E., Mammano, F., Cohen, E. A., and Gottlinger, H. G. (1995). The p6gag domain of human immunodeficiency virus type 1 is sufficient for the incorporation of Vpr into heterologous viral particles. *J. Virol.* **69**, 2759–2764.

Kramer, B., Pelchen-Matthews, A., Deneka, M., Garcia, E., Piguet, V., and Marsh, M. (2005). HIV interaction with endosomes in macrophages and dendritic cells. *Blood Cells Mol. Dis.* **35**, 136–142.

Kremer, M., and Schnierle, B. S. (2005). HIV-1 Vif: HIV's weapon against the cellular defense factor APOBEC3G. *Curr. HIV Res.* **3**, 339–344.

Kulkosky, J., and Bray, S. (2006). HAART-persistent HIV-1 latent reservoirs: Their origin, mechanisms of stability and potential strategies for eradication. *Curr. HIV Res.* **4**, 199–208.

Lapadat-Tapolsky, M., De Rocquigny, H., Van Gent, D., Roques, B., Plasterk, R., and Darlix, J. L. (1993). Interactions between HIV-1 nucleocapsid protein and viral DNA may have important functions in the viral life cycle. *Nucleic Acids Res.* **21**, 831–839.

Lapadat-Tapolsky, M., Gabus, C., Rau, M., and Darlix, J. L. (1997). Possible roles of HIV-1 nucleocapsid protein in the specificity of proviral DNA synthesis and in its variability. *J. Mol. Biol.* **268**, 250–260.

Le Rouzic, E., Mousnier, A., Rustum, C., Stutz, F., Hallberg, E., Dargemont, C., and Benichou, S. (2002). Docking of HIV-1 Vpr to the nuclear envelope is mediated by the interaction with the nucleoporin hCG1. *J. Biol. Chem.* **277**, 45091–45098.

Leblanc, P., Baas, D., and Darlix, J. L. (2004). Analysis of the interactions between HIV-1 and the cellular prion protein in a human cell line. *J. Mol. Biol.* **337**, 1035–1051.

Leblanc, P., Alais, S., Porto-Carreiro, I., Lehmann, S., Grassi, J., Raposo, G., and Darlix, J. L. (2006). Retrovirus infection strongly enhances scrapie infectivity release in cell culture. *EMBO J.* **25**, 2674–2685.

Lee, B. M., De Guzman, R. N., Turner, B. G., Tjandra, N., and Summers, M. F. (1998). Dynamical behavior of the HIV-1 nucleocapsid protein. *J. Mol. Biol.* **279**, 633–649.

Lener, D., Tanchou, V., Roques, B. P., Le Grice, S. F., and Darlix, J. L. (1998). Involvement of HIV-I nucleocapsid protein in the recruitment of reverse transcriptase into nucleoprotein complexes formed *in vitro*. *J. Biol. Chem.* **273**, 33781–33786.

Lever, A., Gottlinger, H., Haseltine, W., and Sodroski, J. (1989). Identification of a sequence required for efficient packaging of human immunodeficiency virus type 1 RNA into virions. *J. Virol.* **63**, 4085–4087.

Levin, J. G., Guo, J., Rouzina, I., and Musier-Forsyth, K. (2005). Nucleic acid chaperone activity of HIV-1 nucleocapsid protein: Critical role in reverse transcription and molecular mechanism. *Prog. Nucleic Acid Res. Mol. Biol.* **80**, 217–286.

Levy, D. N., Fernandes, L. S., Williams, W. V., and Weiner, D. B. (1993). Induction of cell differentiation by human immunodeficiency virus 1 vpr. *Cell* **72**, 541–550.

Li, X., Quan, Y., Arts, E. J., Li, Z., Preston, B. D., de Rocquigny, H., Roques, B. P., Darlix, J. L., Kleiman, L., Parniak, M. A., and Wainberg, M. A. (1996). Human immunodeficiency virus Type 1 nucleocapsid protein (NCp7) directs specific initiation of minus-strand DNA synthesis primed by human tRNA(Lys3) *in vitro*: Studies of viral RNA molecules mutated in regions that flank the primer binding site. *J. Virol.* **70**, 4996–5004.

Liang, C., Rong, L., Morin, N., Cherry, E., Huang, Y., Kleiman, L., and Wainberg, M. A. (1997). The roles of the human immunodeficiency virus type 1 Pol protein and the primer binding site in the placement of primer tRNA(3Lys) onto viral genomic RNA. *J. Virol.* **71**, 9075–9086.

Liu, B., Yu, X., Luo, K., Yu, Y., and Yu, X. F. (2004). Influence of primate lentiviral Vif and proteasome inhibitors on human immunodeficiency virus type 1 virion packaging of APOBEC3G. *J. Virol.* **78**, 2072–2081.

Liu, H. W., Cosa, G., Landes, C. F., Zeng, Y., Kovaleski, B. J., Mullen, D. G., Barany, G., Musier-Forsyth, K., and Barbara, P. F. (2005). Single-molecule FRET studies of important intermediates in the nucleocapsid-protein-chaperoned minus-strand transfer step in HIV-1 reverse transcription. *Biophys. J.* **89**, 3470–3479.

Lopez-Lastra, M., Gabus, C., and Darlix, J. L. (1997). Characterization of an internal ribosomal entry segment within the 5′ leader of avian reticuloendotheliosis virus type A RNA and development of novel MLV-REV-based retroviral vectors. *Hum. Gene Ther.* **8**, 1855–1865.

Lopez-Lastra, M., Rivas, A., and Barria, M. I. (2005). Protein synthesis in eukaryotes: The growing biological relevance of cap-independent translation initiation. *Biol. Res.* **38**, 121–146.

Lori, F., di Marzo Veronese, F., de Vico, A. L., Lusso, P., Reitz, M. S., Jr., and Gallo, R. C. (1992). Viral DNA carried by human immunodeficiency virus type 1 virions. *J. Virol.* **66**, 5067–5074.

Lu, Y. L., Bennett, R. P., Wills, J. W., Gorelick, R., and Ratner, L. (1995). A leucine triplet repeat sequence (LXX)4 in p6gag is important for Vpr incorporation into human immunodeficiency virus type 1 particles. *J. Virol.* **69**, 6873–6879.

Lucas, G. M. (2005). Antiretroviral adherence, drug resistance, viral fitness and HIV disease progression: A tangled web is Woven. *J. Antimicrob. Chemother.* **55**(4), 413–416.

Luo, K., Liu, B., Xiao, Z., Yu, Y., Yu, X., Gorelick, R., and Yu, X. F. (2004). Amino-terminal region of the human immunodeficiency virus type 1 nucleocapsid is required for human APOBEC3G packaging. *J. Virol.* **78**(21), 11841–11852.

Mangeat, B., Turelli, P., Caron, G., Friedli, M., Perrin, L., and Trono, D. (2003). Broad antiretroviral defence by human APOBEC3G through lethal editing of nascent reverse transcripts. *Nature* **424**, 99–103.

Mangeat, B., Turelli, P., Liao, S., and Trono, D. (2004). A single amino acid determinant governs the species-specific sensitivity of APOBEC3G to Vif action. *J. Biol. Chem.* **279**, 14481–14483.

Mansky, L. M., Preveral, S., Selig, L., Benarous, R., and Benichou, S. (2000). The interaction of vpr with uracil DNA glycosylase modulates the human immunodeficiency virus type 1 *In vivo* mutation rate. *J. Virol.* **74**, 7039–7047.

Marsh, M., and Thali, M. (2003). HIV's great escape. *Nat. Med.* **9**, 1262–1263.

Maynard, A. T., Huang, M., Rice, W. G., and Covell, D. G. (1998). Reactivity of the HIV-1 nucleocapsid protein p7 zinc finger domains from the perspective of density-functional theory. *Proc. Natl. Acad. Sci. USA* **95**, 11578–11583.

McBride, M. S., and Panganiban, A. T. (1996). The human immunodeficiency virus type 1 encapsidation site is a multipartite RNA element composed of functional hairpin structures. *J. Virol.* **70**, 2963–2973.

McCarthy, M. (1995). HIV gene arrests cell cycle. *Lancet* **346**, 960.

McMichael, A. J. (2006). HIV vaccines. *Annu. Rev. Immunol.* **24**, 227–255.

Mely, Y., Cornille, F., Fournie-Zaluski, M. C., Darlix, J. L., Roques, B. P., and Gerard, D. (1991). Investigation of zinc-binding affinities of Moloney murine leukemia virus nucleocapsid protein and its related zinc finger and modified peptides. *Biopolymers* **31**, 899–906.

Mely, Y., Jullian, N., Morellet, N., De Rocquigny, H., Dong, C. Z., Piemont, E., Roques, B. P., and Gerard, D. (1994). Spatial proximity of the HIV-1 nucleocapsid protein zinc fingers investigated by time-resolved fluorescence and fluorescence resonance energy transfer. *Biochemistry* **33**, 12085–12091.

Mely, Y., de Rocquigny, H., Sorinas-Jimeno, M., Keith, G., Roques, B. P., Marquet, R., and Gerard, D. (1995). Binding of the HIV-1 nucleocapsid protein to the primer tRNA(3Lys), *in vitro*, is essentially not specific. *J. Biol. Chem.* **270**, 1650–1656.

Mely, Y., De Rocquigny, H., Morellet, N., Roques, B. P., and Gerad, D. (1996). Zinc binding to the HIV-1 nucleocapsid protein: A thermodynamic investigation by fluorescence spectroscopy. *Biochemistry* **35**, 5175–5182.

Meric, A. L., III, Purtell, M. J., and Levy, C. C. (1984). Characterization of a p30 fraction from Rauscher leukemia virus which has an associated ATPase activity. *J. Biol. Chem.* **259**, 12865–12872.

Meric, C., Gouilloud, E., and Spahr, P. F. (1988). Mutations in Rous sarcoma virus nucleocapsid protein p12 (NC): Deletions of Cys-His boxes. *J. Virol.* **62**, 3328–3333.

Miller, V., Stark, T., Loeliger, A. E., and Lange, J. M. (2002). The impact of the M184V substitution in HIV-1 reverse transcriptase on treatment response. *HIV Med.* **3**, 135–145.

Mir, M. A., and Panganiban, A. T. (2005). The hantavirus nucleocapsid protein recognizes specific features of the viral RNA panhandle and is altered in conformation upon RNA binding. *J. Virol.* **79**, 1824–1835.

Morellet, N., Jullian, N., De Rocquigny, H., Maigret, B., Darlix, J. L., and Roques, B. P. (1992). Determination of the structure of the nucleocapsid protein NCp7 from the human immunodeficiency virus type 1 by 1H NMR. *EMBO J.* **11**, 3059–3065.

Morellet, N., de Rocquigny, H., Mely, Y., Jullian, N., Demene, H., Ottmann, M., Gerard, D., Darlix, J. L., Fournie-Zaluski, M. C., and Roques, B. P. (1994). Conformational behaviour of the active and inactive forms of the nucleocapsid NCp7 of HIV-1 studied by 1H NMR. *J. Mol. Biol.* **235**, 287–301.

Morellet, N., Demene, H., Teilleux, V., Huynh-Dinh, T., de Rocquigny, H., Fournie-Zaluski, M. C., and Roques, B. P. (1998). Structure of the complex between the HIV-1 nucleocapsid protein NCp7 and the single-stranded pentanucleotide d(ACGCC). *J. Mol. Biol.* **283**, 419–434.

Morellet, N., Meudal, H., Bouaziz, S., and Roques, B. P. (2006). Structure of the zinc finger domain encompassing residues 13–51 of the nucleocapsid protein from simian immunodeficiency virus. *Biochem. J.* **393**, 725–732.

Muriaux, D., De Rocquigny, H., Roques, B. P., and Paoletti, J. (1996). NCp7 activates HIV-1Lai RNA dimerization by converting a transient loop-loop complex into a stable dimer. *J. Biol. Chem.* **271**, 33686–33692.

Muriaux, D., Mirro, J., Harvin, D., and Rein, A. (2001). RNA is a structural element in retrovirus particles. *Proc. Natl. Acad. Sci. USA* **98**, 5246–5251.

Navarro, F., and Landau, N. R. (2004). Recent insights into HIV-1 Vif. *Curr. Opin. Immunol.* **16**, 477–482.

Negroni, M., and Buc, H. (2001). Mechanisms of retroviral recombination. *Annu. Rev. Genet.* **35**, 275–302.

Ohlmann, T., Lopez-Lastra, M., and Darlix, J. L. (2000). An internal ribosome entry segment promotes translation of the simian immunodeficiency virus genomic RNA. *J. Biol. Chem.* **275**, 11899–11906.

Omichinski, J. G., Clore, G. M., Sakaguchi, K., Appella, E., and Gronenborn, A. M. (1991). Structural characterization of a 39-residue synthetic peptide containing the two zinc binding domains from the HIV-1 p7 nucleocapsid protein by CD and NMR spectroscopy. *FEBS Lett.* **292**, 25–30.

Ono, A., and Freed, E. O. (2004). Cell-type-dependent targeting of human immunodeficiency virus type 1 assembly to the plasma membrane and the multivesicular body. *J. Virol.* **78**, 1552–1563.

Ono, A., Ablan, S. D., Lockett, S. J., Nagashima, K., and Freed, E. O. (2004). Phosphatidylinositol (4,5) bisphosphate regulates HIV-1 Gag targeting to the plasma membrane. *Proc. Natl. Acad. Sci. USA* **101**, 14889–14894.

Ottmann, M., Gabus, C., and Darlix, J. L. (1995). The central globular domain of the nucleocapsid protein of human immunodeficiency virus type 1 is critical for virion structure and infectivity. *J. Virol.* **69**, 1778–1784.

Pager, J., Coulaud, D., and Delain, E. (1994). Electron microscopy of the nucleocapsid from disrupted Moloney murine leukemia virus and of associated type VI collagen-like filaments. *J. Virol.* **68**, 223–232.

Pelchen-Matthews, A., Kramer, B., and Marsh, M. (2003). Infectious HIV-1 assembles in late endosomes in primary macrophages. *J. Cell Biol.* **162**, 443–455.

Perez, O., and Hope, T. J. (2006). Cellular restriction factors affecting the early stages of HIV replication. *Curr. HIV/AIDS Rep.* **3**, 20–25.

Piguet, V., and Sattentau, Q. (2004). Dangerous liaisons at the virological synapse. *J. Clin. Invest.* **114**, 605–610.

Piller, S. C., Ewart, G. D., Premkumar, A., Cox, G. B., and Gage, P. W. (1996). Vpr protein of human immunodeficiency virus type 1 forms cation-selective channels in planar lipid bilayers. *Proc. Natl. Acad. Sci. USA* **93**, 111–115.

Poljak, L., Batson, S. M., Ficheux, D., Roques, B. P., Darlix, J. L., and Kas, E. (2003). Analysis of NCp7-dependent activation of HIV-1 cDNA integration and its conservation among retroviral nucleocapsid proteins. *J. Mol. Biol.* **329**, 411–421.

Poon, B., Grovit-Ferbas, K., Stewart, S. A., and Chen, I. S. (1998). Cell cycle arrest by Vpr in HIV-1 virions and insensitivity to antiretroviral agents. *Science* **281**, 266–269.

Popik, W., and Alce, T. M. (2004). CD4 receptor localized to non-raft membrane microdomains supports HIV-1 entry. Identification of a novel raft localization marker in CD4. *J. Biol. Chem.* **279**, 704–712.

Popov, S., Rexach, M., Ratner, L., Blobel, G., and Bukrinsky, M. (1998). Viral protein R regulates docking of the HIV-1 preintegration complex to the nuclear pore complex. *J. Biol. Chem.* **273**, 13347–13352.

Pornillos, O., Garrus, J. E., and Sundquist, W. I. (2002). Mechanisms of enveloped RNA virus budding. *Trends Cell Biol.* **12**, 569–579.

Prats, A. C., Sarih, L., Gabus, C., Litvak, S., Keith, G., and Darlix, J. L. (1988). Small finger protein of avian and murine retroviruses has nucleic acid annealing activity and positions the replication primer tRNA onto genomic RNA. *EMBO J.* **7**, 1777–1783.

Prats, A. C., Housset, V., de Billy, G., Cornille, F., Prats, H., Roques, B., and Darlix, J. L. (1991). Viral RNA annealing activities of the nucleocapsid protein of Moloney murine leukemia virus are zinc independent. *Nucleic Acids Res.* **19**, 3533–3541.

Prevot, D., Decimo, D., Herbreteau, C. H., Roux, F., Garin, J., Darlix, J. L., and Ohlmann, T. (2003). Characterization of a novel RNA-binding region of eIF4GI critical for ribosomal scanning. *EMBO J.* **22**, 1909–1921.

Priola, S. A., and Vorberg, I. (2006). Molecular aspects of disease pathogenesis in the transmissible spongiform encephalopathies. *Mol. Biotechnol.* **33**, 71–88.

Pustowka, A., Dietz, J., Ferner, J., Baumann, M., Landersz, M., Konigs, C., Schwalbe, H., and Dietrich, U. (2003). Identification of peptide ligands for target RNA structures derived from the HIV-1 packaging signal psi by screening phage-displayed peptide libraries. *Chembiochem* **4**, 1093–1097.

Pyronnet, S., and Sonenberg, N. (2001). Cell-cycle-dependent translational control. *Curr. Opin. Genet. Dev.* **11**, 13–18.

Raja, C., Ferner, J., Dietrich, U., Avilov, S., Ficheux, D., Darlix, J. L., de Rocquigny, H., Schwalbe, H., and Mely, Y. (2006). A tryptophan-rich hexapeptide inhibits nucleic acid destabilization chaperoned by the HIV-1 nucleocapsid protein. *Biochemistry* **45**, 9254–9265.

Ramboarina, S., Srividya, N., Atkinson, R. A., Morellet, N., Roques, B. P., Lefevre, J. F., Mely, Y., and Kieffer, B. (2002). Effects of temperature on the dynamic behaviour of the HIV-1 nucleocapsid NCp7 and its DNA complex. *J. Mol. Biol.* **316**, 611–627.

Ramstrom, H., Bourotte, M., Philippe, C., Schmitt, M., Haiech, J., and Bourguignon, J. J. (2004). Heterocyclic bis-cations as starting hits for design of inhibitors of the bifunctional enzyme histidine-containing protein kinase/phosphatase from Bacillus subtilis. *J. Med. Chem.* **47**, 2264–2275.

Raposo, G., Moore, M., Innes, D., Leijendekker, R., Leigh-Brown, A., Benaroch, P., and Geuze, H. (2002). Human macrophages accumulate HIV-1 particles in MHC II compartments. *Traffic* **3**, 718–729.

Rein, A., Ott, D. E., Mirro, J., Arthur, L. O., Rice, W., and Henderson, L. E. (1996). Inactivation of murine leukemia virus by compounds that react with the zinc finger in the viral nucleocapsid protein. *J. Virol.* **70**, 4966–4972.

Rein, A., Henderson, L. E., and Levin, J. G. (1998). Nucleic-acid-chaperone activity of retroviral nucleocapsid proteins: Significance for viral replication. *Trends Biochem. Sci.* **23**, 297–301.

Remy, E., de Rocquigny, H., Petitjean, P., Muriaux, D., Theilleux, V., Paoletti, J., and Roques, B. P. (1998). The annealing of tRNA3Lys to human immunodeficiency virus type 1 primer binding site is critically dependent on the NCp7 zinc fingers structure. *J. Biol. Chem.* **273**, 4819–4822.

Resh, M. D. (2005). Intracellular trafficking of HIV-1 Gag: How Gag interacts with cell membranes and makes viral particles. *AIDS Rev.* **7**, 84–91.

Rhodes, T. D., Nikolaitchik, O., Chen, J., Powell, D., and Hu, W. S. (2005). Genetic recombination of human immunodeficiency virus type 1 in one round of viral replication: Effects of genetic distance, target cells, accessory genes, and lack of high negative interference in crossover events. *J. Virol.* **79**, 1666–1677.

Rice, W. G., Schaeffer, C. A., Graham, L., Bu, M., McDougal, J. S., Orloff, S. L., Villinger, F., Young, M., Oroszlan, S., and Fesen, M. R. (1993). The site of antiviral action of 3-nitrosobenzamide on the infectivity process of human immunodeficiency virus in human lymphocytes. *Proc. Natl. Acad. Sci. USA* **90**, 9721–9724.

Rice, W. G., Supko, J. G., Malspeis, L., Buckheit, R. W., Jr., Clanton, D., Bu, M., Graham, L., Schaeffer, C. A., Turpin, J. A., Domagala, J., Gogliotti, R., Bader, J. P., *et al.* (1995). Inhibitors of HIV nucleocapsid protein zinc fingers as candidates for the treatment of AIDS. *Science* **270**, 1194–1197.

Rice, W. G., Baker, D. C., Schaeffer, C. A., Graham, L., Bu, M., Terpening, S., Clanton, D., Schultz, R., Bader, J. P., Buckheit, R. W., Jr., Field, L., Singh, P. K., *et al.* (1997a). Inhibition of multiple phases of human immunodeficiency virus type 1 replication by a dithiane compound that attacks the conserved zinc fingers of retroviral nucleocapsid proteins. *Antimicrob. Agents Chemother.* **41**, 419–426.

Rice, W. G., Turpin, J. A., Huang, M., Clanton, D., Buckheit, R. W., Jr., Covell, D. G., Wallqvist, A., McDonnell, N. B., DeGuzman, R. N., Summers, M. F., Zalkow, L., Bader, J. P., *et al.* (1997b). Azodicarbonamide inhibits HIV-1 replication by targeting the nucleocapsid protein. *Nat. Med.* **3**, 341–345.

Roques, B. P., Morellet, N., de Rocquigny, H., Demene, H., Schueler, W., and Jullian, N. (1997). Structure, biological functions and inhibition of the HIV-1 proteins Vpr and NCp7. *Biochimie* **79**, 673–680.

Rous, P. (1910). A transmissible avian neoplasm: Sarcoma for the common fowl. *J. Exp. Med.* **12**, 696–705.

Rudner, L., Nydegger, S., Coren, L. V., Nagashima, K., Thali, M., and Ott, D. E. (2005). Dynamic fluorescent imaging of human immunodeficiency virus type 1 gag in live cells by biarsenical labeling. *J. Virol.* **79**, 4055–4065.

Sabbah, E. N., Druillennec, S., Morellet, N., Bouaziz, S., Kroemer, G., and Roques, B. P. (2006). Interaction between the HIV-1 protein Vpr and the adenine nucleotide translocator. *Chem. Biol. Drug Des.* **67**, 145–154.

Sakaguchi, K., Zambrano, N., Baldwin, E. T., Shapiro, B. A., Erickson, J. W., Omichinski, J. G., Clore, G. M., Gronenborn, A. M., and Appella, E. (1993). Identification of a binding site for the human immunodeficiency virus type 1 nucleocapsid protein. *Proc. Natl. Acad. Sci. USA* **90**, 5219–5223.

Schroeder, R., Barta, A., and Semrad, K. (2004). Strategies for RNA folding and assembly. *Nat. Rev. Mol. Cell. Biol.* **5**, 908–919.

Schuler, W., Dong, C., Wecker, K., and Roques, B. P. (1999). NMR structure of the complex between the zinc finger protein NCp10 of Moloney murine leukemia virus and the single-stranded pentanucleotide d(ACGCC): Comparison with HIV-NCp7 complexes. *Biochemistry* **38**, 12984–12994.

Selig, L., Pages, J. C., Tanchou, V., Preval, S., Berlioz-Torrent, C., Liu, L. X., Erdtmann, L., Darlix, J., Benarous, R., and Benichou, S. (1999). Interaction with the p6 domain of the gag precursor mediates incorporation into virions of Vpr and Vpx proteins from primate lentiviruses. *J. Virol.* **73**, 592–600.

Sheppard, N., and Sattentau, Q. (2005). The prospects for vaccines against HIV-1: More than a field of long-term nonprogression? *Expert Rev. Mol. Med.* **7**, 1–21.

Shehu-Xhilaga, M., Tachedjian, G., Crowe, S. M., and Kedzierska, K. (2005). Antiretroviral compounds: Mechanisms underlying failure of HAART to eradicate HIV-1. *Curr. Med. Chem.* **12**, 1705–1719.

Shirakawa, K., Takaori-Kondo, A., Kobayashi, M., Tomonaga, M., Izumi, T., Fukunaga, K., Sasada, A., Abudu, A., Miyauchi, Y., Akari, H., Iwai, K., and Uchiyama, T. (2006). Ubiquitination of APOBEC3 proteins by the Vif-Cullin5-ElonginB-ElonginC complex. *Virology* **344**, 263–266.

Shubsda, M. F., Paoletti, A. C., Hudson, B. S., and Borer, P. N. (2002). Affinities of packaging domain loops in HIV-1 RNA for the nucleocapsid protein. *Biochemistry* **41**, 5276–5282.

Song, Y., Goel, A., Basrur, V., Roberts, P. E., Mikovits, J. A., Inman, J. K., Turpin, J. A., Rice, W. G., and Appella, E. (2002). Synthesis and biological properties of amino acid amide ligand-based pyridinioalkanoyl thioesters as anti-HIV agents. *Bioorg. Med. Chem.* **10**, 1263–1273.

Soros, V. B., and Greene, W. C. (2006). APOBEC3G and HIV-1: Strike and Counterstrike. *Curr. Infect. Dis. Rep.* **8**, 317–323.

South, T. L., Blake, P. R., Hare, D. R., and Summers, M. F. (1991). C-terminal retroviral-type zinc finger domain from the HIV-1 nucleocapsid protein is structurally similar to the N-terminal zinc finger domain. *Biochemistry* **30**, 6342–6349.

Stephen, A. G., Worthy, K. M., Towler, E., Mikovits, J. A., Sei, S., Roberts, P., Yang, Q. E., Akee, R. K., Klausmeyer, P., McCloud, T. G., Henderson, L., Rein, A., *et al.* (2002). Identification of HIV-1 nucleocapsid protein: Nucleic acid antagonists with cellular anti-HIV activity. *Biochem. Biophys. Res. Commun.* **296**, 1228–1237.

Stote, R. H., Kellenberger, E., Muller, H., Bombarda, E., Roques, B. P., Kieffer, B., and Mely, Y. (2004). Structure of the His44 –> Ala single point mutant of the distal finger motif of HIV-1 nucleocapsid protein: A combined NMR, molecular dynamics simulation, and fluorescence study. *Biochemistry* **43**, 7687–7697.

Strack, B., Calistri, A., Craig, S., Popova, E., and Gottlinger, H. G. (2003). AIP1/ALIX is a binding partner for HIV-1 p6 and EIAV p9 functioning in virus budding. *Cell* **114**, 689–699.

Stuchell, M. D., Garrus, J. E., Muller, B., Stray, K. M., Ghaffarian, S., Mckinnon, R., Krausslich, H. G., Morham, S. G., and Sundquist, W. I. (2004). The human endosomal sorting complex required for transport (ESCRT-I) and its role in HIV-1 budding. *J. Biol. Chem.* **279**, 36059–36071.

Summers, M. F., South, T. L., Kim, B., and Hare, D. R. (1990). High-resolution structure of an HIV zinc fingerlike domain via a new NMR-based distance geometry approach. *Biochemistry* **29**, 329–340.

Summers, M. F., Henderson, L. E., Chance, M. R., Bess, J. W., Jr., South, T. L., Blake, P. R., Sagi, I., Perez-Alvarado, G., Sowder, R. C., III, and Hare, D. R. (1992). Nucleocapsid zinc fingers detected in retroviruses: EXAFS studies of intact viruses and the solution-state structure of the nucleocapsid protein from HIV-1. *Protein Sci.* **1**, 563–574.

Tanchou, V., Gabus, C., Rogemond, V., and Darlix, J. L. (1995). Formation of stable and functional HIV-1 nucleoprotein complexes in vitro. *J. Mol. Biol.* **252**, 563–571.

Temin, H. M. (1991). Sex and recombination in retroviruses. *Trends Genet.* **7**, 71–74.

Thomas, J. A., Shulenin, S., Coren, L. V., Bosche, W. J., Gagliardi, T. D., Gorelick, R. J., and Oroszlan, S. (2006). Characterization of human immunodeficiency virus type 1 (HIV-1) containing mutations in the nucleocapsid protein at a putative HIV-1 protease cleavage site. *Virology* **354**, 261–270.

Tisne, C., Roques, B. P., and Dardel, F. (2001). Heteronuclear NMR studies of the interaction of tRNA(Lys)3 with HIV-1 nucleocapsid protein. *J. Mol. Biol.* **306**, 443–454.

Tisne, C., Roques, B. P., and Dardel, F. (2003). Specific recognition of primer tRNA Lys 3 by HIV-1 nucleocapsid protein: Involvement of the zinc fingers and the N-terminal basic extension. *Biochimie* **85**, 557–561.

Tisne, C., Roques, B. P., and Dardel, F. (2004). The annealing mechanism of HIV-1 reverse transcription primer onto the viral genome. *J. Biol. Chem.* **279**, 3588–3595.

Tompa, P., and Csermely, P. (2004). The role of structural disorder in the function of RNA and protein chaperones. *FASEB J.* **18**, 1169–1175.

Trono, D. (1992). Partial reverse transcripts in virions from human immunodeficiency and murine leukemia viruses. *J. Virol.* **66**, 4893–4900.

Tummino, P. J., Harvey, P. J., McQuade, T., Domagala, J., Gogliotti, R., Sanchez, J., Song, Y., and Hupe, D. (1997). The human immunodeficiency virus type 1 (HIV-1) nucleocapsid protein zinc ejection activity of disulfide benzamides and benzisothiazolones: Correlation with anti-HIV and virucidal activities. *Antimicrob. Agents Chemother.* **41**, 394–400.

Turner, B. G., and Summers, M. F. (1999). Structural biology of HIV. *J. Mol. Biol.* **285**, 1–32.

Turpin, J. A., Song, Y., Inman, J. K., Huang, M., Wallqvist, A., Maynard, A., Covell, D. G., Rice, W. G., and Appella, E. (1999). Synthesis and biological properties of novel pyridinioalkanoyl thiolesters (PATE) as anti-HIV-1 agents that target the viral nucleocapsid protein zinc fingers. *J. Med. Chem.* **42**, 67–86.

Urisman, A., Molinaro, R. J., Fischer, N., Plummer, S. J., Casey, G., Klein, E. A., Malathi, K., Magi-Galluzzi, C., Tubbs, R. R., Ganem, D., Silverman, R. H., and Derisi, J. L. (2006). Identification of a novel gammaretrovirus in prostate tumors of patients homozygous for R462Q RNASEL variant. *PLoS Pathog.* **2**, e25.

Uversky, V. N. (2002). Natively unfolded proteins: A point where biology waits for physics. *Protein Sci.* **11**, 739–756.

Vagner, S., Waysbort, A., Marenda, M., Gensac, M. C., Amalric, F., and Prats, A. C. (1995). Alternative translation initiation of the Moloney murine leukemia virus mRNA controlled by internal ribosome entry involving the p57/PTB splicing factor. *J. Biol. Chem.* **270**, 20376–20383.

Vandevelde, M., Witvrouw, M., Schmit, J. C., Sprecher, S., De Clercq, E., and Tassignon, J. P. (1996). ADA, a potential anti-HIV drug. *AIDS Res. Hum. Retroviruses* **12**, 567–568.

Varin, A., Decrion, A. Z., Sabbah, E., Quivy, V., Sire, J., Van Lint, C., Roques, B. P., Aggarwal, B. B., and Herbein, G. (2005). Synthetic Vpr protein activates activator protein-1, c-Jun N-terminal kinase, and NF-kappaB and stimulates HIV-1 transcription in promonocytic cells and primary macrophages. *J. Biol. Chem.* **280**, 42557–42567.

Vieira, H. L., Haouzi, D., El Hamel, C., Jacotot, E., Belzacq, A. S., Brenner, C., and Kroemer, G. (2000). Permeabilization of the mitochondrial inner membrane during apoptosis: Impact of the adenine nucleotide translocator. *Cell Death Differ.* **7**, 1146–1154.

Vodicka, M. A., Koepp, D. M., Silver, P. A., and Emerman, M. (1998). HIV-1 Vpr interacts with the nuclear transport pathway to promote macrophage infection. *Genes Dev.* **12**, 175–185.

Von Schwedler, U. K., Stuchell, M., Muller, B., Ward, D. M., Chung, H. Y., Morita, E., Wang, H. E., Davis, T., He, G. P., Cimbora, D. M., Scott, A., Krausslich, H. G., *et al.* (2003). The Protein network of HIV budding. *Cell* **114**, 701–713.

Vuilleumier, C., Bombarda, E., Morellet, N., Gerard, D., Roques, B. P., and Mely, Y. (1999). Nucleic acid sequence discrimination by the HIV-1 nucleocapsid protein NCp7: A fluorescence study. *Biochemistry* **38**, 16816–16825.

Wain-Hobson, S., Renoux-Elbe, C., Vartanian, J. P., and Meyerhans, A. (2003). Network analysis of human and simian immunodeficiency virus sequence sets reveals massive recombination resulting in shorter pathways. *J. Gen. Virol.* **84**, 885–895.

Wang, L., Mukherjee, S., Jia, F., Narayan, O., and Zhao, L. J. (1995). Interaction of virion protein Vpr of human immunodeficiency virus type 1 with cellular transcription factor Sp1 and trans-activation of viral long terminal repeat. *J. Biol. Chem.* **270**, 25564–25569.

Wang, L., Mukherjee, S., Narayan, O., and Zhao, L. J. (1996). Characterization of a leucine-zipper-like domain in Vpr protein of human immunodeficiency virus type 1. *Gene* **178**, 7–13.

Wecker, K., Morellet, N., Bouaziz, S., and Roques, B. P. (2002). NMR structure of the HIV-1 regulatory protein Vpr in H2O/trifluoroethanol. Comparison with the Vpr N-terminal (1–51) and C-terminal (52–96) domains. *Eur. J. Biochem.* **269**, 3779–3788.

Wright, P. E., and Dyson, H. J. (1999). Intrinsically unstructured proteins: Re-assessing the protein structure-function paradigm. *J. Mol. Biol.* **293**, 321–331.

Wu, J. Q., Maki, A. H., Ozarowski, A., Urbaneja, M. A., Henderson, L. E., and Casas-Finet, J. R. (1997). Fluorescence, phosphorescence, and optically detected magnetic resonance studies of the nucleic acid association of the nucleocapsid protein of the murine leukemia virus. *Biochemistry* **36**, 6115–6123.

You, J. C., and McHenry, C. S. (1994). Human immunodeficiency virus nucleocapsid protein accelerates strand transfer of the terminally redundant sequences involved in reverse transcription. *J. Biol. Chem.* **269**, 31491–31495.

Yu, Q., and Darlix, J. L. (1996). The zinc finger of nucleocapsid protein of Friend murine leukemia virus is critical for proviral DNA synthesis *in vivo*. *J. Virol.* **70**, 5791–5798.

Zander, K., Sherman, M. P., Tessmer, U., Bruns, K., Wray, V., Prechtel, A. T., Schubert, E., Henklein, P., Luban, J., Neidleman, J., Greene, W. C., and Schubert, U. (2003). Cyclophilin A interacts with HIV-1 Vpr and is required for its functional expression. *J. Biol. Chem.* **278**, 43202–43213.

Zhang, H., Bagasra, O., Niikura, M., Poiesz, B. J., and Pomerantz, R. J. (1994). Intravirion reverse transcripts in the peripheral blood plasma on human immunodeficiency virus type 1-infected individuals. *J. Virol.* **68**, 7591–7597.

Zhang, J., and Temin, H. M. (1993). Rate and mechanism of nonhomologous recombination during a single cycle of retroviral replication. *Science* **259**, 234–238.

Zhao, L. J., Wang, L., Mukherjee, S., and Narayan, O. (1994). Biochemical mechanism of HIV-1 Vpr function. Oligomerization mediated by the N-terminal domain. *J. Biol. Chem.* **269**, 32131–32137.

Zhou, W., Parent, L. J., Wills, J. W., and Resh, M. D. (1994). Identification of a membrane-binding domain within the amino-terminal region of human immunodeficiency virus type 1 Gag protein which interacts with acidic phospholipids. *J. Virol.* **68**, 2556–2569.

Catherine S. Adamson and Eric O. Freed

Virus-Cell Interaction Section, HIV Drug Resistance Program
National Cancer Institute, Frederick, Maryland 21702

Human Immunodeficiency Virus Type 1 Assembly, Release, and Maturation

I. Chapter Overview

A detailed understanding of *human immunodeficiency virus type 1* (HIV-1) assembly, release, and maturation is fundamental to our knowledge of the HIV-1 replication cycle and has the potential to inform the development of new antiretroviral strategies. The structural protein Gag plays a central role in these pathways and drives production of a mature infectious particle through protein–protein, protein–RNA, and protein–lipid interactions. These interactions facilitate multimerization of Gag to form the

Advances in Pharmacology, Volume 55
1054-3589/07 $35.00
DOI: 10.1016/S1054-3589(07)55010-6

structural shell of the particle, encapsidation of the RNA genome, trafficking of the virion components to the site of assembly, acquisition of a lipid bilayer and associated envelope glycoproteins, hijacking host cell machinery to facilitate virus release, and proteolytic maturation of the nascent virion. In this review, we describe the significant progress that has been achieved in understanding these processes and highlight key areas that remain unclear. Finally, we discuss how this knowledge is being applied to develop new anti-HIV drugs, an important research priority due to rapid emergence of HIV-1 isolates resistant to currently approved antiretroviral drugs.

II. Overview of HIV-1 Assembly, Release, and Maturation _____

The process of HIV-1 assembly, release, and maturation results in the production of a mature virus particle capable of infecting a new target cell. The infectious particle is composed of a host cell-derived lipid bilayer in which are embedded the viral envelope (Env) glycoprotein spikes (Fig. 1). Directly beneath, and attached to, the viral membrane is a spherical protein shell composed of the matrix (MA) protein. In the center of the mature particle is a condensed conical core composed of capsid (CA) protein. Inside this core are the viral enzymes reverse transcriptase (RT) and integrase (IN) and the nucleocaspid (NC) protein complexed with dimerized viral genomic RNA. The mature infectious particle is generated not by assembly of the individual protein components but from multifunctional polyprotein precursors Gag, Gag-Pol, and Env. The Gag and Gag-Pol precursor proteins

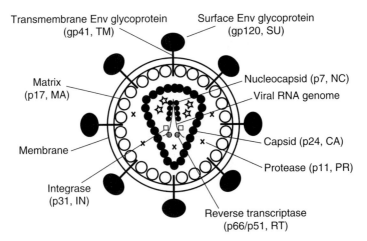

FIGURE 1 Structure of a mature HIV-1 virion depicting the key viral proteins and their arrangement within the virion. Adapted from Freed (1998).

are cleaved by the viral protease (PR) to the mature Gag and Pol proteins after virion assembly; the Env glycoprotein precursor, gp160, is cleaved by a cellular protease during gp160 trafficking from the endoplasmic reticulum (ER) to the plasma membrane. Cleavage of gp160 gives rise to the mature surface (SU) Env glycoprotein gp120 and the transmembrane (TM) glycoprotein gp41.

The Gag polyprotein precursor, known as $Pr55^{Gag}$ (Fig. 2), is the central player in HIV-1 particle formation as it drives assembly through protein–protein, protein–RNA, and protein–lipid interactions, orchestrating the incorporation of each of the major virion components into the assembling particle. $Pr55^{Gag}$ is translated from unspliced viral mRNA on free ribosomes in the cytoplasm and encodes the internal structural components of the virion: MA, CA, and NC along with the C-terminal p6 domain and two spacer peptides SP1 and SP2 (previously referred to as p2 and p1, respectively). $Pr55^{Gag}$ is the only virion-encoded molecule required for the assembly of immature virus-like particles (VLPs); it can self-assemble into VLPs by ordered multimerization of $Pr55^{Gag}$ monomers to produce a spherical shell, which forms the structural framework of the immature virus particle. The molecular interactions necessary for Gag–Gag multimerization occur between multiple domains of $Pr55^{Gag}$. Assembly occurs primarily at the site of virus budding, which in most cell types, including T cells, is the plasma membrane. However, in certain cell types, particularly primary monocyte-derived macrophages, assembly and budding take place in an intracellular late-endosomal compartment, the multivesicular body (MVB). The MA domain of $Pr55^{Gag}$ has been shown to be the major determinant responsible for the targeting and binding of Gag to the membrane. The assembly process is completed on budding of the particle from the plasma membrane, resulting in a released immature virion wrapped in a host-derived lipid bilayer. Budding is catalyzed by components of the cellular endosomal sorting machinery, including the ESCRT-I complex (for endosomal sorting complex required for transport) and associated factors, which are recruited to the site of assembly and release by the P(T/S)AP late domain motif located in the p6 region of $Pr55^{Gag}$ (Fig. 2).

While $Pr55^{Gag}$ is the only virion-encoded molecule required for assembly and release of immature VLPs, production of mature infectious virions requires encapsidation of the viral genomic RNA and incorporation of the Env glycoprotein complex and Gag-Pol precursor ($Pr160^{Gag-Pol}$). $Pr55^{Gag}$ is actively involved in the recruitment of these three components into the assembling particle. During virus assembly, interaction between MA and the Env glycoprotein complex embedded in the cellular membrane is thought to be responsible for active incorporation of the Env glycoprotein complex into the virion lipid bilayer. The NC domain of $Pr55^{Gag}$ is required for the encapsidation of the full-length, unspliced viral genomic RNA into virions. The viral enzymes PR, RT, and IN are incorporated into the assembling virus

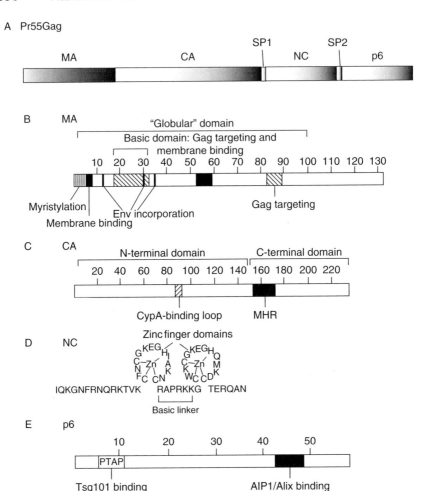

FIGURE 2   Functional map of the Gag precursor protein (Pr55^{Gag}) and mature Gag domains. (Panel A) Linear organization of Pr55^{Gag}, with matrix (MA), capsid (CA), nucleocapsid (NC), and p6 domains and spacer peptides (SP1 and SP2) indicated. (Panels B–E) Schematic representation of each mature protein domain: (B) MA, (C) CA, (D), NC and (E) p6. Functional domains important in HIV-1 assembly, release, and maturation are indicated. Amino acid position is represented numerically. CypA, cyclophilin A; MHR, major homology region. Adapted from Freed (1998) and Freed and Martin (2007), copyright Lippincott Williams and Wilkins, with permission.

particle via molecular interactions between Pr55^{Gag} and the Gag portion of Pr160$^{Gag-Pol}$. During or shortly after virus budding, PR cleaves Pr55Gag and Pr160Gag-Pol into their respective protein domains in a process referred to as maturation. Maturation is essential for virus infectivity and results in a major structural and morphological rearrangement of the immature to the mature particle, which contains the condensed conical core.

In the sections that follow, we will describe in detail the significant progress that has been made in understanding: multimerization of Gag to form the structural framework of the immature virus particle, encapsidation of the viral RNA genome, trafficking virion components to the site of assembly, acquisition of a lipid bilayer and associated Env glycoproteins, virus particle release, and generation of a mature infectious virion. An understanding of HIV-1 particle assembly is crucial for a complete picture of the HIV-1 replication cycle and, as discussed in the last section of this chapter, can be exploited to generate new antiretroviral drugs.

III. Multimerization of Gag to Form the Structural Framework of the Immature Virus Particle

The immature virus particle is a roughly spherical shell composed of ~5000 tightly packed molecules of $Pr55^{Gag}$ (Briggs et al., 2004). As $Pr55^{Gag}$ is the only protein required for VLP assembly (Gheysen et al., 1989), an understanding of how the immature particle assembles requires insight into the molecular interactions necessary for $Pr55^{Gag}$ multimerization, the structure of $Pr55^{Gag}$, and its organization within the assembled particle.

Cryo and high-resolution electron microscopy (EM) have allowed visualization of $Pr55^{Gag}$ within immature VLPs. Individual $Pr55^{Gag}$ molecules are organized in a radial fashion with the N-terminus associated with the membrane and the C-terminus orientated toward the interior of the particle (Fuller et al., 1997; Wilk et al., 2001; Yeager et al., 1998). The $Pr55^{Gag}$ molecules are packed side-by-side in a multimerized lattice which has a hexameric arrangement (Barklis et al., 1998; Briggs et al., 2004; Fuller et al., 1997; Huseby et al., 2005; Nermut et al., 1994, 1998). $Pr55^{Gag}$ appears to be rod-shaped and is composed of four individually folded domains; MA, CA N-terminal and C-terminal domains (NTD and CTD, respectively), and NC, separated by unstructured linker regions (Fuller et al., 1997; Wilk et al., 2001). A high-resolution three-dimensional (3D) structure of $Pr55^{Gag}$ has not been determined due to its large size; however, structures have been solved for the constituent MA (Fig. 3), CA (Fig. 4), SP1, NC (Fig. 5), and p6 domains by X-ray crystallography and nuclear magnetic resonance (NMR) spectroscopy (Berthet-Colominas et al., 1999; Gamble et al., 1996, 1997; Gitti et al., 1996; Hill et al., 1996; Massiah et al., 1994; Momany et al., 1996; Morellet et al., 1992, 2005; Stys et al., 1993; Summers et al., 1992; Worthylake et al., 1999). These structures, in combination with numerous genetic studies, have identified several regions along the length of $Pr55^{Gag}$ that are involved in its multimerization. A number of experimental systems were employed in these studies; mutant forms of $Pr55^{Gag}$ were expressed in cells either as part of infectious HIV-1 clones or as $Pr55^{Gag}$ alone to form VLPs, and a variety of in vitro assembly systems in which individual components can be defined and controlled have also been developed.

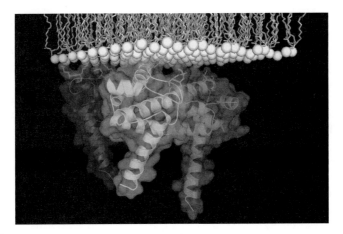

FIGURE 3   Crystal structure of a matrix (MA) trimer (bottom) portrayed interacting with membrane (top). Membrane is represented as a phospholipid bilayer (yellow and gray), basic residues essential for virus replication are clustered on the face of the MA trimer opposing the lipid bilayer (magenta); and the C-terminal helical tail is depicted projecting away from the globular domain. Provided by B. Kelly, C. Hill, and W. I. Sundquist and adapted from Hill *et al.* (1996). (See Color Insert.)

A. Matrix

A region of MA spanning residues 54–68, which corresponds to MA α-helix 4 (Hill *et al.*, 1996; Massiah *et al.*, 1994) has been implicated in assembly (Cannon *et al.*, 1997; Chazal *et al.*, 1995; Freed *et al.*, 1994; Morikawa *et al.*, 1995, 1998; Yu *et al.*, 1992). Amino acid substitutions located on the hydrophobic face of this α-helix abolished particle assembly, a defect that correlated with an inability of MA to form trimers in solution (Morikawa *et al.*, 1998). MA trimer interactions are relatively weak however (Hill *et al.*, 1996; Morikawa *et al.*, 1998), and deletion of MA does not prevent downstream assembly domains in CA, SP1, and NC from driving particle assembly (Accola *et al.*, 2000; Borsetti *et al.*,1998; Lee and Linial, 1994; Reil *et al.*, 1998; Wang *et al.*, 1993, 1998). Thus, although MA may play a structural role in assembly it is not a major determinant in driving Gag multimerization. MA does, however, perform significant functions in Gag trafficking and Env incorporation into virions (see Sections V and VI) (Fig. 2).

B. Capsid and SP1

Major determinants of Gag multimerization are located in the CTD of CA and the adjoining SP1 domain. CA is composed of two independent and largely helical folded domains, the NTD and CTD, which are separated by a short flexible interdomain linker (Berthet-Colominas *et al.*, 1999;

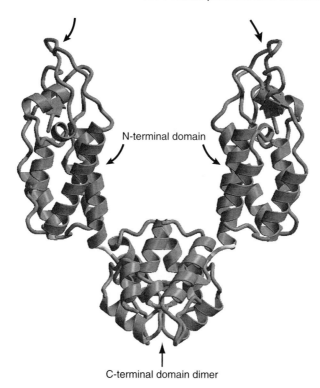

N-terminal domain

C-terminal domain dimer

FIGURE 4 Model of capsid (CA) dimer. The model is a composite from the crystal structures of CA N-terminal domain (NTD, residues 1–145) (top) and C-terminal domain (CTD, residues 148–219) (bottom). Disordered CA residues 146 and 147 link the two structures to generate full-length CA protein in the depicted orientation. The CTD is dimeric. Arrows situated at the top of the NTD indicate the cyclophilin A (CypA)-binding loop. Adapted from Worthylake *et al.* (1999), copyright 1999 IUCr, with permission.

Gamble *et al.*, 1996, 1997; Gitti *et al.*, 1996; Momany *et al.*, 1996; Worthylake *et al.*, 1999) (Figs. 2 and 4). The NTD is not thought to play a significant role in particle assembly, as deletion of the entire domain does not disrupt VLP production (Accola *et al.*, 1998; Borsetti *et al.*, 1998). However, when the NTD is present, point mutations in helices 4–6 impair particle production, suggesting that this region of the NTD forms weak interactions during assembly (von Schwedler *et al.*, 2003a) or that mutations in the NTD can disrupt global CA folding. It has been proposed that NTD–CTD contacts are essential for assembly, as the NTD and CTD must be derived from the same retroviral CA protein for proper assembly to occur (Ako-Adjei *et al.*, 2005).

The CA CTD plays a major role in Pr55^{Gag} multimerization, in particular via its capacity to form dimers (Fig. 4). CTD dimers have been demonstrated both in solution (Gamble *et al.*, 1997; Rose *et al.*, 1992) and within

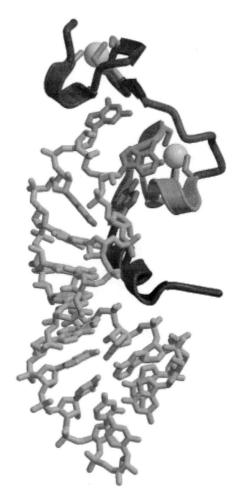

FIGURE 5 Structure showing nucleocapsid (NC) complexed with stem loop 3 (SL3) of the HIV-1 RNA–packaging signal. Zinc ions that bind to the zinc finger motifs are depicted as gray balls. Adapted from Turner and Summers (1999), copyright 1999 Elsevier, with permission.

crystals (Gamble *et al.*, 1997; Worthylake *et al.*, 1999). Dimerization occurs through the parallel packing of CA helix 9 against its symmetry-related mate. Disruption of the dimer interface caused by mutations in residues 184 and 185, which are buried in the core of the interface on helix 9 (Gamble *et al.*, 1997), leads to a significant reduction in particle production (Gamble *et al.*, 1997; von Schwedler *et al.*, 2003a) and reduced intermolecular Pr55^{Gag} interactions *in vitro* (Burniston *et al.*, 1999). As particle assembly is not completely abolished by residue 184/185 mutations (Joshi *et al.*, 2006; Ono *et al.*, 2005; von Schwedler *et al.*, 2003a), the CTD dimer interface is not absolutely required for assembly. The CTD also contains the major homology region (MHR) (Fig. 2), a highly conserved stretch of 20 amino acids found in all retroviral CA proteins (Wills and Craven, 1991). Genetic studies have shown that point mutations in the MHR can lead to defects in assembly, and other aspects of the viral life cycle can also be affected (Mammano *et al.*, 1994; von Schwedler *et al.*, 2003a). The structural contribution of the MHR to the Pr55^{Gag} lattice has not been clearly defined; in the crystal structure it is distinct from the dimer interface and forms an intricate array of hydrogen bonds (Gamble *et al.*, 1997). A new hypothesis for MHR function has recently been proposed based on the high degree of structural homology between the CTD and a mammalian SCAN domain, which forms a domain-swapped dimer (Ivanov *et al.*, 2005; Kingston and Vogt, 2005).

Residues that project from the base of the CTD are thought to be important for creating a tightly closed particle lattice. Mutation of these residues severely impairs particle production but does not completely prevent Pr55^{Gag} multimerization (von Schwedler *et al.*, 2003a). Extending from the base of the CTD is the C-terminal tail of CA composed of the last ~12 residues of CA. This region of CA, along with the adjoining 14-amino acid SP1, is unstructured and highly flexible in Pr55^{Gag} (Gamble *et al.*, 1997; Newman *et al.*, 2004; Worthylake *et al.*, 1999) but may adopt an α-helical conformation which spans the CA/SP1 junction (Accola *et al.*, 1998; Morellet *et al.*, 2005; Newman *et al.*, 2004). The CA/SP1 junction forms a critical assembly domain, as mutations in both the C-terminal residues of CA (Abdurahman *et al.*, 2004; Liang *et al.*, 2002, 2003; Melamed *et al.*, 2004; von Schwedler *et al.*, 2003a) and the N-terminal amino acids of SP1 (Accola *et al.*, 1998, 2000; Krausslich *et al.*, 1995; Liang *et al.*, 2002; Morikawa *et al.*, 2000) disrupt particle production. The CA/SP1 junction has been shown to mediate strong Gag–Gag interactions, leading to higher-order multimerization critical for particle assembly (Guo *et al.*, 2005; Liang *et al.*, 2002, 2003; Morikawa *et al.*, 2000; Ono *et al.*, 2000). The physical properties of this region, particularly the Gly-rich hinge motif in the CA C-terminal tail situated directly before the putative α-helix, have been proposed to confer structural flexibility to the Pr55^{Gag} molecule allowing multiple Gag conformations, which in turn permit the formation of higher-order multimers (Liang *et al.*, 2003).

During assembly, HIV-1 CA binds the cellular protein cyclophilin A (CypA) (Fig. 2) and relatively high levels of this cellular factor are incorporated into released virions (Franke *et al.*, 1994; Luban *et al.*, 1993; Thali *et al.*, 1994). CA interacts with CypA via a well-characterized interaction that involves a Pro-rich loop in the CA NTD (Gamble *et al.*, 1996) (Fig. 4). While the functional significance of CA/CypA binding is still under investigation, it appears that the association of CA with CypA following entry into the target cell may provide some protection from the host restriction factor TRIM5α (Hatziioannou *et al.*, 2005; Nisole *et al.*, 2004; Sayah *et al.*, 2004; Sokolskaja *et al.*, 2004).

C. Nucleocapsid

The interaction (I) domain of Pr55^{Gag}, which is located in NC, plays a major role in Gag multimerization and assembly. The primary structural features of NC are two zinc finger–like motifs flanked by highly basic sequences (Morellet et al., 1992; Summers et al., 1992) (Figs. 2 and 5). The zinc fingers contribute to the specificity of viral genomic RNA encapsidation (see Section IV) but are not required for assembly; instead, it is the basic residues that are primarily responsible for I domain function. The minimal residues required for I domain function have been mapped to a few basic residues at the N-terminus of NC (Sandefur et al., 1998, 2000); however, it is generally thought that multiple basic residues throughout NC contribute to efficient I domain activity (Cimarelli and Luban, 2000; Cimarelli et al., 2000; Dawson and Yu, 1998; Sandefur et al., 2000).

The prevailing view of I domain function is that it promotes Pr55^{Gag} multimerization by binding RNA, which in turn acts as a structural scaffold bringing Gag molecules into a concentrated environment where they can align and interact (Campbell and Rein, 1999; Campbell and Vogt, 1995; Cimarelli et al., 2000; Muriaux et al., 2001). In the context of a bona fide viral infection, NC displays a strong preference for full-length genomic RNA (see Section IV). However, if this RNA species is not available, nonspecific RNA or DNA species of varying lengths can serve to promote assembly (Campbell and Rein, 1999; Campbell and Vogt, 1995; Cimarelli et al., 2000; Muriaux et al., 2001).

IV. Encapsidation of the Viral RNA Genome

During the assembly process two copies of full-length dimeric viral genomic RNA are packaged into the immature virus particle, an event that is not required for assembly but is essential for virion infectivity. The genomic RNA is specifically selected for packaging from the cytosolic environment that contains an excess pool of cellular and spliced viral mRNAs. Packaging is principally mediated by interactions between the NC domain of Pr55^{Gag} and a 5′ segment of the viral genome variously termed the packaging signal, encapsidation element (E), or Ψ site (D'Souza and Summers, 2005; Jewell and Mansky, 2000; Rein, 1994) (Fig. 6).

A. The Role of Nucleocapsid

The NC domain of Pr55^{Gag} regulates both the efficiency and specificity of genomic RNA packaging. The key determinants within NC involved in specific genome packaging are two zinc finger (sometimes referred to as zinc-knuckle) motifs (Aldovini and Young, 1990; Dorfman *et al.*, 1993; Gorelick *et al.*, 1990, 1993; Schwartz *et al.*, 1997; Zhang and Barklis, 1995) (Figs. 2 and 5). The zinc finger motifs are of the CCHC type (Cys-X_2-Cys-X_4-His-X_4-Cys) (Berg, 1986; Covey, 1986) and bind zinc tightly both *in vitro* and *in vivo* (Bess *et al.*, 1992; Morellet *et al.*, 1992; South *et al.*, 1990; Summers *et al.*, 1992). Binding of zinc to NC promotes folding of two independent globular knuckle structures that are brought into proximity by a flexible linker (Morellet *et al.*, 1992, 1994; South *et al.*, 1990; Summers *et al.*, 1992). NMR data indicate that the resulting globular structure interacts directly with viral RNA (Amarasinghe *et al.*, 2000a; De Guzman *et al.*, 1998). Abolition of zinc binding through mutagenesis of zinc-binding residues prevents genome encapsidation and hence infectivity (Aldovini and Young, 1990; Gorelick *et al.*, 1990). The two zinc fingers are not functionally equivalent, as the first zinc finger plays a more prominent role in encapsidation (Gorelick *et al.*, 1993; Schwartz *et al.*, 1997). Although the zinc fingers are necessary for encapsidation, they are not sufficient (Zhang and Barklis, 1995); the basic residues flanking the zinc fingers have also been implicated in nucleic acid binding (Cimarelli *et al.*, 2000; Dannull *et al.*, 1994; De Guzman *et al.*, 1998; Poon *et al.*, 1996; Schmalzbauer *et al.*, 1996) along with the SP1 region of Pr55^{Gag} (Kaye and Lever, 1998).

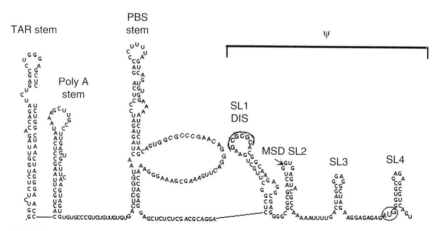

FIGURE 6 Secondary structure of the HIV-1 mRNA 5′ region, which includes the viral RNA–packaging (Ψ) signal. Structural elements involved in RNA encapsidation are depicted from 5′ to 3′: *trans*-acting responsive (TAR) element, poly A hairpin, primer-binding site (PBS), and the Ψ site composed of stem loops 1–4 (SL1–SL4). SL1 contains the dimer initiation site (DIS) and SL2 contains the major splice donor site (MSD). The Gag AUG initiation codon is circled. Reprinted from Freed and Martin (2007), copyright Lippincott Williams and Wilkins, with permission.

B. The Role of the Viral RNA–Packaging Signal (Ψ Site)

The segment of the RNA genome involved in packaging spans hundreds of nucleotides and includes the entire 5′ untranslated region (5′ UTR) and the 5′ half of the *gag* gene (D'Souza and Summers, 2005; Jewell and Mansky, 2000; McBride *et al.*, 1997) (Fig. 6). Within this overall packaging signal is a stretch of ~120 nucleotides (termed the Ψ site), which is involved in mediating packaging via a stable secondary structure consisting of four closely spaced hairpin loops: stem loops 1–4 (SL1, SL2, SL3, and SL4) (Baudin *et al.*, 1993; Clever *et al.*, 1995; Harrison and Lever, 1992; Hayashi *et al.*, 1993; Sakaguchi *et al.*, 1993). Genetic studies suggest that all four stem loop structures play an independent role in RNA packaging (Clever and Parslow, 1997; Harrison *et al.*, 1998; Hayashi *et al.*, 1992; McBride and Panganiban, 1996, 1997). SL2 and SL3 are thought to be the primary determinants driving the interaction with the NC zinc fingers, as they bind NC with high affinity (Amarasinghe *et al.*, 2000a; De Guzman *et al.*, 1998) (Fig. 5). In addition to its role in NC binding, SL2 contains the major splice donor, providing a potential selection mechanism for specific encapsidation of full-length genomic viral RNA, as spliced RNAs lack part of the packaging signal (Amarasinghe *et al.*, 2000b; D'Souza and Summers, 2005; Jewell and Mansky, 2000; Rein, 1994). SL1 and SL4 do not bind NC with high affinity but still function in genome packaging (Amarasinghe *et al.*, 2001; Lawrence *et al.*, 2003). SL1 contains the primary dimer initiation site (DIS) that promotes genomic RNA dimerization, a process that may be linked to packaging (Russell *et al.*, 2004). SL4 has been proposed to contribute to RNA–RNA interactions that stabilize the tertiary structure of the Ψ site (Amarasinghe *et al.*, 2001). A model has been suggested in which the tertiary structure resulting from SL1 dimer formation and SL4 stabilization exposes SL3 and SL4 for high-affinity NC binding (Amarasinghe *et al.*, 2001). Despite the importance of SL1–SL4 in RNA encapsidation, the overall packaging signal maps to a much larger segment of RNA located at the 5′-end of the molecule, which includes three other structural elements, the *trans*-acting responsive (TAR) element, polyA hairpin, and primer-binding site (PBS) (D'Souza and Summers, 2005) (Fig. 6).

V. Trafficking Virion Components to the Site of Assembly _____

Assembly of an HIV-1 particle requires that all virion components converge at the site of assembly. HIV-1 assembly has been shown to occur at two distinct subcellular locations (Fig. 7). In most cell types, including primary CD4$^+$ T lymphocytes and T-cell lines, the primary site of assembly is the plasma membrane (Swanstrom and Wills, 1997). However, in certain other cell types, including monocyte-derived macrophages, assembly and

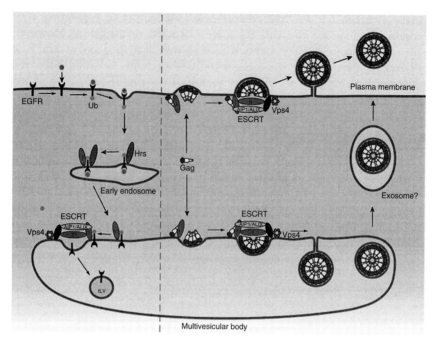

FIGURE 7   Schematic representation of cellular endocytosis and mulitvesicular body (MVB)-sorting pathways (left) and HIV-1 release (right). (Left) An activated growth factor receptor (EGFR) is monoubiquitylated. The ubiquitylated cargo is recognized and sequestered by a complex containing hepatocyte growth factor–regulated tyrosine kinase substrate (Hrs) at the early endosomal membrane. Hrs interacts with Tsg101 to recruit endosomal sorting complex required for transport (ESCRT)-I. ESCRT-I sequentially recruits ESCRT-II and ESCRT-III. AIP1/ALIX is recruited to the assembled complexes and bridges ESCRT-I and ESCRT-III. Following inward budding of intralumenal vesicles (ILV) into the endosomal lumen, vacuolar sorting protein 4 (Vps4) catalyzes ATP-dependent disassembly of the budding machinery. Right: HIV-1 commandeers the cellular budding machinery to facilitate virus release. Virus particles are depicted assembling and budding at the plasma membrane (e.g., in T cells) or assembling at the MVB followed by release through the exosome pathway (e.g., in macrophages). Gag directly binds Tsg101, thereby recruiting ESCRT-I and associated factors to the site of assembly. Adapted from Demirov and Freed (2004), copyright Elsevier, with permission.

budding take place primarily at the membrane of an intracellular compartment and not at the plasma membrane (Gendelman *et al.*, 1988; Orenstein *et al.*, 1988). This compartment has recently been identified as the late endosome/MVB (Nguyen *et al.*, 2003; Ono and Freed, 2004; Pelchen-Matthews *et al.*, 2003; Raposo *et al.*, 2002) (see Section VII).

As assembly can occur at two different locations, the virus must have evolved cell type-dependent strategies for trafficking virion components from the site of synthesis to the site of assembly. Trafficking itineraries of virion components, and the role of host cell factors in regulating viral protein targeting, are currently the subject of active investigation. However, some viral targeting determinants have been well described and several host cell factors identified. Progress is currently being made by using improved microscopy techniques, which allow visualization of trafficking in real time in living cells.

A. Trafficking of Gag

Pr55^{Gag} is synthesized on free cytosolic ribosomes (Swanstrom and Wills, 1997). In cells in which assembly occurs at the plasma membrane, the traditional view of Gag trafficking is that the newly synthesized protein is transported rapidly and directly through the cytoplasm to the plasma membrane. This view has recently been challenged by the proposal that Pr55^{Gag} is first transported to the late endosome/MVB, or to other component(s) of the endocytic pathway, and then carried to the plasma membrane (Dong et al., 2005; Perlman and Resh, 2006; Resh, 2005; Sherer et al., 2003). The pathway taken by Pr55^{Gag} in cells in which assembly occurs at the late endosome/MVB is currently not understood.

Viral determinants that direct Pr55^{Gag} to the plasma membrane are located in the MA domain (Fig. 2). A multipartite plasma membrane-binding signal (M) is located at the N-terminus of MA (also see Section VI). Part of the signal is provided by a myristic acid moiety covalently attached to the N-terminal Gly of MA. Prevention of myristylation by mutating this Gly residue blocks membrane binding and abolishes virus assembly (Bryant and Ratner, 1990; Freed et al., 1994; Gottlinger et al., 1989). A highly basic region between MA residues 17 and 30 provides the second part of the membrane-binding signal (Yuan et al., 1993; Zhou et al., 1994). Mutation of these basic residues causes virus assembly to be redirected from the plasma membrane to intracellular membranes (Ono et al., 2000; Yuan et al., 1993). Similarly, single amino substitutions between MA residues 84 and 88 redirect virus assembly to the same intracellular site (Freed et al., 1994; Ono et al., 2000). The intracellular membrane to which Pr55^{Gag} is retargeted has been identified as the late endosome/MVB, recapitulating the targeting phenotype observed for wild-type Pr55^{Gag} in macrophages (Ono and Freed, 2004). It is noteworthy that although the p6 domain contains sequences that interact directly with components of the MVB machinery (see Section VII), deletion of p6 does not alter the site of Gag targeting (Ono and Freed, 2004; Rudner et al., 2005).

The trafficking of Pr55^{Gag} to different destinations in different cell types implies that host-cell factors regulate the site of assembly. Although these cellular determinants remain to be fully defined, several studies have begun to identify host factors that regulate Gag localization. One such factor is the phosphoinositide phosphatidylinositol (4,5) bisphosphate [PI(4,5)P$_2$], a lipid that regulates plasma membrane localization of several cellular proteins (McLaughlin and Murray, 2005). Alteration of normal PI(4,5)P$_2$ levels retargets HIV-1 assembly from the plasma membrane to the late endosome/MVB and a direct interaction between PI(4,5)P$_2$ and the MA domain of Pr55^{Gag} has been demonstrated (Freed, 2006; Ono *et al.*, 2004; Saad *et al.*, 2006; Shkriabai *et al.*, 2006) (see Section VI). The δ subunit of the clathrin adaptor protein complex AP-3 has also been reported to interact directly with the MA domain of Pr55^{Gag} (Dong *et al.*, 2005). The AP-3 adaptor complex directs intracellular protein trafficking to the MVB (Dell'Angelica *et al.*, 1999; Rous *et al.*, 2002). Disruption of the interaction between AP-3 and MA blocks localization of Pr55^{Gag} to MVBs in HeLa cells, leading to a more diffuse, cytosolic Gag distribution. These results imply a role for AP-3 in Gag targeting to the MVB (Dong *et al.*, 2005).

B. Trafficking of Env Glycoproteins

The Env glycoprotein precursor (gp160) is synthesized by ribosomes associated with the rough ER and is an integral membrane protein anchored to the membrane by a hydrophobic stop-transfer signal in the gp41 domain. Gp160 is transported through the cellular secretory pathway to the plasma membrane. During this process, it undergoes extensive glycosylation, oligomerization into trimers, and proteolytic maturation mediated by a cellular furin-type protease that cleaves it into the mature gp120 and gp41 Env subunits (Freed and Martin, 1995a; Swanstrom and Wills, 1997) (Fig. 1).

The gp120/gp41 complex is rapidly internalized after its transport to the plasma membrane. This rapid internalization is at least partially mediated by a Tyr-X-X-Leu motif in the gp41 cytoplasmic tail (LaBranche *et al.*, 1995; Rowell *et al.*, 1995). Tyr-based motifs are known to regulate endocytosis of cellular plasma membrane proteins by binding the $\mu2$ chain of clathrin-associated AP complexes, and such interactions have been observed with gp41 cytoplasmic domains (Boge *et al.*, 1998; Ohno *et al.*, 1997). Following internalization, the gp120/gp41 complex is transported to an endosomal/lysosomal compartment (Ohno *et al.*, 1997; Rowell *et al.*, 1995). The cytoplasmic domain of gp41 has also been shown to interact with the cellular protein TIP47 (tail-interacting protein of 47 kD). This interaction mediates retrograde transport of Env from endosomes to the *trans*-Golgi network (Blot *et al.*, 2003) and may also be involved in Env incorporation into virions (see Section VI). Therefore, like Pr55^{Gag}, the Env glycoproteins can traffic to either the plasma membrane or internal membranes associated with endosomal/lysosomal compartments; hence, they can be localized to both known sites of HIV-1 assembly.

VI. Acquisition of a Lipid Bilayer and Associated Env Glycoproteins

The cellular membrane acts as a platform for higher-order Gag multimerization, which drives particle assembly and release. Binding of Pr55^{Gag} to the membrane is therefore an essential step in the assembly pathway. Gag multimerization at the membrane forces the membrane to curve outward, forming a roughly spherical particle that eventually pinches off from the membrane. The released particle consists of the Pr55^{Gag} structural shell surrounded by a cell-derived lipid bilayer. Virus-encoded Env glycoprotein spikes that project through the virion lipid bilayer are essential for virion infectivity. Pr55^{Gag} mediates the incorporation of Env into the assembling virus by interactions between the MA domain of Gag and the cytoplasmic tail of gp41.

A. Gag Membrane Binding

Binding of Pr55^{Gag} to the plasma membrane is mediated by the bipartite membrane-binding signal (M), composed of an N-terminal myristate and a highly basic domain located in MA (see Section V) (Fig. 2). Structural studies have shown that the basic residues cluster on a face of an MA trimer that is predicted to be orientated upward toward the membrane, creating a putative membrane-binding surface and positioning the basic residues to make electrostatic interactions with negatively charged phospholipid head groups on the inner leaflet of the plasma membrane (Hill *et al.*, 1996) (Fig. 3). Recently, an NMR study has shown that MA binds to one such negatively charged phospholipid, PI(4,5)P$_2$, which is normally located on the inner leaflet of the plasma membrane (Behnia and Munro, 2005; Freed, 2006; Saad *et al.*, 2006) (see Section V). The inositol head group and 2′ fatty acid chain of the lipid molecule fit into a hydrophobic cleft in MA and the negatively charged phosphates form salt bridges with basic residues in MA, anchoring MA to the membrane.

The MA myristyl group can adopt a conformation in which it is either exposed or sequestered within the MA protein (Tang *et al.*, 2004). Transition between these alternative myristate conformations is known as a myristyl switch (Ames *et al.*, 1996, 1997). The myristyl switch is thought to regulate MA membrane binding at different stages of the viral life cycle. During virus assembly, MA in the context of Pr55^{Gag} is required to bind membrane to undergo higher-order Gag multimerization. However, mature MA (p17) (see Section VIII) may dissociate from the membrane early post-entry in the next round of infection. Therefore, the myristate must be exposed in Pr55^{Gag} to promote hydrophobic interactions with the membrane and sequestered in a preexisting cavity in mature MA to allow membrane dissociation on virus entry into a new cell (Hermida-Matsumoto and Resh, 1999;

Resh, 2004; Spearman *et al.*, 1997; Tang *et al.*, 2004; Zhou and Resh, 1996). Regulation of the myristyl switch was originally proposed to be a consequence of altered MA conformation triggered by proteolytic processing (Hermida-Matsumoto and Resh, 1999); however, recent structural studies have shown that MA does not undergo significant conformational changes following Gag proteolysis. Instead, the myristyl switch appears to be regulated by the multimeric state of the protein, as myristate is sequestered in monomeric MA and exposed in trimeric MA (Tang *et al.*, 2004; Wu *et al.*, 2004). Binding of MA to $PI(4,5)P_2$ is also reported to trigger myristate exposure, thereby facilitating membrane binding (Saad *et al.*, 2006).

As mentioned above, the proposal that the myristyl switch is regulated by $Pr55^{Gag}$ multimerization suggests that membrane binding and Gag multimerization are linked. Although EM images of assembly intermediates at the plasma membrane clearly demonstrate that higher-order Gag multimerization occurs in association with membrane (Swanstrom and Wills, 1997), where and when lower-order Gag multimerization occurs is not clearly understood. $Pr55^{Gag}$ multimerization is, however, required to stabilize membrane binding, as mutagenesis of the CA CTD and SP1 regions of $Pr55^{Gag}$, which are major determinants of Gag–Gag interactions (see Section III), disrupt both membrane binding and virus assembly (Joshi *et al.*, 2006; Liang *et al.*, 2003; Ono *et al.*, 2005). Once bound to the membrane, $Pr55^{Gag}$ is localized to discrete microdomains in the plasma membrane known as lipid rafts (Nguyen and Hildreth, 2000; Ono and Freed, 2001), which are by definition enriched in cholesterol and sphingolipids with saturated acyl chains (Simons and Toomre, 2000; Simons and Vaz, 2004). These microdomains provide a microenvironment that selectively concentrates some proteins while actively excluding others and hence have been proposed to act as concentration platforms for Gag multimerization (Ono *et al.*, 2005, 2007). Although it is not currently known whether $Pr55^{Gag}$ multimerization is a prerequisite for membrane binding, or whether membrane binding is required for Gag multimerization, it seems probable that each reaction promotes the other, thereby catalyzing the assembly process.

B. Incorporation of the Viral Env Gycoproteins

An interaction between the MA domain of $Pr55^{Gag}$ and the long cytoplasmic tail of gp41 is thought to actively promote the incorporation of HIV-1 Env glycoproteins into the assembling virion (Dorfman *et al.*, 1994b; Dubay *et al.*, 1992; Freed and Martin, 1995b, 1996; Lodge *et al.*, 1994; Mammano *et al.*, 1995; Murakami and Freed, 2000a; Owens *et al.*, 1991; Yu *et al.*, 1992) (Fig. 2). This interaction has been shown to be essential for HIV-1 Env incorporation in physiologically relevant cell types, such as T cells and primary monocyte-derived macrophages, as gp41 truncations severely disrupt Env incorporation (Murakami and Freed, 2000b).

However, in some cell types (e.g., HeLa and MT-4), gp41 truncations have little effect on Env incorporation suggesting that the incorporation of Env, like that of cellular membrane-associated proteins, can occur in a relatively nonspecific manner. The observation that the role of the gp41 cytoplasmic domain in Env incorporation is cell type-dependent suggests that host factors play a role in the incorporation process (Murakami and Freed, 2000b). One such host factor, TIP47, has recently been identified. TIP47 binds both the cytoplasmic tail of gp41 and residues 5–16 of MA, potentially serving as a bridge to link Gag and Env during virus assembly (Lopez-Verges *et al.*, 2006). At present it is unknown when and where Gag and gp41 interact. As the Env glycoprotein complex is membrane-bound, the interaction undoubtedly occurs at a membrane; however, at which membrane and at what stage of Gag multimerization remain unclear. It is noteworthy that the Gag–gp41 interaction has been correlated with efficient association of Env glycoproteins with lipid rafts (Bhattacharya *et al.*, 2006).

In addition to the viral Env glycoproteins, the viral lipid bilayer also contains substantial amounts of cellular surface proteins (Cantin *et al.*, 2005; Ott, 1997, 2002; Tremblay *et al.*, 1998). The incorporation of these proteins is likely to be passive and determined by their level of abundance in the region of the membrane from which virus budding occurs. In cells in which assembly occurs at the plasma membrane, incorporated cellular lipids and proteins are largely representative of lipid rafts (Brugger *et al.*, 2006; Nguyen and Hildreth, 2000; Ono and Freed, 2005). Conversely, virions produced from macrophages have been shown to contain high levels of late endosome/MVB-associated proteins (Chertova *et al.*, 2006; Nguyen *et al.*, 2003; Pelchen-Matthews *et al.*, 2003). The significance of these host plasma membrane or MVB-associated proteins to HIV biology is not fully understood.

VII. Virus Particle Release

The assembling virion must be released from the producer cell to enable infection of a new cell. A membrane fission event in which the membrane neck of the budding virion is pinched off implements release of the assembled virus particle. To facilitate this process, HIV-1, along with other enveloped RNA viruses, commandeers host cell machinery that is normally used to create vesicles that bud into the late-endosomal MVBs (Fig. 7). The topology of vesicle budding into the late endosome/MVB is functionally analogous to retrovirus budding from the plasma membrane or into the MVB. The two processes mirror each other by facilitating budding through a membrane away from the cytosol. Therefore, enveloped viruses have evolved the ability to hijack this cellular budding machinery to enable their own release (Demirov and Freed, 2004; Freed, 2002; Morita and

Sundquist, 2004; Pornillos *et al.*, 2002). Viruses assembled at the plasma membrane are released directly into the extracellular space. In contrast, virions released into MVBs have recently been hypothesized to reach the extracellular space by fusion of the MVB with the plasma membrane via the cellular exosome pathway (Gould *et al.*, 2003; Nguyen *et al.*, 2003; Pelchen-Matthews *et al.*, 2003, 2004; Raposo *et al.*, 2002).

A. Late Domains

As Pr55^{Gag} is the only virion component required for particle assembly and release, any cellular factors that promote virus budding must be recruited by Pr55^{Gag}. The region of Gag responsible for mediating HIV-1 release has been mapped to a highly conserved Pro-Thr/Ser-Ala-Pro (PT/SAP) motif situated near the N-terminus of the p6 domain (Gottlinger *et al.*, 1991; Huang *et al.*, 1995) (Fig. 2). In many cell types, particles assembled from PT/SAP mutants display a release defect characterized by an accumulation of virions attached to the plasma membrane by a thin tether or stalk (Demirov *et al.*, 2002a; Gottlinger *et al.*, 1991) (Fig. 8). In macrophages, budding into the MVB lumen is arrested, again with particles attached by a thin tether (Demirov *et al.*, 2002a). In T cells, however, the mutant phenotype is manifested by the release of chains of tethered immature virions. Other retroviruses encode short peptide sequences functionally analogous to the PT/SAP motif of HIV-1 p6. To reflect the role of these motifs in the final stages of viral egress, they have been termed "late" or "L" domains.

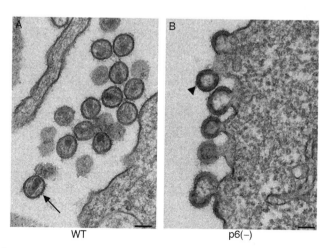

FIGURE 8 Morphology of (A) wild-type and (B) p6-deleted HIV-1. (A) Particles have a mature morphology (arrow) and are released from the cell. (B) Particles are tethered to the cell and have an immature-like morphology (arrow head). Images are visualized by transmission electron microscopy, bar = 100 nm. Micrographs kindly provided by Kunio Nagashima. Reprinted from Freed and Martin (2007), copyright Lippincott Williams and Wilkins, with permission.

Three general classes of late domains have been defined, PT/SAP, PPXY, and $YP(X)_nL$, all of which have been identified in retroviruses (Demirov and Freed, 2004; Freed, 2002; Morita and Sundquist, 2004; Pornillos *et al.*, 2002). Functional late domains have also been identified in a number of other enveloped RNA virus families including the filo, rhabdo, arena, orthomyxo, and paramyxo viruses, suggesting that a wide range of viruses bud via similar mechanisms (Freed, 2002; Morita and Sundquist, 2004; Pornillos *et al.*, 2002). It is noteworthy that many of these viruses contain two different late domain motifs; for example, HIV-1 contains a $YP(X)_nL$ motif near the p6 C-terminus in addition to the well-characterized N-terminal PT/SAP motif (Strack *et al.*, 2003). Similarly, human T-cell leukemia virus (HTLV-I) encodes a bipartite PPPYVEPTAP motif (Bouamr *et al.*, 2003). Although some studies have investigated the role of dual late domains (Bouamr *et al.*, 2003; Gottwein *et al.*, 2003; Heidecker *et al.*, 2004; Licata *et al.*, 2003; Wang *et al.*, 2004), the biological purpose of multiple late domain is not clearly defined. However, as dual late domains have evolved frequently, it is likely that they are functionally significant and it can be hypothesized that they are utilized in cellular environments in which the cellular partner for one of the late domains is unavailable (see below).

B. Host Cell Factors

Late domains exhibit several characteristics of docking sites for host cell factors. These features include the fact that they are small, highly conserved, and can remain functional when moved to different locations in Gag or swapped between viruses that normally use different late domains (Li *et al.*, 2002; Parent *et al.*, 1995; Yuan *et al.*, 2000). Several host proteins have now been identified which mediate virus release; common to all these proteins is a link to the cellular ubiquitylation and endosomal MVB protein–sorting pathway (Demirov and Freed, 2004; Freed, 2002; Morita and Sundquist, 2004; Pornillos *et al.*, 2002). Knowledge of this pathway has been obtained from extensive studies in both yeast and mammalian cells (reviewed by Hurley and Emr, 2006; Katzmann *et al.*, 2002). Briefly, monoubiquitylation serves as a signal to recruit membrane proteins into the pathway; once recruited they are ultimately packaged into vesicles that bud into the lumen of the late endosome/ MVB. Three multiprotein complexes, ESCRT-I, -II, and -III, sequentially recognize the recruited protein and finally Vps4 (vacuolar protein sorting 4) catalyzes their ATP-dependent disassembly (Fig. 7). Overall, the ESCRT complexes and associated proteins function in both cargo sorting and vesicle formation and play a role in many key cellular processes ranging from protein degradation to stimulation of the immune response.

Tsg101, the mammalian homolog of yeast Vps23 and a member of ESCRT-I, has been shown to interact with the HIV-1 p6 PT/SAP motif via its N-terminal UEV domain (Garrus *et al.*, 2001; Pornillos *et al.*, 2002b; VerPlank *et al.*, 2001). Several lines of evidence indicate that this interaction is the primary mechanism by which HIV-1 particle release is mediated: depletion of Tsg101 arrests particle budding at a late stage (Garrus *et al.*, 2001), overexpression of an N-terminal fragment of Tsg101 (TSG-5′) blocks HIV-1 budding (Demirov *et al.*, 2002b), and fusion of Tsg101 to the C-terminus of Gag corrects a late-domain defect (Martin-Serrano *et al.*, 2001). Tsg101 recruitment is thought to provide a link to the rest of the ESCRT protein network, redirecting this cellular machinery to the site of viral budding to facilitate release.

Tsg101-mediated virus release is PT/SAP dependent, as viruses with PPXY and $YP(X)_nL$ motifs are not affected by disruption of Tsg101 (Demirov *et al.*, 2002b; Garrus *et al.*, 2001; Martin-Serrano *et al.*, 2003a; Shehu-Xhilaga *et al.*, 2004). Instead, the PPXY and $YP(X)_nL$ motifs interact with different cellular proteins also connected to the ubiquitylation machinery and endosomal MVB protein–sorting pathway. The $YP(X)_nL$ motif of HIV-1 and equine infectious anemia virus (EIAV) binds the endosomal sorting factor ALIX (or AIP-1) (Martin-Serrano *et al.*, 2003a; Munshi *et al.*, 2007; Strack *et al.*, 2003; von Schwedler *et al.*, 2003b) (Fig. 2). ALIX is not an ESCRT component per se but provides a link between the ESCRT-I and ESCRT-III complexes (Martin-Serrano *et al.*, 2003a; Strack *et al.*, 2003; von Schwedler *et al.*, 2003b) (Fig. 7). Disruption of the EIAV $YP(X)_nL$ motif or ALIX depletion potently inhibits EIAV release (Martin-Serrano *et al.*, 2003a; Puffer *et al.*, 1997; Strack *et al.*, 2003). In the context of HIV-1, however, the PT/SAP motif is the dominant late domain and only in some situations does disruption of the $YP(X)_nL$–ALIX interaction significantly inhibit virus release (Demirov *et al.*, 2002b; Gottlinger *et al.*, 1991; Martin-Serrano *et al.*, 2003a; Munshi *et al.*, 2007; Strack *et al.*, 2002, 2003). The PPXY motifs bind members of the Nedd4 family of E3 ubiquitin ligases; however, the mechanism by which this interaction promotes virus release remains to be defined (Demirov and Freed, 2004; Morita and Sundquist, 2004).

Interaction of different late domains with distinct cellular factors appears to provide viruses with multiple entry points into the endosomal/MVB sorting pathway. Vps4 functions at the final step of this pathway and its disruption universally blocks retrovirus release regardless of the viral late domain utilized, indicating that an intact pathway is required for the release of most if not all retroviruses (Garrus *et al.*, 2001; Martin-Serrano *et al.*, 2003b; Morita and Sundquist, 2004; Shehu-Xhilaga *et al.*, 2004; Tanzi *et al.*, 2003; von Schwedler *et al.*, 2003b). The connection between Gag ubiquitylation and the mechanism of virus release remains to be clearly defined and is the subject of ongoing investigation (Demirov and Freed, 2004; Freed, 2002; Morita and Sundquist, 2004; Pornillos *et al.*, 2002; Vogt, 2000).

VIII. Generating a Mature Infectious Virion _____

During or shortly after virus budding, Pr55^{Gag} and Pr160$^{Gag-Pol}$ are cleaved into their respective individual protein domains by the viral-encoded PR in a process referred to as maturation. As the immature virion matures, MA remains associated with the viral membrane, NC condenses with the dimeric RNA genome, and CA reassembles to form a closed conical capsid shell that surrounds the NC–RNA complex (Figs. 1 and 8). This structural rearrangement results in a mature infectious virion that is capable of disassembly on entry into a new cell, a process essential for virion replication (Swanstrom and Wills, 1997; Vogt, 1996).

A. The Gag Proteolytic Processing Cascade

Retroviral proteases, including HIV-1 PR, are related to the cellular aspartyl protease family as they feature an active site which consists of two apposed catalytic aspartic acid residues, each within a conserved Asp-Thr/Ser-Gly motif, which coordinate a water molecule that is used to hydrolyze a peptide (or scissile) bond in the target protein. Retroviral PRs contain only one Asp-Thr/Ser-Gly motif, and therefore the active enzymes form a dimer with the Asp-containing active site situated near the center and the substrate-binding site located within a long cleft formed between the two monomers (Lapatto et al., 1989; Navia et al., 1989; Wlodawer et al., 1989). PR interacts with a substrate recognition site of at least seven residues termed P4-P3' with the scissile bond lying between the P1 and P1' amino acids. A strict consensus sequence for this target site does not appear to exist; instead, loose amino acid requirements coupled with the degree of cleavage site exposure or accessibility appear to govern the efficiency with which each site in Gag is cleaved. The wide range of cleavage efficiencies results in an ordered stepwise cascade of processing events (Swanstrom and Wills, 1997).

An active PR is generated by dimerization of the PR domain. Enzyme dimerization and activation appear to be functionally linked and must be tightly regulated as premature or excessive PR activity abolishes particle assembly (Adamson et al., 2003; Gheysen et al., 1989; Karacostas et al., 1993; Kräusslich, 1991). It has been suggested that concentration of Gag-Pol molecules inside the assembling particle is the mechanism by which PR is activated (Kräusslich, 1991). However, the factors that control PR activation are not well understood. As PR is expressed as part of the Gag-Pol precursor, initial dimerization occurs while in the context of the polyprotein and that initial cleavages performed by this immature PR are intramolecular (Pettit et al., 2004). PR subsequently liberates itself from the polyprotein and the mature PR dimer is then free to perform all subsequent cleavages.

Proteolytic processing of $Pr55^{Gag}$ follows a sequential series of events, which are kinetically controlled by the rate of cleavage at each individual site in Gag (Erickson-Viitanen et al., 1989; Krausslich et al., 1988; Mervis et al., 1988; Pettit et al., 1994; Tritch et al., 1991; Vogt, 1996; Wiegers et al., 1998). Initial cleavage releases the NC-SP2-p6 fragment from MA-CA-SP1 and is subsequently followed by cleavage at the MA-CA and SP1-p6 sites and finally at the CA-SP1 and NC-SP2 sites. Accurate proteolytic processing of Gag is essential for the production of infectious virions, as mutations that disrupt cleavage of individual sites or alter the order in which sites are cleaved result in aberrant particles that have significantly reduced infectivity (Accola et al., 1998; Kaplan et al., 1993; Krausslich et al., 1995; Li et al., 2003; Pettit et al., 1994, 2002; Wiegers et al., 1998; Zhou et al., 2004).

B. Virion Reorganization on Proteolytic Maturation

The consequences of HIV-1 proteolytic maturation are multifold and prepare the virus for infection of a new cell. Release of mature CA results in a second assembly event in which a proportion of the resultant CA forms a core structure (Benjamin et al., 2005; Briggs et al., 2004). Core formation is essential for virus infectivity, as disruption of core formation or stability blocks steps associated with reverse transcription on infection of a new cell (Freed, 1998; Swanstrom and Wills, 1997). Lentiviral cores are typically cone-shaped; however, a wide variety of related structures, such as tubes, have also been described (Benjamin et al., 2005; Briggs et al., 2003, 2006; Welker et al., 2000). Imaging studies have described the core's structure to be based on the geometric organization of a fullerene cone assembled from a curved hexagonal CA lattice and closed through the inclusion of 12 pentameric defects (Benjamin et al., 2005; Briggs et al., 2003; Ganser et al., 1999; Li et al., 2000) (Fig. 9). The positioning of the pentamers in the hexameric lattice defines the overall shape of the core (Ganser et al., 1999; Ganser-Pornillos et al., 2004).

The mechanism of core formation remains to be fully defined, though it is clear that CA–CA interactions play a central role. Fitting established CA crystal structures onto the conical structural model predicts that the NTD forms hexameric rings (Fig. 9A) and the CTD dimerization domain links adjacent hexamers (Li et al., 2000). In agreement with this model, in vitro studies have implicated helix 1 and 2 of the NTD and the CTD dimer interface in core assembly (Ganser-Pornillos et al., 2004; Lanman et al., 2003). Mutational analyses have demonstrated that the NTD is required for correct core formation (Dorfman et al., 1994a; Fitzon et al., 2000; Reicin et al., 1996; Scholz et al., 2005; Tang et al., 2001; von Schwedler et al., 1998, 2003a). However, mutations in the CTD often affect earlier assembly events (see Section III); therefore, CTD involvement in core formation has been difficult to establish in vivo. A third intersubunit interaction

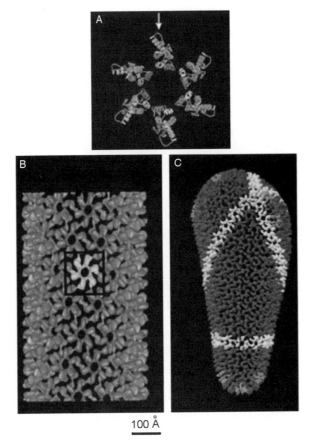

100 Å

FIGURE 9   Image reconstruction of helical assemblies of HIV-1 capsid (CA) protein. (A) Molecular model of the hexameric ring formed by the CA N-terminal domain (NTD). Structural features: β-hairpin (orange), helix 1 (red), helix 2 (yellow), helix 3 (green), helix 4 (cyan), helix 5 (dark blue), helix 6 (red), helix 7 (pink). Cyclophilin A-binding loop (arrow). (B) Exterior view of the assembled tube structure showing the hexagonal CA lattice. A single hexamer is highlighted in yellow. (C) Model of the HIV-1 conical core. A continuous line of hexamers is highlighted in yellow and pentameric defects are shown in pink. Adapted from Li *et al.* (2000). Copyright 2000 Nature Publishing Group, with permission. (See Color Insert.)

between the NTD and CTD of different CA molecules has also been implicated in core formation (Ganser-Pornillos *et al.*, 2004; Lanman *et al.*, 2002, 2003).

Release of CA from Pr55^{Gag} results in the most morphologically significant change during maturation; however, the generation of MA and NC also has important consequences for virus maturation. Mature NC plays a key role in condensation of the ribonucleoprotein complex (RNP) and viral dimeric RNA stabilization, both of which are important for efficient retroviral replication (Paillart *et al.*, 2004; Rein *et al.*, 1998). Mature MA exhibits weak membrane-binding affinity compared to the MA domain of un-processed Gag (Zhou and Resh, 1996), possibly allowing membrane dis-sociation on entry into a new cell. The differential membrane binding of MA may be facilitated by Gag cleavage, which reduces the extent of MA multimerization and consequently induces the myristate moiety to adopt a sequestered conformation (see Section VI). Proteolytic processing of Gag also regulates Env-mediated cell-to-cell fusion, perhaps by altering the inter-action between MA and the cytoplasmic tail of gp41 (Murakami *et al.*, 2004; Wyma *et al.*, 2004) (see Section VI).

IX. HIV Assembly and Maturation as Targets for New Antiretroviral Drugs

This chapter describes the extensive progress that has been made in understanding the molecular basis of HIV-1 assembly, release, and matura-tion. The information gained has highlighted multiple steps in these path-ways that could serve as potential targets for the development of new antiretroviral drugs. The identification of new drugs is a high research priority due to the rapid emergence of isolates resistant to currently ap-proved therapeutics. Therefore, the development of new drugs targeting novel sites of action will be essential for continued successful HIV treatment, but represents a considerable challenge for future research.

A. Assembly Inhibitors

It has been widely speculated that assembly may represent a viable target for therapeutic intervention. It can be envisioned that a small mole-cule that competitively binds a functional surface in Gag and/or CA will disrupt the multiple protein–protein interactions required for assembly (see Sections III and VIII). To date, however, only a few studies have attempted to identify such molecules and assess their ability to inhibit virus assembly (Garzon *et al.*, 2004; Hoglund *et al.*, 2002; Niedrig *et al.*, 1994; Sticht *et al.*, 2005; Tang *et al.*, 2003). The most recent approach used *in vitro* assembly assays to facilitate systematic high-throughput screening of a phage-display random peptide library (Sticht *et al.*, 2005). This strategy successfully iden-tified a peptide (referred to as CAI) that inhibited *in vitro* assembly of both immature VLPs and capsid cores by binding the CA CTD and altering the dimer interface (Sticht *et al.*, 2005). Unfortunately, this peptide was not active in cell-based assays, a problem likely to be inherent to the use of peptides as drugs that require intracellular uptake (Sticht *et al.*, 2005). However, the crystal structure of CAI in complex with CA CTD has been reported (Ternois *et al.*, 2005) and will aid future rational design of small molecules that are more promising as therapeutics (Ternois *et al.*, 2005;

Vogt, 2005). A separate study identified a compound (termed CAP1) that binds to a site on the CA NTD (Tang *et al.*, 2003). CAP1 binding disrupts CA assembly *in vitro*. In cells, this compound inhibits both assembly and maturation. Interestingly, it appears that only a relatively small number of molecules are required to elicit inhibitory activity. While CAP1 may not be clinically viable, other molecules that bind the same site on the CA NTD could in theory provide a therapeutic benefit.

B. Release Inhibitors

The discovery that a number of enveloped RNA viruses, including HIV-1, hijack host cell endosomal sorting machinery to facilitate virus particle release (see Section VII) has created the exciting possibility of developing novel antiviral strategies that target virus budding. Global disruption of the host cell machinery itself is likely to be unfeasible due to cellular toxicity; however, inhibition of essential virus–host protein interactions remains a possibility. A promising target for such an approach is the interaction between the HIV-1 late domain (PT/SAP) and its cellular partner Tsg101, a concept that is supported by the finding that overexpression of an N-terminal fragment of Tsg101 (termed TSG-5′) potently inhibits virus production by blocking efficient virus release (Demirov *et al.*, 2002b). Encouragingly, TSG-5′ inhibits virus release in a PTAP-dependent manner and does not appear to globally disrupt cellular class E Vps machinery (Demirov *et al.*, 2002b; Goila-Gaur *et al.*, 2003; Shehu-Xhilaga *et al.*, 2004). While TSG-5′ is unlikely to be useful as a deliverable therapeutic, small molecule inhibitors that mimic the action of TSG-5′ could be clinically effective. The rational design of such inhibitors will be guided by the structure of Tsg101 in complex with the HIV-1 PTAP motif (Pornillos *et al.*, 2002a).

C. Maturation Inhibitors

HIV-1 PR inhibitors constitute a class of antiretroviral drugs that competitively inhibit PR enzymatic function and hence prevent proteolytic processing at all cleavage sites in Gag and Gag-Pol. Several PR inhibitors are currently approved for clinical use and have proven to be highly effective when used in combination with RT inhibitors. PR inhibitors have been extensively reviewed elsewhere (Emini and Fan, 1997; Temesgen *et al.*, 2006; Wlodawer and Erickson, 1993; Wlodawer and Vondrasek, 1998).

Maturation inhibitors represent an emerging class of antiretroviral drugs that are distinct from competitive PR inhibitors due to a novel mechanism of action. PA-457 [3-0-(3′,3′-dimethylsuccinyl) betulinic acid] is first in class and inhibits HIV-1 infectivity by blocking a late stage in PR-mediated Gag processing; specifically, the release of SP1 from the C-terminus of CA

(Li *et al.*, 2003; Zhou *et al.*, 2004). Blocking CA-SP1 cleavage prevents proper virion maturation and results in noninfectious aberrant particles, which fail to form conical cores and display an electron-dense layer of Gag adjacent to the viral membrane (Li *et al.*, 2003; Wiegers *et al.*, 1998). Mutations that confer resistance to PA-457 all map to the CA-SP1 region of Gag (Adamson *et al.*, 2006; Li *et al.*, 2003; Zhou *et al.*, 2004). Although the mechanism by which PA-457 prevents cleavage of CA-SP1 has not been fully defined, recent data suggest that the compound binds directly the CA-SP1 region of an oligomeric form of Gag within a partially or fully assembled immature particle (Sakalian *et al.*, 2006; Zhou *et al.*, 2005). PA-457's novel mechanism of action permits it to retain full activity against strains of HIV-1 that are resistant to currently approved antiretrovirals (Li *et al.*, 2003; Zhou *et al.*, 2004), making it an excellent drug candidate. PA-457 (or bevirimat) is currently undergoing clinical trials with early favorable results.

Acknowledgments

We thank members of the Freed laboratory for helpful discussions and critical review of the chapter. We also thank authors who granted us permission to reprint Gag structures.

References

Abdurahman, S., Hoglund, S., Goobar-Larsson, L., and Vahlne, A. (2004). Selected amino acid substitutions in the C-terminal region of human immunodeficiency virus type 1 capsid protein affect virus assembly and release. *J. Gen. Virol.* **85**(Pt. 10), 2903–2913.

Accola, M. A., Hoglund, S., and Gottlinger, H. G. (1998). A putative alpha-helical structure which overlaps the capsid-p2 boundary in the human immunodeficiency virus type 1 Gag precursor is crucial for viral particle assembly. *J. Virol.* **72**(3), 2072–2078.

Accola, M. A., Strack, B., and Gottlinger, H. G. (2000). Efficient particle production by minimal Gag constructs which retain the carboxy-terminal domain of human immunodeficiency virus type 1 capsid-p2 and a late assembly domain. *J. Virol.* **74**(12), 5395–5402.

Adamson, C. S., Nermut, M., and Jones, I. M. (2003). Control of human immunodeficiency virus type-1 protease activity in insect cells expressing Gag-Pol rescues assembly of immature but not mature virus-like particles. *Virology* **308**(1), 157–165.

Adamson, C. S., Ablan, S. D., Boeras, I., Goila-Gaur, R., Soheilian, F., Nagashima, K., Li, F., Salzwedel, K., Sakalian, M., Wild, C. T., and Freed, E. O. (2006). *In vitro* resistance to the Human immunodeficiency virus type 1 maturation inhibitor Pa-457 (Bevirimat). *J. Virol.* **80**(22), 10957–10971.

Ako-Adjei, D., Johnson, M. C., and Vogt, V. M. (2005). The retroviral capsid domain dictates virion size, morphology, and coassembly of gag into virus-like particles. *J. Virol.* **79**(21), 13463–13472.

Aldovini, A., and Young, R. A. (1990). Mutations of RNA and protein sequences involved in human immunodeficiency virus type 1 packaging result in production of noninfectious virus. *J. Virol.* **64**(5), 1920–1926.

Amarasinghe, G. K., De Guzman, R. N., Turner, R. B., Chancellor, K. J., Wu, Z. R., and Summers, M. F. (2000a). NMR structure of the HIV-1 nucleocapsid protein bound to stem-loop SL2 of the psi-RNA packaging signal. Implications for genome recognition. *J. Mol. Biol.* **301**(2), 491–511.

Amarasinghe, G. K., De Guzman, R. N., Turner, R. B., and Summers, M. F. (2000b). NMR structure of stem-loop SL2 of the HIV-1 psi RNA packaging signal reveals a novel A-U-A base-triple platform. *J. Mol. Biol.* **299**(1), 145–156.

Amarasinghe, G. K., Zhou, J., Miskimon, M., Chancellor, K. J., McDonald, J. A., Matthews, A. G., Miller, R. R., Rouse, M. D., and Summers, M. F. (2001). Stem-loop SL4 of the HIV-1 psi RNA packaging signal exhibits weak affinity for the nucleocapsid protein. structural studies and implications for genome recognition. *J. Mol. Biol.* **314**(5), 961–970.

Ames, J. B., Tanaka, T., Stryer, L., and Ikura, M. (1996). Portrait of a myristoyl switch protein. *Curr. Opin. Struct. Biol.* **6**(4), 432–438.

Ames, J. B., Ishima, R., Tanaka, T., Gordon, J. I., Stryer, L., and Ikura, M. (1997). Molecular mechanics of calcium-myristoyl switches. *Nature* **389**(6647), 198–202.

Barklis, E., McDermott, J., Wilkens, S., Fuller, S., and Thompson, D. (1998). Organization of HIV-1 capsid proteins on a lipid monolayer. *J. Biol. Chem.* **273**(13), 7177–7180.

Baudin, F., Marquet, R., Isel, C., Darlix, J. L., Ehresmann, B., and Ehresmann, C. (1993). Functional sites in the 5′ region of human immunodeficiency virus type 1 RNA form defined structural domains. *J. Mol. Biol.* **229**(2), 382–397.

Behnia, R., and Munro, S. (2005). Organelle identity and the signposts for membrane traffic. *Nature* **438**(7068), 597–604.

Benjamin, J., Ganser-Pornillos, B. K., Tivol, W. F., Sundquist, W. I., and Jensen, G. J. (2005). Three-dimensional structure of HIV-1 virus-like particles by electron cryotomography. *J. Mol. Biol.* **346**(2), 577–588.

Berg, J. M. (1986). Potential metal-binding domains in nucleic acid binding proteins. *Science* **232**(4749), 485–487.

Berthet-Colominas, C., Monaco, S., Novelli, A., Sibai, G., Mallet, F., and Cusack, S. (1999). Head-to-tail dimers and interdomain flexibility revealed by the crystal structure of HIV-1 capsid protein (p24) complexed with a monoclonal antibody Fab. *EMBO J.* **18**(5), 1124–1136.

Bess, J. W., Jr., Powell, P. J., Issaq, H. J., Schumack, L. J., Grimes, M. K., Henderson, L. E., and Arthur, L. O. (1992). Tightly bound zinc in human immunodeficiency virus type 1, human T-cell leukemia virus type I, and other retroviruses. *J. Virol.* **66**(2), 840–847.

Bhattacharya, J., Repik, A., and Clapham, P. R. (2006). Gag regulates association of human immunodeficiency virus type 1 envelope with detergent-resistant membranes. *J. Virol.* **80**(11), 5292–5300.

Blot, G., Janvier, K., Le Panse, S., Benarous, R., and Berlioz-Torrent, C. (2003). Targeting of the human immunodeficiency virus type 1 envelope to the trans-Golgi network through binding to TIP47 is required for env incorporation into virions and infectivity. *J. Virol.* **77**(12), 6931–6945.

Boge, M., Wyss, S., Bonifacino, J. S., and Thali, M. (1998). A membrane-proximal tyrosine-based signal mediates internalization of the HIV-1 envelope glycoprotein via interaction with the AP-2 clathrin adaptor. *J. Biol. Chem.* **273**(25), 15773–15778.

Borsetti, A., Ohagen, A., and Gottlinger, H. G. (1998). The C-terminal half of the human immunodeficiency virus type 1 Gag precursor is sufficient for efficient particle assembly. *J. Virol.* **72**(11), 9313–9317.

Bouamr, F., Melillo, J. A., Wang, M. Q., Nagashima, K., de Los Santos, M., Rein, A., and Goff, S. P. (2003). PPPYVEPTAP motif is the late domain of human T-cell leukemia virus type 1 Gag and mediates its functional interaction with cellular proteins Nedd4 and Tsg101 [corrected]. *J. Virol.* **77**(22), 11882–11895.

Briggs, J. A., Wilk, T., Welker, R., Krausslich, H. G., and Fuller, S. D. (2003). Structural organization of authentic, mature HIV-1 virions and cores. *EMBO J.* **22**(7), 1707–1715.

Briggs, J. A., Simon, M. N., Gross, I., Krausslich, H. G., Fuller, S. D., Vogt, V. M., and Johnson, M. C. (2004). The stoichiometry of Gag protein in HIV-1. *Nat. Struct. Mol. Biol.* **11**(7), 672–675.

Briggs, J. A., Grunewald, K., Glass, B., Forster, F., Krausslich, H. G., and Fuller, S. D. (2006). The mechanism of HIV-1 core assembly: Insights from three-dimensional reconstructions of authentic virions. *Structure* **14**(1), 15–20.

Brugger, B., Glass, B., Haberkant, P., Leibrecht, I., Wieland, F. T., and Krausslich, H. G. (2006). The HIV lipidome: A raft with an unusual composition. *Proc. Natl. Acad. Sci. USA* **103**(8), 2641–2646.

Bryant, M., and Ratner, L. (1990). Myristoylation-dependent replication and assembly of human immunodeficiency virus 1. *Proc. Natl. Acad. Sci. USA* **87**(2), 523–527.

Burniston, M. T., Cimarelli, A., Colgan, J., Curtis, S. P., and Luban, J. (1999). Human immunodeficiency virus type 1 Gag polyprotein multimerization requires the nucleocapsid domain and RNA and is promoted by the capsid-dimer interface and the basic region of matrix protein. *J. Virol.* **73**(10), 8527–8540.

Campbell, S., and Rein, A. (1999). *In vitro* assembly properties of human immunodeficiency virus type 1 Gag protein lacking the p6 domain. *J. Virol.* **73**(3), 2270–2279.

Campbell, S., and Vogt, V. M. (1995). Self-assembly *in vitro* of purified CA-NC proteins from Rous sarcoma virus and human immunodeficiency virus type 1. *J. Virol.* **69**(10), 6487–6497.

Cannon, P. M., Matthews, S., Clark, N., Byles, E. D., Iourin, O., Hockley, D. J., Kingsman, S. M., and Kingsman, A. J. (1997). Structure-function studies of the human immunodeficiency virus type 1 matrix protein, p17. *J. Virol.* **71**(5), 3474–3483.

Cantin, R., Methot, S., and Tremblay, M. J. (2005). Plunder and stowaways: Incorporation of cellular proteins by enveloped viruses. *J. Virol.* **79**(11), 6577–6587.

Chazal, N., Gay, B., Carriere, C., Tournier, J., and Boulanger, P. (1995). Human immunodeficiency virus type 1 MA deletion mutants expressed in baculovirus-infected cells: Cis and trans effects on the Gag precursor assembly pathway. *J. Virol.* **69**(1), 365–375.

Chertova, E., Chertov, O., Coren, L. V., Roser, J. D., Trubey, C. M., Bess, J. W., Jr., Sowder, R. C., II, Barsov, E., Hood, B. L., Fisher, R. J., Nagashima, K., Conrads, T. P., *et al.* (2006). Proteomic and biochemical analysis of purified human immunodeficiency virus type 1 produced from infected monocyte-derived macrophages. *J. Virol.* **80**(18), 9039–9052.

Cimarelli, A., and Luban, J. (2000). Human immunodeficiency virus type 1 virion density is not determined by nucleocapsid basic residues. *J. Virol.* **74**(15), 6734–6740.

Cimarelli, A., Sandin, S., Hoglund, S., and Luban, J. (2000). Basic residues in human immunodeficiency virus type 1 nucleocapsid promote virion assembly via interaction with RNA. *J. Virol.* **74**(7), 3046–3057.

Clever, J., Sassetti, C., and Parslow, T. G. (1995). RNA secondary structure and binding sites for gag gene products in the 5' packaging signal of human immunodeficiency virus type 1. *J. Virol.* **69**(4), 2101–2109.

Clever, J. L., and Parslow, T. G. (1997). Mutant human immunodeficiency virus type 1 genomes with defects in RNA dimerization or encapsidation. *J. Virol.* **71**(5), 3407–3414.

Covey, S. N. (1986). Amino acid sequence homology in gag region of reverse transcribing elements and the coat protein gene of cauliflower mosaic virus. *Nucleic Acids Res.* **14**(2), 623–633.

D'Souza, V., and Summers, M. F. (2005). How retroviruses select their genomes. *Nat. Rev. Microbiol.* **3**(8), 643–655.

Dannull, J., Surovoy, A., Jung, G., and Moelling, K. (1994). Specific binding of HIV-1 nucleocapsid protein to PSI RNA *in vitro* requires N-terminal zinc finger and flanking basic amino acid residues. *EMBO J.* **13**(7), 1525–1533.

Dawson, L., and Yu, X. F. (1998). The role of nucleocapsid of HIV-1 in virus assembly. *Virology* **251**(1), 141–157.

De Guzman, R. N., Wu, Z. R., Stalling, C. C., Pappalardo, L., Borer, P. N., and Summers, M. F. (1998). Structure of the HIV-1 nucleocapsid protein bound to the SL3 psi-RNA recognition element. *Science* **279**(5349), 384–388.

Dell'Angelica, E. C., Shotelersuk, V., Aguilar, R. C., Gahl, W. A., and Bonifacino, J. S. (1999). Altered trafficking of lysosomal proteins in Hermansky-Pudlak syndrome due to mutations in the beta 3A subunit of the AP-3 adaptor. *Mol. Cell* **3**(1), 11–21.

Demirov, D. G., and Freed, E. O. (2004). Retrovirus budding. *Virus Res.* **106**(2), 87–102.

Demirov, D. G., Orenstein, J. M., and Freed, E. O. (2002a). The late domain of human immunodeficiency virus type 1 p6 promotes virus release in a cell type-dependent manner. *J. Virol.* **76**(1), 105–117.

Demirov, D. G., Ono, A., Orenstein, J. M., and Freed, E. O. (2002b). Overexpression of the N-terminal domain of TSG101 inhibits HIV-1 budding by blocking late domain function. *Proc. Natl. Acad. Sci. USA* **99**(2), 955–960.

Dong, X., Li, H., Derdowski, A., Ding, L., Burnett, A., Chen, X., Peters, T. R., Dermody, T. S., Woodruff, E., Wang, J. J., and Spearman, P. (2005). AP-3 directs the intracellular trafficking of HIV-1 Gag and plays a key role in particle assembly. *Cell* **120**(5), 663–674.

Dorfman, T., Luban, J., Goff, S. P., Haseltine, W. A., and Gottlinger, H. G. (1993). Mapping of functionally important residues of a cysteine-histidine box in the human immunodeficiency virus type 1 nucleocapsid protein. *J. Virol.* **67**(10), 6159–6169.

Dorfman, T., Bukovsky, A., Ohagen, A., Hoglund, S., and Gottlinger, H. G. (1994a). Functional domains of the capsid protein of human immunodeficiency virus type 1. *J. Virol.* **68**(12), 8180–8187.

Dorfman, T., Mammano, F., Haseltine, W. A., and Gottlinger, H. G. (1994b). Role of the matrix protein in the virion association of the human immunodeficiency virus type 1 envelope glycoprotein. *J. Virol.* **68**(3), 1689–1696.

Dubay, J. W., Roberts, S. J., Hahn, B. H., and Hunter, E. (1992). Truncation of the human immunodeficiency virus type 1 transmembrane glycoprotein cytoplasmic domain blocks virus infectivity. *J. Virol.* **66**(11), 6616–6625.

Emini, E. A., and Fan, H. Y. (1997). Immunological and pharmacological approaches to the control of retroviral infections. *In* "Retroviruses" (J. M. Coffin, S. H. Hughes, and H. E. Varmus, Eds.), Chapter 12, pp. 637–708. Cold Spring Harbor Laboratory Press, Plainview, NY.

Erickson-Viitanen, S., Manfredi, J., Viitanen, P., Tribe, D. E., Tritch, R., Hutchison, C. A., III, Loeb, D. D., and Swanstrom, R. (1989). Cleavage of HIV-1 gag polyprotein synthesized *in vitro*: Sequential cleavage by the viral protease. *AIDS Res. Hum. Retroviruses* **5**(6), 577–591.

Fitzon, T., Leschonsky, B., Bieler, K., Paulus, C., Schroder, J., Wolf, H., and Wagner, R. (2000). Proline residues in the HIV-1 NH2-terminal capsid domain: Structure determinants for proper core assembly and subsequent steps of early replication. *Virology* **268**(2), 294–307.

Franke, E. K., Yuan, H. E., and Luban, J. (1994). Specific incorporation of cyclophilin A into HIV-1 virions. *Nature* **372**(6504), 359–362.

Freed, E. O. (1998). HIV-1 Gag proteins: Diverse functions in the virus life cycle. *Virology* **251**(1), 1–15.

Freed, E. O. (2002). Viral late domains. *J. Virol.* **76**(10), 4679–4687.

Freed, E. O. (2006). HIV-1 Gag: Flipped out for PI(4,5)P$_2$. *Proc. Natl. Acad. Sci. USA* **103**(30), 11101–11102.

Freed, E. O., and Martin, M. A. (1995a). The role of human immunodeficiency virus type 1 envelope glycoproteins in virus infection. *J. Biol. Chem.* **270**(41), 23883–23886.

Freed, E. O., and Martin, M. A. (1995b). Virion incorporation of envelope glycoproteins with long but not short cytoplasmic tails is blocked by specific, single amino acid substitutions in the human immunodeficiency virus type 1 matrix. *J. Virol.* **69**(3), 1984–1989.

Freed, E. O., and Martin, M. A. (1996). Domains of the human immunodeficiency virus type 1 matrix and gp41 cytoplasmic tail required for envelope incorporation into virions. *J. Virol.* **70**(1), 341–351.

Freed, E. O., and Martin, M. A. (2007). HIVs and their replication. *In* "Fields Virology" (D. M. Knipe and P. M. Howley, Eds.), Chapter 57, 5th edn., pp. 2107–2185. Lippincott, Williams and Wilkins.

Freed, E. O., Orenstein, J. M., Buckler-White, A. J., and Martin, M. A. (1994). Single amino acid changes in the human immunodeficiency virus type 1 matrix protein block virus particle production. *J. Virol.* **68**(8), 5311–5320.

Fuller, S. D., Wilk, T., Gowen, B. E., Krausslich, H. G., and Vogt, V. M. (1997). Cryo-electron microscopy reveals ordered domains in the immature HIV-1 particle. *Curr. Biol.* **7**(10), 729–738.

Gamble, T. R., Vajdos, F. F., Yoo, S., Worthylake, D. K., Houseweart, M., Sundquist, W. I., and Hill, C. P. (1996). Crystal structure of human cyclophilin A bound to the amino-terminal domain of HIV-1 capsid. *Cell* **87**(7), 1285–1294.

Gamble, T. R., Yoo, S., Vajdos, F. F., von Schwedler, U. K., Worthylake, D. K., Wang, H., McCutcheon, J. P., Sundquist, W. I., and Hill, C. P. (1997). Structure of the carboxyl-terminal dimerization domain of the HIV-1 capsid protein. *Science* **278**(5339), 849–853.

Ganser, B. K., Li, S., Klishko, V. Y., Finch, J. T., and Sundquist, W. I. (1999). Assembly and analysis of conical models for the HIV-1 core. *Science* **283**(5398), 80–83.

Ganser-Pornillos, B. K., von Schwedler, U. K., Stray, K. M., Aiken, C., and Sundquist, W. I. (2004). Assembly properties of the human immunodeficiency virus type 1 CA protein. *J. Virol.* **78**(5), 2545–2552.

Garrus, J. E., von Schwedler, U. K., Pornillos, O. W., Morham, S. G., Zavitz, K. H., Wang, H. E., Wettstein, D. A., Stray, K. M., Cote, M., Rich, R. L., Myszka, D. G., and Sundquist, W. I. (2001). Tsg101 and the vacuolar protein sorting pathway are essential for HIV-1 budding. *Cell* **107**(1), 55–65.

Garzon, M. T., Lidon-Moya, M. C., Barrera, F. N., Prieto, A., Gomez, J., Mateu, M. G., and Neira, J. L. (2004). The dimerization domain of the HIV-1 capsid protein binds a capsid protein-derived peptide: A biophysical characterization. *Protein Sci.* **13**(6), 1512–1523.

Gendelman, H. E., Orenstein, J. M., Martin, M. A., Ferrua, C., Mitra, R., Phipps, T., Wahl, L. A., Lane, H. C., Fauci, A. S., Burke, D. S., Skillman, D., and Meltzer, M. S. (1988). Efficient isolation and propagation of human immunodeficiency virus on recombinant colony-stimulating factor 1-treated monocytes. *J. Exp. Med.* **167**(4), 1428–1441.

Gheysen, D., Jacobs, E., De Foresta, F., Thines, D., and De Wilde, M. (1989). Assembly and release of HIV-1 precursor Pr55Gag virus-like particles from recombinant baculovirus-infected insect cells. *Cell* **59**, 103–112.

Gitti, R. K., Lee, B. M., Walker, J., Summers, M. F., Yoo, S., and Sundquist, W. I. (1996). Structure of the amino-terminal core domain of the HIV-1 capsid protein. *Science* **273** (5272), 231–235.

Goila-Gaur, R., Demirov, D. G., Orenstein, J. M., Ono, A., and Freed, E. O. (2003). Defects in human immunodeficiency virus budding and endosomal sorting induced by TSG101 overexpression. *J. Virol.* **77**(11), 6507–6519.

Gorelick, R. J., Nigida, S. M., Jr., Bess, J. W., Jr., Arthur, L. O., Henderson, L. E., and Rein, A. (1990). Noninfectious human immunodeficiency virus type 1 mutants deficient in genomic RNA. *J. Virol.* **64**(7), 3207–3211.

Gorelick, R. J., Chabot, D. J., Rein, A., Henderson, L. E., and Arthur, L. O. (1993). The two zinc fingers in the human immunodeficiency virus type 1 nucleocapsid protein are not functionally equivalent. *J. Virol.* **67**(7), 4027–4036.

Gottlinger, H. G., Sodroski, J. G., and Haseltine, W. A. (1989). Role of capsid precursor processing and myristoylation in morphogenesis and infectivity of human immunodeficiency virus type 1. *Proc. Natl. Acad. Sci. USA* 86(15), 5781–5785.

Gottlinger, H. G., Dorfman, T., Sodroski, J. G., and Haseltine, W. A. (1991). Effect of mutations affecting the p6 gag protein on human immunodeficiency virus particle release. *Proc. Natl. Acad. Sci. USA* 88, 3195–3199.

Gottwein, E., Bodem, J., Muller, B., Schmechel, A., Zentgraf, H., and Krausslich, H. G. (2003). The Mason-Pfizer monkey virus PPPY and PSAP motifs both contribute to virus release. *J. Virol.* 77(17), 9474–9485.

Gould, S. J., Booth, A. M., and Hildreth, J. E. (2003). The Trojan exosome hypothesis. *Proc. Natl. Acad. Sci. USA* 100(19), 10592–10597.

Guo, X., Roldan, A., Hu, J., Wainberg, M. A., and Liang, C. (2005). Mutation of the SP1 sequence impairs both multimerization and membrane-binding activities of human immunodeficiency virus type 1 Gag. *J. Virol.* 79(3), 1803–1812.

Harrison, G. P., and Lever, A. M. (1992). The human immunodeficiency virus type 1 packaging signal and major splice donor region have a conserved stable secondary structure. *J. Virol.* 66(7), 4144–4153.

Harrison, G. P., Miele, G., Hunter, E., and Lever, A. M. (1998). Functional analysis of the core human immunodeficiency virus type 1 packaging signal in a permissive cell line. *J. Virol.* 72(7), 5886–5896.

Hatziioannou, T., Perez-Caballero, D., Cowan, S., and Bieniasz, P. D. (2005). Cyclophilin interactions with incoming human immunodeficiency virus type 1 capsids with opposing effects on infectivity in human cells. *J. Virol.* 79(1), 176–183.

Hayashi, T., Shioda, T., Iwakura, Y., and Shibuta, H. (1992). RNA packaging signal of human immunodeficiency virus type 1. *Virology* 188(2), 590–599.

Hayashi, T., Ueno, Y., and Okamoto, T. (1993). Elucidation of a conserved RNA stem-loop structure in the packaging signal of human immunodeficiency virus type 1. *FEBS Lett.* 327(2), 213–218.

Heidecker, G., Lloyd, P. A., Fox, K., Nagashima, K., and Derse, D. (2004). Late assembly motifs of human T-cell leukemia virus type 1 and their relative roles in particle release. *J. Virol.* 78(12), 6636–6648.

Hermida-Matsumoto, L., and Resh, M. D. (1999). Human immunodeficiency virus type 1 protease triggers a myristoyl switch that modulates membrane binding of Pr55(gag) and p17MA. *J. Virol.* 73(3), 1902–1908.

Hill, C. P., Worthylake, D., Bancroft, D. P., Christensen, A. M., and Sundquist, W. I. (1996). Crystal structures of the trimeric human immunodeficiency virus type 1 matrix protein: Implications for membrane association and assembly. *Proc. Natl. Acad. Sci. USA* 93(7), 3099–3104.

Hoglund, S., Su, J., Reneby, S. S., Vegvari, A., Hjerten, S., Sintorn, I. M., Foster, H., Wu, Y. P., Nystrom, I., and Vahlne, A. (2002). Tripeptide interference with human immunodeficiency virus type 1 morphogenesis. *Antimicrob. Agents Chemother.* 46(11), 3597–3605.

Huang, M., Orenstein, J. M., Martin, M. A., and Freed, E. O. (1995). p6Gag is required for particle production from full length human immunodeficiency virus type 1 molecular clones expressing protease. *J. Virol.* 69, 6810–6818.

Hurley, J. H., and Emr, S. D. (2006). The ESCRT complexes: Structure and mechanism of a membrane-trafficking network. *Annu. Rev. Biophys. Biomol. Struct.* 35, 277–298.

Huseby, D., Barklis, R. L., Alfadhli, A., and Barklis, E. (2005). Assembly of human immunodeficiency virus precursor gag proteins. *J. Biol. Chem.* 280(18), 17664–17670.

Ivanov, D., Stone, J. R., Maki, J. L., Collins, T., and Wagner, G. (2005). Mammalian SCAN domain dimer is a domain-swapped homolog of the HIV capsid C-terminal domain. *Mol. Cell* 17(1), 137–143.

Jewell, N. A., and Mansky, L. M. (2000). In the beginning: Genome recognition, RNA encapsidation and the initiation of complex retrovirus assembly. *J. Gen. Virol.* **81**(Pt. 8), 1889–1899.

Joshi, A., Nagashima, K., and Freed, E. O. (2006). Mutation of dileucine-like motifs in the human immunodeficiency virus type 1 capsid disrupts virus assembly, gag-gag interactions, gag-membrane binding, and virion maturation. *J. Virol.* **80**(16), 7939–7951.

Kaplan, A. H., Zack, J. A., Knigge, M., Paul, D. A., Kempf, D. J., Norbeck, D. W., and Swanstrom, R. (1993). Partial inhibition of the Human Immunodeficiency Virus Type 1 protease results in abberant virus assembly and the formation of non-infectious particles. *J. Virol.* **67**, 4050–4055.

Karacostas, V., Wolffe, E. J., Nagashima, K., Gonda, M. A., and Moss, B. (1993). Overexpression of the HIV-1 Gag-Pol polyprotein results in intracellular activation of HIV-1 protease and inhibition of assembly and budding of virus-like particles. *Virology* **193**, 661–671.

Katzmann, D. J., Odorizzi, G., and Emr, S. D. (2002). Receptor downregulation and multivesicular-body sorting. *Nat. Rev. Mol. Cell Biol.* **3**(12), 893–905.

Kaye, J. F., and Lever, A. M. (1998). Nonreciprocal packaging of human immunodeficiency virus type 1 and type 2 RNA: A possible role for the p2 domain of Gag in RNA encapsidation. *J. Virol.* **72**(7), 5877–5885.

Kingston, R. L., and Vogt, V. M. (2005). Domain swapping and retroviral assembly. *Mol. Cell* **17**(2), 166–167.

Kräusslich, H.-G. (1991). Human Immunodeficiency Virus Proteinase dimer as a component of the viral polyprotein prevents particle assembly and viral infectivity. *Proc. Natl. Acad. Sci. USA* **88**, 3213–3217.

Krausslich, H. G., Facke, M., Heuser, A. M., Konvalinka, J., and Zentgraf, H. (1995). The spacer peptide between human immunodeficiency virus capsid and nucleocapsid proteins is essential for ordered assembly and viral infectivity. *J. Virol.* **69**(6), 3407–3419.

Krausslich, H. G., Schneider, H., Zybarth, G., Carter, C. A., and Wimmer, E. (1988). Processing of *in vitro*-synthesized gag precursor proteins of human immunodeficiency virus (HIV) type 1 by HIV proteinase generated in *Escherichia coli*. *J. Virol.* **62**(11), 4393–4397.

LaBranche, C. C., Sauter, M. M., Haggarty, B. S., Vance, P. J., Romano, J., Hart, T. K., Bugelski, P. J., Marsh, M., and Hoxie, J. A. (1995). A single amino acid change in the cytoplasmic domain of the simian immunodeficiency virus transmembrane molecule increases envelope glycoprotein expression on infected cells. *J. Virol.* **69**(9), 5217–5227.

Lanman, J., Sexton, J., Sakalian, M., and Prevelige, P. E., Jr. (2002). Kinetic analysis of the role of intersubunit interactions in human immunodeficiency virus type 1 capsid protein assembly *in vitro*. *J. Virol.* **76**(14), 6900–6908.

Lanman, J., Lam, T. T., Barnes, S., Sakalian, M., Emmett, M. R., Marshall, A. G., and Prevelige, P. E., Jr. (2003). Identification of novel interactions in HIV-1 capsid protein assembly by high-resolution mass spectrometry. *J. Mol. Biol.* **325**(4), 759–772.

Lapatto, R., Blundell, T., Hemmings, A., Overington, J., Wilderspin, A., Wood, S., Merson, J. R., Whittle, P. J., Danley, D. E., and Geoghegan, K. F. (1989). X-ray analysis of HIV-1 proteinase at 2.7 A resolution confirms structural homology among retroviral enzymes. *Nature* **342**(6247), 299–302.

Lawrence, D. C., Stover, C. C., Noznitsky, J., Wu, Z., and Summers, M. F. (2003). Structure of the intact stem and bulge of HIV-1 Psi-RNA stem-loop SL1. *J. Mol. Biol.* **326**(2), 529–542.

Lee, P. P., and Linial, M. L. (1994). Efficient particle formation can occur if the matrix domain of human immunodeficiency virus type 1 Gag is substituted by a myristylation signal. *J. Virol.* **68**(10), 6644–6654.

Li, F., Chen, C., Puffer, B. A., and Montelaro, R. C. (2002). Functional replacement and positional dependence of homologous and heterologous L domains in equine infectious anemia virus replication. *J. Virol.* 76(4), 1569–1577.

Li, F., Goila-Gaur, R., Salzwedel, K., Kilgore, N. R., Reddick, M., Matallana, C., Castillo, A., Zoumplis, D., Martin, D. E., Orenstein, J. M., Allaway, G. P., Freed, E. O., et al. (2003). PA-457: A potent HIV inhibitor that disrupts core condensation by targeting a late step in Gag processing. *Proc. Natl. Acad. Sci. USA* 100(23), 13555–13560.

Li, S., Hill, C. P., Sundquist, W. I., and Finch, J. T. (2000). Image reconstructions of helical assemblies of the HIV-1 CA protein. *Nature* 407(6802), 409–413.

Liang, C., Hu, J., Russell, R. S., Roldan, A., Kleiman, L., and Wainberg, M. A. (2002). Characterization of a putative alpha-helix across the capsid-SP1 boundary that is critical for the multimerization of human immunodeficiency virus type 1 gag. *J. Virol.* 76(22), 11729–11737.

Liang, C., Hu, J., Whitney, J. B., Kleiman, L., and Wainberg, M. A. (2003). A structurally disordered region at the C terminus of capsid plays essential roles in multimerization and membrane binding of the gag protein of human immunodeficiency virus type 1. *J. Virol.* 77(3), 1772–1783.

Licata, J. M., Simpson-Holley, M., Wright, N. T., Han, Z., Paragas, J., and Harty, R. N. (2003). Overlapping motifs (PTAP and PPEY) within the Ebola virus VP40 protein function independently as late budding domains: Involvement of host proteins TSG101 and VPS-4. *J. Virol.* 77(3), 1812–1819.

Lodge, R., Gottlinger, H., Gabuzda, D., Cohen, E. A., and Lemay, G. (1994). The intracytoplasmic domain of gp41 mediates polarized budding of human immunodeficiency virus type 1 in MDCK cells. *J. Virol.* 68(8), 4857–4861.

Lopez-Verges, S., Camus, G., Blot, G., Beauvoir, R., Benarous, R., and Berlioz-Torrent, C. (2006). Tail-interacting protein TIP47 is a connector between Gag and Env and is required for Env incorporation into HIV-1 virions. *Proc. Natl. Acad. Sci. USA* 103(40), 14947–14952.

Luban, J., Bossolt, K. L., Franke, E. K., Kalpana, G. V., and Goff, S. P. (1993). Human immunodeficiency virus type 1 Gag protein binds to cyclophilins A and B. *Cell* 73(6), 1067–1078.

Mammano, F., Ohagen, A., Hoglund, S., and Gottlinger, H. G. (1994). Role of the major homology region of human immunodeficiency virus type 1 in virion morphogenesis. *J. Virol.* 68(8), 4927–4936.

Mammano, F., Kondo, E., Sodroski, J., Bukovsky, A., and Gottlinger, H. G. (1995). Rescue of human immunodeficiency virus type 1 matrix protein mutants by envelope glycoproteins with short cytoplasmic domains. *J. Virol.* 69(6), 3824–3830.

Martin-Serrano, J., Zang, T., and Bieniasz, P. D. (2001). HIV-1 and Ebola virus encode small peptide motifs that recruit Tsg101 to sites of particle assembly to facilitate egress. *Nat. Med.* 7(12), 1313–1319.

Martin-Serrano, J., Yarovoy, A., Perez-Caballero, D., and Bieniasz, P. D. (2003a). Divergent retroviral late-budding domains recruit vacuolar protein sorting factors by using alternative adaptor proteins. *Proc. Natl. Acad. Sci. USA* 100(21), 12414–12419.

Martin-Serrano, J., Zang, T., and Bieniasz, P. D. (2003b). Role of ESCRT-I in retroviral budding. *J. Virol.* 77(8), 4794–4804.

Massiah, M. A., Starich, M. R., Paschall, C., Summers, M. F., Christensen, A. M., and Sundquist, W. I. (1994). Three-dimensional structure of the human immunodeficiency virus type 1 matrix protein. *J. Mol. Biol.* 244(2), 198–223.

McBride, M. S., and Panganiban, A. T. (1996). The human immunodeficiency virus type 1 encapsidation site is a multipartite RNA element composed of functional hairpin structures. *J. Virol.* 70(5), 2963–2973.

McBride, M. S., and Panganiban, A. T. (1997). Position dependence of functional hairpins important for human immunodeficiency virus type 1 RNA encapsidation *in vivo*. *J. Virol.* **71**(3), 2050–2058.

McBride, M. S., Schwartz, M. D., and Panganiban, A. T. (1997). Efficient encapsidation of human immunodeficiency virus type 1 vectors and further characterization of cis elements required for encapsidation. *J. Virol.* **71**(6), 4544–4554.

McLaughlin, S., and Murray, D. (2005). Plasma membrane phosphoinositide organization by protein electrostatics. *Nature* **438**(7068), 605–611.

Melamed, D., Mark-Danieli, M., Kenan-Eichler, M., Kraus, O., Castiel, A., Laham, N., Pupko, T., Glaser, F., Ben-Tal, N., and Bacharach, E. (2004). The conserved carboxy terminus of the capsid domain of human immunodeficiency virus type 1 gag protein is important for virion assembly and release. *J. Virol.* **78**(18), 9675–9688.

Mervis, R. J., Ahmad, N., Lillehoj, E. P., Raum, M. G., Salazar, F. H., Chan, H. W., and Venkatesan, S. (1988). The gag gene products of human immunodeficiency virus type 1: Alignment within the gag open reading frame, identification of posttranslational modifications, and evidence for alternative gag precursors. *J. Virol.* **62**(11), 3993–4002.

Momany, C., Kovari, L. C., Prongay, A. J., Keller, W., Gitti, R. K., Lee, B. M., Gorbalenya, A. E., Tong, L., McClure, J., Ehrlich, L. S., Summers, M. F., Carter, C., *et al.* (1996). Crystal structure of dimeric HIV-1 capsid protein. *Nat. Struct. Biol.* **3**(9), 763–770.

Morellet, N., Jullian, N., De Rocquigny, H., Maigret, B., Darlix, J. L., and Roques, B. P. (1992). Determination of the structure of the nucleocapsid protein NCp7 from the human immunodeficiency virus type 1 by 1H NMR. *EMBO J.* **11**(8), 3059–3065.

Morellet, N., de Rocquigny, H., Mely, Y., Jullian, N., Demene, H., Ottmann, M., Gerard, D., Darlix, J. L., Fournie-Zaluski, M. C., and Roques, B. P. (1994). Conformational behaviour of the active and inactive forms of the nucleocapsid NCp7 of HIV-1 studied by 1H NMR. *J. Mol. Biol.* **235**(1), 287–301.

Morellet, N., Druillennec, S., Lenoir, C., Bouaziz, S., and Roques, B. P. (2005). Helical structure determined by NMR of the HIV-1 (345–392)Gag sequence, surrounding p2: Implications for particle assembly and RNA packaging. *Protein Sci.* **14**(2), 375–386.

Morikawa, Y., Kishi, T., Zhang, W. H., Nermut, M. V., Hockley, D. J., and Jones, I. M. (1995). A molecular determinant of human immunodeficiency virus particle assembly located in matrix antigen p17. *J. Virol.* **69**(7), 4519–4523.

Morikawa, Y., Zhang, W. H., Hockley, D. J., Nermut, M. V., and Jones, I. M. (1998). Detection of a trimeric human immunodeficiency virus type 1 Gag intermediate is dependent on sequences in the matrix protein, p17. *J. Virol.* **72**(9), 7659–7663.

Morikawa, Y., Hockley, D. J., Nermut, M. V., and Jones, I. M. (2000). Roles of matrix, p2, and N-terminal myristoylation in human immunodeficiency virus type 1 Gag assembly. *J. Virol.* **74**(1), 16–23.

Morita, E., and Sundquist, W. I. (2004). Retrovirus budding. *Annu. Rev. Cell Dev. Biol.* **20**, 395–425.

Munshi, U., Kim, J., Hurley, J. H., and Freed, E. O. (2007). An ALIX fragment potently inhibits HIV-1 budding: Characterization of binding to retroviral YPXL late domains. *J. Biol. Chem.* **282**(6), 3847–3855.

Murakami, T., and Freed, E. O. (2000a). Genetic evidence for an interaction between human immunodeficiency virus type 1 matrix and alpha-helix 2 of the gp41 cytoplasmic tail. *J. Virol.* **74**(8), 3548–3554.

Murakami, T., and Freed, E. O. (2000b). The long cytoplasmic tail of gp41 is required in a cell type-dependent manner for HIV-1 envelope glycoprotein incorporation into virions. *Proc. Natl. Acad. Sci. USA* **97**(1), 343–348.

Murakami, T., Ablan, S., Freed, E. O., and Tanaka, Y. (2004). Regulation of human immunodeficiency virus type 1 Env-mediated membrane fusion by viral protease activity. *J. Virol.* **78**(2), 1026–1031.

Muriaux, D., Mirro, J., Harvin, D., and Rein, A. (2001). RNA is a structural element in retrovirus particles. *Proc. Natl. Acad. Sci. USA* **98**(9), 5246–5251.

Navia, M. A., Fitzgerald, P. M., McKeever, B. M., Leu, C. T., Heimbach, J. C., Herber, W. K., Sigal, I. S., Darke, P. L., and Springer, J. P. (1989). Three-dimensional structure of aspartyl protease from human immunodeficiency virus HIV-1. *Nature* **337**(6208), 615–620.

Nermut, M. V., Hockley, D. J., Jowett, J. B. M., Jones, I. M., Garreau, M., and Thomas, D. (1994). Fullerene-like organization of HIV gag-protein shell in virus-like particles produced by recombinant baculovirus. *Virology* **198**, 288–296.

Nermut, M. V., Hockley, D. J., Bron, P., Thomas, D., Zhang, W. H., and Jones, I. M. (1998). Further evidence for hexagonal organization of HIV gag protein in prebudding assemblies and immature virus-like particles. *J. Struct. Biol.* **123**(2), 143–149.

Newman, J. L., Butcher, E. W., Patel, D. T., Mikhaylenko, Y., and Summers, M. F. (2004). Flexibility in the P2 domain of the HIV-1 Gag polyprotein. *Protein Sci.* **13**(8), 2101–2107.

Nguyen, D. H., and Hildreth, J. E. (2000). Evidence for budding of human immunodeficiency virus type 1 selectively from glycolipid-enriched membrane lipid rafts. *J. Virol.* **74**(7), 3264–3272.

Nguyen, D. G., Booth, A., Gould, S. J., and Hildreth, J. E. (2003). Evidence that HIV budding in primary macrophages occurs through the exosome release pathway. *J. Biol. Chem.* **278**(52), 52347–52354.

Niedrig, M., Gelderblom, H. R., Pauli, G., Marz, J., Bickhard, H., Wolf, H., and Modrow, S. (1994). Inhibition of infectious human immunodeficiency virus type 1 particle formation by Gag protein-derived peptides. *J. Gen. Virol.* **75**(Pt. 6), 1469–1474.

Nisole, S., Lynch, C., Stoye, J. P., and Yap, M. W. (2004). A Trim5-cyclophilin A fusion protein found in owl monkey kidney cells can restrict HIV-1. *Proc. Natl. Acad. Sci. USA* **101**(36), 13324–13328.

Ohno, H., Aguilar, R. C., Fournier, M. C., Hennecke, S., Cosson, P., and Bonifacino, J. S. (1997). Interaction of endocytic signals from the HIV-1 envelope glycoprotein complex with members of the adaptor medium chain family. *Virology* **238**(2), 305–315.

Ono, A., and Freed, E. O. (2001). Plasma membrane rafts play a critical role in HIV-1 assembly and release. *Proc. Natl. Acad. Sci. USA* **98**(24), 13925–13930.

Ono, A., and Freed, E. O. (2004). Cell-type-dependent targeting of human immunodeficiency virus type 1 assembly to the plasma membrane and the multivesicular body. *J. Virol.* **78**(3), 1552–1563.

Ono, A., and Freed, E. O. (2005). Role of lipid rafts in virus replication. *Adv. Virus Res.* **64**, 311–358.

Ono, A., Demirov, D., and Freed, E. O. (2000). Relationship between human immunodeficiency virus type 1 Gag multimerization and membrane binding. *J. Virol.* **74**(11), 5142–5150.

Ono, A., Orenstein, J. M., and Freed, E. O. (2000). Role of the Gag matrix domain in targeting human immunodeficiency virus type 1 assembly. *J. Virol.* **74**(6), 2855–2866.

Ono, A., Ablan, S. D., Lockett, S. J., Nagashima, K., and Freed, E. O. (2004). Phosphatidylinositol (4,5) bisphosphate regulates HIV-1 Gag targeting to the plasma membrane. *Proc. Natl. Acad. Sci. USA* **101**(41), 14889–14894.

Ono, A., Waheed, A. A., Joshi, A., and Freed, E. O. (2005). Association of human immunodeficiency virus type 1 gag with membrane does not require highly basic sequences in the nucleocapsid: Use of a novel Gag multimerization assay. *J. Virol.* **79**(22), 14131–14140.

Ono, A., Waheed, A. A., and Freed, E. O. (2007). Depletion of cellular cholesterol inhibits membrane binding and higher-order multimerization of human immunodeficiency virus type 1 gag. *Virology* **360**(1), 27–35.

Orenstein, J. M., Meltzer, M. S., Phipps, T., and Gendelman, H. E. (1988). Cytoplasmic assembly and accumulation of human immunodeficiency virus types 1 and 2 in recombinant human colony-stimulating factor-1-treated human monocytes: An ultrastructural study. *J. Virol.* **62**(8), 2578–2586.

Ott, D. E. (1997). Cellular proteins in HIV virions. *Rev. Med. Virol.* **7**(3), 167–180.

Ott, D. E. (2002). Potential roles of cellular proteins in HIV-1. *Rev. Med. Virol.* **12**(6), 359–374.

Owens, R. J., Dubay, J. W., Hunter, E., and Compans, R. W. (1991). Human immunodeficiency virus envelope protein determines the site of virus release in polarized epithelial cells. *Proc. Natl. Acad. Sci. USA* **88**(9), 3987–3991.

Paillart, J. C., Shehu-Xhilaga, M., Marquet, R., and Mak, J. (2004). Dimerization of retroviral RNA genomes: An inseparable pair. *Nat. Rev. Microbiol.* **2**(6), 461–472.

Parent, L. J., Bennett, R. P., Craven, R. C., Nelle, T. D., Krishna, N. K., Bowzard, J. B., Wilson, C. B., Puffer, B. A., Montelaro, R. C., and Wills, J. W. (1995). Positionally independent and exchangeable late budding functions of the Rous sarcoma virus and human immunodeficiency virus Gag proteins. *J. Virol.* **69**(9), 5455–5460.

Pelchen-Matthews, A., Kramer, B., and Marsh, M. (2003). Infectious HIV-1 assembles in late endosomes in primary macrophages. *J. Cell Biol.* **162**(3), 443–455.

Pelchen-Matthews, A., Raposo, G., and Marsh, M. (2004). Endosomes, exosomes and Trojan viruses. *Trends Microbiol.* **12**(7), 310–316.

Perlman, M., and Resh, M. D. (2006). Identification of an intracellular trafficking and assembly pathway for HIV-1 gag. *Traffic* **7**(6), 731–745.

Pettit, S. C., Moody, M. D., Wehbie, R. S., Kaplan, A. H., Nantermet, P. V., Klein, C. A., and Swanstrom, R. (1994). The p2 domain of human immunodeficiency virus type 1 Gag regulates sequential proteolytic processing and is required to produce fully infectious virions. *J. Virol.* **68**(12), 8017–8027.

Pettit, S. C., Henderson, G. J., Schiffer, C. A., and Swanstrom, R. (2002). Replacement of the P1 amino acid of human immunodeficiency virus type 1 Gag processing sites can inhibit or enhance the rate of cleavage by the viral protease. *J. Virol.* **76**(20), 10226–10233.

Pettit, S. C., Everitt, L. E., Choudhury, S., Dunn, B. M., and Kaplan, A. H. (2004). Initial cleavage of the human immunodeficiency virus type 1 GagPol precursor by its activated protease occurs by an intramolecular mechanism. *J. Virol.* **78**(16), 8477–8485.

Poon, D. T., Wu, J., and Aldovini, A. (1996). Charged amino acid residues of human immunodeficiency virus type 1 nucleocapsid p7 protein involved in RNA packaging and infectivity. *J. Virol.* **70**(10), 6607–6616.

Pornillos, O., Alam, S. L., Davis, D. R., and Sundquist, W. I. (2002a). Structure of the Tsg101 UEV domain in complex with the PTAP motif of the HIV-1 p6 protein. *Nat. Struct. Biol.* **9**(11), 812–817.

Pornillos, O., Alam, S. L., Rich, R. L., Myszka, D. G., Davis, D. R., and Sundquist, W. I. (2002b). Structure and functional interactions of the Tsg101 UEV domain. *EMBO J.* **21** (10), 2397–2406.

Pornillos, O., Garrus, J. E., and Sundquist, W. I. (2002). Mechanisms of enveloped RNA virus budding. *Trends Cell Biol.* **12**(12), 569–579.

Puffer, B. A., Parent, L. J., Wills, J. W., and Montelaro, R. C. (1997). Equine infectious anemia virus utilizes a YXXL motif within the late assembly domain of the Gag p9 protein. *J. Virol.* **71**(9), 6541–6546.

Raposo, G., Moore, M., Innes, D., Leijendekker, R., Leigh-Brown, A., Benaroch, P., and Geuze, H. (2002). Human macrophages accumulate HIV-1 particles in MHC II compartments. *Traffic* **3**(10), 718–729.

Reicin, A. S., Ohagen, A., Yin, L., Hoglund, S., and Goff, S. P. (1996). The role of Gag in human immunodeficiency virus type 1 virion morphogenesis and early steps of the viral life cycle. *J. Virol.* **70**(12), 8645–8652.

Reil, H., Bukovsky, A. A., Gelderblom, H. R., and Gottlinger, H. G. (1998). Efficient HIV-1 replication can occur in the absence of the viral matrix protein. *EMBO J.* **17**(9), 2699–2708.

Rein, A. (1994). Retroviral RNA packaging: A review. *Arch. Virol. Suppl.* **9**, 513–522.

Rein, A., Henderson, L. E., and Levin, J. G. (1998). Nucleic-acid-chaperone activity of retroviral nucleocapsid proteins: Significance for viral replication. *Trends Biochem. Sci.* **23**(8), 297–301.

Resh, M. D. (2004). A myristoyl switch regulates membrane binding of HIV-1 Gag. *Proc. Natl. Acad. Sci. USA* **101**(2), 417–418.

Resh, M. D. (2005). Intracellular trafficking of HIV-1 Gag: How Gag interacts with cell membranes and makes viral particles. *AIDS Rev.* **7**(2), 84–91.

Rose, S., Hensley, D. J., O'Shannessy, J., Culp, C., Debouck, C., and Chaiken, I. (1992). Characterisation of HIV-1 p24 self-association using affinity chromatography. *Proteins* **13**, 112–119.

Rous, B. A., Reaves, B. J., Ihrke, G., Briggs, J. A., Gray, S. R., Stephens, D. J., Banting, G., and Luzio, J. P. (2002). Role of adaptor complex AP-3 in targeting wild-type and mutated CD63 to lysosomes. *Mol. Biol. Cell* **13**(3), 1071–1082.

Rowell, J. F., Stanhope, P. E., and Siliciano, R. F. (1995). Endocytosis of endogenously synthesized HIV-1 envelope protein. Mechanism and role in processing for association with class II MHC. *J. Immunol.* **155**(1), 473–488.

Rudner, L., Nydegger, S., Coren, L. V., Nagashima, K., Thali, M., and Ott, D. E. (2005). Dynamic fluorescent imaging of human immunodeficiency virus type 1 gag in live cells by biarsenical labeling. *J. Virol.* **79**(7), 4055–4065.

Russell, R. S., Liang, C., and Wainberg, M. A. (2004). Is HIV-1 RNA dimerization a prerequisite for packaging? Yes, no, probably? *Retrovirology* **1**(1), 23. doi: 10.1186/1742-4690-1-23.

Saad, J. S., Miller, J., Tai, J., Kim, A., Ghanam, R. H., and Summers, M. F. (2006). Structural basis for targeting HIV-1 Gag proteins to the plasma membrane for virus assembly. *Proc. Natl. Acad. Sci. USA* **103**(30), 11364–11369.

Sakaguchi, K., Zambrano, N., Baldwin, E. T., Shapiro, B. A., Erickson, J. W., Omichinski, J. G., Clore, G. M., Gronenborn, A. M., and Appella, E. (1993). Identification of a binding site for the human immunodeficiency virus type 1 nucleocapsid protein. *Proc. Natl. Acad. Sci. USA* **90**(11), 5219–5223.

Sakalian, M., McMurtrey, C. P., Deeg, F. J., Maloy, C. W., Li, F., Wild, C. T., and Salzwedel, K. (2006). 3-o-(3′,3′-dimethysuccinyl) betulinic Acid inhibits maturation of the human immunodeficiency virus type 1 gag precursor assembled *in vitro*. *J. Virol.* **80**(12), 5716–5722.

Sandefur, S., Varthakavi, V., and Spearman, P. (1998). The I domain is required for efficient plasma membrane binding of human immunodeficiency virus type 1 Pr55Gag. *J. Virol.* **72**(4), 2723–2732.

Sandefur, S., Smith, R. M., Varthakavi, V., and Spearman, P. (2000). Mapping and characterization of the N-terminal I domain of human immunodeficiency virus type 1 Pr55(Gag). *J. Virol.* **74**(16), 7238–7249.

Sayah, D. M., Sokolskaja, E., Berthoux, L., and Luban, J. (2004). Cyclophilin A retrotransposition into TRIM5 explains owl monkey resistance to HIV-1. *Nature* **430** (6999), 569–573.

Schmalzbauer, E., Strack, B., Dannull, J., Guehmann, S., and Moelling, K. (1996). Mutations of basic amino acids of NCp7 of human immunodeficiency virus type 1 affect RNA binding *in vitro*. *J. Virol.* **70**(2), 771–777.

Scholz, I., Arvidson, B., Huseby, D., and Barklis, E. (2005). Virus particle core defects caused by mutations in the human immunodeficiency virus capsid N-terminal domain. *J. Virol.* **79**(3), 1470–1479.

Schwartz, M. D., Fiore, D., and Panganiban, A. T. (1997). Distinct functions and requirements for the Cys-His boxes of the human immunodeficiency virus type 1 nucleocapsid protein during RNA encapsidation and replication. *J. Virol.* **71**(12), 9295–9305.

Shehu-Xhilaga, M., Ablan, S., Demirov, D. G., Chen, C., Montelaro, R. C., and Freed, E. O. (2004). Late domain-dependent inhibition of equine infectious anemia virus budding. *J. Virol.* **78**(2), 724–732.

Sherer, N. M., Lehmann, M. J., Jimenez-Soto, L. F., Ingmundson, A., Horner, S. M., Cicchetti, G., Allen, P. G., Pypaert, M., Cunningham, J. M., and Mothes, W. (2003). Visualization of retroviral replication in living cells reveals budding into multivesicular bodies. *Traffic* **4**(11), 785–801.

Shkriabai, N., Datta, S. A., Zhao, Z., Hess, S., Rein, A., and Kvaratskhelia, M. (2006). Interactions of HIV-1 Gag with assembly cofactors. *Biochemistry* **45**(13), 4077–4083.

Simons, K., and Toomre, D. (2000). Lipid rafts and signal transduction. *Nat. Rev. Mol. Cell Biol.* **1**(1), 31–39.

Simons, K., and Vaz, W. L. (2004). Model systems, lipid rafts, and cell membranes. *Annu. Rev. Biophys. Biomol. Struct.* **33**, 269–295.

Sokolskaja, E., Sayah, D. M., and Luban, J. (2004). Target cell cyclophilin A modulates human immunodeficiency virus type 1 infectivity. *J. Virol.* **78**(23), 12800–12808.

South, T. L., Blake, P. R., Sowder, R. C., III, Arthur, L. O., Henderson, L. E., and Summers, M. F. (1990). The nucleocapsid protein isolated from HIV-1 particles binds zinc and forms retroviral-type zinc fingers. *Biochemistry* **29**(34), 7786–7789.

Spearman, P., Horton, R., Ratner, L., and Kuli-Zade, I. (1997). Membrane binding of human immunodeficiency virus type 1 matrix protein *in vivo* supports a conformational myristyl switch mechanism. *J. Virol.* **71**(9), 6582–6592.

Sticht, J., Humbert, M., Findlow, S., Bodem, J., Muller, B., Dietrich, U., Werner, J., and Krausslich, H. G. (2005). A peptide inhibitor of HIV-1 assembly *in vitro*. *Nat. Struct. Mol. Biol.* **12**(8), 671–677.

Strack, B., Calistri, A., and Gottlinger, H. G. (2002). Late assembly domain function can exhibit context dependence and involves ubiquitin residues implicated in endocytosis. *J. Virol.* **76**(11), 5472–5479.

Strack, B., Calistri, A., Craig, S., Popova, E., and Gottlinger, H. G. (2003). AIP1/ALIX is a binding partner for HIV-1 p6 and EIAV p9 functioning in virus budding. *Cell* **114**(6), 689–699.

Stys, D., Blaha, I., and Strop, P. (1993). Structural and functional studies *in vitro* on the p6 protein from the HIV-1 gag open reading frame. *Biochim. Biophys. Acta* **1182**(2), 157–161.

Summers, M. F., Henderson, L. E., Chance, M. R., Bess, J. W., Jr., South, T. L., Blake, P. R., Sagi, I., Perez-Alvarado, G., Sowder, R. C., III, and Hare, D. R. (1992). Nucleocapsid zinc fingers detected in retroviruses: EXAFS studies of intact viruses and the solution-state structure of the nucleocapsid protein from HIV-1. *Protein Sci.* **1**(5), 563–574.

Swanstrom, R., and Wills, J. W. (1997). Synthesis, assembly and processing of viral proteins. *In* "Retroviruses" (J. M. Coffin, S. H. Hughes, and H. E. Varmus, Eds.), pp. 263–334. Cold Spring Harbor Laboratory Press, Plainview, NY.

Tang, C., Loeliger, E., Kinde, I., Kyere, S., Mayo, K., Barklis, E., Sun, Y., Huang, M., and Summers, M. F. (2003). Antiviral inhibition of the HIV-1 capsid protein. *J. Mol. Biol.* **327** (5), 1013–1020.

Tang, C., Loeliger, E., Luncsford, P., Kinde, I., Beckett, D., and Summers, M. F. (2004). Entropic switch regulates myristate exposure in the HIV-1 matrix protein. *Proc. Natl. Acad. Sci. USA* **101**(2), 517–522.

Tang, S., Murakami, T., Agresta, B. E., Campbell, S., Freed, E. O., and Levin, J. G. (2001). Human immunodeficiency virus type 1 N-terminal capsid mutants that exhibit aberrant core morphology and are blocked in initiation of reverse transcription in infected cells. *J. Virol.* 75(19), 9357–9366.

Tanzi, G. O., Piefer, A. J., and Bates, P. (2003). Equine infectious anemia virus utilizes host vesicular protein sorting machinery during particle release. *J. Virol.* 77(15), 8440–8447.

Temesgen, Z., Warnke, D., and Kasten, M. J. (2006). Current status of antiretroviral therapy. *Expert Opin. Pharmacother.* 7(12), 1541–1554.

Ternois, F., Sticht, J., Duquerroy, S., Krausslich, H. G., and Rey, F. A. (2005). The HIV-1 capsid protein C-terminal domain in complex with a virus assembly inhibitor. *Nat. Struct. Mol. Biol.* 12(8), 678–682.

Thali, M., Bukovsky, A., Kondo, E., Rosenwirth, B., Walsh, C. T., Sodroski, J., and Gottlinger, H. G. (1994). Functional association of cyclophilin A with HIV-1 virions. *Nature* 372(6504), 363–365.

Tremblay, M. J., Fortin, J. F., and Cantin, R. (1998). The acquisition of host-encoded proteins by nascent HIV-1. *Immunol. Today* 19(8), 346–351.

Tritch, R. J., Cheng, Y. E., Yin, F. H., and Erickson-Viitanen, S. (1991). Mutagenesis of protease cleavage sites in the human immunodeficiency virus type 1 gag polyprotein. *J. Virol.* 65(2), 922–930.

Turner, B. G., and Summers, M. F. (1999). Structural biology of HIV. *J. Mol. Biol.* 285(1), 1–32.

VerPlank, L., Bouamr, F., LaGrassa, T. J., Agresta, B., Kikonyogo, A., Leis, J., and Carter, C. A. (2001). Tsg101, a homologue of ubiquitin-conjugating (E2) enzymes, binds the L domain in HIV type 1 Pr55(Gag). *Proc. Natl. Acad. Sci. USA* 98(14), 7724–7729.

Vogt, V. M. (1996). Proteolytic processing and particle maturation. *Curr. Top. Microbiol. Immunol.* 214, 95–131.

Vogt, V. M. (2000). Ubiquitin in retrovirus assembly: Actor or bystander? *Proc. Natl. Acad. Sci. USA* 97(24), 12945–12947.

Vogt, V. M. (2005). Blocking HIV-1 virus assembly. *Nat. Struct. Mol. Biol.* 12(8), 638–639.

von Schwedler, U. K., Stemmler, T. L., Klishko, V. Y., Li, S., Albertine, K. H., Davis, D. R., and Sundquist, W. I. (1998). Proteolytic refolding of the HIV-1 capsid protein amino-terminus facilitates viral core assembly. *EMBO J.* 17(6), 1555–1568.

von Schwedler, U. K., Stray, K. M., Garrus, J. E., and Sundquist, W. I. (2003a). Functional surfaces of the human immunodeficiency virus type 1 capsid protein. *J. Virol.* 77(9), 5439–5450.

von Schwedler, U. K., Stuchell, M., Muller, B., Ward, D. M., Chung, H. Y., Morita, E., Wang, H. E., Davis, T., He, G. P., Cimbora, D. M., Scott, A., Krausslich, H. G., et al. (2003b). The protein network of HIV budding. *Cell* 114(6), 701–713.

Wang, C. T., Zhang, Y., McDermott, J., and Barklis, E. (1993). Conditional infectivity of a human immunodeficiency virus matrix domain deletion mutant. *J. Virol.* 67(12), 7067–7076.

Wang, C. T., Lai, H. Y., and Li, J. J. (1998). Analysis of minimal human immunodeficiency virus type 1 gag coding sequences capable of virus-like particle assembly and release. *J. Virol.* 72(10), 7950–7959.

Wang, H., Machesky, N. J., and Mansky, L. M. (2004). Both the PPPY and PTAP motifs are involved in human T-cell leukemia virus type 1 particle release. *J. Virol.* 78(3), 1503–1512.

Welker, R., Hohenberg, H., Tessmer, U., Huckhagel, C., and Krausslich, H. G. (2000). Biochemical and structural analysis of isolated mature cores of human immunodeficiency virus type 1. *J. Virol.* 74(3), 1168–1177.

Wiegers, K., Rutter, G., Kottler, H., Tessmer, U., Hohenberg, H., and Krausslich, H. G. (1998). Sequential steps in human immunodeficiency virus particle maturation revealed by alterations of individual Gag polyprotein cleavage sites. *J. Virol.* 72(4), 2846–2854.

Wills, J. W., and Craven, R. C. (1991). Form, function, and use of retroviral gag proteins. *AIDS* **5**, 639–654.

Wilk, T., Gross, I., Gowen, B. E., Rutten, T., de Haas, F., Welker, R., Krausslich, H. G., Boulanger, P., and Fuller, S. D. (2001). Organization of immature human immunodeficiency virus type 1. *J. Virol.* **75**(2), 759–771.

Wlodawer, A., and Erickson, J. W. (1993). Structure-based inhibitors of HIV-1 protease. *Annu. Rev. Biochem.* **62**, 543–585.

Wlodawer, A., and Vondrasek, J. (1998). Inhibitors of HIV-1 protease: A major success of structure-assisted drug design. *Annu. Rev. Biophys. Biomol. Struct.* **27**, 249–284.

Wlodawer, A., Miller, M., Jaskolski, M., Sathyanarayana, B. K., Baldwin, E., Weber, I. T., Selk, L. M., Clawson, L., Schneider, J., and Kent, S. B. (1989). Conserved folding in retroviral proteases: Crystal structure of a synthetic HIV-1 protease. *Science* **245**(4918), 616–621.

Worthylake, D. K., Wang, H., Yoo, S., Sundquist, W. I., and Hill, C. P. (1999). Structures of the HIV-1 capsid protein dimerization domain at 2.6 A resolution. *Acta Crystallogr. D Biol. Crystallogr.* **55**(Pt. 1), 85–92.

Wu, Z., Alexandratos, J., Ericksen, B., Lubkowski, J., Gallo, R. C., and Lu, W. (2004). Total chemical synthesis of N-myristoylated HIV-1 matrix protein p17: Structural and mechanistic implications of p17 myristoylation. *Proc. Natl. Acad. Sci. USA* **101**(32), 11587–11592.

Wyma, D. J., Jiang, J., Shi, J., Zhou, J., Lineberger, J. E., Miller, M. D., and Aiken, C. (2004). Coupling of human immunodeficiency virus type 1 fusion to virion maturation: A novel role of the gp41 cytoplasmic tail. *J. Virol.* **78**(7), 3429–3435.

Yeager, M., Wilson-Kubalek, E. M., Weiner, S. G., Brown, P. O., and Rein, A. (1998). Supramolecular organization of immature and mature murine leukemia virus revealed by electron cryo-microscopy: Implications for retroviral assembly mechanisms. *Proc. Natl. Acad. Sci. USA* **95**, 7299–7304.

Yu, X., Yuan, X., Matsuda, Z., Lee, T. H., and Essex, M. (1992). The matrix protein of human immunodeficiency virus type 1 is required for incorporation of viral envelope protein into mature virions. *J. Virol.* **66**(8), 4966–4971.

Yuan, B., Campbell, S., Bacharach, E., Rein, A., and Goff, S. P. (2000). Infectivity of Moloney murine leukemia virus defective in late assembly events is restored by late assembly domains of other retroviruses. *J. Virol.* **74**(16), 7250–7260.

Yuan, X., Yu, X., Lee, T. H., and Essex, M. (1993). Mutations in the N-terminal region of human immunodeficiency virus type 1 matrix protein block intracellular transport of the Gag precursor. *J. Virol.* **67**(11), 6387–6394.

Zhang, Y., and Barklis, E. (1995). Nucleocapsid protein effects on the specificity of retrovirus RNA encapsidation. *J. Virol.* **69**(9), 5716–5722.

Zhou, W., and Resh, M. D. (1996). Differential membrane binding of the human immunodeficiency virus type 1 matrix protein. *J. Virol.* **70**(12), 8540–8548.

Zhou, J., Yuan, X., Dismuke, D., Forshey, B. M., Lundquist, C., Lee, K. H., Aiken, C., and Chen, C. H. (2004). Small-molecule inhibition of human immunodeficiency virus type 1 replication by specific targeting of the final step of virion maturation. *J. Virol.* **78**(2), 922–929.

Zhou, J., Huang, L., Hachey, D. L., Chen, C. H., and Aiken, C. (2005). Inhibition of HIV-1 maturation via drug association with the viral Gag protein in immature HIV-1 particles. *J. Biol. Chem.* **280**(51), 42149–42155.

Zhou, W., Parent, L. J., Wills, J. W., and Resh, M. D. (1994). Identification of a membrane-binding domain within the amino-terminal region of human immunodeficiency virus type 1 Gag protein which interacts with acidic phospholipids. *J. Virol.* **68**(4), 2556–2569.

John L. Foster and J. Victor Garcia

Department of Internal Medicine, University of Texas Southwestern
Medical Center, Dallas, Texas 75390

Role of Nef in HIV-1 Replication and Pathogenesis

I. Chapter Overview

Nef is a pathogenic factor of *Human immunodeficiency virus* (HIV). Assessment of the role of Nef in the development of AIDS will require model systems that reflect to a significant degree the anatomical, developmental, regulatory features of the human immune system under assault by HIV-1. Relatively simple *in vitro* HIV-1 infection models include peripheral blood mononuclear cells (PBMCs), T cells, dendritic cell–T cell cocultures, thymic organ cultures, and tonsil cultures. Two general conclusions from investigations with these systems are: (1) A positive Nef effect on viral replication is most obvious in partially activated T cells, and (2) CXCR4 (X4) trophic

Advances in Pharmacology, Volume 55
Copyright © 2000, 2007, Elsevier Inc. All rights reserved.

1054-3589/07 $35.00
DOI: 10.1016/S1054-3589(07)55011-8

virus is more cytopathic than CCR5 (R5) trophic virus. Investigations with the SCID-hu model for HIV-1 infection confirmed and extended work with *in vitro* systems. It was found that Nef is a replication and pathogenesis factor for X4 virus, but largely a replication factor for R5 virus since these viruses are minimally pathogenic in the SCID-hu model. Mechanistically, the enhancement of viral replication and pathogensis by Nef remains obscure, but could involve one or more of the following *in vitro* activities of Nef: (1) CD4 downregulation, (2) activation of cell signaling pathways, (3) MHC I downregulation, and (4) the ability of Nef to enhance virus particle infectivity. Ongoing studies have yielded several mutants of Nef that are specifically defective for the first three of these Nef functions, which will greatly facilitate mechanistic studies. The recent development of mouse/human xenograph models that mimic to a significant extent the intact human immune system together with novel HIV/SIV chimeras that replicate in macaque PBMCs will allow precise correlations between Nef functions and viral replication and pathogenesis. These studies in turn will help define the *in vivo* role of Nef in the development of AIDS.

II. Introduction

Since the first case reports of acquired immunodeficiency syndrome (AIDS) over 20 years ago, great strides have been made in our understanding of the basic molecular mechanisms of its etiological agent, HIV. The enormous effort to understand HIV has been complemented by investigation of other closely related primate lentiviruses. Like all retroviruses, the genomes of primate lentiviruses contain *gag*, *pol*, and *env* genes that encode well-characterized structural and enzymatic proteins essential for proper virus processing and assembly. In addition, primate lentiviruses encode six or seven accessory genes. The two best characterized accessory genes, *tat* and *rev*, encode essential regulators of viral gene expression (Cullen, 1991, 1998; Emerman and Malim, 1998). In contrast, the remaining accessory genes play less well-defined roles in viral replication and pathogenesis. Much ambiguity, for example, remains about the function of the *nef* accessory gene encoded by HIV-1, HIV-2, and *Simian immunodeficiency virus* (SIV).

Nef is a small myristolylated phosphoprotein (varying in size from 25,000 for HIV-1 to 33,000 Da for SIV) that is largely localized in the paranuclear region of the cell with small amounts present at the plasma membrane. It is a major determinant of primate lentivirus pathogenicity, as a large deletion in the *nef* gene greatly reduces the severity of SIV-induced disease in rhesus macaques (Kestler *et al.*, 1991). Furthermore, following intravenous injection of macaques with SIV encoding a *nef* gene with a point mutation giving a premature stop codon, the *nef* open reading frame (ORF) is rapidly restored. This demonstrates that there is significant selective pressure to express Nef (Kestler *et al.*, 1991). In humans, there is also a correlation between infection with *nef*-defective HIV-1 and a dramatically decreased rate of disease progression (Deacon *et al.*, 1995; Kirchhoff *et al.*, 1995; Learmont *et al.*, 1999; Salvi *et al.*, 1998).

Although strong evidence exists that Nef plays a role in pathogenesis *in vivo*, only correlative studies can be done in humans. Studies in SIV models are limited in that SIVs may exhibit fundamentally different mechanisms of pathogenesis than are present in the human disease. Specifically, Schindler *et al.* (2006) have suggested that the absence of CD3 downregulation by Nef is of crucial importance in determining the pathogenesis of primate lentiviruses. SIVs, which are nonpathogenic in their hosts, have Nefs that downregulate CD3 but chimpanzee and human immunodeficiency viruses do not. Schindler *et al.* suggests that the lack of this function makes the chimp/human virus intrinsically pathogenic. This notion of intrinsic pathogenicity of the chimp virus in humans is confirmed by the fact that the minor clades of HIV-1, Group N and O viruses, cause AIDS (Hahn *et al.*, 2000; Roques *et al.*, 2002, 2004).[1] However, the extant chimpanzee virus is nonpathogenic in chimps, therefore, this model would require that earlier forms of the chimpanzee immunodeficiency virus were pathogenic. Subsequently, the pathogenic chimp virus would have adapted to be nonpathogenic by a mechanism independent of Nef-induced CD3 downregulation and therefore specific to the chimpanzee. Thus, the Nef-induced CD3 downregulation model may explain why the human virus is *not* nonpathogenic but offers little direction for determining the actual mechanism of HIV-1 pathogenicity. The obvious need is to study the infection of human cells by human virus in order to determine why the human virus is pathogenic. This is most readily achieved by *in vitro* infection of PBMCs. Efforts to create more complex models that better reflect HIV-1 disease have led to development of several infection systems, including the thymic organ culture (TOC) and the SCID-hu thymic implant models. Results from these models are not

---

[1] Hahn and coworkers (Keele *et al.*, 2006) have recently expanded our knowledge of the origins of HIV-1 by conducting a molecular epidemiological field study of SIV_{cpz} in wild chimpanzees in Cameroon. Isolated chimpanzee communities that harbor virus closely related to HIV-1 Groups M and N were identified and characterized. HIV-1 Group M related chimpanzee virus was found in the extreme southeast of Cameroon and virus closely related to Group N was found in south, central Cameroon. Chimpanzees infected with virus closely related to Group O have yet to be found. Cameroon had been suspected as the geographical source of HIV-1 since all HIV-1 Group M subtypes are located there. That all three Groups of HIV-1 including all subtypes of Group M are pathogenic suggests that the chimpanzee virus is directly pathogenic to humans. Further, it appears that all subtypes of Group M HIV-1 are highly transmissible since all subtypes are found in Kinshasa, Mbandaka, and Mbuji-Mayi, which are cities that are hundreds of miles south and east of Cameroon (Vidal *et al.*, 2000). Why Groups N and O failed to expand beyond the borders of Cameroon is a question of major import since transmissibility is a property of equal significance to pathogenicity for a pandemic virus.

only consistent with the data from macaques of a significant contribution by *nef* to viral pathogenicity, but have also demonstrated a complex interplay between virus-induced pathogenesis, the level of viral replication, and viral tropism that is not yet amenable to mechanistic interpretation.

III. Nef and HIV-1 Infection of PBMCs

The importance of Nef for replication *in vivo* is not always recapitulated *in vitro*. Nef was originally characterized as a negative regulator of HIV replication and was thus named *Negative Factor* (Ahmad and Venkatesan, 1988; Terwilliger *et al.*, 1986). As would occur with many subsequent observations about Nef, however, these eponymous findings were later refuted (Hammes *et al.*, 1989; Kim *et al.*, 1989). Although some still suggest that an unusual Nef isolate may have a negative effect (Fackler *et al.*, 2001), most investigators find that Nef has either no effect or a positive effect on viral replication *in vitro*. *nef* has no effect with quiescent T cells since HIV-1 does not readily infect these cells and the presence or absence of a functional Nef is not relevant. Also in fully activated T cells, viral replication is maximal with or without Nef. For example, Nef generally has no effect on viral replication in T-cell lines, activated PBMC (Hammes *et al.*, 1989; Jamieson *et al.*, 1994; Kestler *et al.*, 1991), or mature dendritic cell–T cell cocultures (Messmer *et al.*, 2000). On the other hand, a significant role for Nef in viral replication has been found in postinfection-stimulated PBMC (Miller *et al.*, 1994; Spina *et al.*, 1994), chronically immune-activated PBMC (Shapira-Nahor *et al.*, 2002), immature dendritic cell–T cell cocultures (Lundquist *et al.*, 2002; Messmer *et al.*, 2000), TOCs (Su *et al.*, 1997), and *ex vivo* tonsil culture systems (Glushakova *et al.*, 1999; Stove *et al.*, 2003). Thus, a positive effect of Nef in virus replication is most obvious in less than fully activated cells.

The pathogenicity of a particular HIV-1 isolate may be determined by HIV-1 genes other than *nef*. This has been clearly documented for *env* by Schweighardt *et al.* (2004) in activated PBMC where Nef has little or no effect on replication. These investigators determined that coreceptor usage can dictate pathogenesis. For these studies, the authors first confirmed that a large majority of PBMCs expressed high levels of CXCR4 (X4) but few (2%) expressed CCR5 (R5). CD3 plus CD28 stimulation of PBMCs was found to strongly activate T cells to divide and induce about 8% of the cells to express CCR5. Despite the discrepancy in the number of target cells, the R5 virus, HIV-1JR-CSF, replicated to comparable levels to the highly infectious X4 virus, HIV-1LAI. Analysis of changes of cell populations in the *in vitro* cultures revealed that LAI rapidly killed the cells of the culture while JR-CSF did not. The results from this simple system provide evidence that reduced or lack of pathogenicity can be an advantage in long-term replication. Therefore, T-cell activation state, coreceptor utilization by the infecting virus, and Nef function must be considered before interpreting the results from HIV-1 infections.

IV. Nef Studies in Human Thymic Systems

HIV-1 infection of SCID mice implanted with human fetal thymus and liver (SCID-hu) can lead to the massive depletion of double positive (DP) thymocytes (Bonyhadi et al., 1993). Although in early studies some primary isolates rapidly proliferated and were highly cytopathic (rapid-high) and some were found to grow slowly and exhibit weak cytopathicity (slow-low) (Kaneshima et al., 1994), other investigators utilizing molecularly cloned virus have demonstrated a dissociation of replication and pathogenesis. Specifically, viruses with an intact *nef* ORF replicate faster, and achieve a higher titer than a *nef* deleted counterpart (Jamieson et al., 1994). This was the case for an X4 virus, HIV-1 NL4-3, and an R5 virus, JR-CSF. (Note: coreceptor usage had not yet been discovered.) In contrast, the pathogenic potential of these two viruses were not the same. It was observed that intact NL4-3 obliterated CD4+/CD8+ DP T cells in the implant by 6 weeks, while NL4-3 with *nef* inactivated had little effect on cell viability. JR-CSF with an intact *nef* gene was weakly cytopathic recapitulating the PBMC results of Schweighardt et al. (2004). It should be noted that the X4 virus, NL4-3, replicated to tenfold higher levels in this system than the R5-utlizing JR-CSF. Thus, as early as 1994 a difference was found between the cytopathogenicity of X4 and R5 viruses even though both were found to efficiently replicate in the SCID-hu model.

Other investigators have taken advantage of the availability of *env* sequences from a virus isolated from a laboratory worker (LW) infected with HIV-1 from the HTLV-IIIB isolate (Lori et al., 1992; Reitz et al., 1994; Weiss et al., 1988). The HTLV-IIIB isolate (X4) was highly attenuated by *in vitro* passage (Chang et al., 1993). This isolate and its derived molecular clone HXB2 replicate in activated PBMCs and T-cell lines but fail to replicate in SCID-hu or TOC (Duus et al., 2001; Su et al., 1997). HXB2 is pathogenic in the Jurkat T-cell line, but weakly pathogenic in purified primary T cells (Cao et al., 1994). *env*-coding sequence was derived from LW at least 2 years after infection and found to still utilize CXCR4 (Miller et al., 2001). When it was incorporated into HXB2 which is defective for *nef* (HXB2/LW) this *nef*-defective chimeric virus was found to be highly competent for replication in thymic cells but not pathogenic in either SCID-hu or TOC (Duus et al., 2001). Repair of the *nef* reading frame in HXB2/LW did indeed result in a pathogenic virus but there was no further enhancement of replication (Duus et al., 2001).

The SCID-hu model for HIV-1 infection represents a major advance in the study HIV-1 replication and pathogenesis. As discussed above, evidence has been presented that Nef is both an important pathogenic and replication factor for X4 viruses in this system. For R5 viruses, Nef may only be a replication factor since these viruses are minimally pathogenic in SCID-hu. Clearly, the studies discussed represent only a few viral isolates and generalizations are tentative. For example, HXB2 and HXB2/LW both utilize X4, but only HXB2/LW will replicate in monocyte-derived macrophages (MDM). A threonine in the V3 loop of LW *env* that is alanine in HXB2 was considered as the reason for this difference, but this T to A mutation in *nef* had no effect on the ability of HXB2/LW to replicate in MDM. Surprisingly, a different result was obtained in SCID-hu and TOC where HXB2/LW also actively replicates but HXB2 does not. The back mutation of the V3 loop T to A abrogates the ability of HXB2/LW to replicate in thymocytes (Miller *et al.*, 2001). Further confusing the situation is the fact that NL4-3 which as mentioned above is pathogenic in the SCID-hu model has alanine (like HXB2) not threonine. Model-specific results are difficult to interpret and point out the complexity of the problem of understanding the mechanism of Nef effects on viral replication and pathogenesis, and suggest that the cytopathic effect of HIV-1 is highly dependent on the lineage of the infected cell.

V. Mechanism of Nef Enhancement of Replication and Pathogenesis

Four *in vitro* activities common to both HIV and SIV Nefs have been clearly demonstrated (Fig. 1). Each or even all of these could be involved in Nef's role in replication and pathogenesis. Specifically, Nef (1) downregulates cell surface levels of CD4 (Aiken *et al.*, 1996; Anderson *et al.*, 1994; Garcia and Miller, 1991; Lundquist *et al.*, 2002; Mangasarian *et al.*, 1997), (2) mediates cellular signaling and activation (Arora *et al.*, 2000; Renkema and Saksela, 2000; Simmons *et al.*, 2001, 2005; Wei *et al.*, 2005), (3) downregulates surface levels of major histocompatibility class I (MHC I) molecules (Blagoveshchenskaya *et al.*, 2002; Kasper *et al.*, 2005; Schwartz *et al.*, 1996; Williams *et al.*, 2005), and (4) enhances virus infectivity by CD4-independent mechanisms (Aiken, 1997; Campbell *et al.*, 2004; Chowers *et al.*, 1994; Luo *et al.*, 1997; Miller *et al.*, 1995). These four functions (Table 1) were reviewed in detail in Arora *et al.* (2002).

Each of these four Nef functions can serve as a basis for possible explanations of Nef's elusive role in replication and pathogenesis. Several reports have suggested the importance of removing CD4 from the surface of infected cells for the production of infectious HIV-1 particles (Arganaraz *et al.*, 2003; Lundquist *et al.*, 2002). Without this Nef function CD4 can bind to Env present on the viral particle and interfere with the production of fully infectious particles. Also, Nef-mediated cellular activation of cell

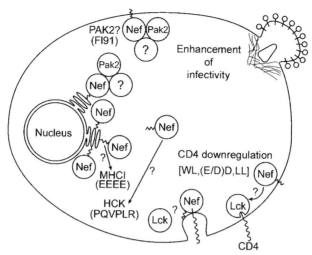

FIGURE 1   Putative cellular locations corresponding to the multiple Nef activities. "Nef" in circles with wavy line represents the myristoylated Nef protein. Multiple Nefs at the Golgi apparatus represent the fact that Nef is predominately localized in the paranuclear region with a small amount bound to the plasma membrane (left). MHCI represents the action of Nef to downregulate MHC I from the cell surface. The "?" indicates that the mechanism of MHCI downregulation remains unknown. EEEE represents amino acids 62–65 of the Nef protein that have been reported to be required for the paranuclear localization of Nef and the downregulation of MHC I proteins. PAK2 represents the activation of Pak2 by Nef by an unknown mechanism at an unknown cellular location (top left). Nef is bound in a membrane-associated complex with Pak2 and an unknown number of other proteins represented by the circles labeled as Pak2 and "?." It is not known on which cellular membrane this activation takes place therefore the Nef–Pak2 activation complex is represented as occurring in either the Golgi or the plasma membrane. F191 represents a Nef residue that when mutated results in Nef specifically defective for Pak2 activation. The role of Nef in enhancement of infectivity of the HIV-1 virion is represented by "Enhancement of infectivity" (top right). One postulated mechanism for this Nef effect is that Nef directly or indirectly facilitates the passage of the viral core through cortical actin. The ball and stick figures represent Env present on the surface of a fusing HIV-1 virion. The thimble-shaped figure represents the viral core of a *nef*[+] HIV-1 virion penetrating the cortical actin sheath. There are no known mutations that specifically inactivate enhancement of infectivity though mutation of PQVPLR or WL exhibit multiple defects including enhancement of infectivity. The ability of Nef to remove CD4 from the cell surface is represented by "CD4 downregulation" (lower right). It is not known if plasma membrane bound Nef interacts with the p56^{lck} bound to the cytoplasmic domain of CD4 as indicated by the arrow and "?." The possibility that Nef interacts with the cytoplasmic tail of CD4 after the displacement of p56^{lck} and during endocytosis of the CD4 molecule prior to targeting for digestion in lysosomes is represented by Nef bound to the cytoplasmic tail of CD4 with a displaced p56^{lck} and a "?." [WL, (E/D)D, LL] represents the specific CD4 downregulation mutations reported to date. Finally, HCK represents the putative binding of cytosolic Nef to Hck and activation of this tyrosine kinase (center). (PQVPLR) represents the putative SH3 binding domain of Nef that binds to Hck.

TABLE I   Summary of Nef Activities

In vitro *activity*	*References*
CD4 downregulation	Aiken *et al.*, 1996; Anderson *et al.*, 1994; Garcia and Miller, 1991; Lundquist *et al.*, 2002; Mangasarian *et al.*, 1997
MHC I downregulation	Blagoveshchenskaya *et al.*, 2002; Kasper *et al.*, 2005; Schwartz *et al.*, 1996; Williams *et al.*, 2005
Cellular signaling and activation	Arora *et al.*, 2000; Renkema and Saksela, 2000; Simmons *et al.*, 2001, 2005; Wei *et al.*, 2005
Infectivity enhancement	Aiken, 1997; Campbell *et al.*, 2004; Chowers *et al.*, 1994; Luo *et al.*, 1997; Miller *et al.*, 1995

signaling pathways could enhance viral replication in partially stimulated T cells. In other words, if Nef functions *in vivo* to elevate the activation level of certain partially activated T-cell populations, then the availability of targets for productive infection would be expanded resulting in greater pathogenicity. Of particular interest in this regard are the memory T cells in the gut that are early targets of HIV-1 and SIV infection, despite the lack of expression of classic T-cell activation markers (Brenchley *et al.*, 2004; Li *et al.*, 2005; Mattapallil *et al.*, 2005). A third possible Nef mechanism is that the downmodulation of MHC I molecules could facilitate HIV immune evasion and thus enhance replication *in vivo*, without effecting replication *in vitro* (Collins *et al.*, 1998; Yang *et al.*, 2002). Finally, the well-documented Nef-dependent enhancement of the infectivity of viral particles would be expected to accelerate the spread of virus *in vivo*. This function of Nef is observed in single-cycle infection assays and is distinct from the role that CD4 downregulation can play in the production of competent HIV-1 virions since it is observed with virus produced in the absence of CD4 (Aiken and Trono, 1995; Luo *et al.*, 1997, 1998; Miller *et al.*, 1995). The mechanism of Nef's enhancement of infectivity remains unknown (Khan *et al.*, 2001; Wei *et al.*, 2003), although one interesting suggestion is that Nef acts directly as an intravirion constituent or indirectly to facilitate the passage of the viral core through cortical actin (Campbell *et al.*, 2004). In addition, Wu and Marsh (2001) have presented data indicating that the Nef effect observed in poststimulation-activated PBMC (Chowers *et al.*, 1994; Miller *et al.*, 1994) is independent of the enhancement of infectivity effect observed in single infection assays. Unfortunately, the lack of understanding of the mechanism of Nef's enhancement of the infectivity of viral particles is compounded by the lack of mutations that specifically block this function (Foster *et al.*, 2001; O'Neill *et al.*, 2006). Considerably more mutational analysis is available on CD4 downregulation, activation of cell signaling pathways, and MHC I downregulation. Further, mutations at least partially specific for each of these last three functions have been described, which allow preliminary structure–function relationships to be addressed. These three Nef functions will now be discussed in greater detail.

A. CD4 Downmodulation by Nef

The first and most extensively characterized function of Nef is its ability to dramatically reduce the steady state levels of CD4 on the cell surface (Garcia and Miller, 1992; Guy et al., 1987). CD4 is downmodulated by almost all Nefs, in all mammalian cell types tested, and under nearly all experimental conditions tested (Anderson et al., 1993; Benson et al., 1993; Garcia et al., 1993; Mariani and Skowronski, 1993). At least two enhancements to virus replication are proposed to result from downmodulation of CD4, the primary receptor for both HIV and SIV. First, Benson et al. (1993) have demonstrated that SIV Nef expression renders human T-cell lines resistant to HIV infection, suggesting Nef prevents disadvantageous superinfection of the host cell. A second role for Nef may be in overcoming the detrimental effects of high cellular CD4 expression in the producer cell that has been shown both to inhibit progeny release and to decrease viral infectivity by sequestration of viral Env (Lama, 2003; Lama et al., 1999; Lundquist et al., 2002; Ross et al., 1999).

Nef-induced CD4 downmodulation involves the internalization of surface CD4 followed by degradation via the endosomal–lysosomal pathway (Anderson et al., 1994; Luo et al., 1996). Consistent with this mechanism Nef increases the number of CD4 containing clathrin-coated pits (Foti et al., 1997). Inhibition of lysosomal acidification blocks Nef-induced CD4 degradation, without restoring CD4 surface expression (Luo et al., 1996; Sanfridson et al., 1994; Rhee and Marsh, 1994). Moreover, Nef-induced CD4 downmodulation is blocked by transdominant-negative dynamin-1 coexpression (Le Gall et al., 2000), as well as pharmacological inhibitors (Luo et al., 2001) of clathrin-coated pit-mediated endocytosis.

Much work is still required in order to elucidate the molecular mediators of Nef-induced CD4 downmodulation and establish a definitive model. Unlike CD4 downmodulation by phorbol esters, Nef-induced downmodulation is independent of phosphorylation of serine residues on the CD4 cytoplasmic tail (Garcia and Miller, 1991). Indeed, current data suggest that Nef acts as a connector between CD4 and elements of the cell's endocytic machinery (Mangasarian et al., 1997). The cytoplasmic domain of CD4 is both necessary and sufficient for Nef-induced CD4 downregulation (Anderson et al., 1994; Garcia et al., 1993). While SIV Nef and HIV Nef utilize distinct residues in the membrane proximal cytoplasmic tail of CD4, both rely on an overlapping region containing a dileucine motif (Hua and Cullen, 1997). Furthermore, NMR and yeast-two-hybrid analysis indicate that the CD4 dileucine motif is necessary for its interaction with Nef (Grzesiek et al.,

1996; Rossi *et al.*, 1996). Nef residues W57 and L58 predicted by NMR to be critical in this interaction (Grzesiek *et al.*, 1996) have also been functionally demonstrated to be important for CD4 downmodulation (Mangasarian *et al.*, 1999) and enhancement of infectivity (Miller *et al.*, 1997). The role of this proposed interaction between Nef and the cytoplasmic tail of CD4 is obscured by the fact that it is weak, but the interaction of p56^{lck} and CD4 is strong and the p56^{lck}–CD4 complex is not subject to rapid endocytosis (Marsh and Pelchen-Matthews, 1996; Pelchen-Matthews *et al.*, 1998).

How Nef connects to the endocytic machinery is unclear but the AP-2 adaptor complexes have been implicated because Nef colocalizes with AP-2 (Greenberg *et al.*, 1997). Moreover, a possible leucine-based sorting motif (L164 and L165) in the C-terminal flexible loop of Nef has also been shown to be important for CD4 downmodulation and for AP-2 colocalization (Bresnahan *et al.*, 1999; Craig *et al.*, 1998; Greenberg *et al.*, 1998). Most data suggest that HIV Nef interacts weakly with AP-2 (Craig *et al.*, 2000). SIV Nef, in contrast, shows a more striking interaction with the μ chain of AP-2 (Bresnahan *et al.*, 1999; Lock *et al.*, 1999; Piguet *et al.*, 1998).

A third pair of Nef amino acids specifically involved in the downregulation of CD4 is E/D174 and D175. However, a mechanistic role remains unknown (Iafrate *et al.*, 1997). Mutation of each of these three amino acid pairs [W57/L58, L164/L165, and (E/D)174/D175] to Ala results in CD4 downregulation-defective Nefs. Stoddart *et al.* (2003) employed these mutations to investigate the role of CD4 downregulation in HIV-1 pathogenesis in the SCID-hu model. In addition, mutation of the putative SH3-binding domain of Nef that is defective in MHC I downregulation, p21-activated protein kinase 2 (Pak2) activation, and enhancement of virion infectivity, but not CD4 downregulation was employed (Stoddart *et al.*, 2003). These mutations were incorporated into the cytopathic NL4-3 (X4) molecular clone and virus produced for injection into SCID-hu implants. At 6 weeks, only small statistically nonsignificant effects on virus replication were observed with virus bearing the above mutations. However, in one experiment with tissue derived from a single donor there was significant diminution of CD4+/CD8+ thymocyte killing with the L164/L165 and W57/L58 mutations but not the SH3-binding domain or (E/D)174/D175 mutations. A second experiment with a different tissue donor gave statistically significant diminution of DP with (E/D)174/D175 mutations but not W57/L58 or SH3-binding domain mutations. Experimental variation was attributed to differences in the response of cells from different donors with regard to optimal dose of virus, time course of the onset of cell death, and susceptibility to infection. These factors have been reported to result in 20- to 30-fold differences in viral production in replicate mice (Rabin *et al.*, 1996). As a result, interpretation of the data in this report is difficult and the role of CD4 downregulation in cell killing by HIV-1 remains to be confirmed. These results do point out the need for models in which continuous monitoring of virus levels can be carried out throughout the course of a single infection.

B. Cellular Activation and Signaling by Nef

A large body of work has investigated Nef-mediated perturbations in cellular signaling (Biggs *et al.*, 1999; Manninen *et al.*, 2001; Muthumani *et al.*, 2005; Simmons *et al.*, 2001, 2005). Although conflicting findings have been reported, convincing evidence implicates Nef in cellular activation. Some of the strongest evidence supporting a role for Nef in T-cell activation comes from experiments using a quiescent IL-2-dependent T-cell line derived from macaques. Infection of these cells with SIV constructs containing either SIV or HIV *nef* not only induces IL-2 production, but also enhances virus replication 8- to 100-fold (Alexander *et al.*, 1997). Microarray analysis using Jurkat cells further demonstrated that Nef activates T cells in a way that mimics T-cell receptor engagement (Simmons *et al.*, 2001). In addition, Nef expression leads to the upregulation of a number of genes whose products are known to activate the HIV LTR (Simmons *et al.*, 2001). In some cases, the upregulated genes express secreted products that have been shown to enhance *in vitro* HIV replication when added to culture media (Simmons *et al.*, 2001). Thus, the paracrine effects of Nef-induced factors may be sufficient to enhance replication. Similar findings have been reported with human macrophages. Supernatants from macrophages infected with adenovirus vectors expressing Nef can facilitate HIV replication in resting lymphoid cultures (Swingler *et al.*, 1999). Interestingly, Nef also upregulates expression of cellular proteins that facilitate the actions of Tat (Simmons *et al.*, 2001). Complementary and confirmatory data in this general respect were obtained using HeLa cells expressing wild-type Nef and two Nefs defective in myristoylation or SH3 binding (Shaheduzzaman *et al.*, 2002). These findings suggest that Nef, which is expressed early in the virus life cycle, may play an important role in optimizing the cellular gene expression profile for virus replication.

A complete signaling pathway directly linking Nef to its reported effects on transcription and cellular activation has not been demonstrated. However, it is very likely that Nef may regulate cellular activation through several kinases including Pak2 (Arora *et al.*, 2000, 2002; Renkema *et al.*, 1999), tyrosine kinases (Ye *et al.*, 2004), MAPKs (Biggs *et al.*, 1999; Muthumani *et al.*, 2005), protein kinase C (PKC) (Smith *et al.*, 1996; Witte *et al.*, 2004), and phosphoinositol 3 kinase (PI3K; Wolf *et al.*, 2001). Pak2 is the best characterized and therefore the most suitable for *in vivo* analysis of all the reported Nef-activated kinases. Substantial agreement exists that Nef forms a complex with Pak2 (Agopian *et al.*, 2006; Pulkkinen *et al.*, 2004). Nef is not only complexed with Pak2 but also induces Pak2 activation (Arora *et al.*, 2000; Raney *et al.*, 2005). The ability of Nef to activate Pak2 suggests that a key role may be mediated by Pak2 in HIV-1 infection because activation of this kinase prior to productive infection is not necessary.

Manninen *et al.* (2001) have shown that, in certain contexts, Nef expression can dramatically alter nuclear factor of activated T cells (NFAT) transcriptional activity and that Nef residues important for Pak2 activation are also important for Nef's effects on NFAT. Moreover, NFAT has been implicated in Nef-induced upregulation of a number of activation-associated genes (Simmons *et al.*, 2001). Thus, a Nef–Pak2 complex may regulate many of Nef's effects on gene transcription.

It has also been demonstrated that Nef activation of Pak2 leads to merlin phosphorylation at Ser518 (Wei *et al.*, 2005). The obvious suggestion that Nef regulates the actin cyotskeleton function is appealing, but not yet investigated. Nor is it clear that HIV-1 infection is in anyway dependent on merlin. Wei *et al.* reported, however, that the mutation of F191 to R in the Nef from HIV-1SF2, blocks Pak2 activation and merlin phosphorylation. This last observation suggests that this mutation could be useful for investigating the possible role of Nef-induced Pak2 activation in HIV-1 replication and pathogenesis.

At this point, none of the other Nef-activated kinases are sufficiently characterized to study *in vivo*. In most cases *in vivo* binding of Nef to a host cell protein has not been clearly demonstrated. One notable exception is the myeloid lineage–specific tyrosine kinase, Hck (Fig. 1). Coexpression of Nef and Hck in Rat-2 fibroblasts leads to cellular transformation (Briggs *et al.*, 1997). Nef moreover tightly binds to the Hck SH3 domain *in vitro* and activates its kinase activity (Moarefi *et al.*, 1997). In Rat-2 cells, enforced dimerization of Nef greatly enhances Hck activation (Ye *et al.*, 2004). Nef has also been shown to modestly activate endogenous Hck and, in turn, the Stat3 transcription factor in myeloid cells (Briggs *et al.*, 2001). Interestingly, Hck is the only cellular activity of Nef known not to require Nef myristoylation (Briggs *et al.*, 2001). In order to activate Pak2, in contrast, Nef must be myristoylated as well as have an intact SH3-binding domain (Wiskerchen and Cheng-Mayer, 1996). Thus, the Nef SH3-binding domain could mediate Pak2 activation when localized to cellular membranes, while cytosolic Nef could activate Hck. However, as Nef expression is not associated with a phenotype that is clearly myeloid specific, it is difficult to speculate on the role of Nef-induced Hck activation.

With regard to other Nef-activated kinases, it is not known if Nef activation of p38 and ERK-1,2 represents separate Nef functions. A further complication is that Nef-deleted viruses exhibit about one-third the activity of Nef-intact virus in activating p38 and upregulating FasL (Muthumani *et al.*, 2005). There are conflicting reports of PKC and PI3K activation by Nef (Linnemann *et al.*, 2002; Smith *et al.*, 1996; Witte *et al.*, 2004; Wolf *et al.*, 2001). Furthermore, structural–functional analyses of these kinase activations by Nef have not been done.

C. MHC I Downmodulation by Nef

Another well-conserved property of Nef is its ability to downmodulate MHC I molecules (Schwartz *et al.*, 1996). As Nef is expressed early after infection, Nef-induced downmodulation of MHC I molecules could help subvert the infected cell to evade the immune system during active viral replication. In support, Collins *et al.* (1998) demonstrated that Nef expression reduces the susceptibility of HIV-infected cells to cytotoxic T lymphocyte (CTL)-mediated lysis *in vitro* (Collins *et al.*, 1998). However, it should be noted that Nef does not render cells completely protected from immune surveillance as there is a strong CTL response to HIV antigens including Nef itself (Betts *et al.*, 2000). Nevertheless, data clearly shows that Nef-expressing proviruses are well adept at avoiding CTLs *in vitro* whereas Nef-defective proviruses are not (Yang *et al.*, 2002). The mechanism by which Nef causes MHC I downregulation is controversial and considerable work remains to be done in this area (Blagoveshchenskaya *et al.*, 2002; Kasper *et al.*, 2005; Piguet *et al.*, 2000; Roeth *et al.*, 2004; Williams *et al.*, 2005).

The best mutation available for studying MHC I downregulation is the mutation of the EEEE sequence at positions 62–65 to AAAA. The specificity of this mutation for MHC I has not been determined other than it does not effect CD4 downregulation. Characterization of the functional defects of this quadruple mutation will be important before the role of MHC I downregulation in HIV-1 replication and pathogenesis can be determined.

VI. Conclusions

At this point there is no unifying hypothesis to explain how HIV Nef achieves any of its effects, in fact all HIV Nef's major activities are genetically separable (Foster *et al.*, 2001; O'Neill *et al.*, 2006). Development of better and more accessible models such as the recently described simian-tropic HIV-1 (Hatziioannou *et al.*, 2006) has the potential of greatly facilitating the study of HIV-1 replication and pathogenesis and in turn the nature of Nef's role. Also of particular significance is the recent development of human–mouse xenograft models that maintain a full repertoire of human lymphoid cells (Ishikawa *et al.*, 2005; Macchiarini *et al.*, 2005; Melkus *et al.*, 2006; Shultz *et al.*, 2005). In addition, some of these models mimic to a significant extent the elements of the intact human immune system that are involved in HIV-1 disease (Ishikawa *et al.*, 2005; Macchiarini *et al.*, 2005; Melkus *et al.*, 2006; Shultz *et al.*, 2005). In principle, these new models will permit the longitudinal analysis of the course of a single infection. This should simplify the determination of which cells are infected and/or killed by X4 and R5 virus and the role of Nef for each type of virus. As structure–function analysis of Nef advances precise correlations for each of the four *in vitro* defined activities to Nef's *in vivo* effects will be possible. The detailed knowledge gained may indicate effective approaches for Nef-based therapies for AIDS.

References

Agopian, K., Wei, B. L., Garcia, J. V., and Gabuzda, D. (2006). A hydrophobic binding surface on the human immunodeficiency virus type 1 Nef core is critical for association with p21-activated kinase 2. *J. Virol.* **80**, 3050–3061.

Ahmad, N., and Venkatesan, S. (1988). Nef protein of HIV-1 is a transcriptional repressor of HIV-1 LTR. *Science* **241**, 1481–1485.

Aiken, C. (1997). Pseudotyping human immunodeficiency virus type 1 (HIV-1) by the glycoprotein of vesicular stomatitis virus targets HIV-1 entry to an endocytic pathway and suppresses both the requirement for Nef and the sensitivity to cyclosporin A. *J. Virol.* **71**, 5871–5877.

Aiken, C., and Trono, D. (1995). Nef stimulates human immunodeficiency virus type 1 proviral DNA synthesis. *J. Virol.* **69**, 5048–5056.

Aiken, C., Krause, L., Chen, Y. L., and Trono, D. (1996). Mutational analysis of HIV-1 Nef: Identification of two mutants that are temperature-sensitive for CD4 downregulation. *Virology* **217**, 293–300.

Alexander, L., Du, Z., Rosenzweig, M., Jung, J. U., and Desrosiers, R. C. (1997). A role for natural simian immunodeficiency virus and human immunodeficiency virus type 1 nef alleles in lymphocyte activation. *J. Virol.* **71**, 6094–6099.

Anderson, S., Shugars, D. C., Swanstrom, R., and Garcia, J. V. (1993). Nef from primary isolates of human immunodeficiency virus type 1 suppresses surface CD4 expression in human and mouse T cells. *J. Virol.* **67**, 4923–4931.

Anderson, S. J., Lenburg, M., Landau, N. R., and Garcia, J. V. (1994). The cytoplasmic domain of CD4 is sufficient for its down-regulation from the cell surface by human immunodeficiency virus type 1 Nef. *J. Virol.* **68**, 3092–3101 [Erratum appears in *J. Virol.* (1994), **68**(7), 4705].

Arganaraz, E. R., Schindler, M., Kirchhoff, F., Cortes, M. J., and Lama, J. (2003). Enhanced CD4 down-modulation by late stage HIV-1 nef alleles is associated with increased Env incorporation and viral replication. *J. Biol. Chem.* **278**, 33912–33919.

Arora, V. K., Molina, R. P., Foster, J. L., Blakemore, J. L., Chernoff, J., Fredericksen, B. L., and Garcia, J. V. (2000). Lentivirus Nef specifically activates Pak2. *J. Virol.* **74**, 11081–11087.

Arora, V. K., Fredericksen, B. L., and Garcia, J. V. (2002). Nef: Agent of cell subversion. *Microbes. Infect.* **4**, 189–199.

Benson, R. E., Sanfridson, A., Ottinger, J. S., Doyle, C., and Cullen, B. R. (1993). Downregulation of cell-surface CD4 expression by simian immunodeficiency virus Nef prevents viral super infection. *J. Exp. Med.* **177**, 1561–1566.

Betts, M. R., Casazza, J. P., Patterson, B. A., Waldrop, S., Trigona, W., Fu, T. M., Kern, F., Picker, L. J., and Koup, R. A. (2000). Putative immunodominant human immuno-deficiency virus-specific CD8(+) T-cell responses cannot be predicted by major histocompatibility complex class I haplotype. *J. Virol.* **74**, 9144–9151.

Biggs, T. E., Cooke, S. J., Barton, C. H., Harris, M. P., Saksela, K., and Mann, D. A. (1999). Induction of activator protein 1 (AP-1) in macrophages by human immunodeficiency virus type-1 NEF is a cell-type-specific response that requires both hck and MAPK signaling events. *J. Mol. Biol.* **290**, 21–35.

Blagoveshchenskaya, A. D., Thomas, L., Feliciangeli, S. F., Hung, C. H., and Thomas, G. (2002). HIV-1 Nef downregulates MHC-I by a PACS-1- and PI3K-regulated ARF6 endocytic pathway. *Cell* **111**, 853–866.

Bonyhadi, M. L., Rabin, L., Salimi, S., Brown, D. A., Kosek, J., McCune, J. M., and Kaneshima, H. (1993). HIV induces thymus depletion *in vivo. Nature* **363**, 728–732.

Brenchley, J. M., Schacker, T. W., Ruff, L. E., Price, D. A., Taylor, J. H., Beilman, G. J., Nguyen, P. L., Khoruts, A., Larson, M., Haase, A. T., and Douek, D. C. (2004). CD4+ T cell depletion during all stages of HIV disease occurs predominantly in the gastrointestinal tract. *J. Exp. Med.* **200**, 749–759.

Bresnahan, P. A., Yonemoto, W., and Greene, W. C. (1999). Cutting edge: SIV Nef protein utilizes both leucine- and tyrosine-based protein sorting pathways for down-regulation of CD4. *J. Immunol.* **163**, 2977–2981.

Briggs, S. D., Sharkey, M., Stevenson, M., and Smithgall, T. E. (1997). SH3-mediated Hck tyrosine kinase activation and fibroblast transformation by the Nef protein of HIV-1. *J. Biol. Chem.* **272**, 17899–17902.

Briggs, S. D., Scholtz, B., Jacque, J. M., Swingler, S., Stevenson, M., and Smithgall, T. E. (2001). HIV-1 Nef promotes survival of myeloid cells by a Stat3-dependent pathway. *J. Biol. Chem.* **276**, 25605–25611.

Campbell, E. M., Nunez, R., and Hope, T. J. (2004). Disruption of the actin cytoskeleton can complement the ability of Nef to enhance human immunodeficiency virus type 1 infectivity. *J. Virol.* **78**, 5745–5755.

Cao, J., Vasir, B., and Sodroski, J. G. (1994). Changes in the cytopathic effects of human immunodeficiency virus type 1 associated with a single amino acid alteration in the ectodomain of the gp41 transmembrane glycoprotein. *J. Virol.* **68**, 4662–4668.

Chang, S. Y., Bowman, B. H., Weiss, J. B., Garcia, R. E., and White, T. J. (1993). The origin of HIV-1 isolate HTLV-IIIB. *Nature* **363**, 466–469.

Chowers, M. Y., Spina, C. A., Kwoh, T. J., Fitch, N. J., Richman, D. D., and Guatelli, J. C. (1994). Optimal infectivity *in vitro* of human immunodeficiency virus type 1 requires an intact nef gene. *J. Virol.* **68**, 2906–2914.

Collins, K. L., Chen, B. K., Kalams, S. A., Walker, B. D., and Baltimore, D. (1998). HIV-1 Nef protein protects infected primary cells against killing by cytotoxic T lymphocytes. *Nature* **391**, 397–401.

Craig, H. M., Pandori, M. W., and Guatelli, J. C. (1998). Interaction of HIV-1 Nef with the cellular dileucine-based sorting pathway is required for CD4 down-regulation and optimal viral infectivity. *Proc. Natl. Acad. Sci. USA* **95**, 11229–11234.

Craig, H. M., Reddy, T. R., Riggs, N. L., Dao, P. P., and Guatelli, J. C. (2000). Interactions of HIV-1 nef with the mu subunits of adaptor protein complexes 1, 2, and 3: Role of the dileucine-based sorting motif. *Virology* **271**, 9–17.

Cullen, B. R. (1991). Regulation of HIV-1 gene expression. *FASEB J.* **5**, 2361–2368.

Cullen, B. R. (1998). HIV-1 auxiliary proteins: Making connections in a dying cell. *Cell* **93**, 685–692.

Deacon, N. J., Tsykin, A., Solomon, A., Smith, K., Ludford-Menting, M., Hooker, D. J., McPhee, D. A., Greenway, A. L., Ellett, A., and Chatfield, C. (1995). Genomic structure of an attenuated quasi species of HIV-1 from a blood transfusion donor and recipients. *Science* **270**, 988–991.

Duus, K. M., Miller, E. D., Smith, J. A., Kovalev, G. I., and Su, L. (2001). Separation of human immunodeficiency virus type 1 replication from nef-mediated pathogenesis in the human thymus. *J. Virol.* **75**, 3916–3924.

Emerman, M., and Malim, M. H. (1998). HIV-1 regulatory/accessory genes: Keys to unraveling viral and host cell biology. *Science* **280**, 1880–1884.

Fackler, O. T., D'Aloja, P., Baur, A. S., Federico, M., and Peterlin, B. M. (2001). Nef from human immunodeficiency virus type 1(f12) inhibits viral production and infectivity. *J. Virol.* **75**, 6601–6608.

Foster, J. L., Molina, R. P., Luo, T., Arora, V. K., Huang, Y., Ho, D. D., and Garcia, J. V. (2001). Genetic and functional diversity of human immunodeficiency virus type 1 subtype B Nef primary isolates. *J. Virol.* **75**, 1672–1680.

Foti, M., Mangasarian, A., Piguet, V., Lew, D. P., Krause, K. H., Trono, D., and Carpentier, J. L. (1997). Nef-mediated clathrin-coated pit formation. *J. Cell Biol.* **139**, 37–47.

Garcia, J. V., and Miller, A. D. (1991). Serine phosphorylation-independent downregulation of cell-surface CD4 by nef. *Nature* **350**, 508–511.

Garcia, J. V., and Miller, A. D. (1992). Downregulation of cell surface CD4 by nef. *Res. Virol.* **143**, 52–55.

Garcia, J. V., Alfano, J., and Miller, A. D. (1993). The negative effect of human immunodeficiency virus type 1 Nef on cell surface CD4 expression is not species specific and requires the cytoplasmic domain of CD4. *J. Virol.* **67**, 1511–1516.

Glushakova, S., Grivel, J. C., Suryanarayana, K., Meylan, P., Lifson, J. D., Desrosiers, R., and Margolis, L. (1999). Nef enhances human immunodeficiency virus replication and responsiveness to interleukin-2 in human lymphoid tissue *ex vivo. J. Virol.* **73**, 3968–3974.

Greenberg, M., DeTulleo, L., Rapoport, I., Skowronski, J., and Kirchhausen, T. (1998). A dileucine motif in HIV-1 Nef is essential for sorting into clathrin-coated pits and for downregulation of CD4. *Curr. Biol.* **8**, 1239–1242.

Greenberg, M. E., Bronson, S., Lock, M., Neumann, M., Pavlakis, G. N., and Skowronski, J. (1997). Co-localization of HIV-1 Nef with the AP-2 adaptor protein complex correlates with Nef-induced CD4 down-regulation. *EMBO J.* **16**, 6964–6976.

Grzesiek, S., Stahl, S. J., Wingfield, P. T., and Bax, A. (1996). The CD4 determinant for downregulation by HIV-1 Nef directly binds to Nef. Mapping of the Nef binding surface by NMR. *Biochemistry* **35**, 10256–10261.

Guy, B., Kieny, M. P., Riviere, Y., Le Peuch, C., Dott, K., Girard, M., Montagnier, L., and Lecocq, J. P. (1987). HIV F/3' orf encodes a phosphorylated GTP-binding protein resembling an oncogene product. *Nature* **330**, 266–269.

Hahn, B. H., Shaw, G. M., De Cock, K. M., and Sharp, P. M. (2000). AIDS as a zoonosis: Scientific and public health implications. *Science* **287**, 607–614.

Hammes, S. R., Dixon, E. P., Malim, M. H., Cullen, B. R., and Greene, W. C. (1989). Nef protein of human immunodeficiency virus type 1: Evidence against its role as a transcriptional inhibitor. *Proc. Natl. Acad. Sci. USA* **86**, 9549–9553.

Hatziioannou, T., Princiotta, M., Piatak, M., Jr., Yuan, F., Zhang, F., Lifson, J. D., and Bieniasz, P. D. (2006). Generation of Simian-Tropic HIV-1 by restriction factor evasion. *Science* **314**, 95.

Hua, J., and Cullen, B. R. (1997). Human immunodeficiency virus types 1 and 2 and simian immunodeficiency virus Nef use distinct but overlapping target sites for downregulation of cell surface CD4. *J. Virol.* **71**, 6742–6748.

Iafrate, A. J., Bronson, S., and Skowronski, J. (1997). Separable functions of Nef disrupt two aspects of T cell receptor machinery: CD4 expression and CD3 signaling. *EMBO J.* **16**, 673–684.

Ishikawa, F., Yasukawa, M., Lyons, B., Yoshida, S., Miyamoto, T., Yoshimoto, G., Watanabe, T., Akashi, K., Shultz, L. D., and Harada, M. (2005). Development of functional human blood and immune systems in NOD/SCID/IL2 receptor {gamma} chain(null) mice. *Blood* **106**, 1565–1573.

Jamieson, B. D., Aldrovandi, G. M., Planelles, V., Jowett, J. B., Gao, L., Bloch, L. M., Chen, I. S., and Zack, J. A. (1994). Requirement of human immunodeficiency virus type 1 nef for *in vivo* replication and pathogenicity. *J. Virol.* **68**, 3478–3485.

Kaneshima, H., Su, L., Bonyhadi, M. L., Connor, R. I., Ho, D. D., and McCune, J. M. (1994). Rapid-high, syncytium-inducing isolates of human immunodeficiency virus type 1 induce cytopathicity in the human thymus of the SCID-hu mouse. *J. Virol.* **68**, 8188–8192.

Kasper, M. R., Roeth, J. F., Williams, M., Filzen, T. M., Fleis, R. I., and Collins, K. L. (2005). HIV-1 Nef disrupts antigen presentation early in the secretory pathway. *J. Biol. Chem.* **280**, 12840–12848.

Keele, B. F., Van Heuverswyn, F., Li, Y., Bailes, E., Takehisa, J., Santiago, M. L., Bibollet-Ruche, F., Chen, Y., Wain, L. V., Liegeois, F., Loul, S., Ngole, E. M., et al. (2006). Chimpanzee reservoirs of pandemic and nonpandemic HIV-1. *Science* **313**, 523–526.

Kestler, H. W., III, Ringler, D. J., Mori, K., Panicali, D. L., Sehgal, P. K., Daniel, M. D., and Desrosiers, R. C. (1991). Importance of the nef gene for maintenance of high virus loads and for development of AIDS. *Cell* **65**, 651–662.

Khan, M., Garcia-Barrio, M., and Powell, M. D. (2001). Restoration of wild-type infectivity to human immunodeficiency virus type 1 strains lacking nef by intravirion reverse transcription. *J. Virol.* **75**, 12081–12087.

Kim, S., Ikeuchi, K., Byrn, R., Groopman, J., and Baltimore, D. (1989). Lack of a negative influence on viral growth by the nef gene of human immunodeficiency virus type 1. *Proc. Natl. Acad. Sci. USA* **86**, 9544–9548.

Kirchhoff, F., Greenough, T. C., Brettler, D. B., Sullivan, J. L., and Desrosiers, R. C. (1995). Brief report: Absence of intact nef sequences in a long-term survivor with nonprogressive HIV-1 infection. *N. Engl. J. Med.* **332**, 228–232.

Lama, J. (2003). The physiological relevance of CD4 receptor down-modulation during HIV infection. *Curr. HIV Res.* **1**, 167–184.

Lama, J., Mangasarian, A., and Trono, D. (1999). Cell-surface expression of CD4 reduces HIV-1 infectivity by blocking Env incorporation in a Nef- and Vpu-inhibitable manner. *Curr. Biol.* **9**, 622–631.

Le Gall, S., Buseyne, F., Trocha, A., Walker, B. D., Heard, J. M., and Schwartz, O. (2000). Distinct trafficking pathways mediate Nef-induced and clathrin-dependent major histocompatibility complex class I down-regulation. *J. Virol.* **74**, 9256–9266.

Learmont, J. C., Geczy, A. F., Mills, J., Ashton, L. J., Raynes-Greenow, C. H., Garsia, R. J., Dyer, W. B., McIntyre, L., Oelrichs, R. B., Rhodes, D. I., Deacon, N. J., and Sullivan, J. S. (1999). Immunologic and virologic status after 14 to 18 years of infection with an attenuated strain of HIV-1. A report from the Sydney Blood Bank Cohort. *N. Engl. J. Med.* **340**, 1715–1722.

Li, Q., Duan, L., Estes, J. D., Ma, Z. M., Rourke, T., Wang, Y., Reilly, C., Carlis, J., Miller, C. J., and Haase, A. T. (2005). Peak SIV replication in resting memory CD4+ T cells depletes gut lamina propria CD4+ T cells. *Nature* **434**, 1148–1152.

Linnemann, T., Zheng, Y. H., Mandic, R., and Peterlin, B. M. (2002). Interaction between Nef and phosphatidylinositol-3-kinase leads to activation of p21-activated kinase and increased production of HIV. *Virology* **294**, 246–255.

Lock, M., Greenberg, M. E., Iafrate, A. J., Swigut, T., Muench, J., Kirchhoff, F., Shohdy, N., and Skowronski, J. (1999). Two elements target SIV Nef to the AP-2 clathrin adaptor complex, but only one is required for the induction of CD4 endocytosis. *EMBO J.* **18**, 2722–2733.

Lori, F., Hall, L., Lusso, P., Popovic, M., Markham, P., Franchini, G., and Reitz, M. S., Jr. (1992). Effect of reciprocal complementation of two defective human immunodeficiency virus type 1 (HIV-1) molecular clones on HIV-1 cell tropism and virulence. *J. Virol.* **66**, 5553–5560.

Lundquist, C. A., Tobiume, M., Zhou, J., Unutmaz, D., and Aiken, C. (2002). Nef-mediated downregulation of CD4 enhances human immunodeficiency virus type 1 replication in primary T lymphocytes. *J. Virol.* **76**, 4625–4633.

Luo, T., Anderson, S. J., and Garcia, J. V. (1996). Inhibition of Nef- and phorbol ester-induced CD4 degradation by macrolide antibiotics. *J. Virol.* **70**, 1527–1534.

Luo, T., Livingston, R. A., and Garcia, J. V. (1997). Infectivity enhancement by human immunodeficiency virus type 1 Nef is independent of its association with a cellular serine/threonine kinase. *J. Virol.* **71**, 9524–9530.

Luo, T., Douglas, J. L., Livingston, R. L., and Garcia, J. V. (1998). Infectivity enhancement by HIV-1 Nef is dependent on the pathway of virus entry: Implications for HIV-based gene transfer systems. *Virology* **241**, 224–233.

Luo, T., Fredericksen, B. L., Hasumi, K., Endo, A., and Garcia, J. V. (2001). Human immunodeficiency virus type 1 Nef-induced CD4 cell surface downregulation is inhibited by ikarugamycin. *J. Virol.* 75, 2488–2492.

Macchiarini, F., Manz, M. G., Palucka, A. K., and Shultz, L. D. (2005). Humanized mice: Are we there yet? *J. Exp. Med.* 202, 1307–1311.

Mangasarian, A., Foti, M., Aiken, C., Chin, D., Carpentier, J. L., and Trono, D. (1997). The HIV-1 Nef protein acts as a connector with sorting pathways in the Golgi and at the plasma membrane. *Immunity* 6, 67–77.

Mangasarian, A., Piguet, V., Wang, J. K., Chen, Y. L., and Trono, D. (1999). Nef-induced CD4 and major histocompatibility complex class I (MHC-I) down-regulation are governed by distinct determinants: N-terminal alpha helix and proline repeat of Nef selectively regulate MHC-I trafficking. *J. Virol.* 73, 1964–1973.

Manninen, A., Huotari, P., Hiipakka, M., Renkema, G. H., and Saksela, K. (2001). Activation of NFAT-dependent gene expression by Nef: Conservation among divergent Nef alleles, dependence on SH3 binding and membrane association, and cooperation with protein kinase C-theta. *J. Virol.* 75, 3034–3037.

Mariani, R., and Skowronski, J. (1993). CD4 down-regulation by nef alleles isolated from human immunodeficiency virus type 1-infected individuals. *Proc. Natl. Acad. Sci. USA* 90, 5549–5553.

Marsh, M., and Pelchen-Matthews, A. (1996). Endocytic and exocytic regulation of CD4 expression and function. *Curr. Top. Microbiol. Immunol.* 205, 107–135.

Mattapallil, J. J., Douek, D. C., Hill, B., Nishimura, Y., Martin, M., and Roederer, M. (2005). Massive infection and loss of memory CD4+ T cells in multiple tissues during acute SIV infection. *Nature* 434, 1093–1097.

Melkus, M. W., Estes, J. D., Padgett-Thomas, A., Gatlin, J., Denton, P. W., Othieno, F., Wege, A. K., Hasse, A. T., and Garcia, J. V. (2006). Humanized mice mount specific adaptive and innate immune responses to EBV and TSST-1. *Nat. Med.* 12, 1316–1322.

Messmer, D., Ignatius, R., Santisteban, C., Steinman, R. M., and Pope, M. (2000). The decreased replicative capacity of simian immunodeficiency virus SIVmac239Delta(nef) is manifest in cultures of immature dendritic cells and T cells. *J. Virol.* 74, 2406–2413.

Miller, E. D., Duus, K. M., Townsend, M., Yi, Y., Collman, R., Reitz, M., and Su, L. (2001). Human immunodeficiency virus type 1 IIIB selected for replication *in vivo* exhibits increased envelope glycoproteins in virions without alteration in coreceptor usage: Separation of *in vivo* replication from macrophage tropism. *J. Virol.* 75, 8498–8506.

Miller, M. D., Warmerdam, M. T., Gaston, I., Greene, W. C., and Feinberg, M. B. (1994). The human immunodeficiency virus-1 nef gene product: A positive factor for viral infection and replication in primary lymphocytes and macrophages. *J. Exp. Med.* 179, 101–113.

Miller, M. D., Warmerdam, M. T., Page, K. A., Feinberg, M. B., and Greene, W. C. (1995). Expression of the human immunodeficiency virus type 1 (HIV-1) nef gene during HIV-1 production increases progeny particle infectivity independently of gp160 or viral entry. *J. Virol.* 69, 579–584.

Miller, M. D., Warmerdam, M. T., Ferrell, S. S., Benitez, R., and Greene, W. C. (1997). Intravirion generation of the C-terminal core domain of HIV-1 Nef by the HIV-1 protease is insufficient to enhance viral infectivity. *Virology* 234, 215–225.

Moarefi, I., LaFevre-Bernt, M., Sicheri, F., Huse, M., Lee, C. H., Kuriyan, J., and Miller, W. T. (1997). Activation of the Src-family tyrosine kinase Hck by SH3 domain displacement. *Nature* 385, 650–653.

Muthumani, K., Choo, A. Y., Hwang, D. S., Premkumar, A., Dayes, N. S., Harris, C., Green, D. R., Wadsworth, S. A., Siekierka, J. J., and Weiner, D. B. (2005). HIV-1 Nef-induced FasL induction and bystander killing requires p38 MAPK activation. *Blood* 106, 2059–2068.

O'Neill, E., Kuo, L. S., Krisko, J. F., Tomchick, D. R., Garcia, J. V., and Foster, J. L. (2006). Dynamic evolution of the human immunodeficiency virus type 1 pathogenic factor, Nef. *J. Virol.* **80**, 1311–1320.

Pelchen-Matthews, A., da Silva, R. P., Bijlmakers, M. J., Signoret, N., Gordon, S., and Marsh, M. (1998). Lack of p56lck expression correlates with CD4 endocytosis in primary lymphoid and myeloid cells. *Eur. J. Immunol.* **28**, 3639–3647.

Piguet, V., Chen, Y. L., Mangasarian, A., Foti, M., Carpentier, J. L., and Trono, D. (1998). Mechanism of Nef-induced CD4 endocytosis: Nef connects CD4 with the mu chain of adaptor complexes. *EMBO J.* **17**, 2472–2481.

Piguet, V., Wan, L., Borel, C., Mangasarian, A., Demaurex, N., Thomas, G., and Trono, D. (2000). HIV-1 Nef protein binds to the cellular protein PACS-1 to downregulate class I major histocompatibility complexes. *Nat. Cell Biol.* **2**, 163–167.

Pulkkinen, K., Renkema, G. H., Kirchhoff, F., and Saksela, K. (2004). Nef associates with p21-activated kinase 2 in a p21-GTPase-dependent dynamic activation complex within lipid rafts. *J. Virol.* **78**, 12773–12780.

Rabin, L., Hincenbergs, M., Moreno, M. B., Warren, S., Linquist, V., Datema, R., Charpiot, B., Seifert, J., Kaneshima, H., and McCune, J. M. (1996). Use of standardized SCID-hu Thy/Liv mouse model for preclinical efficacy testing of anti-human immunodeficiency virus type 1 compounds. *Antimicrob. Agents Chemother.* **40**, 755–762.

Raney, A., Kuo, L. S., Baugh, L. L., Foster, J. L., and Garcia, J. V. (2005). Reconstitution and molecular analysis of an active human immunodeficiency virus type 1 Nef/p21-activated kinase 2 complex. *J. Virol.* **79**, 12732–12741.

Reitz, M. S., Hall, L., Robert-Guroff, M., Lautenberger, J., Hahn, B. M., Shaw, G. M., Kong, L. I., Weiss, S. H., Waters, D., and Gallo, R. C. (1994). Viral variability and serum antibody response in a laboratory worker infected with HIV type 1 (HTLV type IIIB). *AIDS Res. Hum. Retroviruses* **10**, 1143–1155.

Renkema, G. H., and Saksela, K. (2000). Interactions of HIV-1 NEF with cellular signal transducing proteins. *Front. Bios.* **5**, D268–D283.

Renkema, G. H., Manninen, A., Mann, D. A., Harris, M., and Saksela, K. (1999). Identification of the Nef-associated kinase as p21-activated kinase 2. *Curr. Biol.* **9**, 1407–1410.

Rhee, S. S., and Marsh, J. W. (1994). HIV-1 Nef activity in murine T cells. CD4 modulation and positive enhancement. *J. Immunol.* **152**, 5128–5134.

Roeth, J. F., Williams, M., Kasper, M. R., Filzen, T. M., and Collins, K. L. (2004). HIV-1 Nef disrupts MHC-I trafficking by recruiting AP-1 to the MHC-I cytoplasmic tail. *J. Cell Biol.* **167**, 903–913.

Roques, P., Robertson, D. L., Souquiere, S., Damond, F., Ayouba, A., Farfara, I., Depienne, C., Nerrienet, E., Dormont, D., Brun-Vezinet, F., Simon, F., and Mauclere, P. (2002). Phylogenetic analysis of 49 newly derived HIV-1 group O strains High viral diversity but no group M-like subtype structure. *Virology* **302**, 259–273.

Roques, P., Robertson, D. L., Souquiere, S., Apetrei, C., Nerrienet, E., Barre-Sinoussi, F., Muller-Trutwin, M., and Simon, F. (2004). Phylogenetic characteristics of three new HIV-1 N strains and implications for the origin of group N. *AIDS* **18**, 1371–1381.

Ross, T. M., Oran, A. E., and Cullen, B. R. (1999). Inhibition of HIV-1 progeny virion release by cell-surface CD4 is relieved by expression of the viral Nef protein. *Curr. Biol.* **9**, 613–621.

Rossi, F., Gallina, A., and Milanesi, G. (1996). Nef-CD4 physical interaction sensed with the yeast two-hybrid system. *Virology* **217**, 397–403.

Salvi, R., Garbuglia, A. R., Di Caro, A., Pulciani, S., Montella, F., and Benedetto, A. (1998). Grossly defective nef gene sequences in a human immunodeficiency virus type 1-seropositive long-term nonprogressor. *J. Virol.* **72**, 3646–3657.

Sanfridson, A., Cullen, B. R., and Doyle, C. (1994). The simian immunodeficiency virus Nef protein promotes degradation of CD4 in human T cells. *J. Biol. Chem.* **269**, 3917–3920.

Schindler, M., Munch, J., Kutsch, O., Li, H., Santiago, M. L., Bibollet-Ruche, F., Muller-Trutwin, M. C., Novembre, F. J., Peeters, M., Courgnaud, V., Bailes, E., Roques, P., *et al.* (2006). Nef-mediated suppression of T cell activation was lost in a lentiviral lineage that gave rise to HIV-1. *Cell* **125**(6), 1055–1067.

Schwartz, O., Marechal, V., Le Gall, S., Lemonnier, F., and Heard, J. M. (1996). Endocytosis of major histocompatibility complex class I molecules is induced by the HIV-1 Nef protein. *Nat. Med.* **2**, 338–342.

Schweighardt, B., Roy, A. M., Meiklejohn, D. A., Grace, E. J., Moretto, W. J., Heymann, J. J., and Nixon, D. F. (2004). R5 human immunodeficiency virus type 1 (HIV-1) replicates more efficiently in primary CD4+ T-cell cultures than X4 HIV-1. *J. Virol.* **78**, 9164–9173.

Shaheduzzaman, S., Krishnan, V., Petrovic, A., Bittner, M., Meltzer, P., Trent, J., Venkatesan, S., and Zeichner, S. (2002). Effects of HIV-1 Nef on cellular gene expression profiles. *J. Biomed. Sci.* **9**, 82–96.

Shapira-Nahor, O., Maayan, S., Peden, K. W., Rabinowitz, R., Schlesinger, M., Alian, A., and Panet, A. (2002). Replication of HIV-1 deleted Nef mutants in chronically immune activated human T cells. *Virology* **303**, 138–145.

Shultz, L. D., Lyons, B. L., Burzenski, L. M., Gott, B., Chen, X., Chaleff, S., Kotb, M., Gillies, S. D., King, M., Mangada, J., Greiner, D. L., and Handgretinger, R. (2005). Human lymphoid and myeloid cell development in NOD/LtSz-scid IL2R gamma null mice engrafted with mobilized human hemopoietic stem cells. *J. Immunol.* **174**, 6477–6489.

Simmons, A., Aluvihare, V., and McMichael, A. (2001). Nef Triggers a transcriptional program in T cells imitating single-signal T cell activation and inducing HIV virulence mediators. *Immunity* **14**, 763–777.

Simmons, A., Gangadharan, B., Hodges, A., Sharrocks, K., Prabhakar, S., Garcia, A., Dwek, R., Zitzmann, N., and McMichael, A. (2005). Nef-mediated lipid raft exclusion of UbcH7 inhibits Cbl activity in T cells to positively regulate signaling. *Immunity* **23**, 621–634.

Smith, B. L., Krushelnycky, B. W., Mochly-Rosen, D., and Berg, P. (1996). The HIV nef protein associates with protein kinase C theta. *J. Biol. Chem.* **271**, 16753–16757.

Spina, C. A., Kwoh, T. J., Chowers, M. Y., Guatelli, J. C., and Richman, D. D. (1994). The importance of nef in the induction of human immunodeficiency virus type 1 replication from primary quiescent CD4 lymphocytes. *J. Exp. Med.* **179**, 115–123.

Stoddart, C. A., Geleziunas, R., Ferrell, S., Linquist-Stepps, V., Moreno, M. E., Bare, C., Xu, W., Yonemoto, W., Bresnahan, P. A., McCune, J. M., and Greene, W. C. (2003). Human immunodeficiency virus type 1 Nef-mediated downregulation of CD4 correlates with Nef enhancement of viral pathogenesis. *J. Virol.* **77**, 2124–2133.

Stove, V., Naessens, E., Stove, C., Swigut, T., Plum, J., and Verhasselt, B. (2003). Signaling but not trafficking function of HIV-1 protein Nef is essential for Nef-induced defects in human intrathymic T-cell development. *Blood* **102**, 2925–2932.

Su, L., Kaneshima, H., Bonyhadi, M. L., Lee, R., Auten, J., Wolf, A., Du, B., Rabin, L., Hahn, B. H., Terwilliger, E., and McCune, J. M. (1997). Identification of HIV-1 determinants for replication *in vivo*. *Virology* **227**, 45–52.

Swingler, S., Mann, A., Jacque, J., Brichacek, B., Sasseville, V. G., Williams, K., Lackner, A. A., Janoff, E. N., Wang, R., Fisher, D., and Stevenson, M. (1999). HIV-1 Nef mediates lymphocyte chemotaxis and activation by infected macrophages. *Nat. Med.* **5**, 997–1003.

Terwilliger, E., Sodroski, J. G., Rosen, C. A., and Haseltine, W. A. (1986). Effects of mutations within the 3' orf open reading frame region of human T-cell lymphotropic virus type III (HTLV-III/LAV) on replication and cytopathogenicity. *J. Virol.* **60**, 754–760.

Vidal, N., Peeters, M., Mulanga-Kabeya, C., Nzilambi, N., Robertson, D., Ilunga, W., Sema, H., Tshimanga, K., Bongo, B., and Delaporte, E. (2000). Unprecedented degree of human immunodeficiency virus type 1 (HIV-1) group M genetic diversity in the Democratic

Republic of Congo suggests that the HIV-1 pandemic originated in Central Africa. *J. Virol.* **74**, 10498–10507.

Wei, B. L., Arora, V. K., Foster, J. L., Sodora, D. L., and Garcia, J. V. (2003). *In vivo* analysis of Nef function. *Curr. HIV Res.* **1**, 41–50.

Wei, B. L., Arora, V. K., Raney, A., Kuo, L. S., Xiao, G. H., O'Neill, E., Testa, J. R., Foster, J. L., and Garcia, J. V. (2005). Activation of p21-activated kinase 2 by human immunodeficiency virus type 1 Nef induces merlin phosphorylation. *J. Virol.* **79**, 14976–14980.

Weiss, S. H., Goedert, J. J., Gartner, S., Popovic, M., Waters, D., Markham, P., di, M. V., Gail, M. H., Barkley, W. E., Gibbons, J., Giff, F. A., Leuther, M., *et al.* (1988). Risk of human immunodeficiency virus (HIV-1) infection among laboratory workers. *Science* **239**, 68–71.

Williams, M., Roeth, J. F., Kasper, M. R., Filzen, T. M., and Collins, K. L. (2005). Human immunodeficiency virus type 1 Nef domains required for disruption of major histocompatibility complex class I trafficking are also necessary for coprecipitation of Nef with HLA-A2. *J. Virol.* **79**, 632–636.

Wiskerchen, M., and Cheng-Mayer, C. (1996). HIV-1 Nef association with cellular serine kinase correlates with enhanced virion infectivity and efficient proviral DNA synthesis. *Virology* **224**, 292–301.

Witte, V., Laffert, B., Rosorius, O., Lischka, P., Blume, K., Galler, G., Stilper, A., Willbold, D., D'Aloja, P., Sixt, M., Kolanus, J., Ott, M., *et al.* (2004). HIV-1 Nef mimics an integrin receptor signal that recruits the polycomb group protein Eed to the plasma membrane. *Mol. Cell* **13**, 179–190.

Wolf, D., Witte, V., Laffert, B., Blume, K., Stromer, E., Trapp, S., D'Aloja, P., Schurmann, A., and Baur, A. S. (2001). HIV-1 Nef associated PAK and PI3-kinases stimulate Akt-independent Bad-phosphorylation to induce anti-apoptotic signals. [see comment]. *Nat. Med.* **7**, 1217–1224.

Wu, Y., and Marsh, J. W. (2001). Selective transcription and modulation of resting T cell activity by preintegrated HIV DNA. *Science* **293**, 1503–1506.

Yang, O. O., Nguyen, P. T., Kalams, S. A., Dorfman, T., Gottlinger, H. G., Stewart, S., Chen, I. S., Threlkeld, S., and Walker, B. D. (2002). Nef-mediated resistance of human immunodeficiency virus type 1 to antiviral cytotoxic T lymphocytes. *J. Virol.* **76**, 1626–1631.

Ye, H., Choi, H. J., Poe, J., and Smithgall, T. E. (2004). Oligomerization is required for HIV-1 Nef-induced activation of the Src family protein-tyrosine kinase, Hck. *Biochemistry* **43**, 15775–15784.

Susan Peterson, Alison P. Reid, Scott Kim, and Robert F. Siliciano

Department of Medicine, Johns Hopkins University School of Medicine
Baltimore, Maryland 21205

Treatment Implications of the Latent Reservoir for HIV-1

I. Chapter Overview

This chapter explores the definition and mechanism of the latent reservoir, resistance and treatment implications, and the impact of the latent reservoir on future drug development. A viral reservoir is a cell type or anatomic location in which virus or virally infected cells persist with slower replication kinetics and/or turnover rate than that of the main pool of actively replicating virus (Haggerty *et al.*, 2006). A stable reservoir for HIV-1 is created when activated CD4+ T cells that are converting into memory T cells become infected. Viral DNA becomes integrated into the chromosomal DNA of the cell. This stable integration into the genomes of long-lived

Advances in Pharmacology, Volume 55
Copyright © 2000, 2007, Elsevier Inc. All rights reserved.

1054-3589/07 $35.00
DOI: 10.1016/S1054-3589(07)55012-X

memory cells provides a mechanism for the archiving of all major forms of virus that have circulated in an infected individual, including viral variants that have resistance to antiretroviral drugs. This can make treatment decisions difficult particularly in light of the fact that the available resistance assays cannot assess the contents of the latent reservoir. Several approaches to counter these challenges have been explored, including scheduled treatment interruptions, which ultimately proved to be ineffective, development of drugs with higher barriers to resistance, and the development of new drug classes with novel mechanisms of action. Efforts to combat the latent reservoir directly through intensification of highly active antiretroviral therapy (HAART) and activating agents have unfortunately shown only limited success, and novel approaches will likely be needed if eradication is to be achieved.

II. Introduction

The discovery of the latent reservoir for HIV-1 in resting CD4+ T cells fundamentally changed the way in which patients, physicians, and scientists conceptualize the treatment of HIV-1 infection (Chun *et al.*, 1995). The latent reservoir is now widely recognized as a formidable barrier to the cure of HIV-1 infection (Chun *et al.*, 1997b; Finzi *et al.*, 1999; Siliciano *et al.*, 2003; Wong *et al.*, 1997), and antiretroviral therapy is no longer given with the hope of eradicating the infection (Bartlett and Lane, 2006). Instead, lifelong suppression of viral replication has become the therapeutic goal. In addition, this reservoir is responsible for persisting drug resistance in infected patients. This chapter will explore the nature and mechanisms of the HIV-1 latency, drug resistance and treatment implications, and the impact of the latent reservoir on future drug development.

III. What is the Latent Reservoir?

A. Cell Type and Location

The term reservoir is frequently used in the virology literature, but not always in a precise way. It is therefore important at the outset to clarify what exactly is meant by a viral reservoir. A viral reservoir is a cell type or anatomic location in which virus or virally infected cells persist with slower replication kinetics and/or turnover rate than that of the main pool of actively replicating virus (Haggerty *et al.*, 2006). The virus in the reservoir must be replication-competent and is to some extent sheltered from the effects of the immune system, antiviral medications, and biochemical decay. A reservoir for HIV-1 has been identified in resting CD4+ T cells through experiments which recovered replication-competent virus from this cell population (Chun *et al.*, 1997b; Finzi *et al.*, 1997, 1999; Siliciano and Siliciano, 2005; Siliciano *et al.*, 2003; Strain *et al.*, 2003; Wong *et al.*, 1997). It has been hypothesized that other cell types, including those in the monocyte-macrophage lineage, may also serve as a reservoir for the virus (Bailey *et al.*, 2006; Igarashi *et al.*, 2001). In fact, macrophages serve as an important source of virus at late stages of infection when CD4+ T cells have been largely depleted (Igarashi *et al.*, 2003). While infected macrophages appear to release virus continuously, they turnover more slowly than infected CD4+ T cells and can thus be considered a reservoir.

1. Reservoir Versus Compartment

The terms reservoir and compartment are frequently confused. The replication kinetics and turnover rates need not be different in a viral compartment. Instead, there is a barrier between the compartment and the rest of the organism that is only rarely crossed. This leads to divergent evolution between the two viral populations in the compartment and the rest of the body. Examples of compartments include the genital tract and the central nervous system. Phylogenetic criteria can be used to differentiate reservoirs and compartments. Sequences from a reservoir will have increased intrapatient diversity and decreased mean divergence from the most recent common ancestor (Nickle *et al.*, 2003). This reflects the fact that a reservoir contains sequences deposited at different times during infection. This is clearly demonstrated by analysis of the latent reservoir for HIV-1 in resting CD4+ T cells where archival wild-type and drug-resistant variants have been demonstrated to persist (Ruff *et al.*, 2002). This is illustrated in Fig. 1. In contrast, sequences from a compartment will demonstrate reduced diversity and will cluster separately on a phylogenetic tree (Nickle *et al.*, 2003). Drug penetration into these compartments is an important concern when designing an antiretroviral regimen because low drug levels in particular compartments can in principle lead to the development of resistance in the compartments. For example, if one component of a three-drug regimen fails to achieve an appropriate level in the central nervous system, then virus in this compartment would be exposed to only two antiretrovirals, increasing the risk of breakthrough resistance.

2. Mechanism of Latency

HIV-1 appears to have evolved to replicate in activated CD4+ T cells. Many of the host factors needed for replication are poorly expressed or are sequestered in an inactive form in resting CD4+ T cells. Activated CD4+ T cells that are productively infected usually die very quickly as a result of both direct viral and indirect immune effects. However, if an activated CD4+ T cell is in the process of converting to a quiescent memory cell when it becomes infected, HIV-1 can stably integrate into the host cell DNA

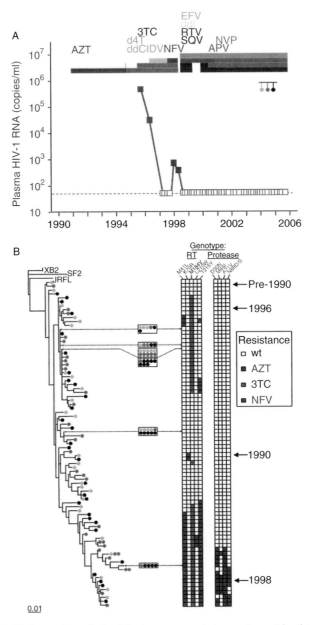

FIGURE I Phylogenetic analysis of the latent reservoir in a patient with a history of prior nonsuppressive therapy. (A) Treatment history of patient 148. Drug regimens are indicated by colored bars. The reservoir was sampled at three time points in 2004 (gray and black circles). (B) Phylogenetic tree of RT sequences from reference strains (HXB2, SF2, JRFL) and from patient 148 (gray and black symbols). Each symbol represents the sequence of virus from a single latently infected CD4+ T cell from the indicated sampling times in 2004. The genotype of

and persist for the lifetime of the cell. HIV-1 most commonly integrates into introns of actively transcribed genes. Thus, latency is not due to inaccessibility of the provirus to the transcriptional apparatus (Han *et al.*, 2004). Rather, latency results from other factors including inadequate levels of host transcription factors and of HIV-1 Tat, a viral protein which normally upregulates HIV-1 gene expression [for a review, see Lassen *et al.* (2004)].

3. HAART

There are currently 21 FDA approved antiretroviral drugs that can be divided into four classes based on their mechanisms of action. HAART consists of combinations of three or more antiretroviral drugs, usually from at least two different classes. The most commonly used HAART regimens consist of two nucleoside reverse transcriptase inhibitors (NRTIs) and either a protease inhibitor (PI) or a nonnucleoside reverse transcriptase inhibitor (NNRTI). Early studies of viral dynamics by Ho and Perelson showed that monotherapy can decrease the viral load in a patient by up to three logs in the first 3 weeks (Ho *et al.*, 1995), and that on HAART the viral load decreases in an exponential, biphasic pattern to undetectable levels in less than 2 months (Ho, 2002; Perelson *et al.*, 1997). Analysis of residual viremia in patients on HAART has shown that HAART slows and in some cases stops viral evolution, but as a result of the existence of stable reservoirs, HAART cannot cure HIV-1 infection (Chun *et al.*, 1997b; Finzi *et al.*, 1999; Persaud *et al.*, 2003; Siliciano and Siliciano, 2004; Siliciano *et al.*, 2003; Strain *et al.*, 2003; Wong *et al.*, 1997).

4. The Latent Reservoir as a Barrier to Cure

In an HIV-1-infected person, $\sim$1 per 10^6 resting CD4+ T cells harbor replication-competent virus (Chun *et al.*, 1997a; Finzi *et al.*, 1999; Siliciano *et al.*, 2003). Thus, the pool of latently infected cells is small. However, the half-life of these latently infected T cells has been calculated to be 44 months. On the basis of this frequency and half life, eradication would take over 73 years of complete suppression of viral replication (Finzi *et al.*, 1999; Siliciano *et al.*, 2003). Shortening this half-life in order to achieve eradication of the latent reservoir has therefore been the goal of a number of different strategies (Section VI.E).

---

each isolate on the phylogenetic tree is indicated in the corresponding horizontal row of boxes on the right. Note that in 2004, the reservoir contained ancestral wild-type viruses (wt), and viruses carrying resistance mutations to zidovudine (AZT), lamivudine (3TC), and nelfinavir (NFV). These drugs were taken 6–13 years previously, before effective suppression of viral replication was achieved. (See Color Insert.)

IV. Resistance: Mechanism of Storage in the Latent Reservoir and Its Clinical Implications _____

A. Development of Resistance

The ultimate goal of antiretroviral therapy is the suppression of plasma virus levels to less than 50 copies/ml, minimizing viral evolution and the emergence of resistance. Common causes of treatment failure and the development of resistance to antiretroviral therapies include nonadherence, the inappropriate use combinations of antagonist drugs, and monotherapy, which was common practice in the early 1990s when there were few drug options available (del Rio, 2006). Suboptimal antiretroviral regimens partially inhibit replication and exert a selective pressure on the wild-type virus allowing resistant variants to become dominant (Clavel and Hance, 2004; Persaud *et al.*, 2003). The problem of resistance is exacerbated by the fact that when a resistant viral quasispecies becomes the dominant population secondary to ineffective therapy, the virus becomes archived in the latent reservoir. This causes the patient to have lifelong resistance to the drugs causing the selective pressure (Persaud *et al.*, 2003; Ruff *et al.*, 2002). In addition, if therapy is discontinued, the more fit wild-type virus reemerges from the latent reservoir as the dominant plasma species, particularly if the replication capacity of the resistant species is significantly impaired by its mutations (Bartlett and Gallant, 2005; Deeks *et al.*, 2001; Ruff *et al.*, 2002).

B. Treatment Interruption

The rapid reemergence of wild-type virus as the dominant plasma species after cessation of antiretroviral therapy led some researchers to believe that resistant variants were transient and easily eliminated in the absence of selection pressure. However, it is now clear that resistant variants are stored in the latent reservoir even when they are no longer detectable in the plasma of patients who interrupt therapy and have a wild-type virus in the plasma. This principle is illustrated by the experience with a therapeutic strategy of *scheduled treatment interruptions* in patients failing therapy (Lawrence *et al.*, 2006). The idea behind these studies was that a treatment interruption would allow the return of wild-type virus, making patients more likely to respond to a salvage regimen. It has since become clear that archived drug-resistant viruses confer lifelong drug resistance and that these variants can reemerge when therapy is restarted. Thus, patients who undergo treatment interruption for this purpose do not respond better to salvage therapy than patients who directly switch to a salvage regimen and demonstrate a higher rate of adverse events related to the loss of viral suppression during the interruption (Lawrence *et al.*, 2006).

C. Blips and the Relationship to the Latent Reservoir

Although antiretroviral drugs can reduce the viral load to levels that are undetectable by ultrasensitive RT-PCR assays, the latent reservoir persists and serves as a stable archive for wild-type virus as well as any resistant variants that may have arisen from prior nonsuppressive therapy. When latently infected resting CD4+ T cells undergo activation, upregulation of viral gene expression can lead to the production of virions that can be detected as low-level viremia. It is now clear that most patients on HAART who have viral loads below the limit of detection of clinical assays actually have continuous residual viremia of <50 copies/ml (Hermankova *et al.*, 2001). This may reflect release of virus from stable reservoirs (Bailey *et al.*, 2006). In addition, some patients have transient elevations of viremia into the detectable range (>50 copies/ml). These are known as blips. With frequent sample, blips may be detected in most patients on suppressive antiretroviral therapy. Clinical studies have demonstrated that these transient increases in viral load are not associated with viral evolution and may represent statistical variation around a mean viral load that is slightly below the limit of detection (Nettles *et al.*, 2005). The finding that there can be viremia without viral evolution suggests that while it may not be possible to cure HIV-1 with current antiretroviral treatment, patients can maintain chronic suppression of viral replication (Siliciano, 2006).

V. Genotypic and Phenotypic Assays: Treatment Implications of the Latent Reservoir _____

Drug resistance is the dominant problem in the management of HIV-1 infection, and it is important to understand how the existence of a latent reservoir for HIV-1 affects clinical decisions regarding the use of antiretroviral drugs in patients who have resistance. Two major types of tests are used to detect resistance and determine the optimal antiretroviral treatment for a patient, the genotypic and phenotypic assays. Neither one detects resistant viruses in the latent reservoir.

A. Genotypic Assays

Clinicians generally request a genotypic assay for resistance when an HIV-1-infected patient is first being evaluated, just prior to the initiation of treatment, during pregnancy, and in the event of treatment failure. This assay involves population level sequencing of the reverse transcriptase (RT) and protease genes to look for resistance mutations present in these regions. Because extensive information is available regarding the correlation between genotype and phenotype, sequencing results can be used to predict the level of resistance to individual antiretroviral drugs. While this assay is relatively inexpensive, quick, and reproducible, it only amplifies the most dominant plasma species and may miss mutations in the less prevalent quasispecies and viruses in the latent reservoir. Additionally, not all resistance mutations are known for newer drugs, and complex resistance profiles require expertise for interpretation (Bartlett and Gallant, 2005).

B. Phenotypic Assays

Phenotypic assays are generally reserved for highly treatment-experienced patients who are failing their current regimen or for those with complex resistance patterns (Wegner *et al.*, 2004). The assay involves the insertion of RT and protease genes from the patient's virus into a backbone reporter virus. Replication is then monitored in single-round assays in transformed cell lines in the presence of a range of different drug concentrations. This assay is considerably more expensive than the genotypic assay. It determines resistance to single drugs rather than combinations and can only detect resistance to dominant species in the plasma. Like the genotypic assay, it requires a plasma viral load of at least 500–1000 copies/ml. However, the interpretation of this assay is far more straightforward, and it allows for the assessment of complex interactions between drug resistance mutations (Bartlett and Gallant, 2005). While this assay provides information that is useful for determining the most effective regimens for a virus with a complex pattern of resistance mutations, there are some concerns that the assay involves laboratory cell lines which do not reflect *in vivo* conditions of infection (Wurtzer *et al.*, 2005). Furthermore, this assay only assesses individual drugs and may not account for the synergistic or antagonistic effects of drug combinations.

C. Latent Reservoir and Drug Sensitivity Assays

Genotypic and phenotypic assays do not necessarily reflect archived resistance in the latent reservoir. Clinicians use these assays to assess the dominant plasma virus population at the time of the assay. However, because viral variants archived in the latent reservoir are not detected by these assays, clinicians are left to rely on the history of the patient's treatment experience as well as their clinical judgment to determine the most effective antiretroviral regimen for a patient.

VI. Drug Development: Taking the Latent Reservoir into Account _____

A. The Problem of Overlap Mutations

When developing new antiretroviral drugs within an established class, it is critical to account for the possible impact of known mutations that confer resistance across the entire class. Prior exposure to drugs in a given class may generate resistance mutations that can persist in the latent reservoir and compromise future responses to agents in the same class. Preexisting mutations that confer resistance to other agents in the same class are known as overlap mutations. The NNRTIs are the most important class to which this applies because there are a number of point mutations that confer complete resistance to all available NNRTIs (Pauwels, 2004). The most promising new NNRTI is etravirine, which is not affected by K103N—one of the most common current NNRTI mutations. Multiple mutations are required for full resistance to this drug (Vingerhoets *et al.*, 2005).

B. High Barrier to Resistance

For an antiretroviral drug, the genetic barrier to resistance depends on the number of mutations necessary to confer drug resistance and how rapidly these mutations develop under selection pressure. Some antiretrovirals such as NNRTIs have a low barrier to resistance, as only one mutation is required for high-level, class-wide resistance. Once an NNRTI resistance mutation such as K103N or Y181C develops, it can be archived in the latent reservoir and confer lifelong resistance to that class of agents. Other antiretrovirals such as the PIs have high barriers to resistance, requiring multiple mutations that characteristically accumulate over long periods of time.

1. Darunavir

The recently approved PI darunavir is being used widely in salvage regimens; its efficacy decreases only with 10 or more general PI mutations or with the accumulation of darunavir-specific mutations (del Rio, 2006). This makes darunavir effective in patients who have failed multiple PI-containing regimens. Recently visualized crystal structures of darunavir in the protease-active site revealed that two different diastereomers bind at two distinct sites simultaneously (Kovalevsky *et al.*, 2006). Darunavir's high barrier to resistance may be related to the fact that the drug acts at two binding sites, thereby requiring simultaneous alteration of both locations for loss of efficacy.

C. Increased Susceptibility

Antiretroviral resistance mutations selected by one drug occasionally confer increased susceptibility to other drugs. There are two main examples of this phenomenon.

1. The AZT–3TC Interaction

The first example is the suppression of resistance to the thymidine analogue zidovudine (AZT) that is induced by the M184V mutation caused by lamivudine (3TC) and emtricitabine (FTC) (Tisdale *et al.*, 1993). When the M184V mutation coexists with thymidine analogue mutations in a resistant strain, the virus continues to be resistant to both FTC and 3TC, but its resistance to AZT is attenuated by the affect of the M184V mutation. A Y181C NNRTI mutation in combination with an M184V mutation is also sufficient to reverse AZT resistance (Byrnes *et al.*, 1994). Subsequent studies have demonstrated that M184V not only attenuates resistance to AZT but also induces hypersusceptibility to AZT in patients without thymidine analogue mutations. This appears to be related to the fact that M184V interferes with the ATP-dependent excision of AZT from the terminated cDNA at the RT active site (Boyer *et al.*, 2002). Other NRTI mutations that have also been shown to induce AZT hypersusceptibility include mutations at positions Q151 and Y115 (Smith *et al.*, 2006).

2. NNRTI Hypersusceptibility

The second example of hypersusceptibility is that which is caused by NRTI mutations. Increasingly, NRTI mutations are being associated with hypersusceptibility to the NNRTIs (Whitcomb *et al.*, 2000). This is presumably due to the fact that mutations that confer resistance to NRTIs are located near the active site of RT and induce conformational changes that may affect the NNRTI-binding site nearby.

3. Hypersensitizing Mutations and the Latent Reservoir

Antiretroviral drug mutations that induce hypersensitivity are archived in the latent reservoir the same way as all other mutations. However, in order to exert their effect on the desired drug, the hypersusceptible virus must be maintained by continued therapy with the inducing drug. For example, many patients on AZT continue to take 3TC (or FTC) even when they have a documented M184V mutation. In this situation, the 3TC maintains selection for the resistant variant. If the 3TC were discontinued, archived variants lacking this mutation might emerge. Although the 3TC resistant virus would also be preserved in the latent reservoir, the advantages related to the reduced fitness and thymidine analogue hypersusceptibility of the M184V variant would be effectively lost.

D. New Classes

For highly treatment-experienced patients failing all current regimens, new classes of drugs are crucial to achieve viral suppression. New classes of drugs such as integrase inhibitors and entry inhibitors are unlikely to be affected by overlap mutations present in plasma virus or virus in the latent reservoir and can offer highly treatment-experienced patients new therapy options. New classes of drugs can also improve side effect profiles and improve compliance with simplified regimens.

I. New Mechanisms

Integrase inhibitors are diketo acids that inhibit the integrase strand-transfer reaction that ligates viral DNA to cellular DNA. Drugs such as T-20 (enfuvirtide) block the fusion reaction mediated by the envelope protein gp41, preventing entry of virions into the cell. Other drugs that are currently under phase I and II trials, including TNX355, SCH-C, and AMD3100 block coreceptors CD4, CCR5, and CXCR4, respectively, ultimately preventing viral entry into the cell (Agrawal *et al.*, 2006).

E. Latent Reservoir as a Target for Future Drug Development

Given that the latent reservoir has been identified as the primary barrier to the cure of HIV-1-1 infection, a number of strategies to reduce reservoir size are currently under investigation.

I. Intensification

The stability of the latent reservoir is most likely due to the inherent stability of memory T cells, and there is no clear evidence that new virus is being stored in the latent reservoirs of patients with suppression of viremia to less than 50 copies/ml. As a result, it is unlikely that simply intensifying a HAART regimen will have a significant impact on the decay of the latent reservoir (Siliciano and Siliciano, 2006).

2. Activating Agents

The use of activating agents such as cytokines has been proposed as a means of forcing virus out of the latent reservoir (Chun and Fauci, 1999). While studies involving IL-2 and IL-12 have not been promising in this regard, studies involving IL-7 have produced a 50–70% decrease in the prevalence of latently infected cells (Brooks *et al.*, 2003; Davey *et al.*, 1999; Wang *et al.*, 2005). Histone deacetylase inhibitors, such as valproic acid, have also been studied in an effort to "flush" virus from the latent reservoir (Ylisastigui *et al.*, 2004). However, the rationale for this strategy was based on the premise that HIV-1 integrates into heterochromatin. In fact, experimental data suggests that HIV-1 integrates into the introns of active genes (Han *et al.*, 2004). A small trial with valproic acid suggests a possible effect in reducing the size of the latent reservoir (Lehrman *et al.*, 2005), although the significance of a minor reduction in the size of the reservoir is not clear (Siliciano *et al.*, 2006). Prostratin, a phorbol ester that stimulates protein kinase C, may also activate latent virus while simultaneously downregulating CD4, CCR5, and CXCR4 receptors (Kulkosky *et al.*, 2001). Exogenous Tat protein has also been used to activate latent virus, and follow-up studies will be necessary to further investigate this effect (Lin *et al.*, 2003). Anti-CD3 agents and IL-2 have also been studied, although these approaches appear to be limited by toxicity associated with global T cell activation (Prins *et al.*, 1999).

It is important to keep in mind that partial eradication of the latent reservoir will be of no benefit to patients because any residual infected cell has potential to rekindle infection. Hence, these approaches to "flushing out" the latent virus are only useful if they provide a thorough elimination of the latent reservoir.

VII. Conclusions

Our knowledge of the latent reservoir and its clinical ramifications is growing rapidly, and this remains an area of active investigation. The existence of the latent reservoir appears to be the main obstacle to the cure of HIV-1 infection, and it functions as a permanent archive for drug resistance mutations. New techniques for identifying archived resistance may provide clinicians with a means of designing optimal HAART for treatment-experienced patients. At present, remarkable advances in antiretroviral development and resistance detection are continuing to offer patients and clinicians new tools for managing HIV-1, despite the challenges of its persistence and evolution. Continuing creativity in drug development as well as dedicated investigation into the mechanisms of HIV-1 latency will continue to be two critical aspects of the ongoing effort to manage the impact of HIV-1 infection.

References

Agrawal, L., Lu, X., Jin, Q., and Alkhatib, G. (2006). Anti-HIV therapy: Current and future directions. *Curr. Pharm. Des* **12**(16), 2031–2055.

Bailey, J. R., Sedaghat, A. R., Kieffer, T., Brennan, T., Lee, P. K., Wind-Rotolo, M., Haggerty, C. M., Kamireddi, A. R., Liu, Y., Lee, J., Persaud, D., Gallant, J. E., *et al.* (2006). Residual human immunodeficiency virus type 1 viremia in some patients on antiretroviral therapy is dominated by a small number of invariant clones rarely found in circulating CD4$^+$ T cells. *J. Virol.* **80**(13), 6441–6457.

Bartlett, J. G., and Gallant, J. (2005). "Medical Management of HIV Infection (2005–2006 edn.)." Johns Hopkins Medicine, Baltimore.

Bartlett, J. G., and Lane, H. C. (2006). Guidelines for the Use of Antiretroviral Agents in HIV-1-Infected Adults and Adolescents. Office of AIDS Research Advisory Council: Panel on Antiretroviral Guidelines for Adults and Adolescents. Department of Health and Human Services.

Boyer, P. L., Sarafianos, S. G., Arnold, E., and Hughes, S. H. (2002). The M184V mutation reduces the selective excision of zidovudine 5′-monophosphate (AZTMP) by the reverse transcriptase of human immunodeficiency virus type 1. *J. Virol.* **76**(7), 3248–3256.

Brooks, D. G., Hamer, D. H., Arlen, P. A., Gao, L., Bristol, G., Kitchen, C. M., Berger, E. A., and Zack, J. A. (2003). Molecular characterization, reactivation, and depletion of latent HIV. *Immunity* **19**(3), 413–423.

Byrnes, V. W., Emini, E. A., Schleif, W. A., Condra, J. H., Schneider, C. L., Long, W. J., Wolfgang, J. A., Graham, D. J., Gotlib, L., and Schlabach, A. J. (1994). Susceptibilities of human immunodeficiency virus type 1 enzyme and viral variants expressing multiple resistance-engendering amino acid substitutions to reserve transcriptase inhibitors. *Antimicrob. Agents Chemother.* **38**(6), 1404–1407.

Chun, T. W., and Fauci, A. S. (1999). Latent reservoirs of HIV: Obstacles to the eradication of virus. *Proc. Natl. Acad. Sci. USA* **96**(20), 10958–10961.

Chun, T. W., Finzi, D., Margolick, J., Chadwick, K., Schwartz, D., and Siliciano, R. F. (1995). *In vivo* fate of HIV-1-infected T cells: Quantitative analysis of the transition to stable latency. *Nat. Med.* **1**(12), 1284–1290.

Chun, T. W., Carruth, L., Finzi, D., Shen, X., DiGiuseppe, J. A., Taylor, H., Hermankova, M., Chadwick, K., Margolick, J., Quinn, T. C., Kuo, Y. H., Brookmeyer, R., *et al.* (1997a). Quantification of latent tissue reservoirs and total body viral load in HIV-1 infection. *Nature* **387**(6629), 183–188.

Chun, T. W., Stuyver, L., Mizell, S. B., Ehler, L. A., Mican, J. A., Baseler, M., Lloyd, A. L., Nowak, M. A., and Fauci, A. S. (1997b). Presence of an inducible HIV-1 latent reservoir during highly active antiretroviral therapy. *Proc. Natl. Acad. Sci. USA* **94**(24), 13193–13197.

Clavel, F., and Hance, A. J. (2004). HIV drug resistance. *N. Engl. J. Med.* **350**(10), 1023–1035.

Davey, R. T., Jr., Chaitt, D. G., Albert, J. M., Piscitelli, S. C., Kovacs, J. A., Walker, R. E., Falloon, J., Polis, M. A., Metcalf, J. A., Masur, H., Dewar, R., Baseler, M., *et al.* (1999). A randomized trial of high- versus low-dose subcutaneous interleukin-2 outpatient therapy for early human immunodeficiency virus type 1 infection. *J. Infect. Dis.* **179**(4), 849–858.

Deeks, S. G., Wrin, T., Liegler, T., Hoh, R., Hayden, M., Barbour, J. D., Hellmann, N. S., Petropoulos, C. J., McCune, J. M., Hellerstein, M. K., and Grant, R. M. (2001). Virologic and immunologic consequences of discontinuing combination antiretroviral-drug therapy in HIV-infected patients with detectable viremia. *N. Engl. J. Med.* **344**(7), 472–480.

del Rio, C. (Rio 2006). Current concepts in antiretroviral therapy failure. *Top. HIV Med.* **14**(3), 102–106.

Finzi, D., Hermankova, M., Pierson, T., Carruth, L. M., Buck, C., Chaisson, R. E., Quinn, T. C., Chadwick, K., Margolick, J., Brookmeyer, R., Gallant, J., Markowitz, M., *et al.* (1997). Identification of a reservoir for HIV-1 in patients on highly active antiretroviral therapy. *Science* **278**(5341), 1295–1300.

Finzi, D., Blankson, J., Siliciano, J. D., Margolick, J. B., Chadwick, K., Pierson, T., Smith, K., Lisziewicz, J., Lori, F., Flexner, C., Quinn, T. C., Chaisson, R. E., *et al.* (1999). Latent infection of CD4+ T cells provides a mechanism for lifelong persistence of HIV-1, even in patients on effective combination therapy. *Nat. Med.* **5**(5), 512–517.

Haggerty, C. M., Pitt, E., and Siliciano, R. F. (2006). The latent reservoir for HIV-1 in resting CD4+ T cells and other viral reservoirs during chronic infection: Insights from treatment and treatment-interruption trials. *Curr. Opin. HIV AIDS* **1**(1), 62–68.

Han, Y., Lassen, K., Monie, D., Sedaghat, A. R., Shimoji, S., Liu, X., Pierson, T. C., Margolick, J. B., Siliciano, R. F., and Siliciano, J. D. (2004). Resting CD4+ T cells from human immunodeficiency virus type 1 (HIV-1)-infected individuals carry integrated HIV-1 genomes within actively transcribed host genes. *J. Virol.* **78**(12), 6122–6133.

Hermankova, M., Ray, S. C., Ruff, C., Powell-Davis, M., Ingersoll, R., D'Aquila, R. T., Quinn, T. C., Siliciano, J. D., Siliciano, R. F., and Persaud, D. (2001). HIV-1 drug resistance profiles in children and adults with viral load of <50 copies/ml receiving combination therapy. *JAMA* **286**(2), 196–207.

Ho, D. D. (2002). HIV and lymphocyte dynamics. *Vaccine* **20**(15), 1933.

Ho, D. D., Neumann, A. U., Perelson, A. S., Chen, W., Leonard, J. M., and Markowitz, M. (1995). Rapid turnover of plasma virions and CD4 lymphocytes in HIV-1 infection. *Nature* 373(6510), 123–126.

Igarashi, T., Brown, C. R., Endo, Y., Buckler-White, A., Plishka, R., Bischofberger, N., Hirsch, V., and Martin, M. A. (2001). Macrophage are the principal reservoir and sustain high virus loads in rhesus macaques after the depletion of CD4+ T cells by a highly pathogenic simian immunodeficiency virus/HIV type 1 chimera (SHIV): Implications for HIV-1 infections of humans. *Proc. Natl. Acad. Sci. USA* 98(2), 658–663.

Igarashi, T., Imamichi, H., Brown, C. R., Hirsch, V. M., and Martin, M. A. (2003). The emergence and characterization of macrophage-tropic SIV/HIV chimeric viruses (SHIVs) present in CD4+ T cell-depleted rhesus monkeys. *J. Leukoc. Biol.* 74(5), 772–780.

Kovalevsky, A. Y., Liu, F., Leshchenko, S., Ghosh, A. K., Louis, J. M., Harrison, R. W., and Weber, I. T. (2006). Ultra-high resolution crystal structure of HIV-1 protease mutant reveals two binding sites for clinical inhibitor TMC114. *J. Mol. Biol.* 363(1), 161–173.

Kulkosky, J., Culnan, D. M., Roman, J., Dornadula, G., Schnell, M., Boyd, M. R., and Pomerantz, R. J. (2001). Prostratin: Activation of latent HIV-1 expression suggests a potential inductive adjuvant therapy for HAART. *Blood* 98(10), 3006–3015.

Lassen, K., Han, Y., Zhou, Y., Siliciano, J., and Siliciano, R. F. (2004). The multifactorial nature of HIV-1 latency. *Trends Mol. Med.* 10(11), 525–531.

Lawrence, J., Hullsiek, K. H., Thackeray, L. M., Abrams, D. I., Crane, L. R., Mayers, D. L., Jones, M. C., Saldanha, J. M., Schmetter, B. S., and Baxter, J. D. (2006). Disadvantages of structured treatment interruption persist in patients with multidrug-resistant HIV-1: Final results of the CPCRA 064 study. *J. Acquir. Immune. Defic. Syndr.* 43(2), 169–178.

Lehrman, G., Hogue, I. B., Palmer, S., Jennings, C., Spina, C. A., Wiegand, A., Landay, A. L., Coombs, R. W., Richman, D. D., Mellors, J. W., Coffin, J. M., Bosch, R. J., *et al.* (2005). Depletion of latent HIV-1 infection in vivo: A proof-of-concept study. *Lancet* 366(9485), 549–555.

Lin, X., Irwin, D., Kanazawa, S., Huang, L., Romeo, J., Yen, T. S., and Peterlin, B. M. (2003). Transcriptional profiles of latent human immunodeficiency virus in infected individuals: Effects of Tat on the host and reservoir. *J. Virol.* 77(15), 8227–8236.

Nettles, R. E., Kieffer, T. L., Kwon, P., Monie, D., Han, Y., Parsons, T., Cofrancesco, J., Jr., Gallant, J. E., Quinn, T. C., Jackson, B., Flexner, C., Carson, K., *et al.* (2005). Intermittent HIV-1 viremia (Blips) and drug resistance in patients receiving HAART. *JAMA* 293(7), 817–829.

Nickle, D. C., Jensen, M. A., Shriner, D., Brodie, S. J., Frenkel, L. M., Mittler, J. E., and Mullins, J. I. (2003). Evolutionary indicators of human immunodeficiency virus type 1 reservoirs and compartments. *J. Virol.* 77(9), 5540–5546.

Pauwels, R. (2004). New non-nucleoside reverse transcriptase inhibitors (NNRTIs) in development for the treatment of HIV infections. *Curr. Opin. Pharmacol.* 4(5), 437–446.

Perelson, A. S., Essunger, P., Cao, Y., Vesanen, M., Hurley, A., Saksela, K., Markowitz, M., and Ho, D. D. (1997). Decay characteristics of HIV-1-infected compartments during combination therapy. *Nature* 387(6629), 188–191.

Persaud, D., Zhou, Y., Siliciano, J. M., and Siliciano, R. F. (2003). Latency in human immunodeficiency virus type 1 infection: No easy answers. *J. Virol.* 77(3), 1659–1665.

Prins, J. M., Jurriaans, S., van Praag, R. M., Blaak, H., van Rij, R., Schellekens, P. T., ten, Berg, I. J., Yong, S. L., Fox, C. H., Roos, M. T., de Wolf, F., Goudsmit, J., *et al.* (1999). Immuno-activation with anti-CD3 and recombinant human IL-2 in HIV-1-infected patients on potent antiretroviral therapy. *AIDS* 13(17), 2405–2410.

Ruff, C. T., Ray, S. C., Kwon, P., Zinn, R., Pendleton, A., Hutton, N., Ashworth, R., Gange, S., Quinn, T. C., Siliciano, R. F., and Persaud, D. (2002). Persistence of wild-type virus and lack of temporal structure in the latent reservoir for human immunodeficiency virus type 1 in pediatric patients with extensive antiretroviral exposure. *J. Virol.* 76(18), 9481–9492.

Siliciano, J. D., and Siliciano, R. F. (2004). A long-term latent reservoir for HIV-1: Discovery and clinical implications. *J. Antimicrob. Chemother.* **54**(1), 6–9.

Siliciano, J. D., and Siliciano, R. F. (2005). Enhanced culture assay for detection and quantitation of latently infected, resting CD4+ T-cells carrying replication-competent virus in HIV-1-infected individuals. *Methods Mol. Biol.* **304**, 3–15.

Siliciano, J. D., and Siliciano, R. F. (2006). The latent reservoir for HIV-1 in resting CD4+ T cells: A barrier to cure. *Curr. Opin. HIV AIDS* **1**, 121–128.

Siliciano, J. D., Kajdas, J., Finzi, D., Quinn, T. C., Chadwick, K., Margolick, J. B., Kovacs, C., Gange, S. J., and Siliciano, R. F. (2003). Long-term follow-up studies confirm the stability of the latent reservoir for HIV-1 in resting CD4+ T cells. *Nat. Med.* **9**(6), 727–728.

Siliciano, J. D., Lai, J., Callendar, M., Pitt, E., Zhang, H., Margolick, J., Gallant, J., Cofrancesco, J., Moore, R. D., Gange, S., and Siliciano, R. F. (2006). Stability of the latent reservoir for HIV-1 in patients on valproic acid. *J. Infect. Dis.* **195**(6), 833–836.

Siliciano, R. F. (2006). "Clinical Care Options; HIV/AIDS Annual Update 2006" (P. Phair, Ed.), pp. 17–28. Clinical care options, Key Biscayne, Florida.

Smith, R. A., Anderson, D. J., and Preston, B. D. (2006). Hypersusceptibility to substrate analogs conferred by mutations in human immunodeficiency virus type 1 reverse transcriptase. *J. Virol.* **80**(14), 7169–7178.

Strain, M. C., Gunthard, H. F., Havlir, D. V., Ignacio, C. C., Smith, D. M., Leigh-Brown, A. J., Macaranas, T. R., Lam, R. Y., Daly, O. A., Fischer, M., Opravil, M., Levine, H., *et al.* (2003). Heterogeneous clearance rates of long-lived lymphocytes infected with HIV: Intrinsic stability predicts lifelong persistence. *Proc. Natl. Acad. Sci. USA* **100**(8), 4819–4824.

Tisdale, M., Kemp, S. D., Parry, N. R., and Larder, B. A. (1993). Rapid *in vitro* selection of human immunodeficiency virus type 1 resistant to 3′-thiacytidine inhibitors due to a mutation in the YMDD region of reverse transcriptase. *Proc. Natl. Acad. Sci. USA* **90**(12), 5653–5656.

Vingerhoets, J., Azijn, H., Fransen, E., De, B. I., Smeulders, L., Jochmans, D., Andries, K., Pauwels, R., and de Bethune, M. P. (2005). TMC125 displays a high genetic barrier to the development of resistance: Evidence from *in vitro* selection experiments. *J. Virol.* **79**(20), 12773–12782.

Wang, F. X., Xu, Y., Sullivan, J., Souder, E., Argyris, E. G., Acheampong, E. A., Fisher, J., Sierra, M., Thomson, M. M., Najera, R., Frank, I., Kulkosky, J., *et al.* (2005). IL-7 is a potent and proviral strain-specific inducer of latent HIV-1 cellular reservoirs of infected individuals on virally suppressive HAART. *J. Clin. Invest.* **115**(1), 128–137.

Wegner, S. A., Wallace, M. R., Aronson, N. E., Tasker, S. A., Blazes, D. L., Tamminga, C., Fraser, S., Dolan, M. J., Stephan, K. T., Michael, N. L., Jagodzinski, L. L., Vahey, M. T., *et al.* (2004). Long-term efficacy of routine access to antiretroviral-resistance testing in HIV type 1-infected patients: Results of the clinical efficacy of resistance testing trial. *Clin. Infect. Dis.* **38**(5), 723–730.

Whitcomb, J., Deeks, S. G., and Huang, W. (2000). Reduced susceptibility to NRTI is associated with NNRTI shypersusceptibility in virus from HIV-1 infected pateints. Seventh Conference on Retroviruses and Opportunistic Infections.

Wong, J. K., Hezareh, M., Gunthard, H. F., Havlir, D. V., Ignacio, C. C., Spina, C. A., and Richman, D. D. (1997). Recovery of replication-competent HIV despite prolonged suppression of plasma viremia. *Science* **278**(5341), 1291–1295.

Wurtzer, S., Compain, S., Benech, H., Hance, A. J., and Clavel, F. (2005). Effect of cell cycle arrest on the activity of nucleoside analogues against human immunodeficiency virus type 1. *J. Virol.* **79**(23), 14815–14821.

Ylisastigui, L., Archin, N. M., Lehrman, G., Bosch, R. J., and Margolis, D. M. (2004). Coaxing HIV-1 from resting CD4 T cells: Histone deacetylase inhibition allows latent viral expression. *AIDS* **18**(8), 1101–1108.

Man Lung Yeung*, Yamina Bennasser*, Shu-Yun Le[†], and Kuan-Teh Jeang*

*Molecular Virology Section, Laboratory of Molecular Microbiology
National Institute of Allergy and Infectious Diseases, National Institutes of Health
Bethesda, Maryland 20892

[†]Center for Cancer Research Nanobiology Program
NCI Center for Cancer Research, NCI, National Insitutes of Health
Frederick, Maryland 21702

RNA Interference and HIV-1

I. Chapter Overview

RNA interference (RNAi) can regulate a variety of biological processes. Recent evidence supports the notion that both cellular and viral miRNAs (vmiRNAs) are able to modulate viral replication. There is also evidence that viruses like HIV-1 have evolved methods to control the cell's RNAi activity. In this chapter, we discuss possible roles for RNAi in the HIV-1 life cycle, and how HIV-1 might use protein and RNA elements to regulate RNA-based viral restriction.

1054-3589/07 $35.00
DOI: 10.1016/S1054-3589(07)55013-1

II. Introduction _____

RNAi, also called "posttranscriptional gene silencing" (PTGS) in plant, was first described as an immune defense against foreign viruses, transgenes, and transposons (Voinnet, 2005). RNAi employs a ribonuclease (RNase) III protein(s) complexed with a small guide RNA for sequence-specific silencing of targeted RNAs. Currently, two types of small RNAs [small interfering RNA (siRNA) and microRNA (miRNA)] have been identified to participate in RNAi.

siRNA and miRNA are first processed from longer precursor RNAs into small RNAs of 18–25 nucleotides (nts) by RNase III proteins termed Dicer and Drosha. An siRNA precursor can be a long linear double-stranded RNA (dsRNA) or a hairpin RNA. Mechanistically, one strand of an siRNA duplex is destined to become a guide RNA which is channeled by Dicer-interacting proteins, PACT and TAR RNA-binding protein (TRBP) (Chendrimada *et al.*, 2005; Gatignol *et al.*, 1991; Haase *et al.*, 2005; Lee *et al.*, 2006) into an RNA-induced silencing complex (RISC). Currently, many RISC components remain uncharacterized; however, it is believed that RISC minimally contains a single-stranded guide siRNA coupled to the Argonaute 2 (Ago2) protein (Liu *et al.*, 2004; Meister *et al.*, 2004). It is envisioned that the guide siRNA hybridizes to its target mRNA based on perfect sequence complementarity. Using such hybridization, the siRNA-guide sequence captures an mRNA target and brings the mRNA into proximity of the Piwi domain of Ago2 for degradation (Fig. 1).

miRNAs constitute a second pathway complementary in function to siRNAs. Although miRNAs also silence gene expression, the genesis and action of miRNAs are different from siRNAs. miRNA precursors (pri-miRNAs) are highly structured RNAs of ~70 nts transcribed generally from noncoding regions endogenous within eukaryotic RNA polymerase II transcribed genes (Lee *et al.*, 2004). Once transcribed, a pri-miRNA is rapidly processed in the cell's nucleus into an imperfect shorter stem-loop structure (pre-miRNA) by the microprocessor, a large multicomponent complex that includes an RNase III protein Drosha and the RNA-binding protein DGCR8 (Han *et al.*, 2004a). Processed pre-miRNAs with 3′ protruded ends are then exported into the cytoplasm by Exportin 5 (Bohnsack *et al.*, 2004; Yi *et al.*, 2003). In the cytoplasm, following the removal of the loop region of pre-miRNA by Dicer, one strand of the resulting double-stranded miRNA is incorporated into RISC.

Differing from siRNAs, miRNA-based target recognition is tolerant of base mismatches. Generally, an miRNA can target an mRNA if the former and the latter show perfect complementarity within nucleotides 2–7 of the 5′ end of the miRNA guide (the seed sequence) while having imperfect complementarity between miRNA and mRNA elsewhere (Lewis *et al.*, 2005; Saetrom *et al.*, 2005). However, the exact mechanism for miRNA-mRNA

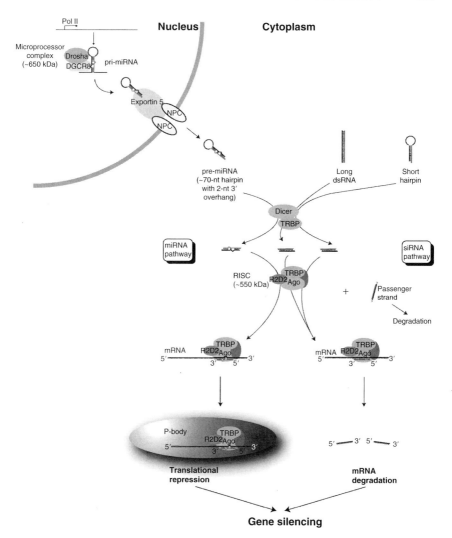

FIGURE 1   miRNA and siRNA pathways. miRNA precursor (pri-miRNA) is first transcribed by RNA Pol II in the nucleus. The highly structured pri-miRNA is recognized by the microprocessor, a complex containing Drosha and DGCR8, and then cropped into an ~70-nt hairpin with two nucleotides in the 3′ overhang (pre-miRNA). With the aid of Exportin 5, the pre-miRNA is exported into the cytoplasm. Processing of pre-miRNA and long dsRNA/short hairpin uses a common pathway which involves the RNA-binding protein TRBP, the RNase III proteins in Dicer and RISC. From a double-stranded small RNA duplex, the passenger strand is removed from the RISC during the process of complex assembly. The remaining strand (guide) is incorporated into RISC and serves for mRNA target recognition. mRNA which have perfect complementary to the guide are hydrolyzed by the Ago2 protein within RISC. The RNase activity of Ago2 is not used when RISC is tagged with an miRNA case. In this setting, mRNAs generally have an imperfect complementarity with the miRNA guide RNA. mRNA–miRNA interaction generally leads to the mRNA being directed into the P-body, a subcellular locale where translation of mRNA fails to occur. NPC, nuclear pore complex.

recognition is still being defined. In general, it is thought that mRNAs captured by miRNAs are not hydrolyzed by Ago2; instead they are ferried by RISC into a ribosome-free translationally silent compartment named Processsing body (P-body; Fig. 1) (Liu *et al.*, 2005a,b; Marx, 2005; Rossi, 2005; Sen and Blau, 2005).

III. siRNA as Anti-HIV Therapy

An obvious use for siRNA is the silencing of viral gene expression (see review Leonard and Schaffer, 2006). Indeed, siRNAs have been extensively tested for anti-HIV-1 properties. siRNAs have been designed to target both HIV-1 coding and noncoding sequences (*nef, tat, gag, vif, env, rev*, LTR) (Boden *et al.*, 2004; Capodici *et al.*, 2002; Coburn and Cullen, 2002; Han *et al.*, 2004b; Jacque *et al.*, 2002; Lee *et al.*, 2002; Novina *et al.*, 2002). These approaches have shown short-term successes; however, HIV's high mutation rates and its possible ability to encode RNAi suppressors (discussed later) challenge the durable success of siRNAs for long-term suppression of virus replication. Indeed, HIV has evolved methods to escape siRNA restriction. Nucleotide substitution and sequence deletion of siRNA-targeted viral sequences by HIV have both been described as ways for this virus to escape siRNA-mediated inhibition (Das *et al.*, 2004). Furthermore, HIV can evolve mutations outside the siRNA recognition site to create a new RNA secondary structure that shields against target access by siRNA and RISC (Westerhout *et al.*, 2005).

HIV's mutational evasion can apparently be blunted by the simultaneous use of multiple siRNAs targeted to different regions of the viral genome. The concept behind this strategy lies in the reasoning that a virus cannot alter many sequences simultaneously and still preserve replication competence. The success of this strategy is supported by data that use of two siRNAs, compared to a single siRNA, significantly delayed HIV-1's mutational escape (ter Brake *et al.*, 2006). Moreover in cells that are stably transduced to express four different HIV-1-targeting siRNAs, no RNAi-resistant virus could be detected up to 60 days after virus infection (Chang *et al.*, 2005; ter Brake *et al.*, 2006). Recent advances in computational modeling provide new insight into predictions as to how HIV-1 might evolve when it is targeted by siRNA (Leonard and Schaffer, 2005). By understanding short-term virus evolution, one can potentially design a larger array of siRNAs to anticipate the "escape" variants.

Another way to combat HIV-1 infection is to use siRNA to knockdown cellular proteins that are essential for the virus life cycle. This approach skirts the ability of viruses to change their viral sequences in order to evade RNAi. Efficient inhibition of virus replication by targeting cellular proteins used for different stages of the HIV-1 life cycle has been demonstrated [see review Yeung *et al.* (2005a) for more details]. However, a longer term concern remains whether there are any cellular genes that can truly be knocked down in a nontoxic fashion for normal cell function(s).

IV. HIV-1 Remodels Cellular miRNA Expression in Infected Cells

The antiviral activity of cellular miRNAs against an infecting virus was first reported by Lecellier *et al.* (2005). These authors demonstrated the ability of miR-32 to restrict primate foamy virus type 1 (PFV-1) replication in cells. PFV-1 counters the cell's miRNA defense by encoding an RNAi suppressor, Tas, which inhibits the processing and maturation of miR-32. Similarly, using a computational approach, five human T-cell miRNAs were predicted to target highly conserved regions across all clades of HIV-1 (Hariharan *et al.*, 2005). If such prediction is correct, then it stands to reason that HIV-1 would want to develop means to avoid being restricted by these human miRNAs. Indeed, we recently reported that the miRNA profile of human cells is dramatically altered after the expression of HIV-1 proteins (Yeung *et al.*, 2005b) with most human miRNAs being reduced in abundance (Fig. 2). We attribute this phenomenon in part to the Dicer-attenuating activity reported for the HIV-1 Tat protein (Bennasser *et al.*, 2005). More recently, the HIV-1 TAR RNA was also shown to be capable of repressing miRNA processing through sequestration of the human cellular dsRNA-binding protein, TRBP, a key cofactor for Dicer (Bennasser *et al.*, 2006b). Because TAR is expressed abundantly in HIV-1-infected cells and because this RNA has high binding affinity for TRBP (Gatignol *et al.*, 1991), one expects that the ability of Dicer to process miRNA precursors would be reduced in the presence of TAR RNA. Hence, like PFV, HIV-1 through a combination of Tat and TAR can apparently reduce the expression of human miRNAs that would otherwise adversely target the virus.

A reduction in miRNA expression may also partially contribute to a higher risk in HIV-1-infected patients to develop neoplasia (Blumenthal *et al.*, 1999; Moulignier *et al.*, 1994; Neal *et al.*, 1996). The most common neoplasm associated with HIV-1 infection is Kaposi's sarcoma (KS), which is caused by *Human herpesvirus 8* (HHV-8, also known as KS-associated herpesvirus, KSHV) (Kempf and Adams, 1996). Notably, immunosuppressed HIV-1 patients have a 70 times higher probability for KS than similar immunosuppression induced by other factors (Beral *et al.*, 1990). It is unclear how HIV-1 assists HHV-8 in this disease. However, because miRNA alterations have been linked to carcinogenesis [see Esquela-Kerscher and Slack (2006) for more detail], one possible speculation, which does not exclude

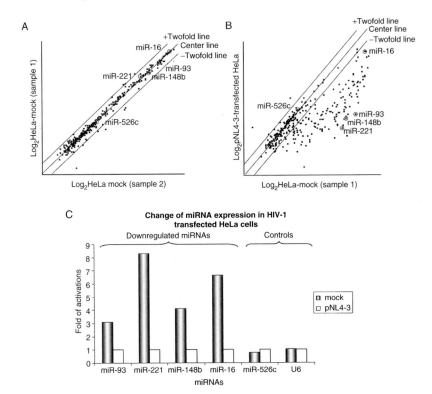

FIGURE 2 The expression profile of human miRNAs is changed by transfection of an HIV-1 molecular clone. (A) Microarray analysis (RAKE, RNA-primed array-based Klenow enzyme) of miRNA expression profile in HeLa cells. (B) Scatter plot analysis of two mock-transfected HeLa cells (sample 1 vs sample 2) suggests that miRNA expression is not affected by the simple act of transfection. In this analysis, each data point represents one miRNA [see Yeung *et al.* (2005b) for more detail]. By contrast, many miRNAs are downregulated in HeLa cells transfected with an HIV-1 molecular clone (pNL4-3). (C) The circled miRNAs were chosen for real-time PCR validation. The fold difference between selected miRNAs from mock- and pNL4-3-transfected HeLa cells are represented in histograms. Samples were first normalized to U6 RNA and an internally unchanged miRNA (miR-526c); and the signals obtained from real-time PCR were then compared.

other possibilities, could be that reduced expression of certain miRNAs in HIV-1-infected cells makes the infected individual more vulnerable to HHV-8-induced sarcomas. More mechanistic data are needed before one can understand the potential role of HIV-1 and miRNAs in cancers like KS. One also has to keep in mind that miRNA contributions must be viewed in the total context of additional, perhaps larger, contributions that arise from immunosuppression.

V. Does HIV-1 Encode miRNAs?

While cellular genomes encode miRNAs, some viruses also carry their own vmiRNAs. Thus far, evidence has been presented to support that more than eight viruses encode miRNA sequences that can be processed inside cells into mature miRNAs (Grey *et al.*, 2005; Omoto and Fujii, 2005; Omoto *et al.*, 2004; Pfeffer *et al.*, 2004, 2005; Sullivan *et al.*, 2005). Although most vmiRNAs' functions remain unknown, expression of some vmiRNAs is thought to be important for establishing latent infections and for permitting infected cells to escape immune surveillance. Examples of self-targeted miRNAs include HIV-1-encoded miRNA (miR-N367) and EBV-encoded miRNA (miR-BART2) which silence *nef* and DNA polymerase (BALF5), respectively (Omoto *et al.*, 2004; Pfeffer *et al.*, 2004). SV40-encoded miRNA (sv40-mir-S1) also inhibits viral transcription (Sullivan *et al.*, 2005). sv40-mir-S1 is expressed late in infection and appears to suppress excessive T-antigen production in SV40-infected cells. In this way, SV40-infected cells are reasoned to be less susceptible to cytotoxic T lymphocyte (CTL) response as well as less potent in stimulating the release of cytokines.

Besides self-targeting, vmiRNAs can also target cellular mRNAs. In Herpes simplex virus type 1 (HSV-1)-infected cells, hsv1-mir-H1, a vmiRNA encoded by the HSV-1 latency-associated transcript (LAT), suppresses transforming growth factor (TGF)-β 1 and SMAD3 proteins and reduces TGF-β-regulated stress-induced apoptosis (Gupta *et al.*, 2006). Thus, vmiRNAs can be used by viruses to change the landscape of host cell gene expression rendering the cellular milieu more favorable for viral replication.

Currently, most identified vmiRNAs are found in DNA viruses. We have developed an algorithm to predict the occurrence of miRNA within a randomly shuffled sequence. Based on this algorithm, we expect three miRNAs can be stochastically present per 100 kb with the assumption SigZscr > 4.0 and $p < 0.00003$ [see Bennasser *et al.* (2006a) for detail]. In a setting of neutral evolution, it seems to us that there should be no bias between the ability of a DNA virus or an RNA virus to encode miRNAs. The empirical data that most reported vmiRNAs are encoded by DNA, rather than RNA, viruses (Table I) would suggest a nonneutral course of evolution (i.e., vmiRNAs is evolutionary favored for DNA vs RNA viruses). While other reasons may be possible, perhaps one reason for a dearth of vmiRNAs in RNA viruses is that the viral genome in RNA form could be a vulnerable substrate for restriction by vmiRNAs. Thus a selective pressure exerted on RNA viral genomes by self-encoded vmiRNA may lead to evolutionary selection against the presence of vmiRNAs in these genomes. Rare preservation of HIV-1-encoded vmiRNAs such as miR-N367 suggests that certain RNA sequences (for unknown reasons) within the HIV-1 genome are poorly

TABLE I   A Summary of Viruses Encoded miRNAs and Their Genome Size

Virus name	No. of miRNAs	Genome size (nts)	No. of miRNA per nts
Simian virus 40	2	5243	2621.50
Epstein–Barr virus	32	171,823	5369.47
Rhesus lymphocryptovirus	22	171,096	7777.09
Kaposi sarcoma-associated herpesvirus	17	135,135	7949.12
Mouse gammaherpesvirus 68	10	119,450	11945.00
Human cytomegalovirus	14	230,287	16449.07
Herpes simplex virus 1	1	152,261	152261.00
Human immunodeficiency virus 1	2	9181	4590.50

mutable despite their presentation within miRNA-like precursor structures. Alternatively, a trivial explanation may simply be that RNA virus encoded vmiRNAs in low abundance which is technically difficult to detect. Time and additional investigation are needed to clarify the picture.

HIV-1 has two candidate viral mi/siRNA sequences (miR-N367 and vsiRNA). HIV-1 also embodies two RNAi suppressors (Tat and TAR) suggesting that this virus employs a complex scheme of gene regulation through small RNAs. Potentially, in a latent HIV-1 infection self-transcripts are targeted by both vmiRNAs and anti-HIV cellular miRNAs (Fig. 3). On productive HIV-1 transcription, Tat protein and TAR RNA inhibit miRNA processing and attenuating vmiRNA- and cellular miRNA-based selection against the virus. This miRNA switch may be one of the factors governing a transition from latent to productively lytic infection.

VI. Future Perspectives

Recent findings suggest that noncoding viral RNAs, other than miRNAs, also function to modulate viral replication. For example, Marek's disease herpesvirus (MDV) encodes a small viral telomerase RNA (vTR) which promotes T-cell transformation by enhancing the telomerase reverse transcriptase (TERT) complex activity (Trapp *et al.*, 2006). Separately, a minus strand HTLV-I basic leucine zipper factor (HBZ) RNA was identified in human T cell leukemia virus type I (HTLV-I)-infected cells (Arnold *et al.*, 2006; Cavanagh *et al.*, 2006; Gaudray *et al.*, 2002). Mutagenesis analyses revealed that a portion of HBZ RNA, not HBZ's protein-coding capacity, likely promote HTLV-1 induced cellular transformation (Satou *et al.*, 2006). Seemingly, different viruses may have developed specific small RNA-based mechanisms to increase their replication. Will another recently discovered class of small ncRNA (Piwi-interacting RNA) (Aravin *et al.*, 2006; Girard *et al.*, 2006) play roles in regulating virus life cycle remains to be addressed.

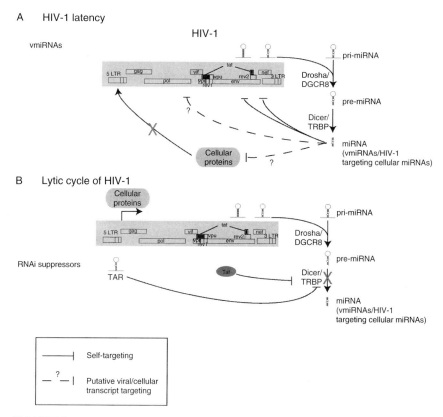

FIGURE 3 A model of how miRNAs could affect the HIV-1 life cycle. (A) HIV-1 encodes shRNA structures which can enter the cell's RNAi processing pathway to generate vmiRNAs (miR-N367 and vsiRNA). Production of vmiRNAs and anti-HIV-1 cellular miRNAs inhibits viral gene expression. These miRNAs may also suppress the expression of some cellular proteins that are essential for HIV-1 transcription. (B) On productive HIV-1 transcription, viral RNAi suppressors (TAR RNA and Tat protein) are produced which attenuate the activity of Dicer/TRBP and moderated the cell's RNAi activity. Attenuation of Dicer/TRBP function leads to inefficient miRNA processing and weakens the cell's miRNA-based restriction of HIV-1.

Also, are there other small ncRNAs encoded by viruses. We have developed a tiling technique that permits us to map all RNAs transcribed from the HIV-1 genome at a resolution of every five base pairs. In coming months, we hope to understand if there is evidence for additional currently unrecognized small HIV-1 viral RNAs.

Acknowledgment

This work was supported through intramural funds from the NIAID and the NCI, NIH.

References

Aravin, A., Gaidatzis, D., Pfeffer, S., Lagos-Quintana, M., Landgraf, P., Iovino, N., Morris, P., Brownstein, M. J., Kuramochi-Miyagawa, S., Nakano, T., Chien, M., Russo, J. J., *et al.* (2006). A novel class of small RNAs bind to MILI protein in mouse testes. *Nature* **442**, 203–207.

Arnold, J., Yamamoto, B., Li, M., Phipps, A. J., Younis, I., Lairmore, M. D., and Green, P. L. (2006). Enhancement of infectivity and persistence *in vivo* by HBZ, a natural antisense coded protein of HTLV-1. *Blood* **107**, 3976–3982.

Bennasser, Y., Le, S. Y., Benkirane, M., and Jeang, K. T. (2005). Evidence that HIV-1 encodes an siRNA and a suppressor of RNA silencing. *Immunity* **22**, 607–619.

Bennasser, Y., Le, S. Y., Yeung, M. L., and Jeang, K. T. (2006a). MicroRNAs in human immunodeficiency virus-1 infection. *Methods Mol. Biol.* **342**, 241–254.

Bennasser, Y., Yeung, M. L., and Jeang, K. T. (2006b). HIV-1 tar RNA subverts RNA interferencein transfected cells through sequestration of tar RNA binding protein, TRBP. *J. Biol. Chem.* **281**, 27674–27678.

Beral, V., Peterman, T. A., Berkelman, R. L., and Jaffe, H. W. (1990). Kaposi's sarcoma among persons with AIDS: A sexually transmitted infection? *Lancet* **335**, 123–128.

Blumenthal, D. T., Raizer, J. J., Rosenblum, M. K., Bilsky, M. H., Hariharan, S., and Abrey, L. E. (1999). Primary intracranial neoplasms in patients with HIV. *Neurology* **52**, 1648–1651.

Boden, D., Pusch, O., and Ramratnam, B. (2004). HIV-1-specific RNA interference. *Curr. Opin. Mol. Ther.* **6**, 373–380.

Bohnsack, M. T., Czaplinski, K., and Gorlich, D. (2004). Exportin 5 is a RanGTP-dependent dsRNA-binding protein that mediates nuclear export of pre-miRNAs. *RNA* **10**, 185–191.

Capodici, J., Kariko, K., and Weissman, D. (2002). Inhibition of HIV-1 infection by small interfering RNA-mediated RNA interference. *J. Immunol.* **169**, 5196–5201.

Cavanagh, M. H., Landry, S., Audet, B., Arpin-Andre, C., Hivin, P., Pare, M. E., Thete, J., Wattel, E., Marriott, S. J., Mesnard, J. M., and Barbeau, B. (2006). HTLV-I antisense transcripts initiating in the 3′LTR are alternatively spliced and polyadenylated. *Retrovirology* **3**, 15.

Chang, L. J., Liu, X., and He, J. (2005). Lentiviral siRNAs targeting multiple highly conserved RNA sequences of human immunodeficiency virus type 1. *Gene Ther.* **12**, 1133–1144.

Chendrimada, T. P., Gregory, R. I., Kumaraswamy, E., Norman, J., Cooch, N., Nishikura, K., and Shiekhattar, R. (2005). TRBP recruits the Dicer complex to Ago2 for microRNA processing and gene silencing. *Nature* **436**, 740–744.

Coburn, G. A., and Cullen, B. R. (2002). Potent and specific inhibition of human immunodeficiency virus type 1 replication by RNA interference. *J. Virol.* **76**, 9225–9231.

Das, A. T., Brummelkamp, T. R., Westerhout, E. M., Vink, M., Madiredjo, M., Bernards, R., and Berkhout, B. (2004). Human immunodeficiency virus type 1 escapes from RNA interference-mediated inhibition. *J. Virol.* **78**, 2601–2605.

Esquela-Kerscher, A., and Slack, F. J. (2006). Oncomirs—microRNAs with a role in cancer. *Nat. Rev. Cancer* **6**, 259–269.

Gatignol, A., Buckler-White, A., Berkhout, B., and Jeang, K. T. (1991). Characterization of a human TAR RNA-binding protein that activates the HIV-1 LTR. *Science* **251**, 1597–1600.

Gaudray, G., Gachon, F., Basbous, J., Biard-Piechaczyk, M., Devaux, C., and Mesnard, J. M. (2002). The complementary strand of the human T-cell leukemia virus type 1 RNA genome encodes a bZIP transcription factor that down-regulates viral transcription. *J. Virol.* **76**, 12813–12822.

Girard, A., Sachidanandam, R., Hannon, G. J., and Carmell, M. A. (2006). A germline-specific class of small RNAs binds mammalian Piwi proteins. *Nature* **442**, 199–202.

Grey, F., Antoniewicz, A., Allen, E., Saugstad, J., McShea, A., Carrington, J. C., and Nelson, J. (2005). Identification and characterization of human cytomegalovirus-encoded micro-RNAs. *J. Virol.* **79**, 12095–12099.

Gupta, A., Gartner, J. J., Sethupathy, P., Hatzigeorgiou, A. G., and Fraser, N. W. (2006). Anti-apoptotic function of a microRNA encoded by the HSV-1 latency-associated transcript. *Nature* **442**, 82–85.

Haase, A. D., Jaskiewicz, L., Zhang, H., Laine, S., Sack, R., Gatignol, A., and Filipowicz, W. (2005). TRBP, a regulator of cellular PKR and HIV-1 virus expression, interacts with Dicer and functions in RNA silencing. *EMBO Rep.* **6**, 961–967.

Han, J., Lee, Y., Yeom, K. H., Kim, Y. K., Jin, H., and Kim, V. N. (2004a). The Drosha-DGCR8 complex in primary microRNA processing. *Genes Dev.* **18**, 3016–3027.

Han, W., Wind-Rotolo, M., Kirkman, R. L., and Morrow, C. D. (2004b). Inhibition of human immunodeficiency virus type 1 replication by siRNA targeted to the highly conserved primer binding site. *Virology* **330**, 221–232.

Hariharan, M., Scaria, V., Pillai, B., and Brahmachari, S. K. (2005). Targets for human encoded microRNAs in HIV genes. *Biochem. Biophys. Res. Commun.* **337**, 1214–1218.

Jacque, J. M., Triques, K., and Stevenson, M. (2002). Modulation of HIV-1 replication by RNA interference. *Nature* **418**, 435–438.

Kempf, W., and Adams, V. (1996). Viruses in the pathogenesis of Kaposi's sarcoma—a review. *Biochem. Mol. Med.* **58**, 1–12.

Lecellier, C. H., Dunoyer, P., Arar, K., Lehmann-Che, J., Eyquem, S., Himber, C., Saib, A., and Voinnet, O. (2005). A cellular microRNA mediates antiviral defense in human cells. *Science* **308**, 557–560.

Lee, N. S., Dohjima, T., Bauer, G., Li, H., Li, M. J., Ehsani, A., Salvaterra, P., and Rossi, J. (2002). Expression of small interfering RNAs targeted against HIV-1 rev transcripts in human cells. *Nat. Biotechnol.* **20**, 500–505.

Lee, Y., Kim, M., Han, J., Yeom, K. H., Lee, S., Baek, S. H., and Kim, V. N. (2004). MicroRNA genes are transcribed by RNA polymerase II. *EMBO J.* **23**, 4051–4060.

Lee, Y., Hur, I., Park, S. Y., Kim, Y. K., Suh, M. R., and Kim, V. N. (2006). The role of PACT in the RNA silencing pathway. *EMBO J.* **25**, 522–532.

Leonard, J. N., and Schaffer, D. V. (2005). Computational design of antiviral RNA interference strategies that resist human immunodeficiency virus escape. *J. Virol.* **79**, 1645–1654.

Leonard, J. N., and Schaffer, D. V. (2006). Antiviral RNAi therapy: Emerging approaches for hitting a moving target. *Gene Ther.* **13**, 532–540.

Lewis, B. P., Burge, C. B., and Bartel, D. P. (2005). Conserved seed pairing, often flanked by adenosines, indicates that thousands of human genes are microRNA targets. *Cell* **120**, 15–20.

Liu, J., Carmell, M. A., Rivas, F. V., Marsden, C. G., Thomson, J. M., Song, J. J., Hammond, S. M., Joshua-Tor, L., and Hannon, G. J. (2004). Argonaute2 is the catalytic engine of mammalian RNAi. *Science* **305**, 1437–1441.

Liu, J., Rivas, F. V., Wohlschlegel, J., Yates, J. R., III, Parker, R., and Hannon, G. J. (2005a). A role for the P-body component GW182 in microRNA function. *Nat. Cell Biol.* **7**, 1261–1266.

Liu, J., Valencia-Sanchez, M. A., Hannon, G. J., and Parker, R. (2005b). MicroRNA-dependent localization of targeted mRNAs to mammalian P-bodies. *Nat. Cell Biol.* **7**, 719–723.

Marx, J. (2005). Molecular biology. P-bodies mark the spot for controlling protein production. *Science* **310**, 764–765.

Meister, G., Landthaler, M., Patkaniowska, A., Dorsett, Y., Teng, G., and Tuschl, T. (2004). Human Argonaute2 mediates RNA cleavage targeted by miRNAs and siRNAs. *Mol. Cell* **15**, 185–197.

Moulignier, A., Mikol, J., Pialoux, G., Eliaszewicz, M., Thurel, C., and Thiebaut, J. B. (1994). Cerebral glial tumors and human immunodeficiency virus-1 infection. More than a coincidental association. *Cancer* **74**, 686–692.

Neal, J. W., Llewelyn, M. B., Morrison, H. L., Jasani, B., and Borysiewicz, L. K. (1996). A malignant astrocytoma in a patient with AIDS: A possible association between astrocytomas and HIV infection. *J. Infect.* **33**, 159–162.

Novina, C. D., Murray, M. F., Dykxhoorn, D. M., Beresford, P. J., Riess, J., Lee, S. K., Collman, R. G., Lieberman, J., Shankar, P., and Sharp, P. A. (2002). siRNA-directed inhibition of HIV-1 infection. *Nat. Med.* **8**, 681–686.

Omoto, S., and Fujii, Y. R. (2005). Regulation of human immunodeficiency virus 1 transcription by nef microRNA. *J. Gen. Virol.* **86**, 751–755.

Omoto, S., Ito, M., Tsutsumi, Y., Ichikawa, Y., Okuyama, H., Brisibe, E. A., Saksena, N. K., and Fujii, Y. R. (2004). HIV-1 nef suppression by virally encoded microRNA. *Retrovirology* **1**, 44.

Pfeffer, S., Zavolan, M., Grasser, F. A., Chien, M., Russo, J. J., Ju, J., John, B., Enright, A. J., Marks, D., Sander, C., and Tuschl, T. (2004). Identification of virus-encoded microRNAs. *Science* **304**, 734–736.

Pfeffer, S., Sewer, A., Lagos-Quintana, M., Sheridan, R., Sander, C., Grasser, F. A., van Dyk, L. F., Ho, C. K., Shuman, S., Chien, M., Russo, J. J., Ju, J., *et al.* (2005). Identification of microRNAs of the herpesvirus family. *Nat. Methods* **2**, 269–276.

Rossi, J. J. (2005). RNAi and the P-body connection. *Nat. Cell Biol.* **7**, 643–644.

Saetrom, O., Snove, O., Jr., and Saetrom, P. (2005). Weighted sequence motifs as an improved seeding step in microRNA target prediction algorithms. *RNA* **11**, 995–1003.

Satou, Y., Yasunaga, J., Yoshida, M., and Matsuoka, M. (2006). HTLV-I basic leucine zipper factor gene mRNA supports proliferation of adult T cell leukemia cells. *Proc. Natl. Acad. Sci. USA* **103**, 720–725.

Sen, G. L., and Blau, H. M. (2005). Argonaute 2/RISC resides in sites of mammalian mRNA decay known as cytoplasmic bodies. *Nat. Cell Biol.* **7**, 633–636.

Sullivan, C. S., Grundhoff, A. T., Tevethia, S., Pipas, J. M., and Ganem, D. (2005). SV40-encoded microRNAs regulate viral gene expression and reduce susceptibility to cytotoxic T cells. *Nature* **435**, 682–686.

ter Brake, O., Konstantinova, P., Ceylan, M., and Berkhout, B. (2006). Silencing of HIV-1 with RNA interference: A multiple shRNA approach. *Mol. Ther* **14**, 883–892.

Trapp, S., Parcells, M. S., Kamil, J. P., Schumacher, D., Tischer, B. K., Kumar, P. M., Nair, V. K., and Osterrieder, N. (2006). A virus-encoded telomerase RNA promotes malignant T cell lymphomagenesis. *J. Exp. Med.* **203**, 1307–1317.

Voinnet, O. (2005). Induction and suppression of RNA silencing: Insights from viral infections. *Nat. Rev. Genet.* **6**, 206–220.

Westerhout, E. M., Ooms, M., Vink, M., Das, A. T., and Berkhout, B. (2005). HIV-1 can escape from RNA interference by evolving an alternative structure in its RNA genome. *Nucleic Acids Res.* **33**, 796–804.

Yeung, M. L., Bennasser, Y., Le, S. Y., and Jeang, K. T. (2005a). siRNA, miRNA and HIV: Promises and challenges. *Cell Res.* **15**, 935–946.

Yeung, M. L., Bennasser, Y., Myers, T. G., Jiang, G., Benkirane, M., and Jeang, K. T. (2005b). Changes in microRNA expression profiles in HIV-1-transfected human cells. *Retrovirology* **2**, 81.

Yi, R., Qin, Y., Macara, I. G., and Cullen, B. R. (2003). Exportin-5 mediates the nuclear export of pre-microRNAs and short hairpin RNAs. *Genes Dev.* **17**, 3011–3016.

Index

Contents of Previous Volumes

Volume 51

Treatment of Leukemia and Lymphoma
Edited by David A. Scheinberg and Joseph G. Jurcic

Kinase Inhibitors in Leukemia
Mark Levis and Donald Small

Therapy of Acute Promyelocytic Leukemia
Steven Soignet and Peter Maslak

Investigational Agents in Myeloid Disorders
Farhad Ravandi and Jorge Cortes

Methodologic Issues in Investigation of Targeted Therapies in Acute
Myeloid Leukemia
Elihu Estey

Purine Analogs in Leukemia
Nicole Lamanna and Mark Weiss

Monoclonal Antibody Therapy in Lymphoid Leukemias
Thomas S. Lin and John C. Byrd

Native Antibody and Antibody-Targeted Chemotherapy for Acute
Myeloid Leukemia
Eric L. Sievers

Radioimmunotherapy of Leukemia
John M. Burke and Joseph G. Jurcic

Immunotoxins and Toxin Constructs in the Treatment of Leukemia
and Lymphoma
Michael Rosenblum

Antibody Therapy of Lymphoma
George J. Weiner and Brian K. Link

Vaccines in Leukemia
Sijie Lu, Eric Wieder, Krishna Komanduri, Qing Ma, and Jeffrey J. Molldrem

Therapeutic Idiotype Vaccines for Non-Hodgkin's Lymphoma
John M. Timmerman

Volume 54

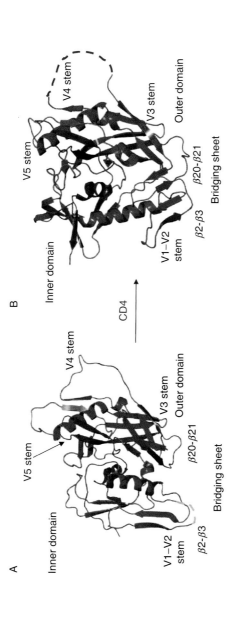

A

Inner domain

V5 stem

V4 stem

V1–V2
stem

β2-β3

Outer domain

V3 stem

β20-β21

Bridging sheet

Unliganded gp120

B

Inner domain

V5 stem

V4 stem

CD4 →

V1–V2
stem

β2-β3

Outer domain

V3 stem

β20-β21

Bridging sheet

Liganded gp120

CHAPTER 2, FIGURE 3 Crystal structures of gp120 core in the unliganded and liganded states. (A) Ribbon diagram of the unliganded SIV gp120 core is shown as in the same orientation of the liganded HIV gp120 structure. The color codes are in rainbow representation from colors blue to red for the N- to C-terminus. The positions of variable loops and bridging sheets are labeled. (B) Ribbon diagram depicting the 3D-structure of HIV gp120 core complexed with the first two domains (D1, D2) of CD4 receptor and the Fab fragment of human monoclonal neutralizing antibody 17b (CD4 and 17b are not shown here). The outer domains (in green and yellow) of liganded and unliganded gp120 are relatively conserved while a dramatic change in the inner domain (blue and cyan) occurs. The bridging sheet that connects inner and outer domains is not formed in the unliganded gp120.

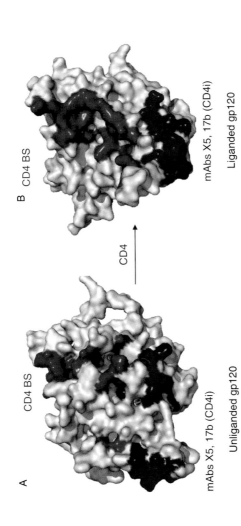

CHAPTER 2, FIGURE 4 Molecular surface diagrams of unliganded (A) and liganded (B) gp120 cores are rendered as viewed from the perspective of CD4 receptor binding. The residues in direct contact with CD4 are in blue; residues contacting the CD4i antibodies, namely, 17b and X5 are in red. The contact residues were selected by limiting interatomic distance of 3.8 Å between gp120 core to the CD4 and CD4i antibodies.

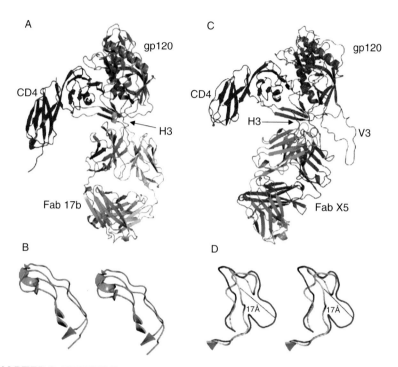

CHAPTER 2, FIGURE 5 Structures of HIV-1 gp120 complexes with CD4 receptor and CD4i antibodies, 17b and X5. (A) HIV-1 gp120 core (green) is bound to the CD4 (orange) and Fab 17b antibody (magenta for heavy and pink for light chains). (B) CDR H3 conformations of antibodies in the free and bound forms are given in stereoviews as crystal structures of 17b and X5 antibodies were available in isolation (PDB codes: 1RZ8 and 1RHH, respectively). (C) HIV-1 gp120 core with an intact V3 (green) is bound to the CD4 (orange) and Fab X5 antibody (blue for heavy and cyan for light chains). CDR H3 loops are labeled and indicated by arrows. The CDR H3 conformations of 17b antibody (C) are similar in free and bound forms. Notably, the H3 of X5 (D) undergoes a large conformational change with the maximum displacement up to 17 Å (blue in bound form and light blue in free form).

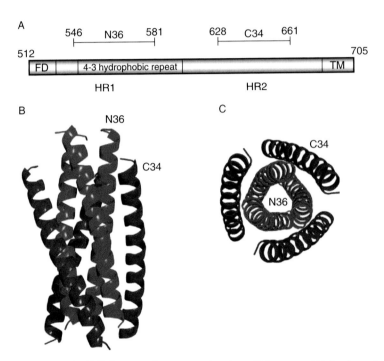

CHAPTER 2, FIGURE 6 Crystal structure trimeric gp41 fragment. (A) A schematic view of gp41 Env showing the locations of functional regions corresponding to the N36 and C34 peptide fragments. (B) The peptides N36–C34 complex forms a stable α-helical domain of six-helix bundle structure. The N36 (green) and C34 (red) helices point to each other in the opposite directions; N36 forms the inner core of the trimeric structure while C34 warps the core. (C) The bottom view of the trimer clearly depicts the arrangement of N36–C34 complex.

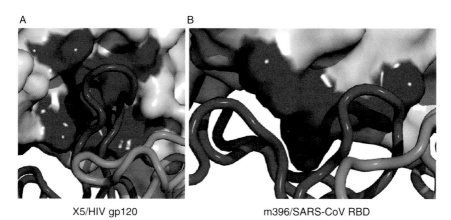

A   B

X5/HIV gp120   m396/SARS-CoV RBD

CHAPTER 2, FIGURE 9 Two different antigen-binding sites and binding modes CDRs. (A) In gp120–Fab X5 antibody interaction, the long CDR H3 protrudes into the CD4i binding site. (B) Conversely, in the SARS Env–Fab m396 antibody interaction, the antibody CDRs form like a canyon around the protruding binding site.

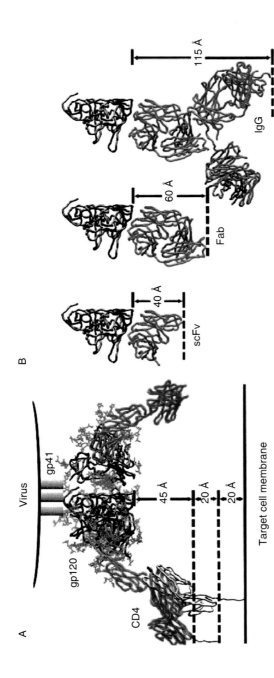

CHAPTER 2, FIGURE 10 Steric restriction of access to CD4i epitopes on CD4 binding. (A) The sketch with molecules shown describes the attachment of HIV-1 from viral membrane to the cell surface CD4 receptor. The binding of CD4 induces conformational changes resulting into the exposure of coreceptor binding site, which is sterically restricted for the CD4i antibodies. Taken into considerations of the dimensions derived from structures of gp120, CD4, and possible flexibility of CD4 molecule, a total distance of about 85 Å between the gp120 and target cell membrane is measured. (B) Dimensions of antibodies in different formats, Fv, Fab, and IgG molecules, are also shown. This clearly shows that CD4i antibodies of scFvs and Fabs have better access to the restricted binding site for competing with the coreceptor than IgGs have.

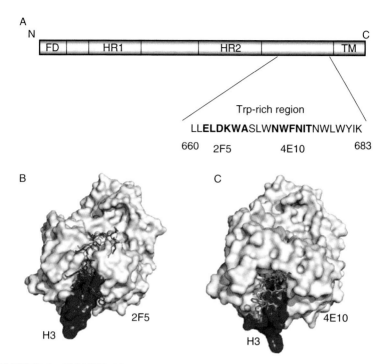

A

N   C

| FD | HR1 | | HR2 | | TM |

Trp-rich region

LLELDKWASLW**NWFNIT**NWLWYIK

660   2F5   4E10   683

B   C

2F5   4E10

H3   H3

CHAPTER 2, FIGURE 11   Antibody interactions at the membrane-proximal region of gp41. (A) Schematic diagram of gp41 shows the different important regions, FD, fusion domain, HR1, HR2-heptad repeats, and TM, transmembrane domain. The location of membrane-proximal region containing the core 2F5 and 4E10 epitopes on the Trp-rich region of gp41 is indicated along with amino acids sequence. Sequence numbering corresponds to HXB2 scheme. Crystal structures of Fab 2F5 (B) and 4E10 (C) in complex with peptides from the MPER. The H3s of the antibodies are shown in green.

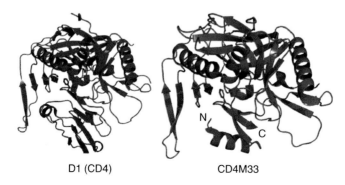

D1 (CD4)   CD4M33

CHAPTER 2, FIGURE 12   Mimicry of receptor CD4 by miniprotein CD4M33. The binding of gp120 (green) to the CD4 (first domain, D1 is only shown) on left and the mini-protein CD4M33 on right are depicted in ribbon diagrams.

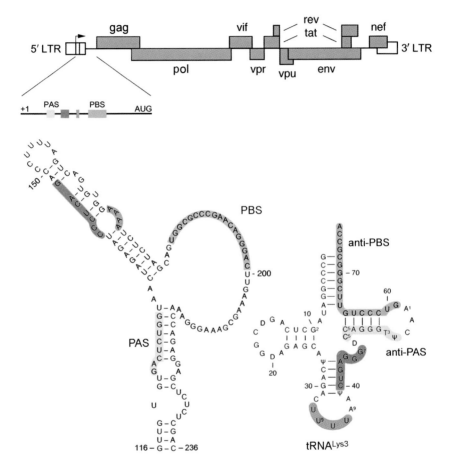

CHAPTER 3, FIGURE 2 The HIV-1 genome and the PBS motif that specify tRNA primer usage. Shown on top is the HIV-1 DNA genome. The 5′ LTR is divided in three segments (U3, R, and U5). Transcription starts at the U3-R border (arrow). A close-up of the untranslated leader of the vRNA is shown (from the transcription start site +1 to the gag start codon AUG). Motifs involved in reverse transcription are color-coded and similarly marked in the secondary structure model shown at the bottom. The cloverleaf structure of the tRNA[Lys3] molecule is also shown. Base modifications in the tRNA molecules are indicated according to standard nomenclature (Sprinzl et al., 1998). Several base-pairing interactions between the primer and the leader have been proposed (color-coded, see text for further details).

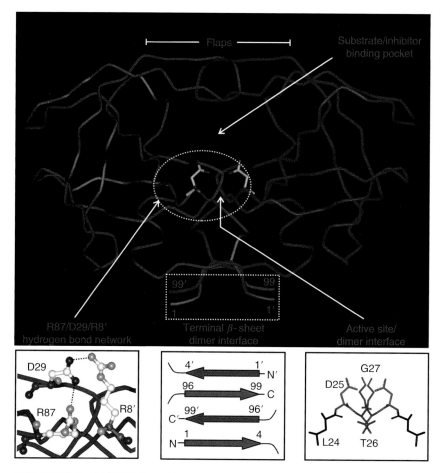

CHAPTER 8, FIGURE I Ribbon drawing of the polypeptide backbone of the HIV-1 protease (PDB accession 1A30) with one protease monomer in green and the other in orange. The two major areas that constitute the dimer interface at the active site and the terminal regions, and the intra- and intersubunit contacts between R87-D29 and D29-R8′ residues, respectively, in the protease are indicated. Residues D25 are represented as stick models. The dotted black lines between R87, D29, and R8′ indicate hydrogen bonds (left bottom panel). A schematic drawing depicting the four-stranded terminal β-sheet of the mature protease dimer and the active site dimer interface hydrogen bond network formed by the triplet D25-T26-G27, also know as the "fireman's grip," are shown in the center and right bottom panels, respectively. The flaps essential for recruiting and binding the substrate or inhibitor are shown in a closed conformation.

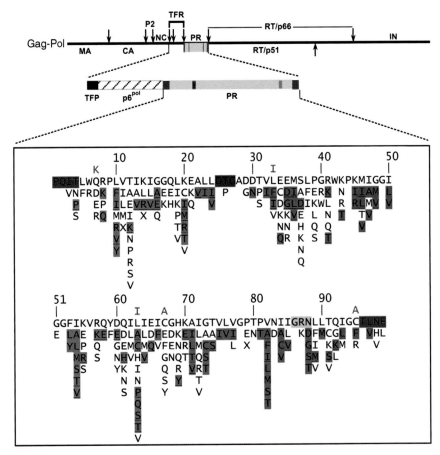

CHAPTER 8, FIGURE 2 Organization of Gag-Pol polyprotein in HIV-1 (top). Straight arrows shown along the Gag-Pol polyprotein indicate specific sites of cleavage by the viral protease. The 99-amino acid protease is flanked at its N-terminus by the transframe region (TFR) consisting of the transframe peptide (TFP) FLREDLAF and 48 amino acids of p6^{pol}. TFP and p6^{pol} are separated by a protease cleavage site. Nomenclature of HIV-1 proteins is according to Leis *et al.* (1988). MA, matrix, CA, capsid; PR, protease; NC, nucleocapsid; RT, reverse transcriptase; RN, RNase; IN, integrase. Natural variation and selected drug-resistant mutations of mature HIV-1 protease (bottom). Natural variations in the protease sequence are listed alphabetically below the HXB2 sequence (wt-PR), selected drug-resistant mutations are indicated in cyan and residues common to both are underlined. The two highly conserved regions, the active site triad (DTG) common to all aspartic proteases and the C-terminal triad (GRN/D) unique to retroviral proteases are highlighted in red and gray, respectively. The N- and C-terminal residues involved in forming the dimer interface β-sheet (see Fig. 1) are highlighted in yellow. The optimized construct (pseudo-wild-type, termed PR) suitable for structural and kinetic studies bears five mutations, three mutations Q7K, L33I, L63I that restrict degradation (autoproteolysis) and two mutations C65A and C95A to avoid Cys-thiol oxidation are shown in red above the HXB2 sequence. TMPR bears only three mutations to restrict autoproteolysis used in some NMR studies.

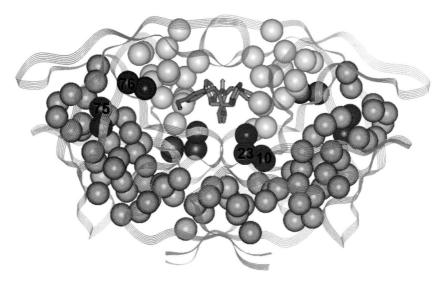

CHAPTER 8, FIGURE 6 Methyl groups in inner (pink spheres) and outer (green spheres) clusters, and a ribbon diagram of the mature protease backbone. Yellow and orange spheres represent methyl groups undergoing motions on sub-ns and ms-μs timescales, respectively. The number on the sphere indicates residue position. The experiment was performed in 20-mM phosphate buffer, pH 5.8, 20 °C (Ishima *et al.*, 2001b).

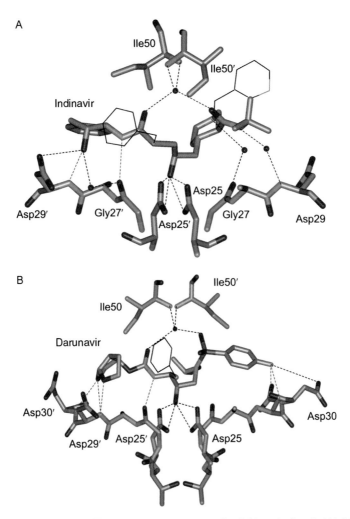

CHAPTER 8, FIGURE 7 Protease interactions with inhibitors indinavir (A) (Liu *et al.*, 2005; Mahalingam *et al.*, 2004) and darunavir (B) (Kovalevsky *et al.*, 2006a,b; Tie *et al.*, 2004). Water molecules are indicated by red spheres. Hydrogen bond interactions are shown as dashed lines. Red lines indicate hydrogen bonds with the main chain atoms of the protease and black lines indicate hydrogen bonds with side chain atoms of the protease or with water.

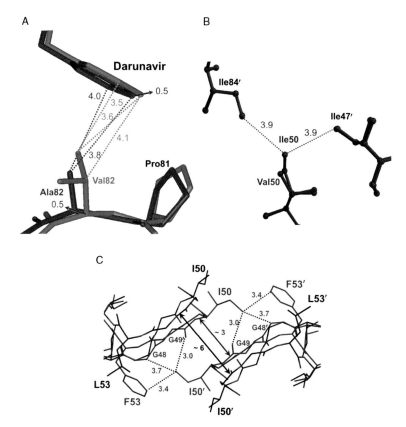

CHAPTER 8, FIGURE 8   (A) Interactions of darunavir with V82 in wt-PR (magenta) and A82 in mutant (cyan). Hydrophobic contacts are indicated by dotted lines with the interatomic separation in angstroms. The structural shift of the C_α atom of residue 82 is shown as a red arrow with distance in angstroms. (B) Intersubunit interactions of I/V50 in crystal structures of I50V mutant (red) and wt-PR (green) with peptide analogue. Favorable van der Waals interactions are shown as dotted lines. Interatomic distances are shown in angstroms. (C) Comparison of intersubunit interactions of residue 53 in unliganded structures of wt (brown) and F53L mutant (black).

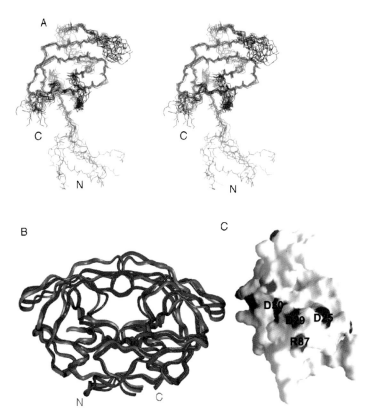

CHAPTER 8, FIGURE 11 Solution structure of the protease monomer (Ishima *et al.*, 2003). (A) Overall stereo view of the PR$_{1-95}$ structure showing the final ensemble of 10 NMR conformers. (B) Comparison of the average NMR structure of PR$_{1-95}$ (blue) with one subunit of two free protease dimer crystal structures shown in green (Lapatto *et al.*, 1989) and yellow (Rick *et al.*, 1998). (C) Electrostatic surface potential of PR$_{1-95}$ (excludes residues 1–10). Note: the crystal structure shown in green has a flap conformation that is more open than the crystal structure shown in yellow.

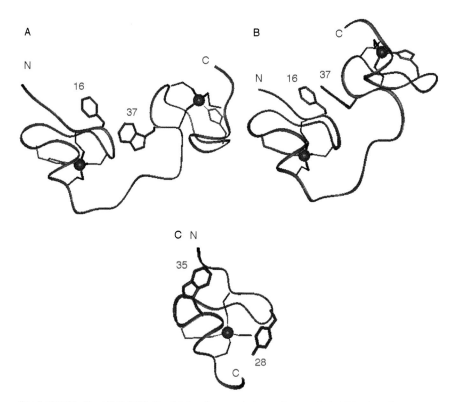

CHAPTER 9, FIGURE 3 Molecular modeling of retroviral NC zinc fingers (I). Figure illustrates the well-conserved ZF backbone (in blue) based on the first ZF of HIV-1 NCp7 (A), in comparison with SIV NCp8 (B) and MuLV NCp10 (C). Aromatic residues essential for NC functions *in vivo* are in red (see numbers) and the N- and C-terminal ends are indicated by orange N and C letters. Zn^{2+} are represented by orange marbles.

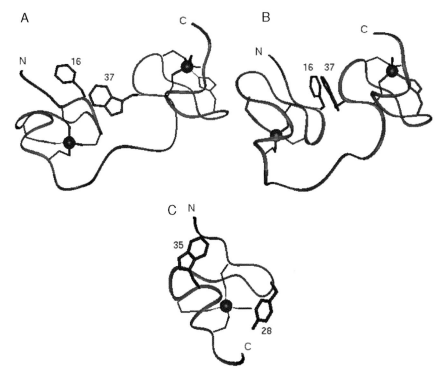

CHAPTER 9, FIGURE 4 Molecular modeling of retroviral NC zinc fingers (II). Figure illustrates the well-conserved ZF backbone (in blue) based on the second ZF of HIV-1 NCp7 (A), in comparison with SIV NCp8 (B) and MoMuLV NCp10 (C). Aromatic residues essential for NC functions *in vivo* are in red (see numbers) and the N- and C-terminal ends are indicated by orange N and C letters. Zn^{2+} are represented by orange marbles.

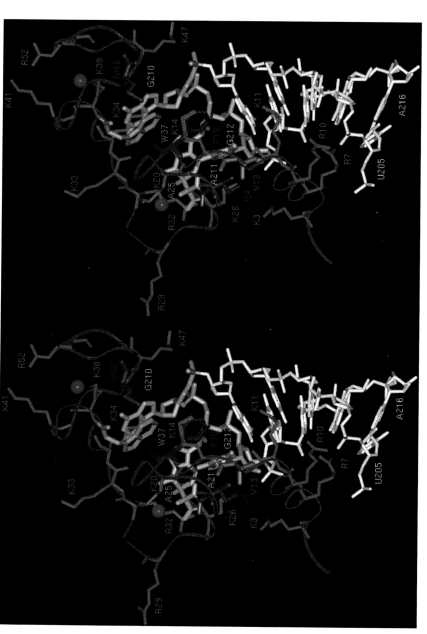

CHAPTER 9, FIGURE 5 HIV-1 NCp7 bound to a small nucleic acid molecule. Stereoview of the NCp7/SL3 complex structure (De Guzman *et al.*, 1998). Only the lysine, arginine, and hydrophobic residues V13, F16, I24, A25, W37, M46, and the 205–216 domain of the HIV-1 SL3 sequence are represented. The zinc ions are in yellow. NCp7 is illustrated as a green ribbon. The nucleotides in interaction with the ZF domain of NCp7 are in light yellow.

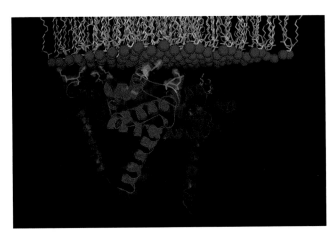

CHAPTER 10, FIGURE 3 Crystal structure of a matrix (MA) trimer (bottom) portrayed interacting with membrane (top). Membrane is represented as a phospholipid bilayer (yellow and gray), basic residues essential for virus replication are clustered on the face of the MA trimer opposing the lipid bilayer (magenta); and the C-terminal helical tail is depicted projecting away from the globular domain. Provided by B. Kelly, C. Hill, and W. I. Sundquist and adapted from Hill *et al.* (1996).

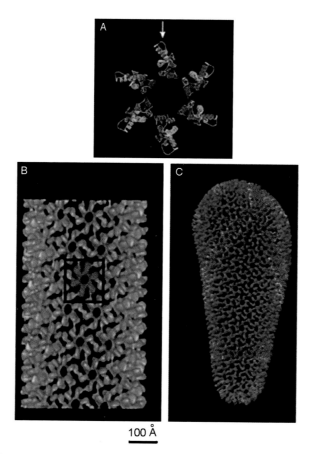

100 Å

CHAPTER 10, FIGURE 9 Image reconstruction of helical assemblies of HIV-1 capsid (CA) protein. (A) Molecular model of the hexameric ring formed by the CA N-terminal domain (NTD). Structural features: β-hairpin (orange), helix 1 (red), helix 2 (yellow), helix 3 (green), helix 4 (cyan), helix 5 (dark blue), helix 6 (red), helix 7 (pink). Cyclophilin A-binding loop (arrow). (B) Exterior view of the assembled tube structure showing the hexagonal CA lattice. A single hexamer is highlighted in yellow. (C) Model of the HIV-1 conical core. A continuous line of hexamers is highlighted in yellow and pentameric defects are shown in pink. Adapted from Li *et al.* (2000). Copyright 2000 Nature Publishing Group, with permission.

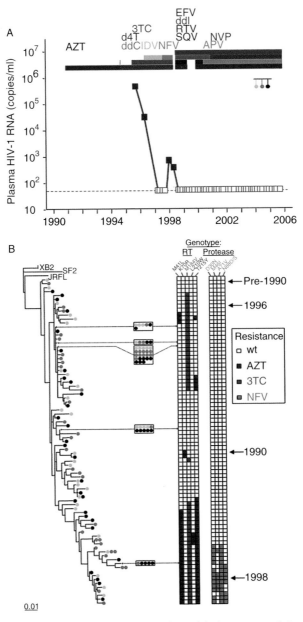

CHAPTER 12, FIGURE 1 Phylogenetic analysis of the latent reservoir in a patient with a history of prior nonsuppressive therapy. (A) Treatment history of patient 148. Drug regimens are indicated by colored bars. The reservoir was sampled at three time points in 2004 (gray and black circles). (B) Phylogenetic tree of RT sequences from reference strains (HXB2, SF2, JRFL) and from patient 148 (gray and black symbols). Each symbol represents the sequence of virus from a single latently infected CD4+ T cell from the indicated sampling times in 2004. The genotype of each isolate on the phylogenetic tree is indicated in the corresponding horizontal row of boxes on the right. Note that in 2004, the reservoir contained ancestral wild-type viruses (wt), and viruses carrying resistance mutations to zidovudine (AZT), lamivudine (3TC), and nelfinavir (NFV). These drugs were taken 6–13 years previously, before effective suppression of viral replication was achieved.